For Harvey B[illegible] M.D.
Neurologist, Schola[illegible], [illegible]tleman,
Colleague and Friend.
Merry Christmas, 1981.
J. C. Cooter, MD

OXFORD MEDICAL PUBLICATIONS

THE DOCTRINE OF THE NERVES

THE DOCTRINE OF THE NERVES

Chapters in the history of neurology

JOHN D. SPILLANE
Formerly Consultant Neurologist to the University Hospital of Wales

Oxford New York Toronto
OXFORD UNIVERSITY PRESS
1981

Oxford University Press, Walton Street, Oxford OX2 6DP

OXFORD LONDON GLASGOW
NEW YORK TORONTO MELBOURNE WELLINGTON
KUALA LUMPUR SINGAPORE JAKARTA HONG KONG TOKYO
DELHI BOMBAY CALCUTTA MADRAS KARACHI
IBADAN NAIROBI DAR ES SALAAM CAPE TOWN

Published in the United States by
Oxford University Press, New York

British Library Cataloguing in Publication Data
Spillane, John David
The doctrine of the nerves. – (Oxford medical publications).
1. Neurology – History
I. Title II Series
616.809 RC338 79-41188

ISBN 0-19-261135-6

Printed in the United States of America

PREFACE

This book is primarily intended to show the newcomer to neurology the lie of the land, historically speaking: to set him on course, as it were, and show him where we neurologists came from. Not that I planned a systematic introduction to the history of neurology like that of my friend McHenry in his valuable *Garrison's History of neurology* (1969). Most clinicians after a lifetime in practice carry in their mind a picture of the growth of their subject: clear perhaps in one area or another, dim in others, and quite obscure in many. Then, the time comes when curiosity increases, dissatisfaction grows, and there is no alternative but to start burrowing in the past among the bookshelves, while one's erstwhile colleagues are busy retooling for the future. The pleasure of it all is undeniable. But what of its worth?

For many years historians have been explaining how invaluable, or indeed indispensable, is the study of history, if the mind is to be cultivated. I suppose no one can fail to see how, for example, a politician could ignore history – but what of the doctor? One of the best general practitioners I have known once told me that he considered medical history 'a waste of time'. I can understand his view that it would not make him any better at the bedside, but when a medical professor nonchalantly proclaims his ignorance I confess to feeling a mite scandalized. I have to remind myself that he is a neoteric historical figure: the chairman–superspecialist. I do not think one can argue profitably about this; it has been tiresomely debated. I have long accepted that, like music and walking, there are some who are not just disinterested in history, they positively dislike it. All I wish to say is that I am on the side of those who believe in the educational value of the history of medicine and who advocate its general incorporation into medical curricula. Meanwhile it looks as if, in the medical school, unlike in the university itself, the teaching of history will remain in the hands of doctors, not historians. Namely, men like myself – game but untrained.

Much of what has passed for medical history *is* 'bunk' and professional historians have been justifiably critical. It is one thing for the enthusiastic amateur to indulge his fancy, hunting down the trail like Nimrod, or virtuously scrutinizing the archives, but it is another matter to analyse, interpret, and exercize historical judgement. Not that such talents are the prerogative of the professional historian, nor that he necessarily excels in the art of writing. His readers may find his meticulous scholarship insufferably dull and his pages more footnotes than text. What he has written may be genuine history, but it will only be read by the votary. Macaulay is still read, not for his views, but because he was a master of narrative. Oh, for a Macaulay of Neurology!

I enter the historian's arena lightly armed but aware of some of the dangers lying in wait for one of my caste. One could not fail to be after reading Clarke's *Modern methods in the history of medicine* (1971). There are the cardinal sins of viewing the past in the light of the present, of seeing analogies which are false, seeing connections which are not significant, inferring influences which are not established, emphasizing or attributing wrongly, and just chronicling where we should be explaining. Not to eulogize may be easy enough; not to be superficial at times, not so easy, but to discuss a concept or trace a train of thought or development – that may require what one does not possess: sufficient knowledge, training, and experience.

I am not sure to what extent I have succeeded in avoiding the snares and pitfalls in my path. I have tried to remember that I, too, am a product of my time. I have not just shaken the tree and rummaged around for fallen fruit, but have chosen a few branches that have attracted me. 'I should like him to hear this', I found myself saying, remembering the newcomer. 'That might liven his day'. But I tread only in the foothills of scholarship, selecting what I thought was important and within my grasp.

Inevitably the approach becomes rather individual, but not, I trust, too idiosyncratic. The desire is to share one's experience with others. There is little biography in the book and only a few portraits and title pages. The latter are often engaging and helpful but take up space, while portraits, although brightening one's pages, are expensive and usually familiar. In his essay 'Of persons one would wish to have seen', William Hazlitt had his friend Charles Lamb decide that Milton would not be one of them as 'I should be afraid of losing some of the manna of his poetry in the leaven of his countenance...'. In any case we have that excellent book *The founders of neurology* (1970), by Haymaker and Schiller.

All who are interested in the anatomical and physiological aspects of the history of neurology have been particularly assisted by major publications such as *The human brain and spinal cord* (1968) by Clarke and O'Malley, *Historical aspects of cerebral anatomy* (1971) by Meyer, and *An illustrated history of brain function* (1972) by Clarke and Dewhurst – a trilogy of incomparable value, from which the author learned a great deal. Emmerson's list of *Translations of medical classics* (1965) is also an admirable aid.

My wish, for the reader, is that in these pages he will catch a glimpse of the past of neurology – its ancient beginnings and long neglect, the sudden advances and the false trails, the happy finds and the laborious toil, the leaps of creative imagination and the cranky theories, the controversies, sedate or venomous, and the characters, noble or otherwise. In so doing he may find that some routine things can be seen in a more significant light.

For help with enquiries I wish to thank Professor A. W. Asscher, Cardiff; Dr. Eric Blackwell, Lubbock, Texas; Dr. Mary A. B. Brazier, Los Angeles; Dr. Craig Burrell, North Caldwell, New Jersey; Dr. Edwin Clarke, London; Professor K. Ekbom, Stockholm; Professor A. S. Duncan, Edinburgh; Dr.

Lester S. King, Chicago; Professor W. I. McDonald, London; Dr. Lawrence C. McHenry Jr., Winston-Salem, North Carolina; and Professor Alfred Meyer, London. Colleagues in Leiden, Göttingen, Heidelberg, and Paris have made my visits happy ones and I wish particularly to acknowledge the kindness and patience of the library staffs at the Royal Society of Medicine, the Wellcome Institute for the History of Medicine, the Royal College of Physicians, the National Hospital for Nervous Diseases, the Welsh National School of Medicine, the National Library of Wales Aberystwyth, and at Dartmouth Medical School, U. S. A.

I am indebted to Mrs. Winifred Mortimer and to my sister-in-law Mrs. Pauline Spillane for transcribing my original typescript and to Miss Patricia Havard for secretarial assistance.

The majority of the illustrations were prepared in the Department of Medical Illustration at the University Hospital of Wales, Cardiff, under the direction of my old friend and colleague Ralph Marshall Ph.D. For some I am obliged to the photographic unit of the Royal Society of Medicine.

Lastly, to my wife, to whom I dedicate my book, I am beholden in many ways. Over the years, for good-naturedly accepting certain journeys and forays which were disguised as holidays, and for her forbearance in the first quinquennium of our retirement, when she could have justifiably skedaddled.

Newport, Pembrokeshire J.D.S.
March 1980

To Joan
For her gift of happiness

ACKNOWLEDGEMENTS

I wish to express my thanks to the following for their kind permission in allowing me to quote passages of translations from their works.

W. L. H. Duckworth: *Galen on anatomical procedures; the later books.* Cambridge University Press (1962).

Margaret Tallmadge May: *Galen on the usefulness of the parts of the body.* Cornell University Press (1968).

Edwin Clarke and C. D. O'Malley: *The human brain and spinal cord.* University of California Press (1968).

R. E Siegel: *Galen's system of physiology and medicine* (1968); *Galen on sense perception* (1970); *Galen on psychology, psychopathology, and function and disease of the nervous system* (1973) S. Karger AG, Basel.

A. J. Brock: *Galen on the natural faculties.* The Loeb classical library, Harvard University Press, William Heinemann, London (1916).

Charles Singer: *Galen on anatomical procedures . . .the surviving books.* Oxford University Press (1956), by permission of the Wellcome Trustees.

R. Walzer: *Galen on medical experience.* Oxford University Press (1946), by permission of the Wellcome Trustees.

John F. Fulton: *Selected readings in the history of physiology*, 2nd ed., Charles C. Thomas, Springfield, Ill. (1966).

Charles Singer: *Vesalius on the human brain.* Oxford University Press, (1952), by permission of the Wellcome Trustees.

C. D. O'Malley: *Andreas Vesalius of Brussels.* University of California Press (1964).

Ruben Eriksson: *Andreas Vesalius' first public anatomy at Bologna.* Almquist and Wilksells, Uppsala (1959).

R. M. Green: *De viribus electritatis by Galvani*, Elizabeth Licht, Cambridge, Mass. (1953).

I am grateful to the editor of the *British Medical Journal* for permission to reproduce my article 'A memorable decade in the history of neurology', **4**, 701 (1974), and to the honorary editors of the *Proceedings of the Royal Society of Medicine* for permission to reproduce my address on 'The birth of American Neurology', **69**, 393 (1976).

I wish to thank the following for permission to reproduce the following illustrations:

Figs. 2, 3 from Charles Singer: *A short history of anatomy and physiology from the Greeks to Harvey.* Dover Publications, N.Y. (1957); Fig. 20 from *Thomas Willis, the anatomy of the brain and nerves*, tercentenary edition. McGill University Press (1964), by permission of William Feindel, editor; Fig. 54: The Lothian Health Board; Fig. 55: Mr. A. J. F. Gogelein, Director of Museum Boeerhaave, Leiden; Fig. 56 from G. Gruber, *Naturwissenschaftliche und medizinische Einrichtungen . . .* Muste-Schmidt, Gottingen (1955); Fig. 148: Russell and Volkening, N. Y.; Figs. 146, 149-151 from Anna Robeson Burr: *Silas Weir Mitchell; his life and letters*, Duffield, N.Y. (1929), with permission of Dodd, Mead and Company Inc, N.Y.; Fig, 168 from *Queen Square and the National Hospital, 1860–1960.* Foreword by Sir Ernest Gowers. Edward Arnold, London; Fig. 71: Musée Carnavalet, Paris; Figs. 80, 81, 109: Musée de l'Histoire de la Médicine, l'Ecole de Médicine, Paris;

Figs. 82, 83: Assistance Publique, Paris; Fig. 105: Musée de l'Homme, Paris; Fig. 147 from G. W. Adams: *Doctors in Blue*. Henry Schuman, N.Y. (1952); Fig. 47: Royal Swedish Academy of Sciences, Stockholm; Fig. 6b: Vesalius frontispiece, New York Academy of Medicine; Fig. 19: Royal Library, Windsor Castle, Inv. No. 12603 recto. Reproduced by gracious permission of Her Majesty Queen Elizabeth II.

CONTENTS

PART I

The foundations of neurology: Galen, Vesalius, and Willis

INTRODUCTION

There are forerunners in all disciplines but few would disagree that the foundations of neurology rest mainly on the works of three men – Galen, Vesalius, and Willis – the first a pagan of the Roman Empire, the second a Catholic of the European Renaissance, and the third an orthodox Anglican of seventeenth-century England. Galen of Pergamon (AD 130–200) was the first experimental physiologist; Andreas Vesalius (1514–64) was the founder of anatomy; Thomas Willis (1621–75) was 'The first inventor of the Nervous System' and he coined for us the word 'Neurologie'.

Galen's voluminous treatises were written over a period of fifty years and those extant comprise twenty-two large volumes, an estimated two and a half million words, exceeding those of Aristotle or Plato.[1] His writings 'smothered the medicine of antiquity'; if the Hippocratic books are omitted, 'Galen represents at least five-sixths of all the medical writings surviving from antiquity'.[2] He was born in Pergamon (now Bergama, in Turkey) on the Mediterranean shores of Asia Minor, a city which was then one of the world's leading centres, famous for its libraries, schools, and medical temple of Asklepio (Latin: *Aesculapius*). The latter was as well known as the temple of Diana at Ephesus, or of Apollo at Delphi. It was at Pergamon that parchment or *charta pergamena*, made from animal skin, was first used as a writing material. His medical education began there and was continued in other cities of learning – Smyrna, Corinth, and then Alexandria, where he spent five years. He travelled widely, visiting Cyprus, Lemnos, Thessaly, Anatolia, and Syria, and when he was thirty-one he settled in Rome. But he left there a few years later, during a pestilence of some kind, returned to Pergamon for five years, and then went back to Rome. He became physician to the Emperor Marcus Aurelius and remained there for the next twenty-five years, practising, teaching, dissecting, experimenting, and, ceaselessly, writing. He finally returned to Pergamon when he was sixty-two years old in AD 192, dying there eight years later. There is no authentic coin or statue to tell us what he looked like and his grave is unknown.

His treatises of most neurological interest are *De usu partium* (On the usefulness of the parts of the body) and *De anatomicis administrationibus* (On anatomical procedures). *De facultatibus naturalibus* (On the natural functions), *De locis affectis* (On the diseased parts), and *Placita* (Commentaries on Plato and Hippocrates) also contain neurological material.

Vesalius was only twenty-eight years of age when he completed his immortal work *De humani corporis fabrica libri septem* (Seven volumes on the structure of the human body), saying 'I am aware that by reason of my age ... my efforts will have little authority'. He was born in Brussels of a medical family and spent three years in Paris and one year in Louvain before completing his education in Padua, which he considered 'the most famous university of the whole world'. On graduation in 1538 he was appointed to the chair of surgery and anatomy there. His *De fabrica* was completed in three or four years and published in Basle in 1543. Then, inexplicably, he left Padua forever and spent the rest of his life as a court physician in the service of Emperor Charles V and his son Phillip II, mainly in Spain and the Netherlands. He died obscurely on the island of Zante (Zakinthos) in the Ionian Sea, off the Peloponnesian coast, at the age of fifty, when returning by ship from a pilgrimage to Jerusalem. His grave is unknown but it was probably in the churchyard of Santa Maria della Grazie, subsequently destroyed in an earthquake.

Willis was forty-three when the *Cerebri anatome* (Anatomy of the brain and nerves) was published in London in 1664. He was born in the village of Great Bedwyn, Wiltshire, probably of yeoman stock, and he studied medicine at Oxford, graduating in 1646. He remained in Oxford for the next twenty-one years, obtaining a chair in natural philosophy and becoming a Fellow of the newly created Royal Society of London. In addition to *Cerebri anatome* Willis also published other works of a neurological nature. The best known is *De anima brutorum* (Two discourses of the soul of brutes which is the vital and sensitive soul of man) which combines an account of comparative anatomy and a dissertation on disorders of the mind. Willis also wrote books on convulsions, hysteria, and hypochondriasis. He moved to London in 1667, dying there in 1675, at the age of fifty-four. He was buried in Westminster Abbey.

All three of these men were famous in their lifetime. Galen remained so for fourteen hundred years – 'divine' and infallible – but he created no school and none of his pupils continued his work. He was the last of the Ancients and with his death there ended eight hundred years of Greek science – one of the greatest mysteries of all time. Vesalius's inheritance in anatomy and physiology was entirely Galenic and, in one sense, the *De fabrica* may be viewed as a corrected, expanded, and illustrated version of Galen's anatomy, with a questionable acceptance of his physiology. Vesalius's fame rests on a single book. In the case of Willis, initial fame was followed by a decline in estimate of his worth, and it is only in this century that he has come into his own.

Although their lives were so different their declared aims were similar. Galen dedicated his *De usu partium*, which he called 'a sacred discourse', as a 'true hymn of praise to our creator'. Vesalius's preface was addressed to the Emperor Charles V, in whose service his family had been employed, and in it he said that anatomy was 'the chief branch of natural philosophy which, since it includes the description of man, ought rightfully to be considered the very beginning and foundation of medicine'. Willis's *Epistle dedicatory* was addressed to Gilbert Sheldon, Archbishop of Canterbury, from whom it was (and still is) possible to obtain a doctorate of medicine, and who was apparently responsible for Willis's election to a university chair. Willis wrote 'I had resolved to unlock the secret places of Man's mind and to look into the living and breathing Chapel of the Deity.'

And all three were pious men who made it clear that they did not wish to offend theologians or to question the divinity of man. In the final passages of *De usu partium*, Galen wrote that he hoped his book would be 'the source of a perfect theology, which is a thing far greater and far nobler than all medicine'. Vesalius said 'Nothing could be produced more pleasing or acceptable to your majesty than an account from which we may learn about the body and mind and, furthermore, about a certain divine power arising from a harmony of both – indeed about ourselves, that which in truth is the study of man.' Willis wrote 'I am not ignorant how great the labour is that I undertake; for it hath been a long while accounted as a certain school-house of atheism to search into nature; as if whatever reasons we grant to philosophy, should derogate religion. . . .'

A modern neurologist may now read, in English, many of the works of these three geniuses, as translations from the original Greek, and Latin, continue to be made available. Indeed one of Galen's books, *On medical experience*, was discovered in Istanbul only forty-five years ago. *De usu partium* was first translated into English as recently as 1968. Similarly, in the past fifty years, Vesalian and Willisian scholars have furnished us with invaluable accounts of their researches.

Never before was a neurologist so well placed to learn of the beginnings of his subject – of the *Great Triumvirate* of neurology.

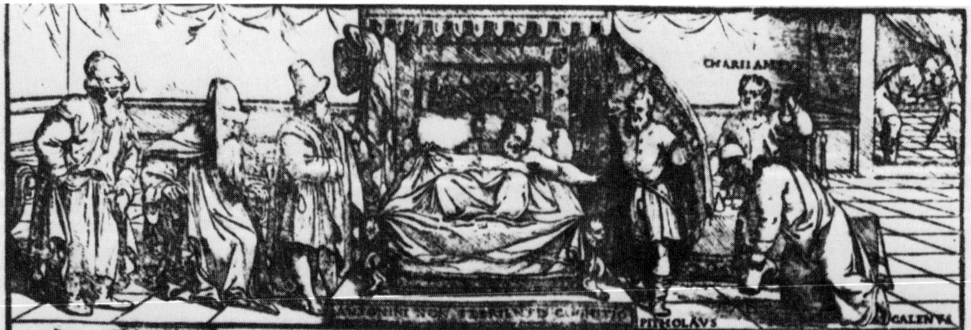

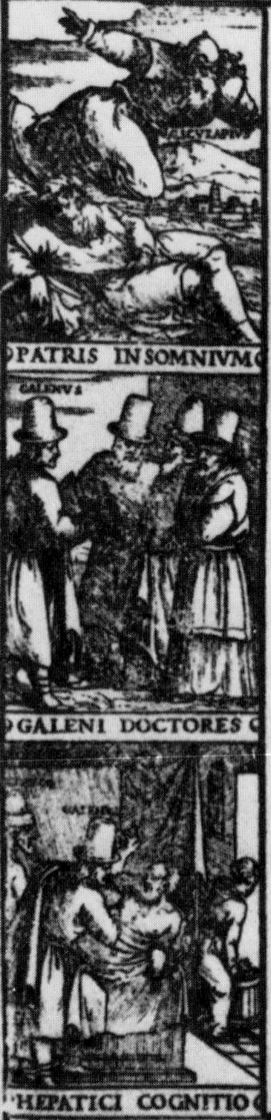

GALENI
OMNIA OPERA

NVNC PRIMVM IN VNVM CORPVS redacta: quorũ alia nunq̃ antea latinitate donata fuerãt, alia aut nouis interpretationibus, aut accuratis recognitionibus sunt illustrata: singula summo studio excusa, atq; e manuscriptis græcorũ uoluminibus infinitis penè locis restituta.

LIBRORVM INDICEM ET DILIGENTIAM PROXIMVS QVATERNIO DEMONSTRABIT.

ἰατρικὴ τέχνη

Cum Decreto Summi Pont. Senatusq; Veneti per annos XV. prout folio VIII legitur.

Apud heredes Lucæantonij Iuntæ Florentini

VENETIIS M. D. XLI.

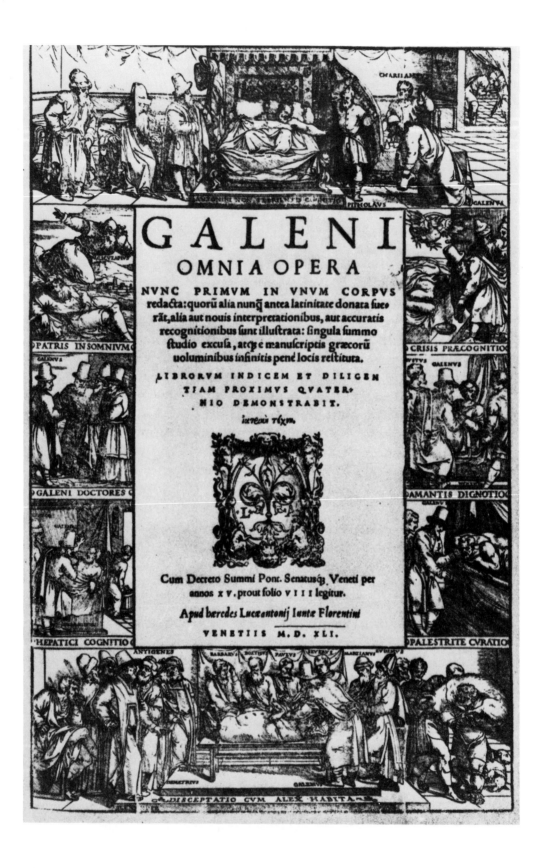

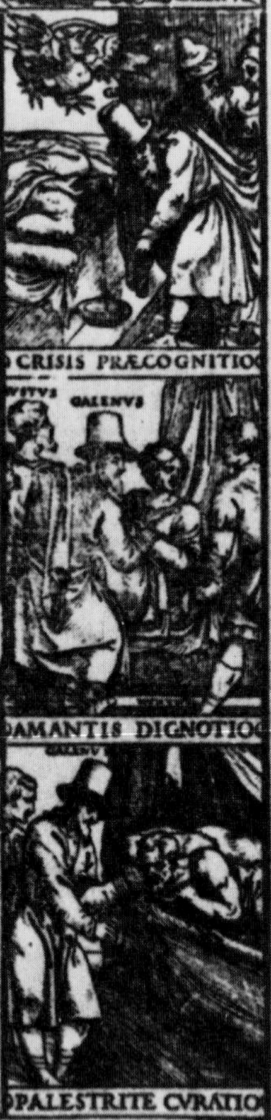

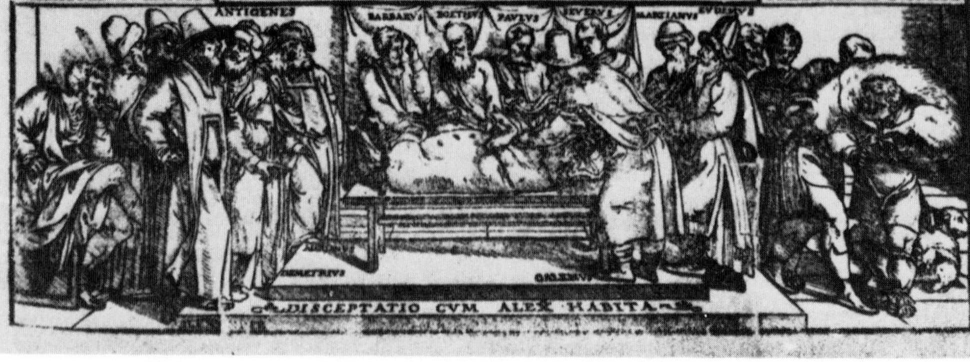

CHAPTER 1

GALEN AND THE NERVOUS SYSTEM

In the second century of the Christian era, the empire of Rome comprehended the fairest part of the earth, and the most civilised portion of mankind.

The opening sentence of Edward Gibbon's *Decline and Fall of the Roman Empire*. 1776–88.

INTRODUCTION

It is generally agreed that examination of the human body after death only came to be undertaken when the ancient Greeks began to overcome the fear of dead bodies and when the hypothesis of a rational soul was evolved.[1] Of course, from time immemorial, exposure of parts of the human body because of injury or disease must have led to many sporadic observations. Some acquaintance with the contents of the human body must also have been obtained in the process of embalming, when the Egyptians removed the brain through the nose, while the lungs, liver, stomach, and intestine were extracted through an incision in the side, pickled, and then returned to the body. Greek sculpture of the fifth century BC certainly disclosed a knowledge of surface musculature, but the Hippocratic physicians made no serious study of anatomy, although observations on fractures, dislocations, and head wounds were made. Despite Aristotle's extensive studies of many species of animals, ranging from the embryo chick to the elephant, there is no evidence that he performed adult human dissection and for some strange reason, theoretical or otherwise, he thought the human brain did not fill the cranial cavity and that there was a space in the occipital region, as in the turtle and some other reptiles.[2] But what seriously retarded progress was his teaching that the heart, and not the brain, was the seat of intellect. He thought the brain was bloodless and without sensation, but that it did possess an important role in cooling the heart. This idea of the supremacy of the heart persisted for centuries. Since a body grew cold when the heart stopped it is not surprising that men thought the heart generated heat. Then, too, speech came from the thorax, and speech presupposes thought, so that the organ of thought must lie in the thorax. What more likely than the heart? William Harvey, in his anatomical lectures of 1616, debated whether heart or brain was the more 'honourable' organ. 'The brain', he wrote, 'is deemed the prince of all the parts. However, there is no disputing the heart because its sway is wider, for the heart is seen in those creatures that want a brain.' But he appreciated that 'man has his brain whereby he excels all other animals . . . And so the head is the richest member of the body'.[3]

Yet, a century before Aristotle, another Greek, a Hippocratic physician,

FIG. 1 (*facing*). The splendid title-page of the first volume of the Giunta edition of Galen of 1541, to which Vesalius, Thomas Linacre, and Jacobus Sylvius contributed. The eight scenes depicted are: Top Galen doffing his tall hat and bowing as he approaches the bedside of a distinguished patient. Right: Prognosticating a crisis; diagnosing love-sickness; venesection. Left: Aesculapius inspiring Galen's father in a dream to send his son into medicine; Galen and his teachers; palpating the liver. Bottom: Galen demonstrating the recurrent laryngeal nerve in a pig.

author of the book *On the sacred disease* (epilepsy), asserted marvellously, in words that still ring fresh and noble, that

> Men ought to know that from the brain, and from the brain only, arises our pleasures, joys, laughter and jests, as well as our sorrows, pains, griefs and tears. Through it, in particular, we think, see, hear, and distinguish the ugly from the beautiful, the bad from the good, the pleasant from the unpleasant . . . It is the same thing which makes us mad or delirious, inspires us with dread or fear, whether by night or by day, brings sleeplessness, inopportune mistakes, aimless anxieties, absentmindedness, and acts that are contrary to habits. These things that we suffer all come from the brain when it is not healthy. . . .[4]

And across the sea, in Alexandria, other physicians thought the brain and not the heart was the seat of intelligence. Here, in Ptolemaic Egypt, human dissection was first systematically pursued by Herophilus and Erasistratus in the third century BC. Their works are entirely lost and what we know of them is largely through Galen. They were among the first to distinguish between arteries (which they thought normally contained not blood, but air) and veins, between cerebrum and cerebellum, and, in general, between sensory and motor nerves, although they often confused the latter with tendons and ligaments. They described the meninges, the cerebral ventricles, including the fourth, and the choroid plexus, and Herophilus described the 'retiform plexus' at the base of the brain, probably in a sheep. Herophilus also named the 'calamus scriptorius', which Vesalius considered very appropriate, explaining in some detail what the Alexandrian had actually meant by a 'scribe's quill'. The 'torcular Herophili' was described in the following words: 'On the crown of the head the doublings of the meninges meet, converging and conveying the blood to an empty space like a cistern', which he therefore called the 'wine-press' (Latin: *torcular*).[5] It was Erasistratus, said Galen, 'who first derived the sensory nerves, which he regarded as hollow, from the meninges; the motor nerves from the brain and cerebellum. Later, however, he traced all nerves to the brain . . .'.[6]

To these Alexandrian physicians sudden death without obvious cause was due to heart weakness. Twitchings and cramp were muscular or nerve affections, and paralysis was the result of a lack of 'nerve force'. They appreciated that sensation and motion could be separately affected.

And it was to Alexandria that Galen came to study in the second century AD, some four to five centuries after Hippocrates, Aristotle, Herophilus, and Erasistratus. Alexandria was then in decline and the practice there of human dissection had already ceased. This was a circumstance which had dire effects on the history of medicine.

THE CLINICIAN

Galen was a physician who accepted the Hippocratic pathology of the 'humours', but although he was the most famous and widely travelled doctor of his day he did not leave much in the way of clinical description. Most of his accounts of patients seem more directed to impressing the reader with his superiority over others and in stressing the near miraculous nature of his cures. He enjoyed giving spectacular prognoses. There is a smug account of his success in treating the Emperor Marcus Aurelius who had a gastro-intestinal upset. 'The case was quite wonderful', he said, and afterwards the emperor 'never stopped lauding me'.[7] Of neurological interest is his mention, during a discussion about the faculties of imagination, reason, and memory, of the sick physician Theophilus. Galen appreciated that these faculties could be separately affected.

Theophilus who, although he otherwise conversed sagaciously and recognised those present, believed that there were pipers in the corner of the house where he was lying ... producing music ... Later, after he had convalesced and recovered ... he told everything which each visitor had said and done, and he remembered the appearance of the pipers.[8]

He described the case of a person who fell from a height and injured his thoracic spinal cord so that, although his upper limbs were spared, his lower limbs were paralysed in a few days.[0] There was complete loss of voice, but no apnoea or dyspnoea because 'the thorax was still kept in motion by the diaphragm and by the six upper muscles since these derive their nerve from the cervical spinal cord. But all the nerves supplying the intercostal muscles which produce expiration were affected.' He deduced that the loss of voice was a consequence of the paralysis of the intercostal muscles because he had produced aphonia in animals by ligating these nerves.

In another case of a man with numbness of the fingers of one hand he learned that the patient had fallen and struck his back at the cervicodorsal junction against a projecting stone. There was sharp local pain for a week which then subsided and was followed by numbness and dysaesthesiae. When Galen saw him it had persisted for thirty days and involved the inner fingers.

I therefore inferred that he had acquired a schirrous affection which came on as the result of the inflammation of the part around the exit of the nerve which proceeds from the spinal cord beyond the eighth cervical vertebra. This I knew because I realised from my knowledge of anatomy that the nerves ... are in reality multiple at their immediate origin, these roots being held and bound together by a common investment which is derived from the meninges. The lower part of this nerve, which has its origins in the nerves in the neck, extends to the little fingers and it is distributed to the skin that covers these fingers, supplying half the middle finger as well.[9]

Galen said that other attending physicians were perplexed by this. Whether or not we consider that Galen had deduced there were motor and sensory roots to each spinal nerve, it is nevertheless an example of the way he applied his anatomical studies to his clinical problems.

A great Roman lady, wife of Justus, suffered from an insomnia which Galen was able to trace to an unhappy affection for a dancer called Pylades. Mention of his name caused tachycardia and agitation.[10, 11]

He described headaches, chronic and remittent, hemicrania, vertigo, syncope, which he thought could arise from heart or brain disorders, and various forms and degrees of impairment of consciousness. In some cases of coma the eyes were closed; in others they were open. He described forms of catalepsy in which there was stiffness of the limbs 'as if frozen' and the eyes, though open, did not blink. These could have been cases of encephalitis, hysteria, or schizophrenia; akinesia with mutism. Siegel[12] wondered whether some of such patients were suffering from Parkinsonism and recalled that James Parkinson, in his 'Essay on the Shaking Palsy', quoted Galen. But Parkinson was not referring to cataleptic posture but to the nature of the tremor. When discussing tremor Galen said it arose spontaneously during voluntary movement but that another type of trembling, palpitation (palmos), was independent of movement and much coarser. It could be seen in a limb at complete rest. It was this distinction that impressed Parkinson. He said 'The separation of palpitation of the limbs (Palmos of Galen, Tremor Coactus of de la Boë) from tremor, is the more necessary to be insisted on, since the distinction may assist in leading to a knowledge of the seat of the disease.'[13]

Galen thought epilepsy was a disorder of the brain due to an accumulation there of thick humours. The convulsion was a reaction – a shaking of the origins of nerves. He viewed voluntary movements as involving some sort of mechanical element in the nerves; convulsive movements were also mechanical, but involuntary. He likened nerves to the chords of a lyre; they might act abnormally if they were unduly dry or wet. Epilepsy could arise directly from a disease of the brain; or the brain could be affected from a disorder of the stomach (from whence the 'aura' or breeze commonly arose); or, thirdly, epilepsy could arise because the brain was affected by some disorder in another part of the body. So he clearly recognized that epilepsy could be idiopathic or secondary. He described focal epilepsy when he recorded the case of a boy in whom 'the condition started in the calf, went up to the thigh, then to the flank and ribs of the same side, and finally to the neck and head. As soon as it reached the latter he became unconscious . . .'.[14]

In all this, as elsewhere in his studies of neurology, Galen, having performed no autopsies, had no notion of brain lesions and consequently could not begin to understand the function of the brain nor gain any glimpse of the problem of cerebral localization. As Siegel[15] remarked, it is all the more extraordinary that he should have concluded that apoplexy involved brain matter but that epilepsy represented only a disturbance of brain function. He deduced this presumably because apoplexy was fatal or disabling, whereas in epilepsy recovery was complete.

Galen observed the effect of light upon the pupil. 'When one eye is closed, the pupil of the other eye becomes larger. But when the (first) eye is opened again, the (other) pupil instantly assumes its natural size.' This did not suggest reflex action; its very speed, he interpreted, could only be that of a 'spirit'.[12]

THE WRITER

Galen's writings remained unknown to the West until the thirteenth century when surviving Greek and Arabic texts began to be translated into

Latin, an important development which was more or less completed by the sixteenth century. Since then French and German readers have had more complete translations at their disposal than the English. An Arabic translation of the fifteen books of Galen's Anatomy (*On anatomical procedures*) was discovered in the Bodleian Library at Oxford as recently as 1844. It contained the missing six books (9 to 15) and had apparently once belonged to Golius, an Arabic scholar in Leyden, then to Bartholinus the elder, Professor of Anatomy at Copenhagen, and finally to Narcissus Marsh, Archbishop of Dublin, who died in about 1697. The anonymous writer in the *London Medical Gazette* announcing 'this valuable discovery' lamented that he feared it would be 'better understood and more justly appreciated in France and Germany than in Great Britain.'[16]

An epitome of Galen's texts in English was prepared by Coxe in 1846.[17] In 1917 Singer[18] appealed for a complete English translation of Galen's works. It is not yet available. At present we have the following books in English translations: *Galen on the natural faculties*,[19] *Galen on medical experience*,[20] *Galen on anatomical procedures*, [21, 22]† and *Galen on the usefulness of the parts of the body*.[23]

Then there are the following extracts from Galen's works which have been translated into English: 'On the Diseased Parts',[24] 'On the Motion of Muscles',[25] 'On the Anatomy of Muscles for Beginners',[26] and 'On the Anatomy of Nerves'.[27]

Galen's accounts of the cranial nerves and the autonomic nervous system have recently been freshly studied in both the Greek and Arabic texts by Emilie Savage Smith.[28] In her interpretations she has taken into account the chronology of Galen's writings and has made new translations. This excellent study deals with that part of his work which had previously presented many difficulties and sources of confusion.

For general reading there is the whole series of papers by Joseph Walsh[29] on 'Galen's Writings and the Influences Inspiring Them', which appeared in the nineteen-thirties, and are listed in the references at the end of this book. There is a biography, *Galen of Pergamon*, by Sarton[30] and three recent books by Siegel: *Galen's system of physiology and medicine* (1968),[15] *Galen on sense perception* (1970),[31] and *Galen on psychology, psychopathology, and function and diseases of the nervous system* (1973).[12]

Lastly, there is Temkin's monograph *Galenism: rise and decline of a medical philosophy*.[32] Galen continues to fascinate not only doctors of medicine, but also biologists, philosophers, theologists, sociologists, and historians.

Although he was clearly an acute observer, a careful dissector, and an imaginative experimentalist, Galen was no literary genius. Many of his books are unnecessarily bulky. He is windy and repetitious, often mocking the work of others and boasting about his own. He never tires of explaining that his biological discoveries only served to demonstrate the wisdom of creation.‡ His errors were gross, but his successes were splendid. It is just as wrong for us to recall only his errors as it was for medieval man to assert his infallibility.

† The reader would scarcely guess that this text had passed through three translations; from Greek to Arabic, to German, and finally to English.

‡ Reminding one of the libretto of Haydn's Creation.

The book *On medical experience* is not what one might anticipate from such a title – an account by a senior physician of his clinical experience. Galen wrote it when he was only twenty years of age and it consists of a polemical debate between an Empiricist and a Dogmatist†; a disputation between two schools of medicine. The Empiricist, whom Galen opposes, is challenged as to the manner in which he collects and evaluates his clinical knowledge. At the beginning, Galen writes,

> and now let the Dogmatist speak first, as if he were before the judge in a Court of Law, ridiculing the arguments of the empiricist, his opponent, in the following manner.

Then follows an argument about methods. Clinical experience must surely be unreliable, because there is such an endless variety of symptoms, which present in different ways and in different sequence; because diseases themselves are so heterogeneous; and because the patients afflicted also differ one from another. 'How can a person determine whether what he sees at this moment is identical with that which someone has seen before or is something quite different, unless he himself has seen both?' What significance should be attached to a difference in the *order* in which symptoms present?

> If, for example, convulsion follows fever, this is a sign of death, and if fever follows convulsion this is a sign of safety. So, too, when lethargy precedes trembling, it is not a sign of death, but if it follows trembling it is a very bad sign. [p. 90]

The empiricist discusses the question of bloodletting in certain diseases. In phrenitis (delirium) the dogmatist considers that it would only weaken the person because in delirium 'the atoms are not found in their proper place in the pores of the cerebral membranes and if you empty out the blood from the veins, it would not be of any use' (p. 136). Also in loss of memory (stupor) speaking to the patient is contraindicated because 'this disease is due to inflammation of the cerebral membranes, and motion is not good for any inflamed organ'. In reply, the empiricist says that those are 'statements about invisible things' and that many physicians, while not actually contesting them, have found that in delirium bloodletting may help, but not always; and that in stupor 'if we did not rouse him and keep him awake, he was worse'.

It is in this book that Galen made his well-known statement:

> I am a man who attends only to what can be perceived by the senses, recognising nothing except that which can be ascertained by the senses alone with the help of observation and retention in the memory, and not going beyond this to any other theoretical construction. [p. 152]

This youthful affirmation, admittedly made in reference to clinical practice, was belied by his later researches and forms the basis of a general criticism which can be levelled at Galen. On the same page, however, he redeems himself to some extent when he says,

> It is likely that the same thing happens to me which often happens to others, namely, that I fail to attain my object and make mistakes in my medical practice, and do not always act correctly, since my knowledge is not true knowledge based on full

† At that time the term 'Dogmatist' carried no stigma of rigidity or narrow-mindedness. The Dogmatists were the orthodox practitioners, followers of Hippocrates. Likewise, the term 'Empiricist' carried no taint of the charlatan. The Empiricists based their knowledge on the light of experience only, in contrast to the Dogmatists who laid most stress on the powers of reasoning.

investigation of the whole of mankind, but knowledge acquired haphazardly and which falls short of the truth.

We should remember, when we are reading Galen, that his writings were spread over a period of fifty years. They were influenced by age, as well as experience, and throughout his life observations were affected by his theories and philosophies.

THE ANATOMIST

Galen's anatomy, we now know, was based on a study of a variety of species, both living and dead; cats, dogs, mice, weasels, sheep, pigs, apes of various species, and at least one elephant. There is no evidence that he ever performed a human dissection although Singer[33] concluded that he knew more about human anatomy than he cared to disclose. He probably did most of his dissection on tailed apes, but his favourite type was the tailless Barbary ape.

> The ape that most resembles man is the one that has a very round face, small canine teeth, a flat sternum, and longer clavicles, and that has the least hair and stands well erect so that it can walk properly and run swiftly.[34]

When he described the skeletal system he referred to two opportunities that had come his way to examine a human skeleton. One had been washed from its grave by a flooding river and was 'ready for inspection, just as though prepared by a doctor for his pupil's lesson', while the other was that of a robber left unburied on a mountainside and scavenged by birds of prey 'ready, as it were, for anyone who cared to enjoy an anatomical demonstration.'[35] He advised his students to go to Alexandria so that they could see human skeletons or else 'you must choose apes which most resemble man'. So, faced with the proscription of human dissection in Rome it is not surprising that Galen's anatomy should turn out to be simian, porcine, bovine, and canine. His neuroanatomy was based largely on the ox and his myology on the ape. 'Ox brains,' he said, 'ready prepared and stripped of most of the cranial parts, are generally on sale in the large cities. If you think more bone than necessary adheres to them, order its removal by the butcher who sells them.'[36]

Galen considered that the three central organs of the body were the liver, the heart, and the brain. 'Nature had three principal aims in constructing the parts of the animal, for she made them either for the sake of life (the brain, heart, and liver), or for a better life (the eyes, ears, and nostrils), or for the continuance of the race (the pudenda, testes, and uterus).'[37] Galen made the fundamental discovery that arteries contained blood and not air, as had been taught for three hundred years. He did this by first ligating the femoral artery in a live animal in two places. He then opened it between the ligatures and inserted a hollow tube. On relaxing the ligatures the flow of blood reappeared. When he repeated this experiment after placing a third ligature nearer the heart, he found that releasing the first two ligatures did not result in a return of blood flow.

Despite this he did not think the heart was formed of muscle, because its fibres were oblique and not longitudinal as in those of the limbs. He could not therefore conceive it as a pump. He thought its function was to produce 'innate heat' and he imagined the pits he saw in the interventricular septum were actually pores which allowed blood to seep through from the right to the left.

These can be seen for a great part; they are like a kind of fossae with wide mouths and they get constantly narrower; it is not possible, however, actually to observe their extreme terminations, owing both to the smallness of these and to the fact that when the animal is dead all the parts are chilled and shrunken.[38]

He did not visualize the auricles as a part of the actual heart, and his carotid arteries arose from a single stem. Blood was formed in the liver and flowed in the veins.

The arteries do not distend (pulsate) because they are filled from the heart, but the arteries are filled with blood because they (actively) distend.[30]

His doctrine of the pulse was one of his gross errors.

His osteology is generally considered to be good; he numbered twenty-four vertebrae. His myology included the description of some three hundred muscles and the identification of the levator of the eyelid, the platysma and the pterygoids and the lumbricals and interossei. He gave full accounts of the muscles of the eyes, the face, lips, tongue and larynx, neck, trunk, and limbs. Moreover he recognized the difference between skeletal and smooth muscle because they not only looked different, but had a different texture and taste. Skeletal muscles reacted to command while smooth muscles acted involuntarily.

Throughout *De usu partium* Galen makes it clear that he wanted his readers to understand how the body worked so that they could better appreciate the ills that could befall it. Nature was a sublime creator; everything had a purpose. The way things were fashioned could not be understood unless their functions were known. 'The spinal medulla was formed to be like a second brain for the parts below the head.'[40] Nerves 'have both faculties (I mean both sensation and motion) the other parts receiving them are not moved at the bidding of the will, but only feel, such parts, that is, as the skin, membranes, tunics, etc. . . .'[41] Again, 'the muscles at the point of the shoulder extend the whole arm and need a strong nerve, since they lift a very large part up and sometimes lift it very high.'[42] And 'no muscle anywhere is united with the skin without a reason, but this union is found only in those places where it serves a necessary purpose . . .', like the eyebrows, ears, and eyelids. Even the eyelashes 'are set like a palisade before the open eyes so that no small bodies may fall into them', while the 'eyebrows provide shelter like a wall and be the first to receive all that flows down from the head'.[43]

Though never tiring of extolling the superiority of the human body he did not refrain from recognizing the ingenious nature of parts of animal creation. To Galen, both the human penis and the elephant's trunk were marvellous contrivances.

In the opening pages of the first volume of *De usu partium* which is on 'The Hand,' he says,

Come now, let us investigate this very important part of Man's Body, examining it not simply to determine whether it is useful or whether it is suitable for an intelligent animal, but whether it is in every respect so constituted that it would not have been better had it been made so differently.[44]

The reader will be confronted with this attitude on page after page, but he will soon find that his annoyance passes. He will find himself smilingly anticipating the old heathen's arguments and admiring his ingenuity and zeal. There are many entertaining digressions. The following eugenic lines, for example, appear in the chapter on the tongue, an instrument which Nature made perfect, without error.

How frequently in the fathers that beget and the mothers that bear us it must not be error that is rare but right-doing. For drunkards consort with drunkards, and men that do not know their own whereabouts from repletion with women in the same state. Hence in this way the very beginning of our procreation is faulty, and then come the unspeakable errors of the pregnant woman, her indifference to proper exercise, her gluttony, passions, drunkenness, bathing and untimely indulgence in love. ... This is not the way in which farmers sow wheat and barley, or plant grapevines or olive trees; for first they see to it in advance that the soil to which they entrust their seeds shall be in good condition, and then take no little care that the seed shall not be deluged with too much water and rot, or withered by droughts, or killed by frost. No one, however, takes such great care in implanting a human being or in nourishing a human embryo ... they are careless of the first generation itself ...[45]

Without doubt there are duller tomes on present day students' bookshelves.

Here are some extracts from the chapter on 'The Hand'.

But when Nature placed the thumb in opposition to the other fingers, she realised that the lateral movements of the fingers in the direction of the thumb would be very advantageous. And if we must spread them apart as far as possible when we are attempting to handle a very large body, it is useful for the four fingers to move toward the outside (in the direction of the little finger) and the thumb towards the inside (extension). For this reason she gave the thumb a rather large tendon (of extensor pollicis longus) to control its motion toward the inside, but she limited the size of the other tendons (of lumbricals) not only because an intelligent workman properly makes nothing superfluous but also because she would have weakened the opposing motion (toward the little finger) if she had balanced it with another of equal force.[46]

When the fingers are flexed by the large tendons the small tendons are carried along by the force of the movement. For in general, whenever a body is subjected to two principles of motion acting at an angle to one another, if one of them is much the stronger, the other is inevitably nullified, but if the difference between them is slight or they are of equal strength, the resultant motion of the body is compounded of both of them.[47]

If you compute the total number of insertions in the ten fingers, you will find one hundred and twenty of them, obtaining this result because there are thirty joints and four insertions into each. But since there is one lacking in each of the thumbs, the total number will be one hundred and eighteen. Now by the Gods! When you can find no fault in these many attachments ... do you maintain that such things have all been done at random and without skill? Certainly, if we flexed this joint (of the thumb) in the same way as the others, I know that you would then criticise harshly and vehemently the uselessness of Nature's labour in creating an unserviceable motion and a tendon that was superfluous.[48]

Men call this finger (the thumb) the antihand, since in their opinion it is itself the equivalent of a whole hand. For they see that the actions of the hand are destroyed to an equal degree by cutting off either the four fingers or only the thumb. ... Tell me, O noble sophists and clever accusers of Nature, have you ever seen in the ape this finger that is called the antihand and that Hippocrates calls the great finger? And if you have not seen the ape's thumb, will you have the effrontery to say that it is just like the human thumb? If you have indeed seen one, I suppose you saw it was short, slender, distorted and altogether ridiculous, just as the ape's whole body is.[49]

Galen then enquires if anyone has seen an ape play the flute or write.[49]

Why were all the fingers made unequal, with the middle one the longest? Was it not because their tips would fall in the same line when they grasp large bodies or try to hold small objects? ... it is the evenly-balanced opposition of the finger tips to one another all around an object that makes them grasp more firmly and throw more vigorously. The same thing is to be seen, I think, in triremes, where the ends of the oars reach to the same line although the oars themselves are of different lengths, for in this case too, the middle ones are made longest for the same reason.[50]

The following extracts are from 'The Wrist and Arm':

Once, when one of these physicians and I were examining a young man who could touch the inner [medial] side of his shoulder with his hand, but not the outer [lateral] side when he flexed his forearm, this doctor could not recognise in which muscle the trouble lay. ... When these two muscles [biceps brachii and brachialis] act together, they flex the forearm in exactly a straight line; when one acts without the other, the forearm is inclined slightly to one side or the other. ... Since, then, the muscles cause the forearm to deviate in opposite directions from perfectly straight flexion, it was logical to make the muscle that moves it inward [biceps] stronger than the one that moves it outward [brachialis]. It was also logical to make the opposing muscles [triceps] correspond, each to its fellow. ...[51]

Now, at the shoulder joint the humerus can be not only extended and flexed but also moved circularly in any direction; for its head is rounded, the ligaments are lax, and the concavity of the neck of the scapula is shallow everywhere, regular in shape, like the head of the humerus. The joints at the wrist and elbow, however, being bound tightly on all sides cannot vary their motion or move in a circle, and so, since they cannot, and since diversity of movement must not be entirely disregarded, Nature made the articulation at both places a double one so that in each case the additional articulation might supply the deficiencies of the first. Thus circular and lateral movements are provided for these members, at the upper joint by the articulation of the radius with the humerus, and at the lower by the articulation of the carpus with the slender apophysis of the ulna (styloid process).[52]

Here follow some extracts from 'The Foot and Leg':

Man is the only one of all the animals to have been provided with hands, instruments suitable for an intelligent animal; likewise, of animals that go afoot he alone was made biped and erect for the reason that he had hands. ... In the dog, deer, horse and similar animals, the forelimbs were made legs like the hind limbs, and this conduces to swiftness. In man, however, the forelimbs became hands; for one who was to take the horse with his skilful hands had no need to be swift himself, and in place of speed it was far better for him to be provided with instruments necessary for all the arts. But why then was he not given four legs and hands as well, like the centaur? The reason is that, in the first place, a commingling of such widely different bodies was impossible for nature.[53]

Galen then goes on to explain the difficulties that would arise in the act of procreation, in feeding (human food for the upper, and horse food for the lower parts), in locomotion (the centaur could not climb a ladder or up the side of a ship), and in sitting down ('What sort of lap would he have for a book?'). 'Man is the only one to sit'.

So if Pindar as a poet accepts the myth of the centaur, we should be indulgent ... knowing the muse of poetry needs the marvellous more than all her other ornaments, we concede you, O Pindar, the right to sing and recount legends; for you wish not to teach, I suppose, but to astonish, charm and enchant your hearers.

Now, as I have said, the human leg is an instrument, not of simple locomotion, but of the kind of locomotion suitable for an intelligent animal. ... Locomotion takes place when one leg is moved around the other which is supported on the ground. Support is furnished by the foot, but the motion is the work of the whole leg, and so locomotion is accomplished by support and motion, and the foot is the instrument of one element and the whole leg of the other.[54]

Galen then describes what happens after the loss of the feet (in a 'plague' that occurred, and also when some pirates had chopped them off), and after the loss of the toes (as in frostbite). The former 'could stand but not walk', the latter

... could stand, walk, run, at least on smooth, level ground ... but if they had to traverse rough ground, particularly if it were precipitous, they not only fell behind, but were entirely helpless and unable to compete.

Here indeed is that extra feature in the construction of the human leg ... it is the division of the feet into toes, together with the concavity of the middle part (of the sole) ... to enable him to walk in all sorts of places by fitting the concavity over the convexities beneath his feet ... and by using the toes particularly in places that are precipitous, oblique or sloping.[55]

Galen stresses that some degree of prehension is to be found in the human foot; he tells the reader to watch a man climb a ladder and notice how he grips the rungs with his feet.

Here, in these selections from *De usu partium*, the reader catches a glimpse of Galen the observer and analyser, his mind free of dogma and uncluttered by theories. In his book *On anatomical procedures* he actually expressed his fear that anatomical studies 'may perish, because of the little regard my contemporaries have for the arts and sciences.' Of his pupils, he said, 'Should they die suddenly after me, these studies will die with them.'[56] How prophetic!

Neuroanatomy

The climate of the Mediterranean was not one in which autopsy could be performed in a leisurely manner. Decomposition of viscera required the dissector to examine first the abdominal and then the thoracic contents. Mondino was to write, in 1316, that dissection should begin with the abdomen because 'these members are foetid, and on this account we should make a start with them, in order that we may be able to throw them away as soon as possible.'[57] But even the enclosed brain – oozing like porridge from the skull on a battlefield, in a gladiator's arena – or even when delivered promptly with the severed head from the executioner, was not an easy organ to examine. Its shape, configuration, and relationships, its vessels and membranes, together with the contained cavities and communications must have presented a most mysterious object of exploration. We know now, of course, that only when the technique of hardening the brain in alcohol was developed in the eighteenth century that adequate dissection was made possible. If Western civilization had sprung up in the icy north – say in Finland, Iceland, or even in the north of Scotland – it is not inconceivable that initial examination of the human body would have progressed more speedily. Actually, the first hint that the cortex of the brain had a laminar structure came from a naked-eye observation on a frozen brain by Gennari in 1776.[58] It is said that the brain was artificially frozen, an uncommon practice in all likelihood in view of its rare mention in the accounts which have come down to us. Francis Bacon (1561 – 1626) is said to have died of a chill caught while experimenting on refrigeration by stuffing a fowl full of snow.

But, to return to Galen's neurology, which most agree is the best feature of all his work. Nature, he said, invested the brain with bone, shaped like a helmet, and made it porous, with sutures that served not only as articulations but as channels through which gaseous products could escape. The sutures were 'very much like that of two saws set against one another with their teeth fitting accurately together'.[59] Galen said the term 'suture' derived from the resemblance to the 'seams' of a sewn garment. He described the procedures he adopted in dissecting a brain, noting the dura mater and pia mater, the convolutions, bisecting the falx, separating the hemispheres, cutting sections, and elevating the fornix to expose the ventricles, choroid plexuses, and the pineal gland. 'The usefulness of that vault-shaped body (fornix) should be assumed to be no different from that of actual vaults in buildings . . . (it) holds up without distress all that portion of the encephalon that lies above it.'[60]

He described the corpus callosum, the lateral, third, and fourth ventricles, the corpora quadrigemina, the infundibulum, and the pituitary gland. He examined the communications between the ventricles and described our foramina of Monro. Opinions differ on whether he identified the acqueduct of Sylvius. Singer and Duckworth, on the basis of their translations of the *Anatomical procedures*, concluded that he had; the problem is discussed by Woollam.[61, 62] May thinks that the account Galen gave in *De usu partium* makes it impossible, for there he said 'The left and right walls of the canal are formed by these bodies [the corpora quadrigemina] . . . it is covered by a thin, though certainly not weak membrane [the arachnoid], attached on both sides to the gloutia [corpora quadrigemina].'[63] This account and his use of a probe which he passed from the third to the fourth ventricle rather suggests that his canal was not deep in the centre of the mid-brain, but more dorsally placed.

Galen did not think the pineal was part of the brain itself, 'like the pylorus is of the stomach',[64] and he did not subscribe to the notion that it served as a valvular mechanism, in regulating the passage of pneuma from the third ventricle. Instead, he thought the cerebellar vermis used an antero-posterior rocking motion to control its entry and exit from the fourth ventricle, which suggests to Siegel that he may have seen the foramen of Magendie.[65]

Galen recommended 'the brain of a starved and emaciated animal . . . it is necessary that the substance of the brain be exceptionally hard and dessicated'. Yet, he can hardly have observed that malnutrition caused cerebral atrophy. He thought the brain's texture was softer anteriorly, and harder posteriorly, including the cerebellum. He similarly classified nerves as more or less hard and soft. Motor nerves emerged from the brain posteriorly and were harder; sensory nerves were softer, so that they could more easily receive sense impressions, and they mainly emerged from the anterior parts of the brain.

Galen did not agree with Aristotle's belief that the brain served to cool the heart. 'For the supposition that the brain was formed for the sake of the heat in the heart, to cool it and bring it to a moderate temperament, is utterly absurd, since in that case Nature would not have placed the brain so far from the heart.'[66]

But what really intrigued him were the meninges and the ventricular cavities. Woollam considers that the most striking of all his descriptions is that of the blood-vessels and meninges, and he questions whether the doctrine of ventricular localization of function, which dominated thought about the brain for so many centuries, may have simply arisen because the hollowness of the brain was such an obvious feature in an otherwise amorphous mass.[67]

In describing the cerebral venous system he noted the differing surfaces of the veins and the sinuses and spoke of the superior and inferior sagittal sinuses as 'sanguineous aqueducts'. Woollam has pointed out that Galen's great cerebral vein was correctly described as running downward, as it does in the ox, and not horizontally, as in man.

The cranial nerves. Galen listed seven pairs of cranial nerves, although he actually described nine, a classification which lasted until the seventeenth century. 'Whoever does not know this is, as the proverbial expression goes, like a seaman who navigates out of a book. Thus he reads the books on anatomy, but he omits inspecting with his own eyes . . .'.[68] Vesalius must have read this as in the preface to the *De fabrica*, when he was deriding his contemporary academic dissectors, he said they 'haughtily govern the ship from a manual'.[69] Galen said that 'The dissection of the [cranial] nerves is a toilsome and difficult matter' and that the basal foramina could only be seen by careful inspection of a dried skull. It was because of poorly prepared skulls that some anatomists were able to assert that 'some skulls have no sutures'.[70] He did not consider that the olfactory bulbs and tracts, 'two long horn-like processes', constituted nerves for 'nerve tissue is not like that', and they did not leave the skull.[71]

Galen's first cranial nerve was the optic. This pair was arranged like 'the Greek letter Chi, which is written like this; X', to form the chiasm. 'Neither of the two processes passes to the opposite side ... the nerve which originates from the right side of the brain gets to the right eye and the nerve which originates from the left side of the brain gets to the left eye.' There 'they break up and each of them becomes the retinal covering.'[72] The optic nerve, he said, contains a hollow, which would admit a hog's bristle. 'In these nerves alone, before they enter the eye, there is within a clear perceptible pore; whence some anatomists have called them canals, not nerves.'[73] Galen was possibly referring to the central artery of the retina. But, elsewhere, he said 'I believe that not all nerves have a central canal.'[74]

His second nerve was the oculomotor, in which some think he included the abducens. He did not identify the trochlear. His third and fourth pairs were the modern trigeminal; he noted the maxillary and mandibular branches, but probably not the ophthalmic. He traced the sensory fibres of the trigeminal to the face and teeth and 'to the membranes which invest the tongue'; its motor fibres went to the temporalis, masseter, and pterygoid muscles, and also, he thought, to the platysma.

The fifth pair were the combined facial and auditory nerves. 'They come off close together but their passage out from the skull is not through a single aperture. Therefore, one might well assume that this is not a single pair, but rather two pairs.' Galen said that another anatomist, Marinus, had already treated them as a single pair, and he was not prepared to disagree with him.[75]

The sixth pair were the combined glossopharyngeal, vagus, and accessory nerves. The vagus he traced to the 'sheath of the lungs', the pericardium and heart, the larynx, oesophagus and stomach, and 'to all the abdominal viscera'.

His seventh cranial nerve was our hypoglossal and it supplied the tongue, so that 'one half of the tongue immediately loses its mobility when one cuts through one of these nerves'. He deduced that the tongue played no part in laryngeal movement because he observed that after hypoglossal section, an animal's 'larynx is drawn and moved upwards while the tongue is doing nothing', if the animal is allowed to take a drink.[77]

Galen's description of the sympathetic nerve trunks has been universally recognized as an early fundamental contribution to anatomy. He described their emergence from the skull with the carotid arteries through the canals in the petrous temporal bones, their course through the neck and thorax, and he noted the three cervical ganglia, the carotid plexus, and the intermingling with the vagus and spinal nerves in the abdomen to form the coeliac plexus. Criticism has usually been offered on two points. First, that he made different statements at various times, and second, that the different animals he dissected had common vago-sympathetic trunks of different lengths.[78, 28] Consequently there has been some difference of opinion about his actual observations but Smith[28] has concluded from her examination of both the Greek and Arabic texts that Galen recognized that the sympathetic nerve was a separate nerve once it emerged from the skull. Although he did not discover its cephalic portion he thought it arose from his third and fourth cranial pairs, and not from the sixth.

Clear separation of the vagus and sympathetic nerves in man was not even established by Vesalius in the sixteenth century.

The recurrent laryngeal nerves. There is a memorable description of these nerves, which he named, and which he perceived to take different courses on the two sides, looping around the arch of the aorta on the left side and the subclavian artery on the right.

I call these two nerves 'the recurrent nerves' and 'those that come upward and backward' on account of a special characteristic of theirs which is not shared by any of the other nerves that descend from the brain.[79]

In the passage of the nerves across the thorax a branch reascends on each side by the same pathways which it took before in descending; thus it accomplishes a double course . . . it reascends from there to the larynx where the nerves insert themselves into the muscles in question . . . it is the same as in that instrument made for the leg (glossocomion); there the origin of the movement arises from our hands around the axis and carries along the motion of the principal springs and pulleys; and from these the motion returns from the top downwards from the pulleys towards the part of the leg which is in the course of being stretched. The nerves of the larynx behave in the same way; the bundle of nerves issuing from the brain is like the axis, the origin of the motion. The part of the thorax whence the nerves commence to retrace their course is like the pulley.[80]

Galen likened the action of these nerves both to the mechanism of a pulley and to 'the runner in the stadium' (there was a double course in the spina at the circus maximus[81]). Singer's illustration depicts Galen's analogy between this nerve and a limb extension apparatus (glossocomion) and he points out how lack of nomenclature made such explanatory comparisons necessary.[82]

Galen studied the function of the laryngeal nerves. He noted that 'animals which possess no voice have no larynx either', and that animals with a loud voice, such as the pig, have a large larynx. 'As one cuts these nerves, or bruises them, or compresses them with the fingers or by a ligature, the voice of the animal is damaged, and its resonance is lost.'[83] Recovery of voice occurred after temporary compression but not if both nerves were severed completely. Galen also mentions two instances in which there was accidental injury to the laryngeal nerves by surgeons removing goitres. Both patients were children; in one both nerves were severed and the infant was rendered 'mute'. In the second patient one nerve was spared and he was 'half-mute'.[84]

It is not surprising that Galen, seeing the strange course of these two nerves, should have concluded that they acted in some mechanical manner. He had no inkling that in the growth of the human embryo they were affected by the descent of the aortic arches.

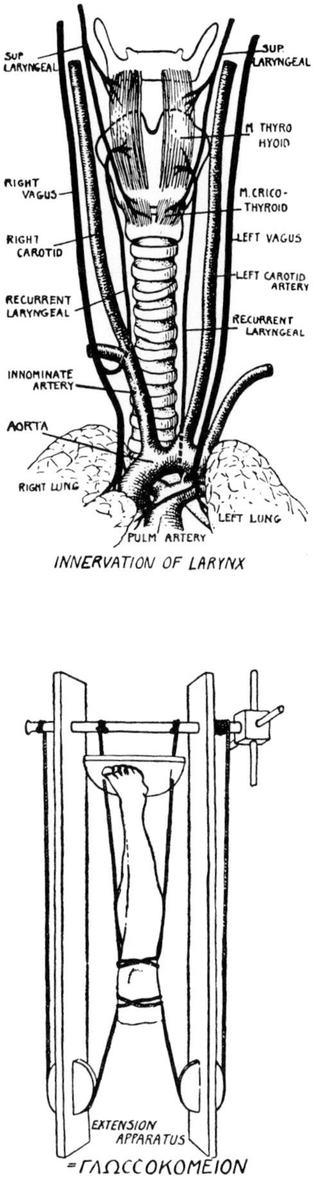

FIG 2. The course of the recurrent laryngeal nerves. Galen compared these in their action to the *glossokomeion*, an extension apparatus then in use by surgeons. Turning the screw tightened the ropes, which pulled in opposite directions. Galen thought that likewise the two branches of the vagus (superior laryngeal and recurrent laryngeal nerves) pulled in opposite directions on the larynx (after Singer[82]).

The special senses. Galen was convinced that the brain was the organ of sensation. 'All the instruments of the senses... communicate with the encephalon.' He disagreed with Aristotle who taught otherwise.

> Aristotle! What a thing for you to say! Does not a nerve . . . enter each ear? Does not a portion of the encephalon . . . come to each side of the nose? Do not one soft nerve [optic] and one hard nerve [occulomotor] come to each eye, the former inserted into its root and the latter into the muscles moving it? Are there not four nerves extending to the tongue, two [lingual] of them soft . . . and two [hypoglossal] hard?[85]

> The tongue has been observed to be deprived sometimes of its motion and sometimes of its power to distinguish and apprehend flavours.[86]

> Unless the alteration in each sense instrument comes from the encephalon and returns to it, the animal will still remain without perception. You could learn this by observing persons stricken with apoplexy, whose sense instruments are all uninjured, but who, for all that, receive no benefit from them in distinguishing sensations.[87]

In the last quotation it appears as if Galen believed that sensation, as well as motion and thought, *began* in the brain. This becomes clearer when he considers the faculty of vision.

To Galen the eyeball could be represented by seven concentric circles comprising the lens, the vitreous, the retina, the choroid, the sclera, the ocular aponeuroses, and the conjunctiva with the bulbar fascia.

The optic nerve 'upon reaching the eyes themselves is resolved again, flattens out, embraces the vitreous humour like a tunic, and is inserted into the crystalline humour [the lens] . . . [the latter] is the principal instrument of vision'.[88]

There were four principal movements of the eyes that were carried out by the four recti, but 'since it was better that the eye should also rotate, Nature made two other muscles that are placed obliquely, one at each eyelid'. (Galen also described a muscle lacking in man, called the retractor bulbi, at the root of the eye.)[8]

In *De usu partium*, the problem of how opening and closing the eyes were effected, puzzled him.

> Every part moved by the will needs at least two muscles set to oppose one another and capable the one of extending, the other of flexing it . . . no muscle can perform both movements . . . if this is so, how will the eyelids be moved?' [0]

After this hint of the phenomenon of reciprocal innervation he concluded that as far as the lower eyelid was concerned it was without motion because it was small and did not require it. In the upper eyelid he described two slips of muscle, a transverse medial and an oblique lateral. But he was dissatisfied with the workings of these and promised he would investigate the matter at a later date. In his subsequent book *On anatomical procedures* (p. 46) he gave the first known account of the levator palpebrae superioris.

When he came to consider the faculty of vision itself Galen displayed his accustomed ingenuity and also his knowledge of geometry, of which he was very proud. He said 'the essence of the visual faculty is of the nature of light'. He mentions how intense light can blind a person as when one gazes at the sun in a partial eclipse, and he quotes the experiences of Xenophon's soldiers in the snow, and the prisoners of Dionysius when brought up from the dungeons. He noticed that failing sight in the elderly may be accompanied by wrinkling of the cornea or narrowing of the pupils.[91] He made observations showing that he appreciated the existence of parallax, and the difference between uniocular and binocular perception, thus:

You have seen the rays of the sun escaping through a narrow opening, advancing without being deflected or bending at any point, and pursuing a path that was perfectly straight and undeviating. Consider, please, the path of the visual rays to be like that too.[92]

Therefore,

... each object seen appears not alone or isolated but always accompanied by something else, because the visual rays surrounding it fall sometimes on objects beyond the body at which one is looking and sometimes on objects near it.[93]

A thing seen by the right eye alone appears somehow to lie more to the left side when it is close by, and more to the right side when it is farther off; that if it is seen with the left eye alone, it will appear to lie more to the right when it is nearer and to the left when it is farther away; and that if it is seen by both eyes, it will appear to lie in the space between.[94]

If the pupil of one of the eyes is pressed or displaced either upward or down, objects hitherto seen to be single appear to be double.
If he stands near a pillar and closes each eye in turn, some of the things seen by the right eye on the right side of the pillar will not be visible to the other eye (and vice versa) ... but when he opens both eyes together, he will see both sides.[95]

The binocular field of vision could also be appreciated.

For if you care to place longitudinally on your nose between your eyes a small piece of wood, your own hand, or anything else that can prevent external objects lying before them from being seen by both eyes, you will see dimly with each eye, but much more clearly if you close one eye, as if the faculty hitherto divided between the two were now coming to the other eye.[96]

Siegel[31] has made a detailed study of Galen's concepts on visual perception and points out that Galen had a twofold approach. One was physiological and the other geometrical. There was an ancient idea of an outgoing emanation from the eye to an object. Galen visualized emission of pneuma from the brain via the optic nerves and retina to the lens and thence through space to the object of vision. The pneuma returned to the brain by the same route. The lens and retina were thus parts of a conductive apparatus. It was not known of course that the lens had refractive properties and that the retina was the light-sensitive structure.

Siegel concluded that Galen's main guide in devising his geometrical approach to vision was the writings of Euclid, who lived in Alexandria some five centuries before Galen. Euclid had shown that light rays travelled in straight lines. Galen inferred that the central ray of a visual cone travelled in a direct line through the centre of the lens to the optic nerve head. He had not appreciated the correct, off-centre position of the latter. The difficulties encountered in trying to explain how rays which only travelled in a straight line, pursued their path through the optic nerve and chiasm, and into the ventricles of the brain, were never overcome until Kepler's day.

Galen thought that the optic nerve arrangement in the chiasm was so that their canals could unite, facilitating the exchange of pneuma, and ensuring fusion of images. He did not, of course, know of the decussation itself. Of the optic nerves, he said,

> . . . as soon as they have touched each other inside the skull they unite their central canals: they then separate immediately . . . as if to show simply and solely that they only came into contact in order to unite their canals.[31]

The notion of beams of 'light' emanating from the eyes and Galen's conjectures about the visual process suggest that he would have been interested in Willis's patient who could see in the dark after drinking alcohol. Willis said he knew 'an ingenious man with an active brain who said that after an extra good bout of wine he could see to read print clearly on a very dark night'.[97] He was postulating the existence of some 'vital fire' that could escape vision.

The rete mirabile. The rete mirabile (wonderful net) was first described by Herophilus[5]; he called it a 'retiform plexus' and throughout the Middle Ages it was usually referred to in words of admiration, as something very precious, mysterious, and delicate – like the 'thin-spun gossamer' of the poets. It is certainly not a normal human anastomosis and Galen presumed its existence in man, although he did not mention its absence in the monkey. It is present in sheep, cats, goats, oxen, and pigs. Since the development of intracranial angiography the term has been misused at times to denote discrete basal anastomotic areas which have been revealed between the internal and external carotid circulations. In a recent review it has been pointed out that such collaterals have neither the gross anatomical characteristics, nor the histological features of *the rete mirabile* of certain animals.[98]

Galen's own words about this structure follow.

> The plexus called retiform by anatomists is the most wonderful of the bodies located in this region. It encircles the gland [pituitary] itself and extends far to the rear . . . it is not a simple network but [looks] as if you had taken several fishermen's nets and superimposed them . . . the meshes of one layer are always attached to those of another, and it is impossible to remove any one of them alone . . . on account of the delicacy of the members composing it and the closeness of its contexture, you could not compare this network to any man-made nets, nor has it been formed from any chance material. Nature appropriated the material for this wonderful network the greatest part [internal carotid arteries] of the arteries ascending from the heart to the head.[99]

Thus Galen observed that the *rete* was derived from the carotid circulation. The internal carotid arteries entered the head,

> . . . and when they have passed beyond the cranium, in the space between it and the thick meninx they are first divided into many very small, slender arteries, and then they are interwoven and pass through one another, some toward the front of the head, some toward the back, and others to the left and right, giving the other

opposite impression, namely, that they have forgotten the route to the encephalon. However, this is not true either; for, as roots combine to form a trunk, so from these many arteries there arises another pair of arteries [anterior cerebral] . . . and so these now enter the encephalon through the perforations in the thick meninx.

Well, what is this wonderful thing, and for what purpose has it been made by a Nature who does nothing in vain?[99]

Then, Galen's readers are subjected to the familiar story – everything was there for a purpose, Nature was an infallible Creator, the *rete* was admirably suited to perform the function which Galen had devised for it, namely the manufacture of his 'animal spirit', the activating agent of all nervous activity. He was terribly pleased.

We do not know if Galen ever saw the circle of Willis. It is absent in oxen, which he used for studies of the brain, but present in dogs and horses. Some species of animals possess both a *rete* and a circle of Willis. Siegel[100] has stressed that the *rete* is below the dura mater, while the circle of Willis is above it.

The effluent ducts. Ventricular drainage was important to Galen's conception of cerebral function and he thought he had identified passages by which residues could escape. Gaseous products could escape upward through the sutures of the skull, and liquid ones trickled downward via two routes. The first of these was through the apertures in the cribriform plate into the nose. The second was through a bifid channel from the base of the third ventricle to the infundibulum, pituitary gland, and nasopharynx. These discharges were called *pituita* (phlegm).

In *De usu partium*, he says

Since there are two kinds of these residues, one vaporous and fuliginous, tending naturally upward, the other watery and slimy, so to speak, which sinks down of its own weight, she [Nature] cut two kinds of channels for their elimination . . . for the former she bored . . . certain fine apertures [the sutures] . . . [and for the latter] visible orifices [in the palatine and ethmoid bones]. . . . It is not always possible to see clearly the elimination of the vaporous residues . . . for it sometimes escapes the sight because they are so thin.[101]

In *Anatomical procedures*, on the same topic, he has some very special pleading to make.

It is not here my purpose to derive the knowledge of the nature of things which I wish to understand by analogy; for this is not the aim of anatomy. Rather I am simply trying to give an account of those things which manifest themselves to the eyesight. And it is not possible for you to perceive with the eye how the canals leading from the brain to the nose terminate. For the matter is, as I explained, that is to say, in this region the brain is soft.[102]

Similarly, writing of the perforations in the dura mater over the cribriform plate, he said 'they are not accessible to the eye', although sunlight could penetrate the lifted dura there 'as if there were fine perforations . . . that a man can surmise'. This line of thought was to become familiar in the history of anatomy. A structure could be too small to be seen clearly or consistently, and post-mortem changes might be imagined to have concealed it. In the seventeenth century Leeuwenhoek, using his primitive microscope, at first found no hollows in nerves. Later, he concluded that they had closed up when the tissues dried. Even today one can understand the difficulties of electron microscopists.

In defence of Galen, Woollam[103] has pointed out that in the ox brain there is a huge *massa intermedia* traversing the third ventricle, so Galen may have thought the two channels so created were, in fact, exit ducts. It is likely that, as elsewhere in Galen's writings, there was at work a combination of genuine misinterpretation, artefactual observation, and inventive theorizing. He had, after all, an extraordinary collection of data, myth, and theory to bring together.

The spine and spinal cord. In the twelfth book of *De usu partium* when he begins to discuss the spine, Galen says 'Nature has made the spine for animals to be like the keel of the body that is necessary for their life.'[104] There were four functions of the spine.

It serves as a base or foundation stone for the instruments necessary to life; second, as a pathway for the spinal medulla; third, as a safeguard; and fourth, as an instrument of motion for the animal's back. Hence it had to be hard, hollow and articulated.[105]

All the outgrowths, the junctions of the joints, the unions, the ligaments, and all the foramina have been marvellously constructed for both action and resistance to injury. . . . The spinal medulla was formed to be like a second encephalon for the parts below the head. . . .[106]

He was probably referring to the intervertebral discs, as pointed out by May,[107] when he wrote,

As the vertebrae withdraw towards the rear from their junction in front, they gradually separate and have all the space between them full of a white viscous humour very like that interspersed in nearly all joints. Indeed the usefulness of such a juice is common to all parts which must move readily. Men smear axles of wagons and chariots with a moist viscous juice.

(May reminds us that in the ape the spine is usually ventroflexed in the thoracic and lumbar regions, and does not have a lumbar lordosis.)

Galen commented on the use of the term 'marrow'. He said 'Plato applies the term "marrow" to the spinal cord, which he calls "vertebral marrow", and to the brain also, which he calls "cranial marrow" . . . but as for the marrow contained in the bones, no nerve takes its origin from that.' He went on, 'When you boil the bones you find, after cooking, the bone marrow very swollen and sweet, whereas in the cranial marrow, that is, the brain, and in the vertebral marrow, that is, the spinal cord, that [alteration] is not found.'[113]

He noted the variable size and shape of the intervertebral foramina at different levels, and how they were formed 'by notches cut out of adjacent vertebrae'. Curiously, he did not mention the termination of the cord in the lumbar region, and the cauda equina, nor the cervical and lumbar expansions of the cord. He listed twenty-nine pairs of spinal nerves but he did not establish without any doubt that each nerve had two roots. He said that 'The nerves grow out of the spinal medulla right at the point where the lateral parts of the vertebrae come to an end.' However, Siegel has discovered the following statement in *De locis affectis*.

> The physicians do not even know that there is a special root at the origin of the nerves which are distributed to the entire hand and from which sensation arises; [nor do they know] that there is another [root] for the nerves moving the muscles.[109]

In describing (in the monkey) the distribution of the cervical and the first and second thoracic nerves to the forelimb, Galen noted that the upper fibres went to the shoulder and upper arm, and the lower fibres to the forearm and hand. So he was probably the first anatomist to note what we now call segmental innervation.

He said

> Much of them is distributed to the muscles of the arm and forearm; what remains is distributed to the tip of the hand. The rule especially is for the last of the origins mentioned to send nerves to the hand, but those to the forearm are from the one above this, and those to the arm and those to parts still higher to reach the scapula, from the highest pairs as a rule.[27]

The nerves. Tracing the course of the spinal nerves Galen noted 'the blending and union' at the brachial and lumbosacral levels, and that 'they are not always arranged in the same pattern in all apes.'[110] Of the nerves themselves he said;

> Hippocrates named the nerves collectively from the Greek 'tenon' . . . which means 'to stretch' . . . [because] some individuals believe that the nerve stretches . . . the term is used because the limbs of animals extend and flex themselves in this or that direction primarily by means of the nerves, since it is the nerves alone, when they have joined the muscles and grown into them, which bestow upon them voluntary movements.[111]

Galen also mentions the terms 'ligaments' and 'tendons', which resembled 'nerves', so that 'you must retain the significance of these names quite distinctly in your memory and remind yourself constantly that when we say 'nerve' we only mean that which springs from the brain or the spinal marrow . . .'.[111] Tendons sprang from muscles, and ligaments from bones. But Galen thought that when a motor nerve entered a muscle its branches merged with those of the ligaments. At the muscle insertion a tendon is formed by this union of nerve and ligamentous fibres. This tendon becomes the principal instrument of motion. The belly of the muscle is merely a mass of protective flesh. Hence, it was not the muscle which contracted, but its tendon and the nerve branches within it.

Galen carefully dissected the course of nerves, noting how they buried themselves between the muscles of the limbs, and hid in grooves in the bones. He observed the vulnerability of the ulnar nerve at the elbow and how the median nerve Nature 'carefully threaded through the middle of the diarthrosis in the deepest part of this region between the ulna and radius'.[112]

In analysing the mechanisms involved in opening and closing the eyelids it was pointed out that Galen caught a glimpse of the phenomenon of reciprocal innervation. He developed it more fully when studying the coordination of movements of a limb. In '*De motu musculorum*' he wrote:

> ... for, since each limb, set in motion by muscles – as though by reins – has to divide its activity between two sides, has one muscle tense and relaxed alternately. The contracted muscle pulls towards itself, while the relaxed muscle is pulled along with its part; therefore both muscles move during the performance of each of the two movements (but they are not both active) for activity consists in tension of the part which moves, and not in the action of obeying; and a muscle obeys when it is pulled in a passive state, just like any other part of the limb.[113]

He could not, of course, draw on the concept of reflex action to explain this, and he did not know that motor and sensory nerve impulses were conducted in fibres bound together in nerves. He could not therefore appreciate that excitatory and inhibitory signals could be transmitted simultaneously.

When Sherrington[114] wrote on the history of the word 'tonus' as a physiological term he referred to Galen's use of the term 'tonic action', meaning 'tense'. Galen said 'Let us see how the legs behave in standing ... although there is in them no visible action of the muscles, all of the muscles are of a truth in motion and action ...'. Galen perceived that there were several types of muscle action and he endeavoured to analyse them by clinical observation, by dissection and by experiment.

There are two common misconceptions about Galen's descriptions of the nerves. First, that he confused them with tendons; second, that he showed they were hollow. The first view arose because of his confused account of the mode of action of the nerve – muscle junction. The second belief was also understandably the consequence of his description of the canals in the optic nerves and his *assumption* of invisible channels in peripheral nerves. The doctrine of the hollow nerve was universally accepted throughout the ancient world and antedates Galen. It persisted throughout the Middle Ages and Vesalius was one of the first Renaissance anatomists to question it. Willis likened the porosity of nerves to the structure of sugar cane. The doctrine survived to the end of the eighteenth century and the identification of the axon. But the twentieth-century discovery of the viscosity of axoplasm, and the dynamic features of our modern concept of nerve transmission, do serve to recall the ancient interpretation. As Clarke has put it, 'Yet another Greek biological concept has been to some extent correct, but for the wrong reasons.'[115]

THE VIVISECTIONIST

Commenting on his predecessors' lack of interest in the function of dissected parts Galen asked 'Did they ever take the trouble to make a section themselves, or themselves to put a ligature around parts in the living animal in order to learn which function is injured?'[116]

He performed operations on the brains of living unanaesthetized animals.

He preferred a pig or goat as 'you avoid seeing the unpleasing expression of the ape when it is vivisected'.[117] He observed that 'The whole brain, so long as the animal does not cry out, rises and sinks slightly with a movement which resembles that of the pulsation of all beating bloodvessels ... and if the animal does cry out then you see that the brain heaves itself up further.' He said 'In very old animals the brain is much too small to fill the cavity of the skull', thereby recording senile cerebral atrophy.[118] Elsewhere, he said, with reference to movement of the brain, 'This meninx, the dura mater, undergirds the skull, but the brain, expanding and contracting, approaches and withdraws from (the skull) in the empty space between.'[119] Movement of the brain, not clearly attributed to pulsation, was to become a popular notion.

In his operations on the living brain Galen came to be impressed by the importance of the ventricles.

And when one presses down on that ventricle which is found in the part of the brain lying at the nape of the neck, then the animal falls into a very heavy and pronounced stupor. This is also what happens when you cut into the ventricles, except that if you do cut into them, the animal does not revert to its natural condition as it does when you press upon them.[120]

When an incision was made into the fourth ventricle 'then the animal seldom returns to its normal condition ...'. But he found that if only the roof of this ventricle were quickly incised, 'You then see how the animal blinks with its eyes', but if you then press on the anterior ventricle 'the animal ceases to blink ... and the eye on the side which you are pressing becomes like the eyes of blind men.'

When Galen debates the question of the supremacy of heart or brain he also said 'If you press so much upon a (cerebral) ventricle that you wound it, immediately the living being will be without movement and sensation, without spirit and voice ... this does not happen if we press the naked heart.'[121]

In his *Commentaries on Hippocrates and Plato* Galen discusses the problem of the seat of the soul and favoured the idea that it lay, not in the ventricles, but in the substance of the brain. He concluded from his experiments that injury penetrating to the ventricles did not actually destroy life and mind, although they were paralysing. But the ventricles 'prepared the instruments of the soul', namely, the animal spirits which flowed into the nerves and which also penetrated the substance of the brain. For an admirable discussion of this confusing subject the reader is referred to Siegel's *Galen's system of physiology and medicine*.[15] Galen's influence in the evolution of the doctrine of ventricular localization of cerebral function is not at all clear. But whatever Galen thought on this topic, he could not have been very impressed by the convolutions, structures which Erasistratus said were so complex in man because of his superior intelligence. Galen said of them, 'Even donkeys have an exceedingly complex encephalon, whereas, judging by their stupidity it ought to be perfectly simple and uncomplicated.'[122] Vesalius was to quote this some fourteen hundred years later.

But Galen's most famous experiments were made on the spinal cord. The Hippocratic writers knew that the spinal cord was an extension of the brain and injury to it could cause paralysis and urinary retention. 'Such patients are more apt to lose the power of their legs and arms, to have torpor of the body, and retention of urine.'[123] They also knew that the level of injury determined the distribution of paralysis. Galen was the first to study the function of the spinal cord and he did this in live apes and monkeys by making various sections, horizontal, complete, and partial, at different levels. He also made longitudinal sections.

On exposing the spinal cord Galen first noted that:

> ... were you to expose this sheath around the spinal marrow then no harm would befall the animal on that account, or even if you made a longitudinal cut in the spinal marrow itself, since all the respective nerves branch off at the places where the vertebrae meet one another at the sides ...[124]

But if the cord was completely severed,

> ... in all the nerves which lie below that place where the transection has been made, both the two potentialities are lost, I mean the capacity of sensation and the capacity of movement, and also all the bodily parts of the animal in which they are distributed become insensitive and motionless, a result which is inevitable, clear and intelligible ...[124]

In the sacral region, where experiments should begin,

> ... the first structure which paralysis affects and which will be deprived of movement, are the ends of the legs; the second, next to the end, are the parts which come in front, then the parts of the thigh and hips ...[125]

In the lumbar region he found that the cord can be transected without injuring the emerging nerves 'because these travel obliquely downwards'. In the thoracic region, in addition to paralysis, there is impairment of respiration and voice.

In the cervical region he discovered the following:

> 1. ... should the spinal marrow that lies between the skull and the first vertebra be severed ... then at once the whole body of the animal becomes deprived of movement.
>
> 2. ... as for the incision which is made behind the first vertebra, it inflicts on the animal just the same manifestations, not because it lays open the first ventricle [our fourth] but because it paralyses the feet of the animal, and arrests the whole of its respiration. And this is found also with regard to the incision which is made behind the second, third and fourth vertebrae ... .
>
> 3. Transection of the spinal marrow behind the fifth vertebra paralyses all the remaining parts of the thorax, and arrests their movements, but the diaphragm remains almost unscathed.
>
> 4. [In transection] behind the sixth vertebra ... the diaphragm meets with less damage.
>
> 5. [In transection below the seventh and eigth vertebra] the whole of the mobility of the diaphragm remains unscathed.[126]

Galen also performed hemisection of the spinal cord.

You have also seen during dissection that transverse incisions of the cord that reach only its centre (hemisection) do not paralyse all the lower parts situated directly below the incision; the right when the right is cut, and the left when the left is cut.[127]

In these experiments Galen noted that the paralysis was both motor and sensory when the section of the cord was complete, but when it was incomplete he said nothing about sensory loss. There were virtually no additions to this knowledge until the nineteenth century, but Brown-Séquard was wrong when he said (see p. 268) that Galen made no reference to sensory loss in complete transection of the cord.

Galen also operated upon nerves and muscles. He noted that when a muscle was cut through, its distal portion was paralysed, but that some degree of motion remained if the section was not complete.

When a nerve is cut, pinched, contused or tied by a ligature, or hardened, all motion and sensitivity is suspended . . . whatever is above the section and continuous with the brain, this still will preserve the activity from its source; but what is lower will be unable to exercise sensation or motion.[128]

He sectioned the intercostal nerves and noted the effect not only upon the respiratory movements but also on the voice. He deduced that the vocal cords vibrated as a consequence of the passage of air upward in the larynx. He sectioned the phrenic nerves and observed the paralysis of the diaphragm.

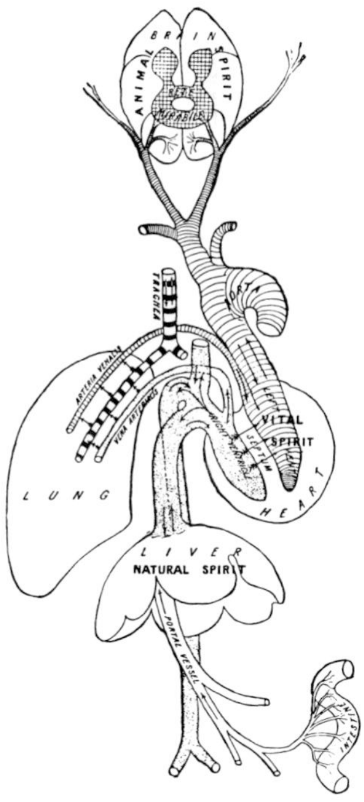

FIG 3. Galen's physiological system (after Singer[82]).

THE PHYSIOLOGIST

Galen's physiology, like Ptolemy's astrology and geography, rested partly on observation and partly on certain philosophical principles. Ptolemy was a contemporary of Galen in Alexandria, and his geography became just as canonical as Galen's physiology. Their teaching was accepted until the years of Christopher Columbus and Andreas Vesalius, respectively.†

To the ancient Greeks the vital principle of living things – plants, animals, and man – was the *pneuma* (air) that was drawn in from the cosmos. Man's physiology was designed to adapt this external pneuma for the purposes of growth, locomotion, and thought.

Galen's ingenious physiological system has been presented in diagrammatic form by Singer (Fig. 3).[129] Nutrition is derived from the alimentary tract and conveyed by the portal vein to the liver where it is elaborated into venous blood and imbued with *natural spirit* (an invention of Galen's). Blood so prepared passes via the vena cava to the right side of the heart, and there impurities are carried off by the pulmonary vessels to be exhaled by the lungs. Cleansed blood from the right ventricle ebbed back again into the general venous system. However, a smaller, but important quantity of blood took another course – through the pores he imagined existed in the interventricular septum – into the left ventricle. There the blood was given a *vital spirit* (invented by Erasistratus) derived from the external pneuma. From thence it was distributed to the organs of the body, including the

† *The Crime of Clausius Ptolemy* by R. Newton (Johns Hopkins University Press, 1977), reveals that Ptolemy fiddled his results on a truly formidable scale.

brain. There it was converted to *animal spirit* by the *rete mirabile*, undergoing final refinement in the ventricles. This was the substance that was transmitted through nerves in which, with the exception of the optic nerve, he could see no hollows. Galen explained that Herophilus termed them 'conduits'. They supplied motion and sensation. Impurities in the cerebral ventricles escaped as we have described.

Thus, blood was manufactured in the liver, and carried in the veins to various parts of the body. Arteries carried the vital spirit in the blood. Having failed to conceive the idea of a circulation of the blood, despite his careful dissection of the heart, the arteries, and the veins, Galen could not know that the cerebrospinal fluid, which he observed but misinterpreted as a residue, was secreted by the choroid plexus, which he had also described. (Sherrington was not really correct in saying that Galen thought the cerebrospinal fluid was the 'vehicle' of the spirits.[130]) Galen was trapped when he accepted the general idea of an all-embracing vital pneuma. The carotid arteries were so named after the Greek word for torpor (*karos*), which ensued on their compression, because they carried the *vital spirit* to the brain. He did not interpret the effects of asphyxia and of cerebral anoxia as indicating that in inhaled air and also in arteries there was a vital substance. But then, gases were unknown.

Although Galen distinguished between motor and sensory paralysis, and between motor and sensory nerves, he thought all messages travelled in an efferent direction. When dealing with vision he postulated something streaming outward from the eyes. Similarly, with common sensation, the flow was centrifugal. Thus, he said, 'Through some nerves the brain transmits the power of sensation to the parts below, through others voluntary movement. It is intelligible that all the nerves should have both these powers, but the soft are more suited for sensation, the hard for movement.'[131]†

When he came to consider the nature of the actual nerve impulse he saw there were several possibilities. He wrote

> We cannot absolutely pronounce whether the power flows from the brain through the nerves to the limbs and the essence of the spirit reaches the feeling and moving parts; or whether it in some way or other strikes the nerves so as to induce in them a powerful change which is propagated to the parts to be moved; whether there is in each nerve an innate spirit belonging to it, and which is struck by something coming as a sort of messenger from the first principle; or whether the spirit flows from the brain to parts, on every occasion, when we will to move them; or whether in the third place there is merely a change in the qualities of parts contiguous to each other (which appears to me to be hinted at by some who say that the influence is a power without a substance) I am not able easily to determine.[132]

This important statement of Galen was translated into English by John Cooke in his *Treatise on nervous diseases* in 1820, so Siegel's[133] claim in 1973 that it had never previously been translated into a modern language is incorrect, but quite understandable. It was at the end of this passage that Galen referred to his qualitative change in a nerve as being 'like a certain quality of the sunlight [which] is propagated into the surrounding air and

† Singer mistakenly wrote 'He [Galen] thinks of sensory nerves as carrying something to the brain.' See Ref. 21, p. 244, note 65.

penetrates into every part of it'. He thus felt that transmission might be mechanical, or induced only when volition was willed, or else it depended on a signal modifying some inherent quality in a nerve.

The nerve-impulse which thus perplexed Galen in the second century AD remained mysterious until the end of the eighteenth century, when, before Galvani was able to reveal its electrical nature, von Haller said that 'it is known to us only by its effects', a statement that would surely have elicited a nod from Galen!

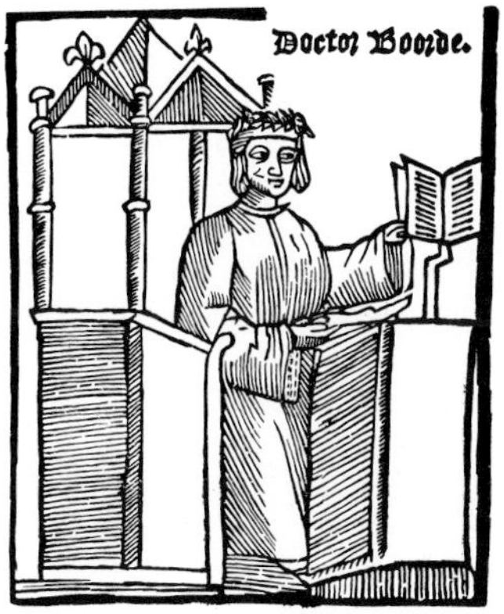

FIG 4. Title-pages from Dr Andrew Boorde's (1490–1549) *A compendyous regyment or a dietary of helth*. A much-travelled Englishmen who took up medicine at forty, after twenty years as a Carthusian monk, saying, 'I am nott able to byd the rigorosite off your relygyon.' The woodcut 'Galien, Prince of Phisycke' is typical of Medieval treatises.

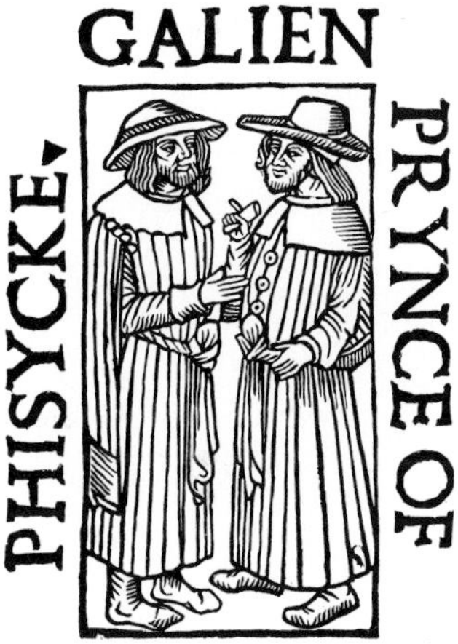

GALEN'S INFLUENCE

There is a long-standing conventional belief that Galen shackled medical thought for a thousand years. While it is true that his anatomy was not human, his physiology exceptionally conjectural, that he tended to argue too much by analogy and was obsessed by the teleological viewpoint, that beginning as a scientist he became a philosopher–theologian, and that after he died there was virtually no study of anatomy or physiology until the time of Vesalius – can we really hold Galen responsible?

His teaching was encyclopaedic and although he was a pagan it appealed to Christian, Moslem, and Jew, because he repeatedly stressed the wonder of creation, and so provided scientific confirmation of their beliefs. His teaching was preserved by the Arabs and it was not his fault that it was turned into a bible. William Harvey himself began his *Disquisition* by referring to Galen, whom he called 'Divine', saying that 'Doctrine once sown strikes deep its roots and respect for antiquity influences all men.' (Sarton[134] said that it was 'pathetic to see Harvey trying to conciliate the Galenists in his immortal book'.)

In general, historians have found the best of Galen to have been his neurology, but his influence as a whole, disastrous. Garrison[135] thought that 'The effect of his dogmatism and infallibility upon after-time was appalling.' Although Allbutt[136] regarded Galen as 'the greatest master of scientific method from the second century to Roger Bacon' he nevertheless felt that 'he fastened his yoke upon Europe'. To Brazier,[137] Galen's effect was 'almost paralysing'.

Soury,[138] on the other hand, thought that 'Recognition of his relative mediocrity as a philosopher is merely to emphasise his originality in basing clinical method on anatomy and pathology.' Souques,[139] another French historian of neurology, also felt that Galen's decline was unjustified. Neither his philosophical arguments, nor his errors in anatomy and physiology, could deprive him of recognition as the first experimental physiologist and 'the greatest neurologist of the ancient world', a view endorsed by Singer[140] who called Galen 'the first modern experimental physiologist'.

In recent times there have been some revisory judgements on Galen. Cole,[141] in his *History of comparative anatomy*, concluded that 'a new generation of commentators have laboriously re-examined the *Corpus galenicum*, and demonstrated the truly great part it has played in the evolution of biological learning'. Sarton,[134] in his life of Galen, said that

'Galenism was a creation of his disciples rather than of the master himself'. Lester King[142] felt that 'we cannot support the idea that Galen, whatever his errors, was responsible for lack of progress thirty or forty generations after his death'. Clarke and O'Malley[143] concluded that Galen's reasoning and experiments cannot fail to evoke respect today and that various attempts to minimize his contributions are unjustified.

As for Galen's 'spirits', no theory in the history of science has had a longer innings. Langley[144] wrote

> The death of a theory is often not due to its being definitely disproved, but to the general progress of scientific knowledge which robs it of its credibility; it was in this way that the theory of 'animal spirits' died.

Sherrington[145] once wrote that Galen's spirits were 'a half-way house between a thing and a thought'. Like protoplasm 'it was an entity and a will-o-the-wisp. The spell of Galen was in fact over life still, in act though not in name.' Sherrington said 'We speak of nerves *for* doing this and that. This is the Galen in us. To do so comes naturally to the lips. And Galen in this was thinking as everyone thinks and was speaking for Mr Everyman, not merely of his own time but for practically ever since.'

Temkin[146] concluded his scholarly study of Galenism with these words,

> Gently and quietly, but none the less resolutely, Galen was handed over to classicists, Arabists, and historians for disposal in the cemetery of the great dead. The great dead are notoriously restless in their graves and ever ready for resurrection. Prognostications about their future are, therefore, futile. So much, however, can be said; the Galenism which began its rise in late antiquity, which flourished in Byzantium, the Arabic East, and the Latin West, which saw its acme and incipient decline in the sixteenth century, its scientific downfall and weakening practical influence in the seventeenth, and which lingered on into the nineteenth century, this Galenism came to an end a hundred years ago.

As a clinician I can understand how Farrington,[147] in his *Greek Science*, came to write of Galen that 'the practising physicians who have written of him in modern times rank him higher than the academic critics'.

CHAPTER 2

VESALIUS AND THE NERVOUS SYSTEM

To the discovery of the outward world the Renaissance added a still greater achievement, by first discerning and bringing to light the whole full nature of Man.

Jacob Burckhardt in *The Civilisation of the Renaissance in Italy*, 1860.

INTRODUCTION

The tragic decline in anatomy following the death of Galen was but one manifestation of a more general decline in intellectual curiosity, particularly about the natural world, which characterized the next eight hundred years. The Christian doctrine that man's body was but a temporary receptacle for his immortal soul made it an object unworthy of study. The great physical encyclopaedias of the thirteenth century, such as those of Vincent of Beauvais and Bartholomew the Englishman, contain little evidence of direct observation of nature.[1] One encyclopaedia of learning, the *Margarita philosophica* of Gregor Reisch, published in Germany in 1503, was used in the instruction of the young Vesalius at Louvain University. It contained a certain number of hideous anatomical representations of a primitive nature characteristic of the German press of the day, and also one displaying the location of the senses in the brain to which Vesalius alluded and which we shall mention later.

The first practical manual of anatomy after Galen's was that of Mondino of Bologna. It was issued in 1316 but not printed until 1478. Entitled the *Anothomia*, it depicted in a famous woodcut (Fig. 5) the academic scene of a dissection. More than thirty editions of this work were published and until the sixteenth century it remained the only work wholly devoted to anatomy. Mondino's views were essentially Galenic but he also accepted the old Aristotelian idea that the brain served to cool the heart.

Some two hundred years later, in 1521, another professor at Bologna, Berengario da Carpi, went one step further by combining text and illustrations in such a way that they were complementary. The latter were not just decorative. He improved Mondino's text, making additions and corrections, and very importantly, he directed anatomy toward the science of observation.[2] Hitherto, dissection had been largely ceremonial and invariably employed to demonstrate traditional teaching. The professor in his high chair (cathedra), would read from a text what should be found and this was demonstrated by his assistants. Hence the academic title 'Reader'. This was more like preaching than teaching and Vesalius scathingly commented on the professors 'like jackdaws aloft in their high chair, with

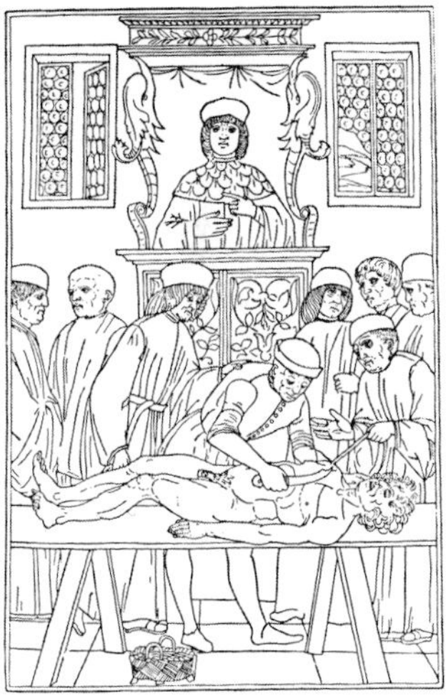

FIG 5. A lesson in dissection, Padua, from the *Fasciculo di Medicina*, 1493. The robed professor in his high chair reads from a book (not visible) while the dissector and demonstrator below perform their tasks. This was the procedure which Vesalius transformed.

egregious arrogance croaking things they have never investigated ... '.[3] Berengario began the process of more accurate recording and he found himself unable to confirm the existence of a human *rete mirabile*, or a multicelled uterus, or Aristotle's third heart ventricle. But he did not find the courage to deny the existence of Galen's pores in the interventricular cardiac septum. It was left to Harvey to cry 'But, damme, there are no pores ... '.[4]

It was in Italy also, during the fifteenth and sixteenth centuries, that the importance of anatomy gained ground through the artistic genius of men like Leonardo da Vinci, Michelangelo, and Raphael, all of whom studied dissection. Italian artists were the first to paint the nude figure before covering it with drapery. And in Germany, Durer, having travelled to Italy in 1506 to learn 'the secret art of perspective', made use of this new approach to the study of the human form, producing a book on human proportions.

Thus, the art of dissection was being reborn. 'In the great felicity of this age,' wrote Vesalius, 'with all studies greatly revitalised, anatomy has begun to raise its head from profound gloom.' In the Universities of Northern Italy, not far from the papal throne, human dissection was beginning to be practised, although in other distant Catholic countries – Spain, France, and Belgium – it still remained a questionable undertaking.[5]

Vesalius decided that anatomy 'ought to be recalled from the region of the dead'. Lamenting the passing of ancient anatomy and the loss of Alexandrian texts he said that of Galen's anatomical books 'scarcely a half have been saved from destruction'. He had recently participated in the publication of a revised Latin edition of Galenic texts, the *Opera galeni* of 1541, and one of his distinguished associates in this work was Thomas Linacre, the first President of the Royal College of Physicians of London. It had a splendid title page depicting in a series of woodcuts various scenes from the life of Galen (Fig. 1). Vesalius's contributions to this work were concerned with the treatises entitled *On anatomical procedure*, *On the dissection of the nerves*, and *On the dissection of the veins and the arteries.*

Vesalius's anatomical inheritance was thus unequivocally Galenic. Galen's name appears on the first page of the preface to the *De fabrica* and repeatedly in subsequent pages. There are at least 265 references to him in the incomplete index.[6] But although he called Galen 'The prince of professors of dissection' and protested his loyalty 'to the author of all good things' he found much to criticize. Galen, he said, 'was deceived by monkeys – although he did have access to two dried human cadavers'. But even with his monkeys he thought Galen could not be relied upon. 'How many incorrect observations you will find in Galen, even regarding his monkeys ... it is very astonishing that Galen noticed none of the many and infinite differences between the organs of the human body and of the monkey except in the fingers and the bend of the knee.' He had counted over two hundred instances in which Galen's human anatomy was in error.

Vesalius recalled the perfunctory nature of the presentation of anatomy that he had been offered in Paris so that 'I had to put my own hand to the matter'. He said 'To the best of my ability I have organised my fullest knowledge of the parts of the human body in these seven books, just as I should normally discuss it before a group of learned men in this city or in Bologna.' In arranging his material he said 'I have followed the opinion of Galen who believed that, after the description of the muscles, the anatomy of the veins, arteries, nerves and then of the viscera ought to be considered.'

He stressed the importance of illustrations saying, 'How greatly pictures assist the understanding of these matters and place them more exactly before the eyes than even the most precise language, no student of geometry and other mathematical disciplines can fail to understand.' He said 'The books contain illustrations of all the parts, inserted in the text of the discourse in such a way that they place the dissected body before the eyes of the students of nature's work.'

That eminent medical historian and authority on Vesalius, Charles Singer, once said that in the 'High Renaissance' the four great factors that determined the course of anatomical development all took form within half a century.[7] 'First was the rise of the science of perspective. Second was the intimately related development of skill in exact representational drawing. Third was the publication of the ancient anatomical texts from which the new anatomy could take its start. Fourth was the perfection of the art of book illustration, so that the anatomist could at last present his findings graphically and acceptably to a wide audience.'

These achievements were personified in the young Vesalius. Destiny may be a concept difficult for historians to admit or dismiss but in Vesalius we surely have a striking example. He was 'The Luther of Anatomy'.[8]

A picture of Vesalius at work is provided by the notes of a student who attended his dissections in 1540. He witnessed the dissection of three human bodies, six dogs, and other animals.[9]

This afternoon he did the anatomy of the head, brain, its ventricles, seven pairs of cranial nerves and all its parts. To ensure better understanding he first spoke at length on Galen's *De anatomicis adminstrationibus*, IX ... (then he exposed the brain) ... next, before he cut into the ventricles, he showed them on the head of a sheep, in which we could see them better ... the middle ventricle was like a passage from the front to the back of the brain. In the back part he also showed us some substance of the brain like a worm [vermis]. He put it on a paper; it was white and had the form of the great white worms that grow in wood. Under the mass of the brain he showed us some white callous substances [corpus callosum] to which go the superfluous fluids of the brain. At each side cavities go down through which he said the superfluous fluids pass to their common receptacle, close to the palate and the nostrils. After we had seen this [the non-existing channels!] he lifted the substance of the brain higher, proceeding to the seven pairs of nerves. He showed the first pair that runs from the brain to the nostrils, and there the true instrument of smell, namely two nerves near the orifices in the cranium from the nostrils. ...

Does this mean that in 1540, three years before *De fabrica* was published, Vesalius considered the olfactory was the first cranial nerve? In *De fabrica* he agreed with Galen that the 'nerve like processes which minister to the organ of smell' were not the first pair. But the student's account of the remaining seven pairs is confusing although he did say that

Vesalius did not tell us their order, which you can see in books on anatomy, because he was very confused, owing to the noise and disorder of the students. Therefore, being upset, as he was very choleric, he hurried on this dissection to get through it anyhow. Eventually he showed us the network of arteries around the *rete mirabile*. . . .

We should not be too surprised that this student thought he had seen structures in the human brain that do not exist. Many a medical student has 'seen', 'heard', 'palpated', or 'percussed' things which his teachers assured him were present. But nevertheless this comment on the olfactory nerve is intriguing.

THE *DE FABRICA*

His *Libri septem* Vesalius arranged as follows. Book I, the skeleton; Book II, the muscles; Book III, the blood-vessels; Book IV, the nerves, cranial and spinal; Book V, the abdomen; Book VI, the thorax; Book VII, the brain. They were illustrated with more than two hundred woodcuts, twenty-two of them occupying a whole page each. These include the famous 'posed' skeletons (three) and 'muscle' figures (sixteen), the latter flayed and dissected, and depicted against a rural and urban background, which, when arranged in series, has been identified as a landscape view of the Colli Euganei region near Padua.[10] Illustrations and text are closely linked in an effective manner, amply justifying his pedagogic claim. He provided an elaborate scheme of cross references and thousands of marginal notes, differing according to their placement in the inner or outer margins of the printed page.

But Vesalius did not intend the *De fabrica* to be just an atlas. He had already provided his students with that in his *Tabulae anatomicae* in 1538. This was intended to illustrate Galen's statements and consisted of a short text with six large woodcuts. Three are diagrams illustrating Galenic physiology, said to be drawn by Vesalius, and three are skeletal figures, drawn by the chief *Fabrica* artist Joannes Stephanus of Calcar. 'The first serious attempt to expound graphically the physiology and anatomy of the human body.'[11] Neither Vesalius's anatomy nor Calcar's plates are of the standard reached in the *De fabrica* and the comparison between the two productions has been the source of endless debate concerning both author and artist. Singer and Rabin concluded that the metamorphosis of Vesalius, between the years 1538 and 1543 was 'the period of gestation for the idea that science is research'.[12]

In the year of publication of the *De fabrica* Vesalius also had published a briefer *Epitome*. This was translated into German the same year, proving popular with students and surgeons, and into English in 1553.

Vesalius was no theologian or philosopher like Galen and he was not for ever harping on the perfection of man's form. But in choosing the title 'Fabrica' it is clear he wished to portray the 'workings' of man's body. It seems we must not translate his title as 'Fabric' or 'Mechanism'. In classical usage 'fabric' means 'an artisan's workshop', where something is going on.[13] The German *Fabrik* and the French *Fabrique* mean both the process of making and the place where things are made. Thus, when he was dealing

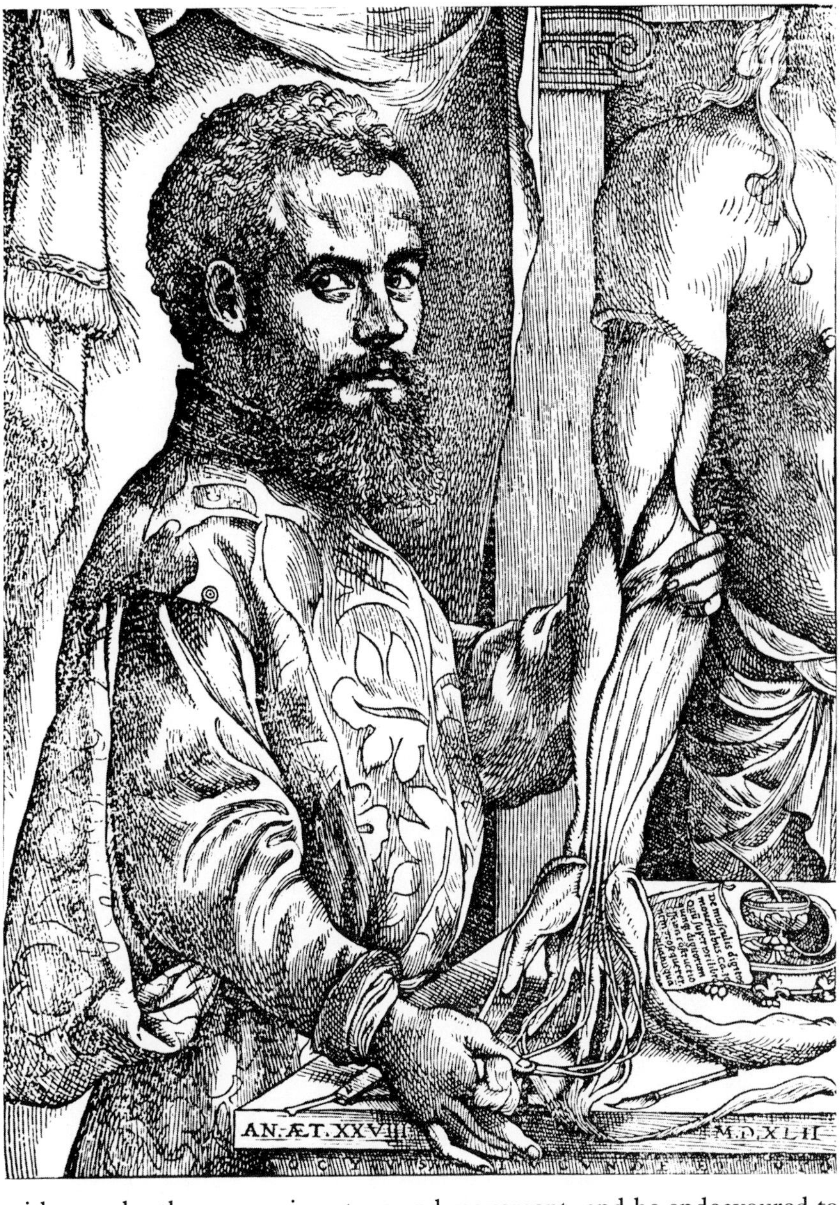

FIG. 6a. Portrait of Vesalius as he appeared in the *De fabrica*. He was only 28 years of age. The poor perspective and the disproportions (large head, short arm of Vesalius, and the gigantic arm of the female cadaver) have intrigued scholars. The writing on the scroll is an innacurate transcript of sentences in *De fabrica* where Vesalius was correcting Galen's account of the flexors of the wrist. Singer (*J. Anatomy* 77, 261 (1943)) concluded that the head was composed by a good artist, and that a woodcutter fitted it on to the trunk. Note that the year is 1542, one year before publication, and Vesalius's age is recorded.

with muscles they were given tone and movement, and he endeavoured to illustrate their function. A muscle is depicted in its normal position and also raised from its origin and allowed to hang from its point of insertion.

He gave precise instructions to the student in how to go about the examination of the musculature.

It will not be enough to observe some muscle on one plate, even if I shall have noted it by a letter, but to see where each one originates or terminates, you must investigate throughout and in particular notice where the whole of it is seen ... when you inspect that [muscle] in the illustration, do not fail to observe what that muscle you are looking at rests upon and what it lies under ... when all things have been correlated, it is clear to anyone in what region each muscle may be found ...[14]

He recalled Galen's view of the nature of muscle but correctly came to the

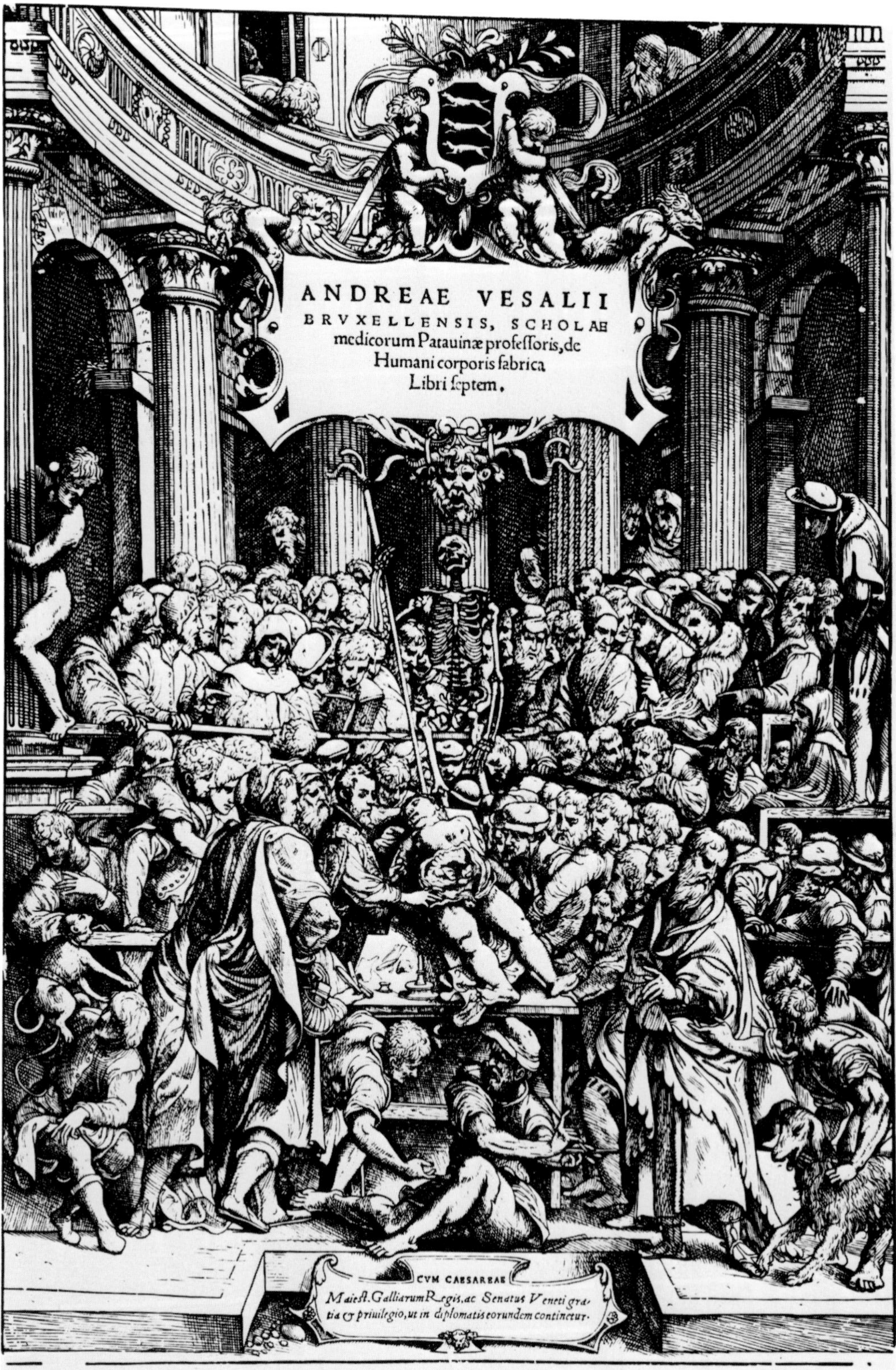
ANDREAE VESALII
BRVXELLENSIS, SCHOLAE
medicorum Patauinæ professoris, de
Humani corporis fabrica
Libri septem.
CVM CAESAREAE
Maiest. Galliarum Regis, ac Senatus Veneti gra-
tia & priuilegio, ut in diplomatis eorundem continetur.

BASILEAE.

conclusion that Galen's 'flesh' was 'the particular organ of motion and not merely the stuffing and support of the fibres'.[15] He identified the four recti and the two oblique muscles of the eye, but, like Galen, included the non-human retractor bulbi. He also thought the eyelids were raised by the orbicularis oculi muscles.

Similarly with the skeleton, he provided three distinct views so that a true picture of the many bones and joints could be obtained. The disproportions which marred the plates of the *Tabulae anatomicae* were largely corrected. He noted the variations in shape of the human skull, actually categorizing five types, believing, with Galen, that there was only one 'natural' form of skull, variants therefrom being abnormal.

Vesalius said, in the second edition of *De fabrica* (1555), that 'most nations claim for themselves a peculiar shape of the head', but he thought that binding the infant head by midwives, and the customary positioning of the infant in the cot, were likely factors. Also in the second edition he mentions two cases of hydrocephalus. In one, a girl of two years, the head was larger than any man's head he had ever seen. The fluid 'had not collected between the skull and the exterior membrane ... but in the cavity of the brain itself'. Her senses were normal and there was no paralysis but toward the end passive movements of her head evoked cough, difficulty in breathing, and in flushing of the face. At autopsy he obtained nine pounds of water from the ventricles; 'the cerebellum and the whole base of the brain were normal'. 'I marvelled at nothing more than that such amount of water had for so long collected in the ventricles of the brain without greater symptoms.'[16]

The cribriform plate of the ethmoid bone, he said, 'Galen described incorrectly, writing that it is perforated like a sieve or sponge to transmit the pituita from the brain'. Vesalius found 'its surface wholly unbroken and solid'.

The spine, he said, in true Galenic fashion, was constructed 'in the form of a keel and foundation' ... with 'a passage suitable for the descent of the dorsal marrow' and articulated 'from many bones (twenty-four) ... for many different motions'. He noted the varying size and shape of the vertebrae and of the spinal canal. He gave the name 'atlas' to the first cervical vertebra, and analysed the complex movements of the neck. Unfortunately the figures failed to demonstrate the natural curvature of the spine, due it is thought to his manner of mounting skeletons. He used a rigid iron bar to support the spinal column.[17]

I have not been able to discover whether he noted at what level the spinal cord terminated but he certainly did not describe the two roots of each spinal nerve.

In describing the nerves as 'long, rounded organs without any apparent internal cavity ... slipping from the skull or dorsal vertebrae ...' he makes the distinction between ligaments and tendons. He agreed with Galen's classification of the cranial nerves, denied the crossing of the optic nerves in the chiasm, and illustrated the base of the brain in a manner which has been generally criticized (Fig. 14). He did not establish the correct emergence of

FIG. 6b. The frontispiece of the *De fabrica* depicting Vesalius conducting a public anatomy in Padua. Vesalius stands to the right of a female cadaver with his left index finger raised, commanding attention. There is a mixed audience of some eighty persons, arranged in tiers – assistants, students, monks and nuns, bearded patriarchs, a man with spectacles, another using a lens, a monkey, and a dog. Above the cadaver is a skeleton sitting on a rail. Vesalius's coat of arms depicts three weasels, indicating that his name is derived from the place Wesel, the Flemish for weasel. (O'Malley said they looked more like coursing greyhounds.) Note Vesalius's title of Professor at Padua and his gratitude to his Imperial Majesty and the Venetian Senate.

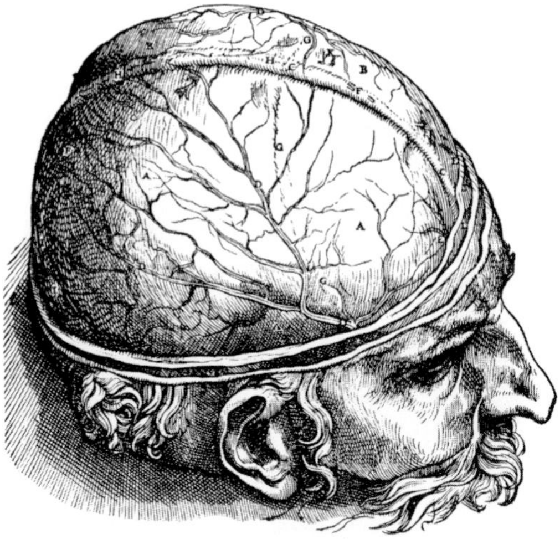

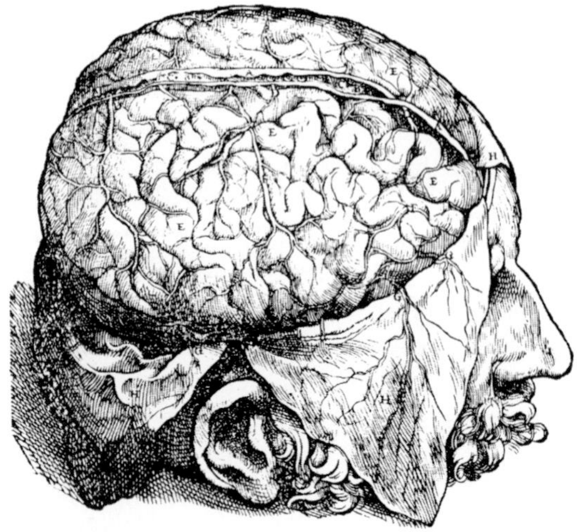

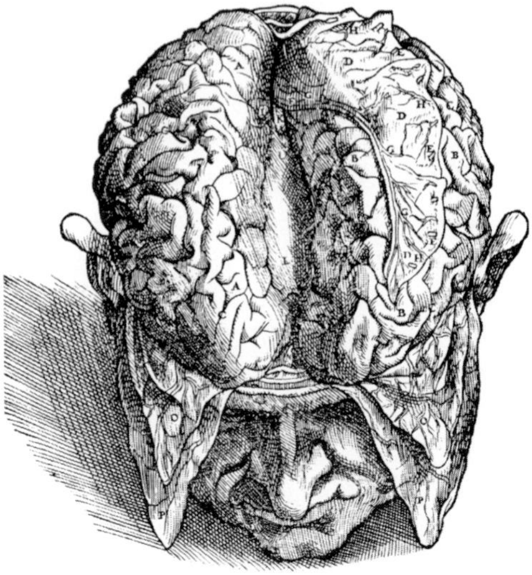

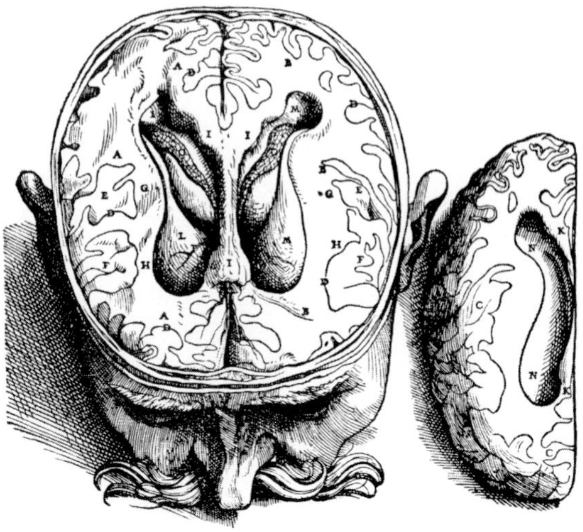

FIG. 7 (*top left*). The first of the twenty-five figures illustrating the dissection of the brain. Here we see the dura mater and middle meningeal vessels, the superior sagittal sinus and adjacent arachnoidal granulations, and the indicated position of the coronal suture.

FIG. 8 (*top right*). The superior sagittal sinus is opened and the entry points of the superior cerebral veins are indicated. The dura is reflected and the pia mater 'closely enveloping the brain and showing beautifully its array of vessels' can be seen. But the convolutions are quite inaccurate.

FIG. 9 (*left*). The meninges are removed, the falx is reflected to the left, revealing the inferior sagittal sinus in its lower edge, and the origin of the vein of Galen (K). The hemispheres are separated to show the underlying corpus callosum (LL). 'The bendings and windings' of the convolutions are seen.

FIG. 10 (*right*). The first of the horizontal sections of the brain with the upper portion of the left hemisphere inverted on the right. This shows the ventricles, choroid plexuses, the corpus callosum, and the demarcation between the white matter and the 'yellowish-grey' of the cortex.

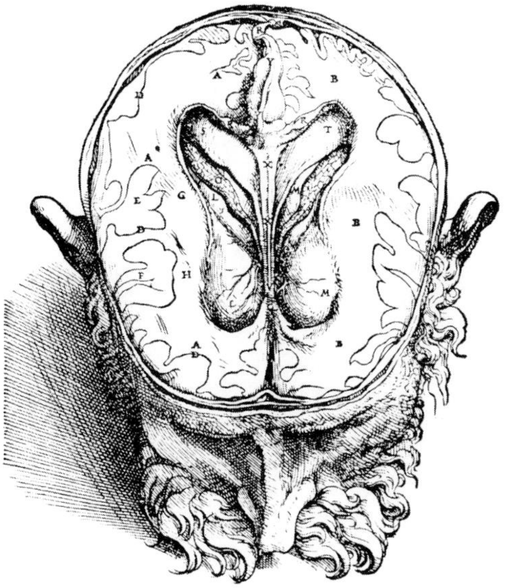

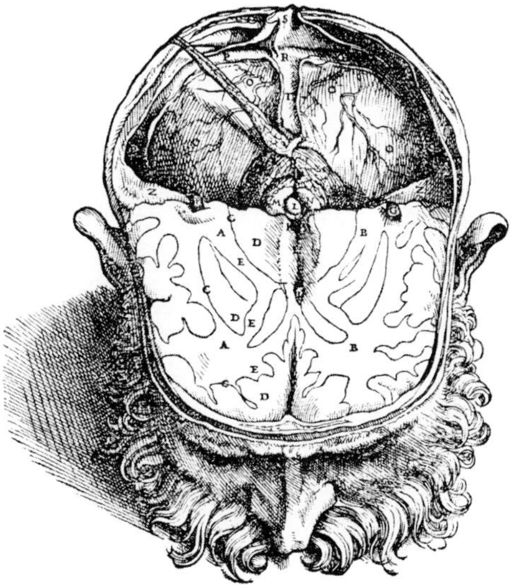

FIG. 11 (*left*). Here the corpus callosum is reflected posteriorly, the septum pellucidum incised, and the fornix (tortoise-like body) disclosed.

FIG. 12 (*right*). The posterior portion of each hemisphere has been removed exposing the cerebellum (X), the confluence of the sinuses (torcular, R), the tentorium, the pineal gland (L), and the nates and testes (M, N, corpora quadrigemina). K, is the aqueduct and H the infundibular recess of the third ventricle. The dissection exposes 'the hardest bone of the body (petrosal) which contains the organ of hearing'. Anteriorly, in the horizontal section are shown the optic thalamus, the caudate and lenticular nuclei, the internal and external capsules, and an outline of the island of Reil.

the roots of the cranial nerves, nor the proper shape and relationships of the pons. Neither did he identify the circle of Willis, presumably because he did not employ arterial injection.

He observed atrophy of the right optic nerve in two corpses. In one 'the right eye had withered away from an early age' and in the other, 'it had been plucked out by the executioner a year before'![18]

When he described the recurrent laryngeal nerves he adopted the same teleological posture of the Galen he criticized.

> With what great industry the fathomless Framer of our bodies has laboured in these convolutions, you may see from dissection itself, from the present precise account of the distribution of the nerves, and from the figure which we have shown above. Nevertheless I advise you to consult Galen who rightly prides himself on having been the very first to find these looped courses of the nerves.[19]

Of 'hollow' nerves in general, he said

> I can assert that I never found any passage of that sort even though I dissected the optic nerves of live dogs and other large animals for this purpose, and the head of a man as yet warm and scarcely a quarter hour after his decapitation.[20]

His illustration of the sixth pair of cranial nerves (Galen's classification) shows the vagus and cervical sympathetic nerves combined in one trunk (Fig. 15). The text is said to reveal little more than the diagram it accompanies, and French[21] points out that Vesalius made no distinction between the jugular foramen, from which the vagus emerges, and the carotid canal containing the sympathetic nerve. It is possible, though unlikely, that such errors were a consequence of injury to the neck sustained in the acts of hanging or decapitation – for the majority of his cadavers were of executed criminals.

Galen's *rete mirabile*, which he had seen in the ox and the pig, Vesalius

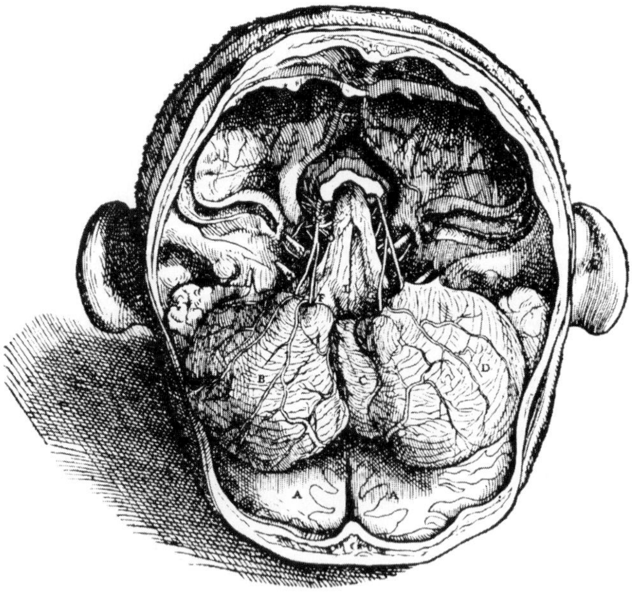

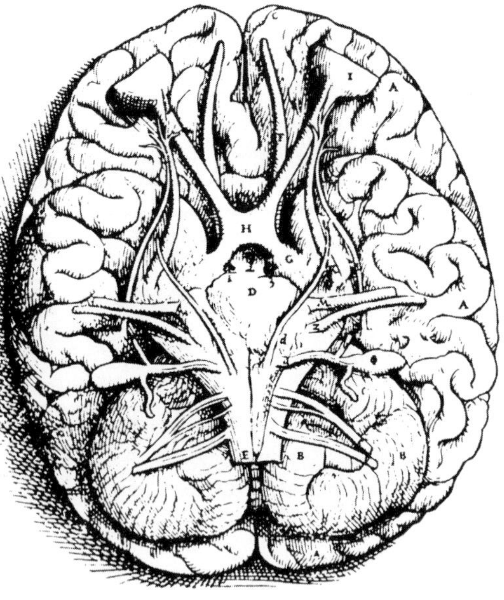

FIG. 13 (*left*). Here the cerebellum is lifted up out of the posterior fossa and allowed to hang downward on the forebrain. It exposes the foramen magnum, the medulla, and lower cranial nerves; F and G are the inferior cerebellar peduncles. I is the floor of the fourth ventricle. C is the vermis.

FIG. 14 (*right*). The base of the brain and the roots of the cranial nerves. Not a good example of dissection or draughtsmanship. A fair general configuration but a quite inaccurate brain stem, with a strangely shaped pons seemingly attached to the temporal lobes. A confused delineation of Galen's cranial nerve pairs.

first acknowledged in the *Tabulae*, but in the *De fabrica* he came to deny its existence in man. Of his original error, he said 'I cannot sufficiently marvel at my own stupidity'.[22]

Book VII, on the brain, surpassed anything previously published. It contains a series of detailed illustrations of horizontal sections of the brain revealing the successive steps of dissection (Figs. 7–14). The text was translated into English in 1952 by the late Charles Singer, in *Vesalius on the human brain*.[34] Well described are the venous sinuses and meninges, the falx cerebri and tentorium cerebelli, the ventricles, and the choroid plexuses. There are accounts of the corpus calsum (which he named), the fornix and the septum pellucidum (which he said resembled 'mica' or the 'wafer' used in the Mass), the corpora quadrigemina, and the pineal gland. Some structures not mentioned in the text may nevertheless be clearly seen in the illustrations, as, for example, the internal and external capsules (but not the claustrum), the thalamus, putamen and globus pallidus, the lenticular and caudate nuclei, and the cerebral peduncles.[23, 24]

Generally speaking he found the brain 'flattened at its base ... moulded by protuberances (of the skull) ... cleft into two parts ... with cerebellar convolutions which do not penetrate so deeply as those of the cerebrum'. The substance of the brain was not all white; near the convolutions it was grey or yellowish in colour. He recalled how Erasistratus likened the convolutions to 'coils of small intestine' and, like Galen, he was not impressed by them, for they were seen in the brains of asses, horses, oxen, and other creatures. He said that philosophers disputed 'whether men have understanding through them or not'.

Despite his errors, some of which were gross, Vesalius succeeded in demonstrating that the brain, although little or nothing was known of how it functioned, did possess an anatomical structure, admittedly complicated, which a methodical process of dissection would reveal. Moreover, he showed that his methods and findings could be taught, illustrated, and reproduced. Most authorities agree that, no matter who the artists were, or who the woodcutters, the general conception of the work with its programme of illustrations is entirely attributable to Vesalius. He created a work of science that is also a work of art. Ivins has expressed a contrary view; he concluded that the hero of the *De fabrica* was not Vesalius but the artist Calcar.[25]

In his *History of medical illustration* Herrlinger wrote 'it remains one of the most astonishing phenomena in the history of medicine that not until 1538 was an anatomical object as accessible as the bones of the body drawn 'correctly – that is from nature . . . '.[26] Vesalius gave meticulous attention to his plates, even, finally, exhorting his printer in Basle that 'particular pains must be used in printing the engravings, since these are not made in the common or ordinary manner and as it were in outline only; neglect nowhere the matter of the picture (even if you do occasionally omit the text on which the illustrations are based)'.[27]

The precious packages of text and woodcuts were dispatched across the Alps, probably via the St. Gotthard pass, which was the most frequent route from Northern Italy to Basle.[28]

Wars finally destroyed some of these artistic treasures of the Renaissance. A vellum copy of the *De fabrica* was lost in the destruction of the Louvain library in 1914, but 230 of the original woodblocks were rediscovered in a box in an attic in the library of the University of Munich in 1932.[29] They included nearly the whole collection used for the first edition of 1543 with the exception of the portrait of Vesalius, one muscle figure, and twenty small blocks. They were found to be made of pear wood, probably previously treated with hot linseed oil, and in an excellent state of preservation, free, miraculously, of worm. In 1934 the blocks were used in The New York Academy of Medicine's publication entitled *Andreae Vesalii Bruxellensis Icones Anatomicae*. They retained the beauty which shone from them four hundred years previously – but ten years later, when Munich in turn suffered bombing, the blocks were destroyed.

A handsome facsimile reproduction of the *De fabrica* with all its illustrations was issued in 1964.†

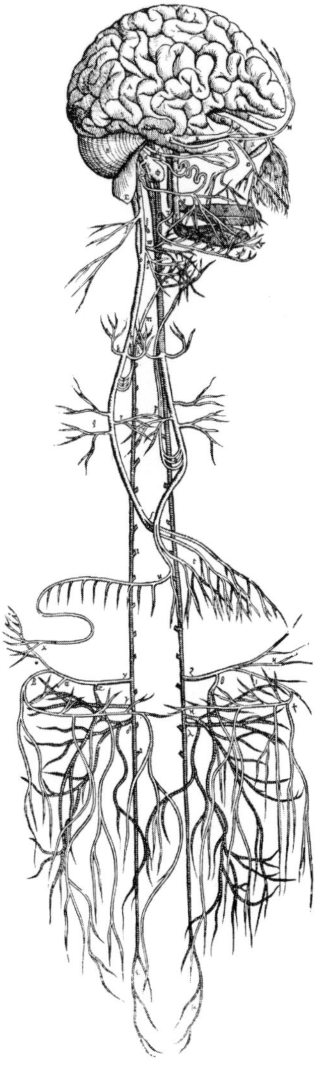

FIG. 15. The distribution of the cranial nerves, in which there is much confusion. With a magnifying lens one can see the olfactory tract, F; the optic nerve, G; the retina, I; the oculomotor nerve, K (connected to the outside of the temporal lobe); the supraorbital branch of the trigeminal, N; and a perplexing arrangement of the remaining nerves. Φ is the 'auditory organ'; Z and Y are the palate and tongue, respectively; the sympathetic branches off from the vagus.

THE VIVISECTIONIST

In the final pages of the *De fabrica*, in a chapter entitled '*On Dissection of the Living*,' Vesalius stresses the value of vivisection which 'clearly demonstrates at once the function itself . . . and the reason for the existence of parts'. He studied the action of ligaments, muscles, nerves, and of the spinal cord and he made observations on the action of the heart and lungs, the relation of the pulse beat to the heart, and the vascular supply of the brain. He sectioned the recurrent laryngeal nerves and noted the effect on the voice. He was thus repeating the experiments of Galen.

† By Culture et Civilisation, 115 Avenue Gabriel, Lebon, Bruxelles.

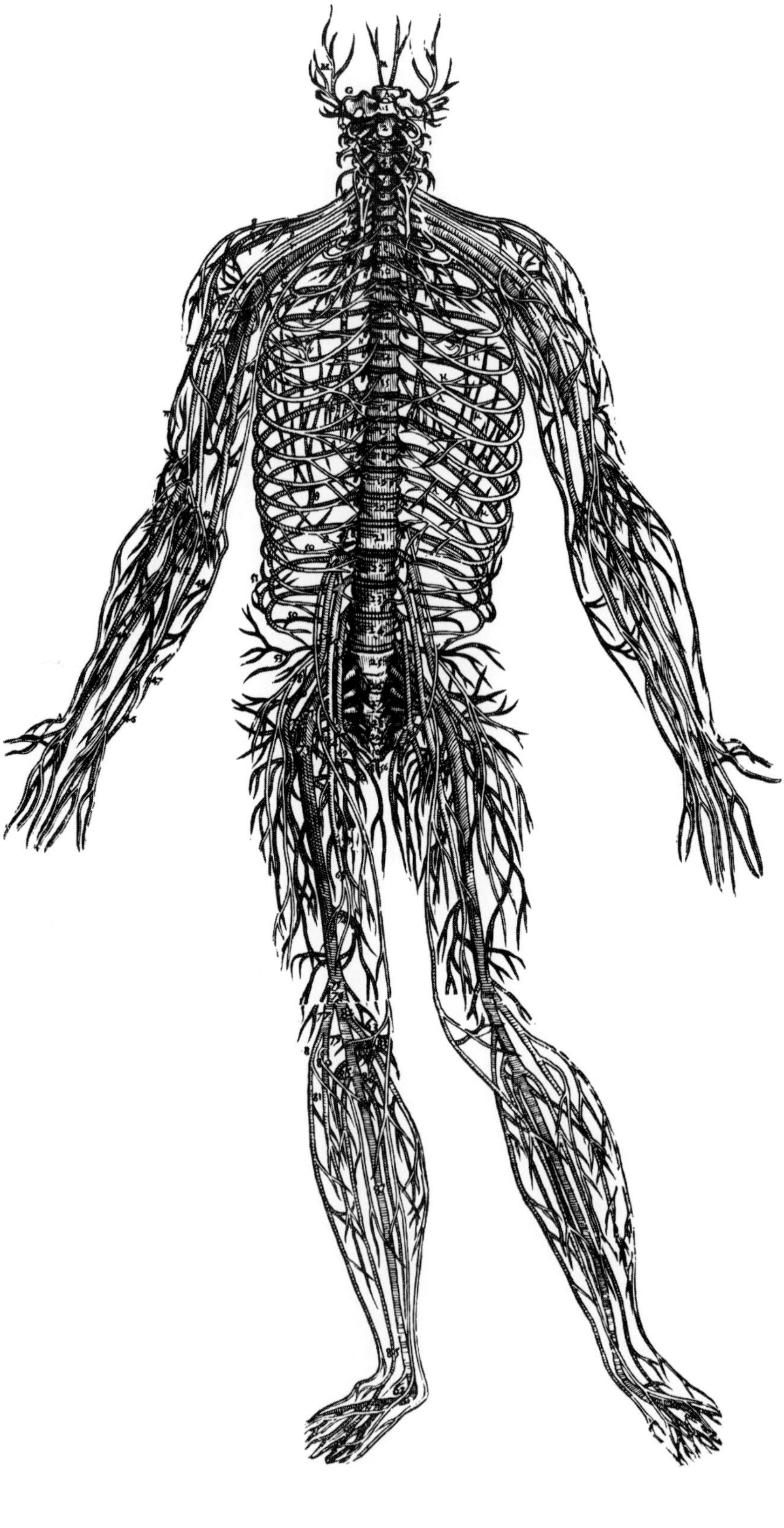

FIG. 16. The 'nerve-man', 'a naked delineation of the thirty pairs of nerves which take origin from the dorsal medulla contained in the backbone'. It shows the occipital nerves, the cervical plexus, with the upper limb nerves, and the phrenic and intercostal nerves; the lumbosacral plexus and nerves to the lower limbs.

He generally used dogs. In the case of the muscles he said 'notice during their own action they contract and become thick', lengthening on relaxation.

When you divide the belly of a muscle straight through you will observe that the muscle draws together and contracts in one part toward its insertion, in the other portion towards its origin.[30]

He ligated motor nerves and recorded the muscles and movements that were affected; he compared temporary ligation with complete section. In the foreleg of the dog he obtained paralysis of flexion or extension according to which nerve he divided. The phrenic and intercostal nerves were also studied.

In the case of the spinal cord, he recorded:

It will be permitted anyone to fasten a dog or to bind it to a block of wood in a way that one stretches out the back and neck. Therefore some of the spines of the vertebrae can be cut in front with a large knife and then the dorsal medulla can be laid bare in its bed, when anyone will get a view of the medulla about to be cut – for nothing is easier than thus to see that movement and sensation are abolished in the parts subjected to the section.[31,32]

These experiments, though not original, indicated his appreciation of the physiological approach and he repeated and modified them in subsequent years, making some additions in the second edition of the *De fabrica*. They are also of great historical significance because, after all, they were the only physiological experiments of any consequence between those of Galen and Harvey.

THE PHYSIOLOGIST

Although he could not confirm the hollowness of nerves Vesalius generally accepted Galen's ideas of nerve function. He did consider that the sutures of the skull 'facilitated the purging of the brain's fuliginous excrement' and, like Galen, he identified passages from the ventricles which excreted phlegm. But he could not find a passage from the pituitary to the nose, nor could he see how phlegm could escape through the cribriform plate. He also said, rather mysteriously, there were 'many other foramina, unknown to other professors of dissection, to the cavity of the nose'. In this section on Galenic cerebral excretory activity Vesalius was at his most evasive and imaginary. This was 'The neurology of effluvia', to quote Wightman.[33]

Vesalius also seems to have accepted Galen's notion of movement of the brain, one which, as we have seen, was probably derived from the observation of cerebral pulsation. But its association with arterial pulsation came to be disregarded, and in some way the movements were thought to arise from meningeal contraction. Writing of the dura, he said that if it were attached to the brain, then the latter 'could not be distended or contracted ... and since the dura is not linked to the tenuis (pia-arachnoid), save by sparse and widely distributed vessels, it does not impede free movement of the brain ... '.[34] Still, it is possible that he was thinking of a pulsatile movement.

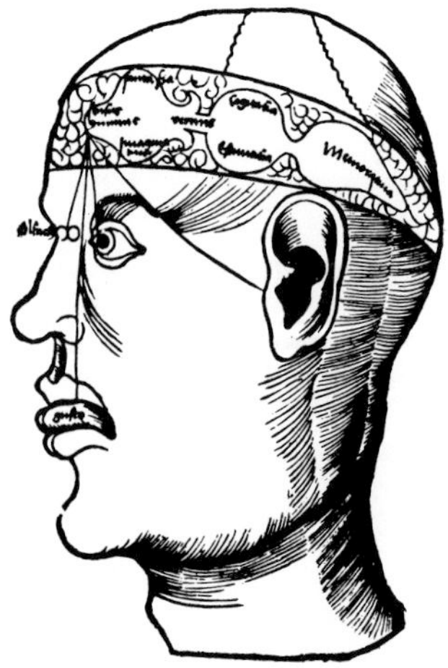

FIG. 17. The ventricles of the brain as depicted by Reisch in *Margarita philosophica* (1503), to which Vesalius scoffingly referred in *De fabrica*. The three communicating ventricles with their designated functions – common sense, cogitation, and memory. Lines from the special senses pass to the first ventricle. Vermis is here placed between first and second ventricle.

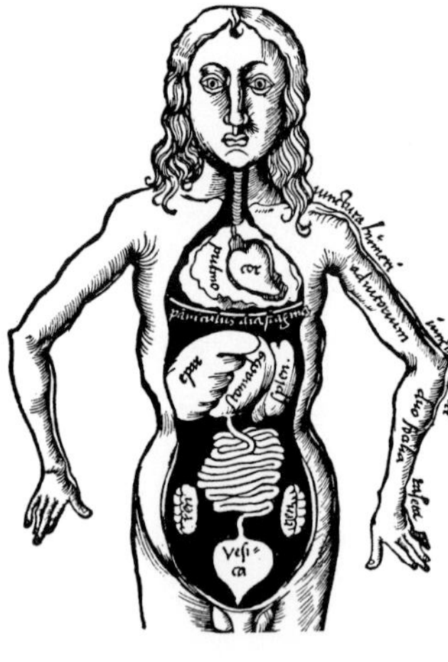

FIG. 18. The viscera of the human body as shown in *Margarita philosophica*.

With regard to the ventricles he made some caustic yet interesting remarks

I well remember when in the University of Louvain ... I gave my efforts to philosophy ... the brain was said to have been equipped with three ventricles. The first was in front, the second in the middle, the third behind, with names according to their position and other names derived from their functions.[35]

The first, or frontal, said to lie toward the forehead, was the ventricle of 'common sense' (sensus communis) since, as they believed, from it the nerves of the five senses pass to their instruments. It was by these nerves that smell, colour, taste, sound and touch were said to be led to the ventricle. Accordingly, the main use of this first ventricle was to receive the objects of the five senses of the kind that we generally call 'Common Sense'.

This ventricle was linked to the second ventricle by a certain passage through which these objects pass. Thus the second ventricle could imagine, meditate and consider the objects in question; for to this ventricle Thought and Reason were ascribed.[35]

The third ventricle was dedicated to Memory. The second ventricle would, according to its nature, pass to it all those things which it wished to be entrusted thereto, namely those objects upon which it had thoroughly meditated.[35]

Vesalius went on to say 'that we students were advised that we should follow up more in detail the items which we were thus taught; we were shown a figure from some Philosophic Pearl (the *Margarita philosophica*) which presented to the eyes the ventricles so discussed. This figure [Fig. 17] we pupils portrayed, each according to his skill as a draughtsman, adding to it our notes'.[36]

This well-known figure of Reisch is a characteristic representation of the medieval doctrine of the ventricles. Its origins are wrapped in mystery. Galen, as we have seen, had disagreed with Herophilus that the ventricles contained the soul; Galen favoured the brain substance. In medieval manuscripts the ventricles were usually depicted as circles within the head, with their functions appropriately labelled.[37] There were many variations, for speculation was a way of life, but most popular were those that placed imagination and common sense in the first, reasoning in the second, and memory in the third. Even Leonardo da Vinci drew them in this way (Fig. 19), although he was later to make a wax cast of the ventricles, presumably of the ox, in 1504. Shakespeare spoke of 'the ventricles of memory'.[37]

All this ventricular mythology drew scorn from Vesalius. 'Such are the inventions of those who never look into our Maker's ingenuity in the building of the human body! How such people err in describing the brain will be demonstrated in our subsequent discussion.'[36]

Concerning the function of the ventricles Vesalius said '... I ventured to ascribe no more to the ventricles than that they are cavities and spaces in which the inhaled air, added to the vital spirit from the heart, is, by power of the peculiar substance of the brain, transformed into animal spirit' for distribution to the nerves. 'Now', he continued, 'I do not deny that the ventricles bring the animal spirit into being, but I hold that this explains nothing about the faculties of the Reigning Soul.'[38] (The latter was a term used to signify the mental faculties.)

'But', he went on, 'how the brain performs its functions in imagination, in reasoning, in thinking, and in memory . . . I can form no opinion whatever. Nor do I think that anything more will be found out by anatomy. . . .' It is accordingly difficult to agree with Foster[39] that Vesalius 'nursed in secret the belief that future enquiry would make clear the hidden meaning of the complicated structure of the brain, and show how its several parts were concerned in the different activities of the soul'.

Vesalius's words that 'the animal spirit . . . is by far the brightest and most delicate and indeed is a quality rather than a thing' recalls those of Sherrington[41] in *Man on his nature*, when he said 'The animal spirits of Galen are for him the medium. They are a halfway house between a thing and a thought' (p. 40). Vesalius considered that the spirits were distributed by the nerves serving 'the same purpose to the . . . brain that the great artery does to the heart . . . and hence may be regarded as the busy attendants and messengers of the brain'. There are passages which reveal how his doubt about the hollowness of the nerves became a conviction. 'We will not too anxiously discuss whether the spirit is carried along certain hollow channels of the nerves, as the vital spirit is carried by the arteries, or whether it passes through the solid material of the nerve, as light passes through air.'[42] Again, 'I scarcely dare to deny the hollowness of the nerve although I have never seen a channel even in the optic nerve.'[43]

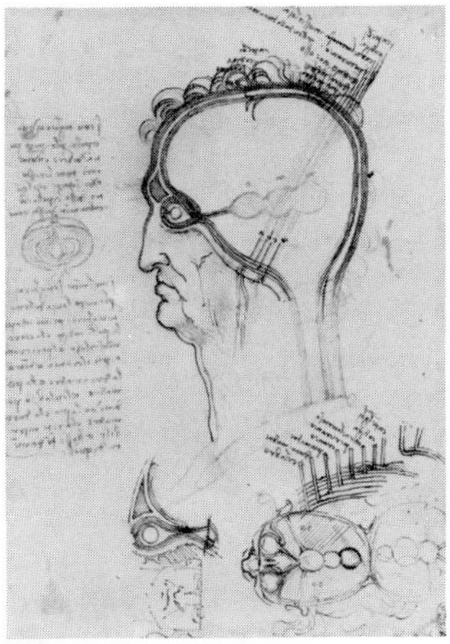

FIG. 19. Leonardo da Vinci's drawing (1490) of the three cerebral ventricles, shown in sagittal and horizontal sections. The eyes and ears communicate with the first ventricle. Later he was to make a wax cast of the ox ventricles.

THE PHYSICIAN

O'Malley[44] and O'Malley and Saunders[45] have translated ten of Vesalius's medical opinions, which were usually in the form of letters in answer to enquiries, some about patients he had not actually seen. A few possess neurological interest.

1. *Failing eyesight*.[46] A male, age 27 years. Eyesight was poor from an early age, one side being 'completely destroyed' and on the other 'he is also bothered because he sees now midges, now bugs, and other things of that sort, which we commonly call vision-blockers and fancied images . . .'. The blind eye 'had lost is natural colour and the pupil appears tinted by a diffuse glaucus and white colour'. Vesalius wished to known 'whether things far removed (are seen) better than others that are nearer and of equal size', and 'whether he sees more poorly in a bright light, such as sunshine, than in the shade'. Only 'full examination' could determine whether the lesion was 'obstruction of the optic nerve, injured eye, enlarged crystalline humor or dried wrinkled and thickened corneal tunic'. Moreover, he said 'we understand that he sees those things that are placed very near but not those that are remotely distant, and those that are small but not those that are large. Furthermore, it will have to be observed whether or not with one eye closed the pupil of the other is dilated. These are two very sure indications of a lack of spirit and argue an obstruction of the optic nerves.' Vesalius suggested needling the eye so we can assume he made a diagnosis of cataract.

2. *Focal epilepsy*.[47] 'It is apparent that this disease is epilepsy, or as it is called in Latin, morbus comitialis, or the sacred disease . . . it has arisen from an obstruction in the brain extending to those processes at the origins of nerves . . . a certain aura or vapour is always felt to be carried from the leg through the hip, then the scapula, upward to the head; then the left leg is agitated by the vehemence of the disease and convulsed more than the other parts, so we may decide that the leg itself is the primary author of the present evil.'

3. *Deformity of the foot* (Talipes equinovarus).[48] Youth, who from an early age 'displayed a contraction in the tendons of the right foot' so that 'only the external side of the sole of the foot rests on the ground in walking, while the inner side with the middle of the sole is drawn upward and removed from the ground'. There was a 'slenderness observed in the lower leg which is said to be more slender below the knee than the whole foot'. Vesalius wondered whether 'corrective bindings with braces and other apparatus would promote straightness'.

4. *Acute polyneuritis or myelitis*.[49] 'A youth suffered a heavy flow of blood from the nostril and was attacked by a continuous fever. Finally, when he had recovered from that and began to be restored to health, his legs suffered such an ailment that he could move his lower legs and feet only with great pain and was not able to stand on them except with difficulty; in addition, sensation was in large part lost in those regions'. No mention is made of the upper limbs. Vesalius thought the legs 'ought to be exercised constantly, even in bed, whether this be done by the patient or in some other way by those assisting him . . .', if possible 'he should constantly move about with canes, for nothing renders even a healthy vigorous type so infirm . . . '.

5. *A fatal head injury in a king*.[50] The patient was King Henry II of France, age 40 years, who sustained a penetrating injury of the right orbit, from a lance, during a jousting match. The joust was witnessed by the English Ambassador to France.[51] 'He managed to keep his saddle . . . dismounted . . . showed loss of consciousness, although he later ascended the steps to his chamber with hardly a totter.' He developed fever and was delirious and 'a large quantity of pituitous blood flowed from the wound . . . and signs occurred which began to indicate more fully damage to the brain'. Ambroise Paré was there with Vesalius, trephination was contemplated but decided against and 'before death (on the eleventh day) the left arm and leg became paralysed while a convulsion of long duration was plainly observed on the whole of the right side'. At autopsy Vesalius found that 'the membranes of the brain and the brain itself at the forehead . . . appeared quite unharmed, and the dural membrane appeared everywhere uninjured'. But at the vertex there was subdural suppuration and cerebral compression.

6. *A non-fatal head injury in a prince*.[52] The patient was Prince Don Carlos of Spain, age 17 years, 'who in hasty following of a wench, daughter to the keeper of the house, fell down a pair of stairs and broke his head'. Thus wrote the English Ambassador to Queen Elizabeth I. But although the prince was concussed 'and the pericranium laid bare' from a wound in the occipital region, exploration of the wound revealed no fracture. However, he

developed erysipelas of the face and scalp, and was delirious and semiconscious for a time. He nearly died. The account of this case, wrote O'Malley, 'is one of the fullest pictures we have of the medical procedure of that age.' In all there were fifty consultations among the attending physicians, fourteen of which took place in the presence of the King. They were formal, elaborate, and lasted two to four hours each.

THE ACHIEVEMENT

It is no exaggeration to say that this great masterpiece, the *De fabrica*, has largely gone unread. It has never been printed in a language other than Latin, and is known to most of us through its illustrations, excellent copper plates of which were produced in England by Geminus as early as 1545, with English captions added in 1553.[53, 54] While William Harvey's little book of seventy-two pages, *De motu cordis*, translated into English within twenty-five years of publication, has been widely available in various translations during the past hundred years, Vesalius's book was familiar only to scholars. It is an enormous tome of some 700 folio pages, each of about 58 lines and 760 words, 'vast, verbose, repetitious, a very torrent of words',[55] monotonously unrelieved by paragraphing, and written in a complicated classical style of Latin.[56] A terrifying task of translation for any scholar.

In the English speaking world the contents of the *De fabrica* have only been widely appreciated during the last fifty years. In 1918,[57] Cullen spoke of Vesalius's 'undeserved oblivion'. The Belgian-inspired monument which was to have been erected to his memory on the island of Zante (Zakinthos), to mark the quatercentenary of his birth, was never completed. It was planned for August 1914. It is true there existed Roth's German biography of Vesalius, published in 1892, and in 1900 Professor Michael Foster wrote about Vesalius, providing a translation of some of his more significant passages in his *Lectures on the history of physiology during the 16th, 17th and 18th centuries*. But it is more recent books which have served to disseminate knowledge of Vesalius and his work.

The preface to *De fabrica* was translated by Farrington in 1932[58] and Hotchkiss in 1942.[59] Harvey Cushing's *Bio-bibliography* was published in 1943.[60] The *Tabulae anatomicae* was presented by Singer and Rabin in 1946, in their *Prelude to modern science*.[61] Lind's translation of the *Epitome* appeared in 1949,[62] while Saunders and O'Malley published *The illustrations from the works of Vesalius*, with a biographical sketch, in 1950.[63] Neurologists, in particular, became indebted to Singer in 1952 for his *Vesalius on the human brain*, which, as already mentioned, included a translation of Book VII of the *Fabrica*.[64] Then, to the delight of all Vesalian enthusiasts, came the discovery in 1959 of the notebook of a German student, Baldasar Heseler, who in 1540 attended Vesalius's dissections in Bologna. They were translated, edited, and published by Dr Ruben Eriksson in Stockholm.[65, 66] A vivid picture emerges of Vesalius at work, dissecting, and lecturing during the course of twenty-six demonstrations.

Lastly, in 1964, marking the four hundredth year after Vesalius's death,

Professor C. D. O'Malley, the foremost authority on Vesalius, published his long awaited definitive biography *Andreas Vesalius of Brussels*.[67] This was a task that occupied him during twelve years and in his book he included a hundred pages of translation from *De fabrica* and a wealth of exhaustive notes.

Thus, the contemporary doctor has the opportunity of learning more about Vesalius than did the majority of his teachers.

Men who have known the *Fabrica* have praised it highly. The Italian medical historian, Castiglioni,[68] said that 'There are books which play in history the role of battles'; *De fabrica* was one. Osler said it was 'the greatest medical work ever printed', a phrase he inscribed on a copy he presented to the library of the New York Academy of Medicine. Foster[69] said it did for anatomy what *De motu cordis* did for physiology, and that, moreover, 'Harvey's great work was the direct outcome of Vesalius's teaching, the direct outcome and yet one reached by successive steps, taken by men of the Italian School, of which Vesalius was the founder and father'. To his biographer, O'Malley, Vesalius's work was 'an unprecedented blending of scientific exposition, art and typography',[70] while Singer concluded that the *Fabrica* was 'one of the great achievements of the human spirit'.[71] I do not know whether Goethe ever turned its pages but I feel he would have thought it 'a hymn of praise'. Goethe was fascinated by the shapes assumed by life and, as Sherrington said, he gave us the word 'morphology' – 'the studying of living shape'.[72]

Discovering Vesalius is a voyage to be remembered. For me it began forty years ago, in the spring of 1939, at Yale, where, armed with a letter of introduction to Harvey Cushing from Paul D. White, in whose department I was then working, I gazed for the first time on the folios and plates of Andreas Vesalius. Cushing was then busy bringing together his collection of Vesaliana, which had occupied him for a lifetime. Vesalius was Cushing's 'Patron Saint', said Fulton. Cushing's fatal anginal attack came that autumn after he had been shifting a heavy Vesalius folio.

For the neurologist, the importance of Vesalius may be emphasized by a quotation from O'Malley. 'There was virtually no knowledge of the brain as the result of dissection and observation before the third decade of the sixteenth century.'[73]

CHAPTER 3

WILLIS AND THE NERVOUS SYSTEM

Almost everything that distinguishes the modern world from earlier centuries is attributable to science, which achieved its most spectacular triumphs in the seventeenth century.

Bertrand Russell in *History of Western Philosophy*, 1946.

INTRODUCTION

In the history of science the seventeenth century has been called the '*insurgent century*.'[1] The astonishing display of genius which characterized the Italian Renaissance, typified in the work of Vesalius, gradually spread north, taking various forms, but having in common a new sense of curiosity and enquiry. The Laws of Nature were being discovered.

There was a flow of epic treatises which portray the transformation of outlook that was taking place. In England it began in 1600 with the publication of the country's first major scientific contribution. This was William Gilbert's (1546–1603) *De magnete – On the magnet and on magnetic bodies and concerning that great magnet, the earth, a new physiology*. Gilbert, then President of the Royal College of Physicians, conducted his enquiries in an objective manner, made experiments, argued inductively, and pleaded for fresh, unbiased approaches. He gave us the word 'electricity', from *elektron*, the Greek for amber, which he used to produce frictional electricity.

In his preface to *De magnete*, Gilbert wrote,

> I know how difficult it is to give freshness to old things, brilliancy to the antiquated, light to the dark, space to the despised, credibility to the doubtful; how much more difficult it is to obtain and establish some authority for things new and unheard of, and which are opposed to all the beliefs of men.[2]

Gilbert was physician to Queen Elizabeth I and it was her former Lord Chancellor, Francis Bacon (1561–1626), who published the second classic text of the century in 1605. This was entitled *Of the proficience and advancement of learning, divine and humane*, commonly known as *The advancement of learning*,[3] and described by Hazlitt as 'a noble chart of the human intellect'. He urged inquirers to direct their attention to the examination of nature, and he explained the processes involved in the inductive method of reasoning.

Bacon lamented that the ancient authors 'had long slept in libraries' but noted that now they 'began generally to be read and revolved.'[4] But he condemned the teleological explanations so loved by Galen, quoting Galen's reference, as an example, that 'the hairs about the eyelids are for safeguard of the sight.'[5] He considered that 'Man's body is the most extremely compounded' and so is 'an instrument easy to distemper.'[6] 'The office of medicine is to tune this curious harp of man's body and to reduce it to harmony.'[7]

Bacon had a comprehensive view of many branches of science but he seems to have known little of anatomy and physiology. He does not mention Vesalius and although William Harvey was his physician he does not mention Harvey's researches. Of anatomists, he said 'I find much deficience; for they enquire of the parts . . . but not of the diversities of the parts . . . nor much of the footsteps of diseases.'[8]

But he advocated vivisection; 'the dissection of beasts alive' was likely to show 'the passages and pores . . . shut and latent in dead bodies.'[9] He also suggested that pathological findings deserved study 'with reference to the diseases and symptoms which resulted from them . . .'. He seemed to realize that minute examination of the body was destined to be important, saying that 'mean and small things' should be examined, for, as Gilbert had shown, 'electricity was found in needles of iron, not in bars of iron'.[10] Gilbert 'had made a philosophy out of the observations of a loadstone.'[11] Nevertheless Bacon did not accept much of what had been discovered about magnetism and electricity.

It is surprising that he did not write of Vesalius's contribution. *The epitome* had been published in English by Geminus in 1545, and it included splendid copper-engraved reproductions of the *De fabrica* illustrations. This book of Geminus was the first to be printed in English for which copper plates were used.[12]

Although Bacon underestimated the value of the deductive process and the framing of hypotheses his work probably had a considerable influence. He would surely have been delighted with Harvey's conclusion that only the concept of the circulation of the blood could explain the facts. 'In spite of all his faults' wrote Medawar, 'scientists still incline to think Francis Bacon their first and greatest spokesman.'[13] Izaak Walton called him 'The Great Secretary of Nature'.

A second 'scientific' philosophical treatise came from the pen of a physician, toward the end of the century. This was John Locke's (1632–1704) *Essay concerning human understanding* (1690). He had been a pupil of Willis at Oxford and later he was apprenticed to Thomas Sydenham in London.[14] Locke's empiricism permeated both his practice of medicine and his philosophy. He called for the examination of 'Nature at Liberty', 'Nature in her errors', and 'Nature in constraint' – the normal, the abnormal, and the experimental. Like Bacon he also saw the significance of morbid anatomy.[15]

It is not without interest, in these days when standards of literacy are under discussion, that in 1917 Sir William Osler, speaking to a mixed lay and medical audience in the village of Fenny Stratford, Buckinghamshire, felt able to say this about Locke's *Essay*. 'There is no one in the room who would not be improved by a careful study of this book over a period of several years.' The occasion was a patronal festival in honour of Thomas Willis, begun in 1734 by his grandson, Browne Willis, who had erected a

FIG. 20. Thomas Willis (1621–75). This portrait by Vertue, 1742, was based on an engraving made in 1666 when Willis was forty-five years of age. He was said to have been 'a plain Man, a Man of no Carriage, little Discourse, Complaisance or Society'. The open book is not *Cerebri anatome* but *Pharmaceutice rationalis* (1674), his last work, in which he described diabetes mellitus, asthma, pleurisy, and cardiospasm – all classic accounts. The illustration in the open book depicts the structure of the lungs. (Courtesy of Dr William Feindel, Montreal.)

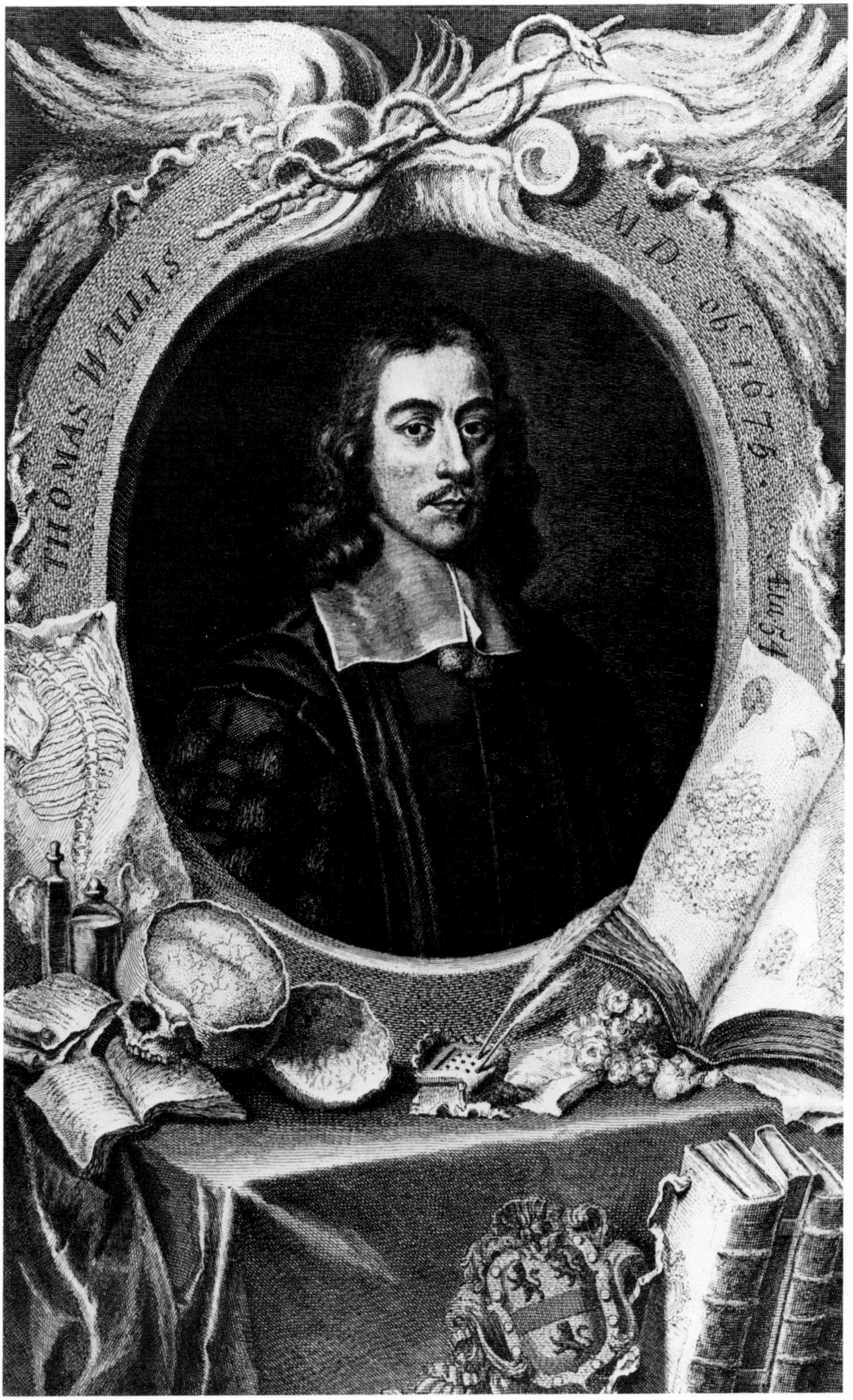
THOMAS WILLIS M.D. ob. 1675.
Ætat 54

church in the village in memory of his grandfather.[16]

In the field of science Robert Boyle's (1627–91) the *Sceptical chymist* (1661) inaugurated the modern period of chemistry. The age of scientific determinism was ushered in by Isaac Newton's (1642–1727) *Principia* in 1687. For physicians there were William Harvey's (1578–1657) *De motu cordis* (1628) and Thomas Willis's (1621–75) *Cerebri anatome* (1664).

Flaws have always been discernible in the imposing oversimplification of eras in terms such as 'renaissance', 'revolution', and 'enlightenment', but it is difficult to avoid using them. And, as every schoolboy knows, or used to know, this was the 'Age of the Enlightenment'.

Throughout the seventeenth century we see the growth of collaboration in study and experiment, increasing objectivity of criticism, and, most importantly, the invention of new instruments and techniques.[17, 18] Willis's book was based on a joint study in which he was clearly the central figure. He warmly acknowledged the assistance he had received in dissection, experiment, and discussion with three colleagues. There was Richard Lower,[19] 'the edge of whose knife and wit I willingly acknowledge'; Christopher Wren 'who delineated with his own most skilful hands, many Figures of the Brain and Skull'; and Thomas Millington, 'a most Learned Man, to whom I from day to day proposed privately my Conjectures and Observations'. Willis felt 'hem'd in by the plentiful assistances of these Illustrious Men'.

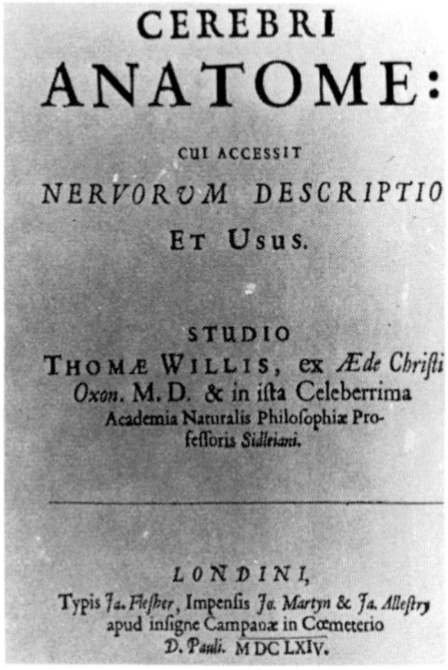
CEREBRI
ANATOME:
CUI ACCESSIT
NERVORUM DESCRIPTIO
ET USUS.
STUDIO
THOMÆ WILLIS, ex *Æde Christi* *Oxon.* M. D. & in iſta Celeberrima Academia Naturalis Philoſophiæ Profeſſoris *Sidleiani.*
LONDINI,
Typis *Ja. Flesher*, Impenſis *Jo. Martyn* & *Ja. Allestry* apud inſigne Campanæ in Cœmeterio *D. Pauli.* MDCLXIV.

FIG. 21. The title page of the *Anatomy of the brain and the description and use of the nerves* (1664).

We also know that Robert Hooke (1635–1703), of *Micrographia* fame, worked as an assistant to Willis, who in turn recommended him to Boyle.[20] Wren's accomplishments were many; 'The learned and ingenious Sir Christopher Wren ... was the first author of that noble experiment of injecting liquors into the veins of animals, first exhibited to the meetings at Oxford, about the year 1656. ...'[21, 22] Wren was one of the first to make drawings of microscopical observations. Willis used the microscope, and injected arteries, veins, and bronchi. Like Harvey he also made observations on embryology, comparative anatomy, and morbid anatomy. All this he did, we should not forget, while he was busy in clinical practice. He had the highest income in Oxford – three hundred pounds per annum.[23–25]

Nevertheless a modern reader of *Cerebri anatome* might well feel that today Lower's name would probably figure on the title page as a co-author. This notwithstanding, his continued devotion to Willis and his defence of him in print suggest that he suffered no sense of grievance. The allegations that it was Lower, and not Willis, who was the principal investigator have been disproved.[26–29]

It is clear that scientific observations and ideas were being fervently discussed in increasingly wider circles. Private gatherings, conversaziones, clubs, and academies multiplied. Traditional authority was being dethroned. The Royal Society, of which Willis was an original, though not an ardent, member, began its publications in the same year that saw the appearance of *Cerebri anatome*. *Nullius in verba* ('On the word of no man'), from lines by Horace,[30] appeared on the Society's crest. But in that same year of 1664 two witches were hanged in Suffolk and the celebrated physician Sir Thomas Browne was one of the witnesses for the prosecution.

As science became fashionable and international communication grew, an author could choose to publish his work in another country. Harvey chose Frankfurt and Willis's book appeared simultaneously in London and Amsterdam.

Criticism, although often trenchant, became more pertinent and appropriately expressed. It lost much of the venom and scurrility attached to it in former years. No one was more critical of Willis than the Danish anatomist Steno (Stensen, 1638–86), but he admitted that 'The best diagrams of the brain that we have to date are those given us by M. Willis.'[31] Willis, in later writings, found himself able to refer to 'the most learned' and 'famous' Steno. What an advance on the reaction of Vesalius's teacher in Paris, Jacobius Sylvius, to his pupil's new anatomy. 'Honest reader,' Sylvius wrote, 'I urge you to pay no attention to a certain ridiculous madman, one utterly lacking in talent who curses and inveighs impiously against his teacher.'[32]

It is generally agreed that 'Galenism, dominant in 1600, was vanquished by 1700'.[33, 34] Bertrand Russell wrote 'In 1700 the mental outlook of educated men was completely modern; in 1600, except among a very few, it was still largely medieval.'[35] And yet Willis, the astute observer and practical clinician, who claimed in 1659 in his essay on *Fermentation* that 'I am content to know what the external senses provide to the reasoning mind; to wit, I readily profess that I do not want to fabricate or to dream of a philosophy',[36] proceeded in 1672, in *On the soul of brutes*, to speculate in an extraordinary fashion about the workings of the nervous system. One cannot fail to recall the similar words of the young Galen in his book *On medical*

FIG. 22 (*left*). The opening lines from the first page of Chapter 1 of the *Anatomy of the brain*. Willis first explains the difficulties he faces, the extraordinary complexity of the brain, and how he proposes a 'Method of Dissection itself, or of Anatomical Administration', which will serve to construct 'a compendious Catalogue'.

FIG. 23 (*right*). The concluding page of the *Anatomy of the brain*. Willis promises his readers that if encouraged by the reception of the present work, he will undertake another, on psychology and comparative anatomy. This he did, in *De anima brutorum* (1672).

THE

ANATOMY

OF THE

BRAIN.

CHAP. I.

The Method or Anatomical Adminiſtration of Diſſecting the Brain is propoſed.

AMong the various parts of an animated Body, which are ſubject to Anatomical diſquiſition, none is preſumed to be eaſier or better known than the Brain; yet in the mean time, there is none leſs or more imperfectly underſtood. All of it that appears, and is commonly deſcribed in the fore-part or forehead, is beheld almoſt at a ſight or two after ſome rude cutting up; but if you ſeek what lyes hid in the receſſes for that end, new boſoms and productions of Bodies, before hid, are every where laid open: yea the parts of the Brain it ſelf are ſo complicated and involved, and their reſpects and habitudes to one another ſo hard to be extricated, that it may ſeem a more hard taſk to inſtitute its perfect Anatomy, than to delineate on a plain, the flexions and Meanders of ſome Labyrinth: Becauſe,

THE

CONCLUSION.

THUS much for the Anatomy of the Brain and Cerebel, and of their Appendix, both Medullar and Nervous, and of the Uſes and Offices of all the ſeveral Parts, of which we have largely treated. There yet remains, after we have viewed, not only the outward Courts and Porches of this Fabrick, as it were of a certain Kingly Palace, but alſo its intimate Receſſes and private Chambers, that we next inquire into, what the Lady or Inhabitant of this Princely place may be, in what part ſhe doth chiefly reſide, and by what Rule and Government ſhe diſpoſes and orders her Family. Then we ought to take notice, what defects and irregularities happen to it, or to its parts and powers; then to what injuries of changes or Diſeaſes this Building or Houſe, to wit, the Brain and nervous Stock, may be obnoxious. For indeed I am as it were bound, by reaſon of the Work it ſelf, and the promiſe I made before, that for the Crown of the Work, a certain Theory of the Soul of Brutes ſhould be added after the naked Anatomical Obſervations and Hiſtories of Living Creatures, and of their animated Parts. Truly it is but juſt and equal, that we enter upon this Diſcourſe of the Soul, and that other task of *Pathologie*, to wit, that the Aſperities and hard ſence of our already inſtituted *Anatomy* may be ſweetned with thoſe kind of more pleaſant Speculations, as it were cloathing the Skeleton with fleſh; and that the Reader being wearied by a long and troubleſom Journey, may be a little refreſhed and recreated. For in truth, whatſoever of our Work is performed without form or beauty, may ſeem as the Foundation of a Building only placed on the ground, in which no elegancy or neatneſs doth yet ſhine, but that all things appear rude, and as yet built of rough and unpoliſhed ſtones. A Superſtructure indeed may be promiſed to be put upon this Foundation, perhaps fair and beautiful, whereby the minds of the Beholders may be pleaſed and inſtructed. But truly this kind of work may be too hard and great to be performed by our weakneſs: neither doth it become me to proceed in my undertakings, before theſe have undergone the Cenſure and chance to which they are ſubject. For I fear, leſt this Foundation, but now laid, ſhould become too weak and feeble for the ſuſtaining an higher Fabrick, at leaſt until this hath for ſome time undergone the tryal, by lying open to winds and ſtorms.

experience which I quoted on p. 12. It is a familiar human failing – to begin to be more heedful of ideas than of facts. The late Sir Francis Walshe once told me that neurologists, in particular, seemed rather susceptible to this trait; 'A concept at fifty, try and avoid!'

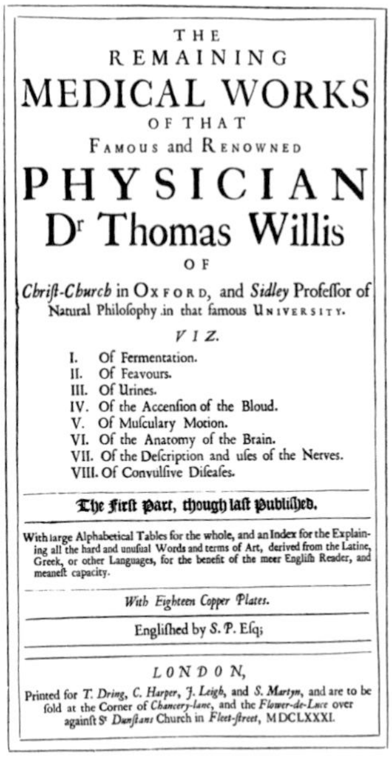

THE
REMAINING
MEDICAL WORKS
OF THAT
FAMOUS and RENOWNED
PHYSICIAN
Dr Thomas Willis
OF
Christ-Church in OXFORD, and *Sidley* Professor of Natural Philosophy in that famous UNIVERSITY.

VIZ.

I. Of Fermentation.
II. Of Feavours.
III. Of Urines.
IV. Of the Accension of the Bloud.
V. Of Musculary Motion.
VI. Of the Anatomy of the Brain.
VII. Of the Description and uses of the Nerves.
VIII. Of Convulsive Diseases.

The First Part, though last Published.

With large Alphabetical Tables for the whole, and an Index for the Explaining all the hard and unusual Words and terms of Art, derived from the Latine, Greek, or other Languages, for the benefit of the meer English Reader, and meanest capacity.

With Eighteen Copper Plates.

Englished by *S. P.* Esq;

LONDON,

Printed for *T. Dring*, *C. Harper*, *J. Leigh*, and *S. Martyn*, and are to be sold at the Corner of *Chancery-lane*, and the *Flower-de-Luce* over against St *Dunstans* Church in *Fleet-street*, MDCLXXXI.

FIG. 24. Title page of the first part of a collected edition of Willis's writings in 1681. The second part had already appeared in 1679 under the title *Pharmaceutice rationalis*. The title *Dr Willis's practice of physick* was later used for the collected edition of 1684.

WILLIS'S WRITINGS

Willis published six books: *On fermentation, fevers and urine* (1659), *Cerebral anatomy* (*Cerebri anatome*) (1664), *Cerebral pathology, convulsive diseases* (1667), *On hysteria, hypochondria, motion of muscles* (1670), *On the soul of brutes* (*De anima brutorum*) (1672), and *Pharmacology* (*Pharmaceutice rationalis*) (1674).

An English translation of *Cerebri anatome* was published in 1681 and of his collected works in *Dr. Willis's practice of physick* in 1684.†

The tercentenary edition (1965) of *Cerebri anatome* consists of two vellum-covered volumes, with paper bearing Willis's crest.[37] In his introduction, William Feindel, the editor, presents an account of Willis's life, his circle of friends, and of Pordage, his English translator. Feindel describes Willis's first use of the term *Neurology* and summarizes the contents of *Cerebri anatome*. There are portraits of Willis and his friends, and, in addition, for comparative purposes there are excellent reproductions of illustrations of the base of the brain from the works of Vesalius, Vesling, and Casserius, showing what they had noted of the arterial circle there. The second volume contains a facsimile of *Cerebri anatome*, 'Englished' by Pordage, with its celebrated plates. One can only agree with Keele, in his review of this publishing 'event' that 'its greatest danger lies in its seductive beauty, which may result in its abduction' into the secret closets of collectors' pieces.[38] I used to peer into it from time to time; now I have leisure to pore over it.

Not that reading Pordage's translation is an easy task. Nomenclature in neuroanatomy, as we have seen when reading of Galen and Vesalius, had presented many difficulties. Translation of Latin texts into a vernacular language also posed problems. In Willis's case the reader will also soon realize that seventeenth-century English, although robust and colourful, is hardly familiar to his eyes and ears. Then, too, Willis himself, especially in *De anima brutorum*, is often vague and heedlessly repetitious. So the going is hard, but completing the course is immensely satisfying.

We are all familiar with the custom of describing the corpora quadrigemina as the nates and testes, the pineal gland as the penis, but where is the 'vulva' or the 'arse-whole' of the brain? And the 'cranklings and windings and turnings about' of what transpires to be the convolutions, reminds one of Oliver Cromwell's wish to put an end to the 'turnings and windings' of the past, when he summoned an Assembly in Parliament in 1653. The 'oblong Marrow' will be recognized as the medulla oblongata, but its extent will not be readily visualized when it is referred to as 'the Kings Highway, [(which)] leads from the Brain, as the Metropolis, into many Provinces of the nervous stock, by private recesses and crossways'. The oblong medulla

† Quotations from Willis's works are from *The anatomy of the brain and nerves* (A.B.), 1965 tercentenary edition; and from *The practice of physick* (1684); *Soul of brutes* (S.B.); *Convulsive diseases* (C.D.); *Motion of muscles* (M.M.); *Pharmacology* (Ph. Rat.).

reached up into the corpus callosum, while the cerebellum, to Willis, included the pons (the annular protuberance) and the inferior cerebellar peduncles. It is important to appreciate this when considering Willis's contribution to the origins of the cranial nerves and the discovery of the autonomic nervous system.

It was in Pordage's edition of *Cerebri Anatome*, in 1681 that the term 'Neurology', or 'Neurologie', first saw the light of day. To Willis it meant the 'Doctrine of the Nerves', or the study of the brain and nerves. Over the centuries the term has come to mean something very much more than its originator intended.

THE CLINICIAN

Living in a fever-ridden, and, for a time, an England at civil war, Willis was inevitably preoccupied with infectious diseases, endemic and epidemic. He recorded his observations in his first book, as his contemporary Sydenham also did. Willis described pleurisy, influenza, asthma, and whooping cough (which Osler said in his textbook was 'a much better description' than that of Sydenham). He gave the first description of epidemic typhoid fever[30] and epidemic cerebrospinal (meningococcal) fever,[40] and the first account of an epidemic of typhus in England.[41, 42] In one epidemic 'whereby men were grievously affected in their brains and nervous stock' he described what may have been epidemic encephalitis.[43] He referred to a 1661 'Soporiferous Epidemical Fever', citing the case of a ploughman taken ill at his plough who slept for days, but recovered. An Oxford gardener 'drowsed' for days, was 'foolish' for two months, but eventually recovered although he never had the 'same vigor'.

Such studies led Creighton (1891) in his *A history of epidemics in Britain*, to write that

> The account by Willis of three consecutive epidemics in the autumn of 1657, the Spring of 1658, and the autumn of 1658 is of peculiar interest for the reason that it is the first systematic piece of epidemiology written in England, and that the middle epidemic of the three was one of influenza.[44]

Willis also described and named puerperal fever, 'the putrid fever of women in child-bed'. Garrison,[45] Rolleston,[46] and others have suggested that it was the first account of this disease, but Hippocrates, no less, can rightly claim this distinction. His patient is well described in Book I, Case IV of *Of the epidemics* (the patient was seized with fever and headache fourteen days after delivery, followed by vomiting, insomnia, spasms, rigors, delirium, stupor, coma and death on the twentieth day).[47]

Concerning diseases of the lungs it is generally agreed that one of the earliest descriptions of emphysema was that of Floyer (1649–1734)[48] but Hierons[49] was able to quote that Willis, twenty years earlier, wrote 'We have known some to have died Asthmatic or shortwinded, whose lungs being free from an Ulcer, or any more grievous wound, have swelled so much, that they wanted room for their motion within the cavity of the chest.' Miller,[50, 51] in two papers in 1922 and 1923, that were probably the first of the modern

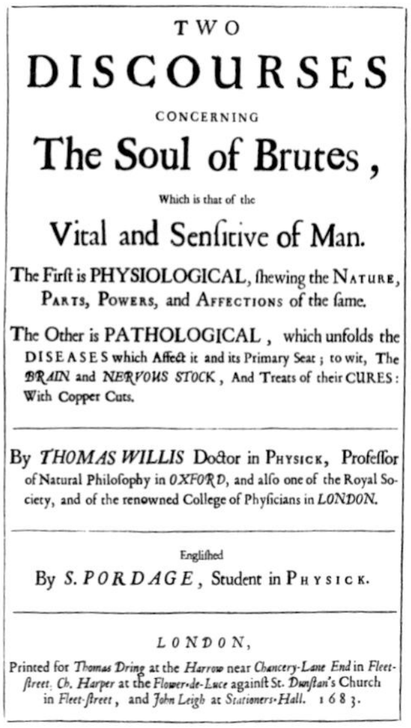
TWO
DISCOURSES
CONCERNING
The Soul of Brutes,
Which is that of the
Vital and Senſitive of Man.
The Firſt is PHYSIOLOGICAL, ſhewing the NATURE, PARTS, POWERS, and AFFECTIONS of the ſame.
The Other is PATHOLOGICAL, which unfolds the DISEASES which Affect it and its Primary Seat; to wit, The BRAIN and NERVOUS STOCK, And Treats of their CURES: With Copper Cuts.

By *THOMAS WILLIS* Doctor in PHYSICK, Profeſſor of Natural Philoſophy in *OXFORD*, and alſo one of the Royal Society, and of the renowned College of Phyſicians in *LONDON*.

Engliſhed
By *S. PORDAGE*, Student in PHYSICK.

LONDON,
Printed for *Thomas Dring* at the *Harrow* near *Chancery-Lane End* in *Fleet-ſtreet*. *Ch. Harper* at the *Flower-de-Luce* againſt St. *Dunſtan's* Church in *Fleet-ſtreet*, and *John Leigh* at *Stationers-Hall*. 1683.

FIG. 25. Title page of *Two discourses concerning the soul of brutes* (1683).

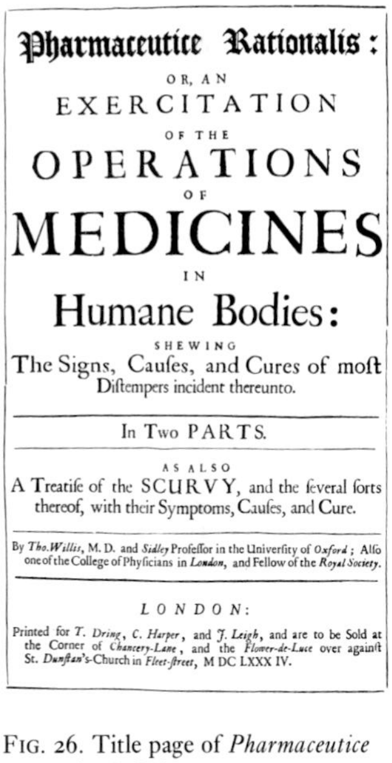
Pharmaceutice Rationalis:
OR, AN
EXERCITATION
OF THE
OPERATIONS
OF
MEDICINES
IN
Humane Bodies:
SHEWING
The Signs, Cauſes, and Cures of moſt Diſtempers incident thereunto.

In Two PARTS.

AS ALSO
A Treatiſe of the SCURVY, and the ſeveral ſorts thereof, with their Symptoms, Cauſes, and Cure.

By *Tho. Willis*, M. D. and *Sidley* Profeſſor in the Univerſity of *Oxford*; Alſo one of the College of Phyſicians in *London*, and Fellow of the *Royal Society*.

LONDON:
Printed for *T. Dring*, *C. Harper*, and *J. Leigh*, and are to be Sold at the Corner of *Chancery-Lane*, and the *Flower-de-Luce* over againſt St. *Dunſtan's*-Church in *Fleet-ſtreet*, M DC LXXX IV.

FIG. 26. Title page of *Pharmaceutice rationalis*. (1684).

studies aimed at restoring Willis's reputation, has shown how important were Willis's writings on the lungs. There are accounts in *Pharmaceutice rationalis* of acute and chronic tuberculosis, asthma, pulmonary abscess and empyema, and anatomical, microscopical, and injection studies of the lungs which furthered knowledge of their detailed structure. He actually described and illustrated the superficial lymphatics of the lung, asserting, apparently justifiably, that this was an original contribution – a claim he did not make for his account of the arterial 'circle'.

We all know that he was the first physician in England to note the sweetness of urine† in some patients with polyuria but Hierons[52] has pointed out that some of his diabetic patients also suffered from 'flying running pains through their whole Bodies' with weakness of their limbs – possibly examples of diabetic polyneuritis. Lastly, in this summary of Willis's clinical accounts of general interest, mention must be made of the patient with 'almost perpetual vomiting . . . that growing hungry he would eat until the *Oesophagus* was filled up to the Throat . . . and he languished away for hunger, and every day was in danger of Death'. Willis treated this patient with cardiospasm, or achalasia of the cardia, with the passage of a bougie made of 'whale Bone, with a little round Button of Sponge fixed to the top of it'. The patient was still using it fifteen years later.

If we turn for a moment to that familiar and serviceable old friend, Major's *Classic descriptions of diseases* (1948, 3rd edn.)[53] we find no less than six original entries under Willis's name (asthma, cardiospasm, diabetes, pleurisy, typhoid fever, and typhus fever), one more, actually, than those attributed to Sydenham (gout, influenza, measles, rheumatic fever, and scarlet fever). Neurological selections were intentionally omitted, but if we add chorea to Sydenham's contributions we perhaps gain some measure of Willis's general clinical ability alongside 'The English Hippocrates'.

Most of Willis's clinical neurology is to be found recorded in *De anima brutorum*. In his preface addressed to the reader, Willis wrote 'I have here given you what I have long promised, the Pathology of the Brain and Nervous Stock . . .'. It is a large work of about 175,000 words and arranged in two parts: (I) physiological and (II) pathological. In Part I he discourses on the various conceptions of the soul in man and animals, seemingly accepting the old doctrines of the four humours and Galen's animal spirits. He brings to their discussion the notions of both the iatrochemical and the iatrophysical schools. He then proceeds to describe his interpretations of the functions of motion and sensation, and of the special senses, normal and abnormal sleep, and states of disturbed consciousness. There are chapters on neurological symptomatology and pathology including accounts of headache, vertigo, epilepsy, convulsions in general, paralysis, and apoplexy. Willis finally comes to a consideration of psychiatric disturbances in four chapters entitled 'Delirium and Phrensie' 'Melancholy', 'Madness', and 'Stupidity and Foolishness'.

Dr Willis's *Practice of physick* did indeed constitute a medical library for the day.

† Moliere's doctors who drank specimens of urine at the bedside were examples of lavatory humour rather than allusions to the diagnosis of diabetes (Hall, H.G. *Proc. Soc. Med.* **70**, 425 (1977)).

Neurological complaints

Headache. Willis recognized different forms of headache – 'within or without the skull', 'universal or particular', 'short', 'continuing' or 'intermittent', 'wandering', 'uncertain', 'before, behind or the side', and 'occasional or habitual'. He said 'The pain of the head is wont to be accounted the chiefest of the Diseases of the Head.' Indeed, it was 'so common that it is become a Proverb as a sign of a more rare and admirable thing *That his head did never ake*' – an observation which should interest those who think migraine is a peculiarly modern ill. He thought there were immediate and remote causes of headache. It was frequently hereditary; it could follow injury or an emotional upset; it often began in the morning. Hierons[54] suggests that Willis may have been the first to record a case of migrainous neuralgia or cluster headaches in the lady who began to suffer every afternoon at about 4 o'clock from severe recurrent daily headaches for some five weeks. Liveing,[55] in 1873, commented on Willis's observation that hunger might precede migraine, and on his theory of 'nerve storms'. Willis noted that polyuria may be associated with an attack of migraine; 'I have observed in many, a watery and a very plentiful urine, either to precede or accompany the fits of the disease'.[56] Both he and Harvey treated Anne, Countess of Conway, who had the most famous headache of the century.[57, 58]

Sir Charles Symonds,[59] in 1955, drew attention to Willis's record of the patient with left-sided headache in whom at autopsy occlusion of the right carotid artery was found. Willis thought that the headache was a consequence of the resulting compensatory dilatation of the left carotid artery. This was one of Willis's reasons for concluding that his circle served an anastomotic function.

He appreciated that headache could be a sinister symptom of brain disorder such as inflammation or tumour. He mentioned the question of trephining; 'The opening of the skull cry'd up by many, but rarely or never attempted ... This our most ingenious Harvey endeavoured to persuade a Noble Lady, labouring with a most grievous inveterate headache, promising a cure from thence, but neither she nor any other would admit that administration.' Willis doubted whether anything would have been disclosed for if a tumour were present there would have been other symptoms such as 'sleepy distempers' or 'deadly convulsions'. But he also wondered whether the headache could be meningeal in origin 'beset with little whelks, a Schirrous or Callous Tumor', although, even then, 'I think opening of the skull will profit little or nothing'.[60]

He concludes his chapter on headache with a summary of eight case histories ranging from bouts of migraine to fatal brain tumour and autopsy. We catch a fine glimpse of Willis the physician in these pages.

Vertigo. This consisted of a 'turning around of the head'. It was 'an affection or distemper, in which the visible objects seem to turn round, and the sick feel a perturbation ... [and might] fall ... though when they shut their eyes they still perceive as it were a turning round, like the turning around of a Mill, in the Brain'. Sometimes the symptom was a minor ill, felt only by some folk when on a height or bridge, or after taking alcohol. 'But it could be a disease of itself which being raised up in the middle part of the brain' was hard to alleviate. It could also arise 'from some other distemper, placed sometimes within the brain, and sometimes without it'. He spoke of 'primary' and 'symptomatick' vertigo.

Vision, hearing, smell and taste. In the chapter 'On Sight' Willis[62] explains the action of the six ocular muscles (four 'straight' and two 'oblique') and the 'sympathy' which exists between them so that 'squinting' is avoided. The muscles are named according to the emotional implication of the direction of movement. Thus we have *upward* 'holy, devout – as in prayer'; *downward*, as in the 'humble, pious'; *outward*; as in 'indignation or aversion'; *obliquely*, 'amatory, because lovers behold one another obliquely or sideways'. *Inward* movement was like the 'squinting drunkard'.

Vision itself was perplexing. He wondered whether the rays of light were 'particles streaming from a lucid body' or whether they were 'unkindled particles of nitro-sulphureous air'. Light rays travelled in a straight manner 'whether reflected or refracted'. He compared flame with light, noting the differences.

Of the senses of taste and smell he noted that 'loss of one of them, oftentimes brings in the defect of the other'. The faculty of taste was practically confined to the tongue: the palate and 'Upper part of the Throat' also contributed. Loss of taste impaired the appetite.[63] In the chapter on hearing he talks of deafness resulting from 'looseness of the drum', and of 'the three little bones (hammer, anvil and stirrup)' and he identifies the cochlea as the organ of hearing:

> As to the Shell, the use of it seems to be, that the audible Species being brought thorow such turning and winding Labyrinths, and so receiving an augmentation by reflection, and manifold refraction, it may become more clear and sensible; then further, that every Impression, carried about by this winding and very narrow way, may come more distinct to the Sensory; because by this means, care is taken, that many confused Species together, may not be brought in ... Further, there is another use of the Shell, no less noted, to wit, that the audible species may be impressed on the Fibres and the ends of the Sensible Nerves, inserted in this place, not at once or at large, but by little and little, and as it were in a just proportion and dimension.[64]

He noted two branches of the auditory nerve, one into the 'shell' and the other 'into the next chamber of the shell'.

It is in this chapter on hearing that we encounter his notable lines on that form of perversion of hearing – paracusis.

> ... I heard from a Credible Person, that he once knew a woman 'tho she were deaf yet so long as a drum was beaten in her chamber, she heard every word perfectly; wherefore her Husband kept a drummer on purpose for his servant, that by that means he might have some converse with his wife. Also I was told of another deaf person, who living near a Ring of Bells, as often as they all rung out, he could easily

hear any word, and not else. Without doubt the reason of these is, that the drum of itself being continually loose, by the impulse of a more vehement sound, is compelled to its due tensity or stretching forth, by which it might in some measure be able to perform its office.[65]

Disorders of sleep and consciousness.[66] He discussed sleeping and waking, pathological forms of sleep, sleep walking, and nightmares. He thought 'lethargy' was a disorder of the 'shell of the brain', or 'cortical part'. Some people were 'afraid to sleep . . . for as soon as they shut their eyes, presently leaping up, they would cry out they would go mad, with a multitude of confused phantasms, so that they were necessitated to abstain from sleep'. He described what we would term hypnagogic hallucinations.

Critchley[67] drew our attention to Willis's account of restless legs (Ekbom's syndrome).

Wherefore to some, when being a Bed, they betake themselves to sleep, presently in the arms and leggs, leapings and contractions of the tendons, and so great a restlessness and Tossings of their members ensue, that the diseased are no more able to sleep, than if they were in a Place of the greatest Torture.[68]

He also referred to 'waking in melancholick people'.

The function of sleep was to ensure rest for the animal spirits in that part of the brain concerned with voluntary functions, 'but not those procreated in the Cerebel', which was concerned with 'vital and nutritive functions'. The 'beginning of sleep was in the cortical part of the brain, which is also the seat of memory'.[69]

'Sleepy distempers' were graded according to the degree of impairment of consciousness. There were 'somnolency, coma, and Caros' (deprivation of the senses). Lethargy arose 'from the cortex not the ventricles. In hydrocephalus there is no lethargy'. Caros arose from lesions 'a little deeper in the brain'.[70] We see here Willis's clinical experience contributing to his conclusion, contrary to Descartes, that it was the brain itself, not its ventricles, that was the important structure, and where the animal spirits were formed. Narcolepsy was identified from the following passages about 'sleepy distempers', by Lennox in 1939.[71]

Most authors call this [sleepiness] not a Disease, but an evil habit, or a sleepy disposition, for the distemper'd, as to other things, are well enough; they eat and drink well, go abroad, take care well enough of their domestick affairs, yet whilst talking, or walking, or eating, yea their mouths being full of meat, they shall nod, and unless rouzed up by others, fall fast asleep; and thus they sleep continually almost, not only some days or months, but (as it is said of Epemenides) many years; wherefore we ought to believe this a Disease, and worthy of Cure, which defrauds one of more than half his life.[72]

No one would question that the first part of this quotation suggests narcolepsy; but when such episodes are linked by Willis to prolonged periods of 'sleep', lasting days or months, one can only think that Willis was grouping his patients with narcolepsy with others suffering from various forms of hypersomnia. He was, we should remember, dealing with a group of patients who suffered from 'sleepy distempers' and they were clearly a heterogeneous category. But he proceeds to some delineation.

It differs not only from the Lethargy, but the Coma also; for in the Distempers which we described, though continual sleep presses on them, yet 'tis easily broken off; then besides, being fully awakened they remember many things, and converse with their friends, though immediately prone again to sleep; whence it appears that the cause of this Disease sticks only in the outer border of the Brain, nor does it enter deep into its compass, as other sleepy distempers do.[73]

Willis considered this disorder relatively benign; it might cease spontaneously or persist indefinitely and sometimes the patients became 'neurotic' – all observations which a modern neurologist would not question.

This Distemper, as I have described in many, is not very dangerous, for as it often happens, it is wholely Cured, or at least remaining for many years, without the Carus or Apoplexy (which is wont to be feared) it doth not become mortal or terrible. The cure of this Disease often happens, the seat of it being changed, to wit, when clearing the Brain, the Morbific Matter is transferred to the Cerebel, which coming thither, produces tremblings of the Heart, the Asthma, loss of Spirits and other troublesome Symptoms, commonly taken for Hypochondriacal.[74]

Willis did not mention cataplexy but, characteristically, he did not hesitate to speculate about the nature of the responsible brain disorder. He envisaged cerebral oedema, vascular stasis, and the penetration of 'Narcotick particles' into the brain substance. However, on a practical plane, he found coffee beneficial. 'At eight of the clock in the Morning, and at five in the Afternoon, let them drink a draught of coffee.' But he advocated coffee for many disorders; it is not that he found it specific for narcolepsy.

Lennox[75] quoted another of Willis's case reports which he thought suggested narcolepsy, but it could equally be one of recurring hepatic stupor.

A certain Gentleman of a Sanguine Complexion, and when he was young, of a sharp and cunning wit, but afterwards growing aged, being given to idleness and drunkeness, became dull and stupid, and also Dropsical, with a great paunch, and his thighs and legs swelled. Yet from these Diseases (which he frequently fell into) when he abstained at any time from drinking, and took Physick, he oftentimes quickly grew well. But at length, though he was freed from the Dropsie, he was opressed with so heavy a sleepiness, and that almost perpetually, that in what place soever he was, or whatever he was doing he would sleep; then being awakened by his Servants or Friends, his mind appeared well enough, and for a few minutes he would discourse of any thing well enough, then immediately fall again to sleep.[76]

Cerebrospinal rhinorrhoea.[77] Willis knew that Schneider (1614–80) had shown that nasal mucus did not originate in the pituitary but he still believed that some watery discharges in the nose came from the brain. He mentioned patients in whom he thought this happened; some of them may possibly have had genuine cerebrospinal rhinorrhoea.[78]

Not long since, a Virgin living in this City, was afflicted a long time with a most cruel headache, and in the midst of her pain much and thin yellow Serum daily flowed out from her Nostrils; the last Winter this excretion stopped for some time, and then the sick party growing worse in her Head, fell into cruel convulsions, with a stupidity; and within three days dyed Apoplectical. Her Head being opened, that kind of yellow Latex overflowed the deeper turnings and windings of the Brain, and its interior Cavities or Ventricles.

I knew a Gentlewoman that was wont to be infested with a most cruel headache, also with a Vertigo, and a frequent melting of the animal spirits, or swooning away; who when she began to be better, after a grievous Fit, felt at first a creeping motion in the top of her Brain, as it were sliding down of water; then that motion passing a little more forwards and downwards, at length many drops of clear water distilled from her Nostrils. This Symptom she used to have so ordinarily, that the sick Gentlewoman did not doubt that this water stilled out from the brain itself.

Many neurologists, I am sure, can recall patients who proved to have spontaneous cerebrospinal rhinorrhoea but in whom initially the diagnosis was not suspected or actually rejected.

Epilepsy. Willis first discussed 'convulsive diseases' in general, explaining that spasms, contractions, and convulsions could arise from various causes, including peripheral irritation. 'We have clearly observed in the dissection of a living whelp, that the knife being put upon the naked ends of the spinal Nerves, presently both themselves and the Bodies of the Muscles in which they were inserted, were hauled'[79] an observation which would have interested Bell and Magendie. He also quoted the case of a patient in whom an ulcer had exposed the tendons and muscles of an arm so that 'when touched by the Surgeons Instrument, caused in the patient a certain rigor through his whole body, and forthwith a Concussion arising, made him to quake for a good space'.

But although convulsive movements could arise 'from the extremities of the nerves', they arose 'most often from the head itself'. This 'is to be imputed to the fault both of the Blood sending, and of the Brain receiving'. Illnesses could result in 'morbifick matter' being carried in the bloodstream to the brain. But convulsions arose only if there was some constitutional predisposition. 'As long as the parts [of the brain] are well made, and are full of vigour, they defend themselves, and what belongs to them; and the doors being shut, they admit nothing [harmful].' He goes on 'but if the passages and pores of the Brain are too lax, or the door-keeping spirits leave, or are called off from their watches . . .' then 'Morbifick matter creeps in together with the Nervous juice'.[80] We might see here a breach of what we now term the blood–brain barrier.

'The evil disposition of the brain is either hereditary or acquired.' Injury, 'prolonged intemperance', or chronic illness might initiate epilepsy. If the 'morbifick matter' remains in the brain epilepsy is likely to be permanent. But often no traces of it can be identified so that an 'evil spirit' may deservedly be suspected. Willis betrays the nature of the times he lived in when he wrote 'the Devil is not able to draw more cruel Arrows from any quiver, or to show miracles by any better Witch than by the assaults of this monstrous Disease'.[81]

The manifestations of epilepsy were sometimes slight – 'only a giddiness and lighter spasms'; the patient did not necessarily lose consciousness or fall.[82] Sometimes 'a Convulsion begun in the bottom of the belly, or at the foot, or hand, creeps by degrees to the upper parts, and for the most part, to the head itself'. It did not necessarily signify that the epigastric aura meant that the disorder originated in the stomach. Indeed he clearly described seizures beginning locally.

We meet with many examples of Epilepticks, in whom the fit being just coming upon them, a spasm is felt with a numness in the hand or toe, or other particular member, which presently from thence as it were with a pricking or tingling, creeps towards the head, which when it hath attained, immediately the sick party falls flat on the earth, and is hurried into insensibility . . .[83]

In the fit itself he noted how 'in the twink of an Eye [it] casts them on the ground, deprived of sense and understanding'. Patients who 'do not only fall, but are flung down with a certain force, are often injured. The teeth are clenched; there is foam at the mouth, a thrusting out of arms and thighs and convulsive movements.' After a time 'sometimes shorter, sometimes longer', the movements cease, 'the sick come to themselves and recover their senses'. But there may be headache, dullness of mind, or perhaps giddiness.[84]

Common aurae were 'heaviness of the head', 'a brightness of the eyes', 'a tingling of the ears', 'a spasm or cramp in a limb'.

Epilepsy particularly affects children and young people, but older ones may also succumb. It may subside or persist indefinitely. Mental deterioration may follow in long-standing cases.

Thus, Willis affirmed that epilepsy was a disorder of the brain. Now, he had come to the opinion, after studying Gassendi (1592–1655), that normal muscular contraction was brought about by an 'explosion'. Particles in the muscles and particles in the blood entering the muscles were ignited by nerve action, like gunpowder. He said 'if anyone shall be displeased at the word *Explosion*, not yet used in Philosophy or Medicine' he would understand.[85] But he thought that similar explosions in the nervous system were the cause of epilepsy. Epilepsy did not arise in the meninges, by some form of contraction, as they were fastened too securely to the skull, and he had seen patients with wounds, abscess, or tumour of the meninges, and also one 'who had the Dura Mater very much torn by the instrument of an unskilful surgeon' who suffered no convulsions. In addition he thought that those epileptics who did not lose consciousness 'would perceive the membranes to be so contracted'.[86] Neither did he think it arose in the ventricles. He concluded that it arose in the brain and he favoured 'the middle of the brain'.

The cerebral explosion could be 'transmitted into various parts of the nervous system'. He likened the spread of the discharge 'as if grains of Gunpowder were laid in a long train to be fired successively'.[87]

It is tempting to see in this explosive concept of epilepsy an extraordinary anticipation of the electrical nature of the 'discharging lesion'. But this would be somewhat of an over-statement. Willis belonged to the school of iatrochemists, who were seeking chemical foundations of normal and disordered bodily function. Many of their ideas, including Willis's, were chimerical. What Willis did was to take one such notion, as applied to muscle action, and apply it to brain function. No doubt one could debate this point at length.

Basal ganglia syndromes. In 1967, Hierons[88] made the interesting suggestion that a few of Willis's case histories recall disorders such as paralysis agitans, torsion dystonia, palilalia, and hepatolenticular degeneration. Disorders of movement were among the first neurological illnesses depicted by physicians of the Middle Ages and many seem to have been forms of hysteria. It is exceedingly difficult, and frequently impossible, to make a diagnosis on the scanty data bequeathed us, but the following is strongly suggestive of torsion dystonia.

> I have known some who have had all the Muscles and Tendons through their whole Body afflicted with contractions and leapings without intermission; I have known others whose Thighs, Arms and other Members, were perpetually forced into various bendings and distortions.[89]

Willis also observed patients with various permanent contractures. Some of these are described in his account of convulsive diseases and give some indication of how widely certain terms were used in clinical description.

> As when one part, or more, being contracted or distorted with a constant stretching, are detained for some time in the same preternatural posture; so when the Muscles, or a Member, suppose the Eyes, Lips, Cheeks, are distorted from their right position, nor cannot easily be presently reduced; the cause of which is sometimes a resolution, or Palsie in some other Muscles, which when they are loosened, the opposite do too strongly act, and draw forcibly the whole part towards themselves. ... The sick sometimes are not able to extend any Member or Joynt, but they are contracted round like a Globe ... in the back [there may be] a gibbousness, or bending out of the Body.[90]

Paralysis. Willis begins discussion 'Of the *Palsie*'[91] by first reminding his readers that the seat of both apoplexy and epilepsy was 'the middle of the brain'. But the seat of the palsy was 'the streaked bodies' (the corpus striatum), 'the medullary trunks' (in the brain stem and spinal cord), and the 'Nerves'. Paralysis could affect motion or sensation 'after two manner of ways'. These modalities could be 'perverted' or 'abolished'. Perversion of motion caused 'Cramps and Convulsions'; perversion of sensation caused 'Pain'. When these functions were abolished or 'hindred', separately or together, 'Palsie' arose. The responsible lesion caused either 'an obstruction of the ways' or an 'impotency of the Animal Spirits'. The lesions could affect mainly 'the beginnings, or middle processes, or in their extreme ends, i.e. the Nervous Fibres', but most commonly the lesion was to be found in the corpus striatum. They were of various kinds; 'blood flowing out of The Vessels', 'some Tumor lying upon them', or injury from a 'wound or bruise'.

The distribution of the paralysis was determined by the site of the lesion. It may be bilateral ('Universal') or unilateral ('hemiplegia or paralysis of one side'). The muscles of the eyes, face, and mouth were often spared in a 'Universal' palsy, 'because the Nerves delineated to the aforesaid Muscles' arose at a lower level than the lesion. Paralysis from spinal cord lesions 'most often happens from a compression or a breaking of the unity' by haemorrhage, abscess, or 'hard tumor'. Tetraparesis, such as occurs in polyneuritis, he describes:

I have sometimes observed in a Palsie, coming after a grievous fit of some other Disease, that all the moving parts, of either side, have been loosened after a more light manner; For though they were not able to perform the more strong motive endeavours, yet for the most part they could extend, bend, yea and move their members hither and thither ...[92]

But he thought that in such cases the lesion 'could be diffused abroad, thorow both the streaked bodies' and not actually peripheral.

Lesions of the brain stem sometimes 'stir up frequent Vertigoes, and mists before the eye, and sometimes in the motive parts short numnesses ... they may bring forth either an half Palsie, or a loosening of some members, sometimes the superior, sometimes the inferior'[93] Willis had thus seen patients with probable transient ischaemic episodes affecting the vertebro-basilar territory, followed by brachial or crural monoplegia.

He was curious to understand why in some cases of paralysis, sensation might be spared. His explanation is rather intriguing.

If it be demanded, why sense is not always hindred as well as motion in every *Palsie*, since as it seems either is performed by the same Nerves and Fibres, within the same Medullary tracts, so that one faculty is only the inversion of the other? As to this we may say, that as light beams thorow glass, when wind is excluded, so also sense being safe, oftentimes motion is lost.[94]

He also thought that sensation did not require so much activity of the animal spirits as motor function, and so was less prone to disturbance.

There were 'Diverse Kinds' of palsy and one category he called 'Spurious'. It was when writing of these that he described myasthenia gravis, an observation which, so far as I know, was first noted by Guthrie in 1903.[95]

Nevertheless, those labouring with a want of spirits, who will exercise local motions, as well as they can, in the morning are able to walk firmly, to fling about their arms hither and thither, or to take up any heavy thing; before noon the Stock of the spirits being spent, which had flowed into the Muscles, they are scarce able to move Hand or Foot. At this time I have under my charge a prudent and honest Woman, who for many years hath been obnoxious to this sort of spurious *Palsie*, not only in her Members, but also in her tongue; she for some time can speak freely and readily enough, but after she has spoke long or hastily, or eagerly, she is not able to speak a word, but becomes as mute as a Fish, nor can she recover the use of her voice under an hour or two.[96]

That he said this patient was 'a prudent and honest Woman' suggests that he thought her ailment was genuine. But there were other patients with 'spurious palsie' who seemed to him to be 'functional'.

Yea, some without any notable sickness, are for a long time fixed in their Bed, as if they were every day about to dye; whilst they lye undisturbed, talk with their Friends, and are cheerful, but they will not, nor dare not move or walk; yea they shun all motion, as a most horrid thing.[97]

Willis's explanation of myasthenic paresis was of some fault in the animal spirits and in the 'explosion' which activated muscles. Keynes[98] has suggested that this 'looks like an inspired anticipation of the modern theory of the action of acetylcholine, the chemically explosive link between nerve and muscle'. But here again, as in the explanation of epilepsy, Willis is merely applying his explosive theory of nervous and muscle function. Too much can be read into these theories. But this does not in anyway diminish the importance of the clinical observations. The next known account of myasthenia gravis was not published until 1877 – by Wilks.[99]

Apoplexy.[100] 'The *Theory* of this Disease seems to be very exactly delivered by the famous Webfer', Willis wrote. Wepfer, as his name is now spelt, published his account of four cases of apoplexy with autopsies in 1658. In each he found a cerebral haemorrhage. He had some knowledge of the route of the circulation of the blood within the cranium and of the arterial connections at the base. Willis quoted him as showing that 'the principal places affected are not the greater Ventricles, but the middle marrowy substance of the Brain and Cerebel'. Wepfer had concluded that apoplexy could arise from obstruction within the carotid or vertebral arteries, from compression of them, or from rupture of their branches within the skull.

It was at this point that Willis stressed the significance of the anastomotic arrangement of the arterial circle, thereby justifying, as Symonds has said, the eponymic title which history subsequently bestowed. Willis wrote,

> And in the first place, though we grant that the flowing in of the blood, may be sometimes denyed to the Brain; yet we do not believe, that it only happens after the aforesaid ways, nor that, for that reason, the *Apoplexy* doth arise. We have everywhere showed, that the *Cephalick* arteries, viz. the *Carotides*, and the *Vertebrals*, do so communicate one with another, and all of them in several places, are so ingrassed one in another mutually, that if it happen, that many of them should be stopped or pressed together at once, yet the blood being admitted to the Head, by the passage of one artery only, either the *Carotid* or the *Vertebral*, it would presently pass thorow all those parts both exterior and interior; which indeed we have sufficiently proved by an experiment, for that Ink being squirted in the trunk of one Vessel, quickly filled all the sanguiniferous passages, and every where stained the Brain it self. I once opened the dead carcase of one wasted away, in which the right Arteries, both the *Carotid* and the *Vertebral*, within the skull, were become bony and impervious, and did shut forth the blood from that side, notwithstanding the sick person was not troubled with the astonishing Disease; wherefore it may be doubted, whether the blood excluded from the Brain, by reason of some Arteries being obstructed or compressed, doth bring forth this Disease. Certainly there is more of danger, that the cause of the Apoplexy, should be from its too great incursion and extravasation within the Brain. . . .[101]

For many years apoplexy meant cerebral haemorrhage. Cerebral ischaemia and infarction were nineteenth-century concepts. In this celebrated passage Willis was demonstrating his grasp of the importance of combining various methods of studying disease – anatomy, physiology, experiment, clinical observation, and pathological examination. Here we can excuse him all his fanciful notions and flights of ideas. Here he was modern.

Willis goes on to explain, however, that not all apoplexy was of cerebral origin. 'There is a twofold *Apoplexy*, one in the Brain, the other proper to the Cerebel.'[102] He was not referring to cerebellar haemorrhage or infarction, but to cases of sudden loss of consciousness or '*Syncopy*', when 'the action of the Heart is stopped or hindred'. Cardiac arrest, he thought, was neurogenic in origin, the cardiac nerves arising in the cerebellum (in which he included parts of the brain stem).

> ... the Cardiack Nerves being Distemper'd with a convulsion ... in which the sick lie for some time without motion or sense, with a small or seldom beating Pulse as if dead ... it seems most likely, that the motion of the Heart is often supressed or inhibited by reason of the Animal Spirits, destinated to the vital function ... to wit, within the Cerebel ... I have known sometimes those distemper'd, to be stiff and cold, Pulse and breathing to be thought quite gone, and to be indeed esteemed quite dead, and put in to their Coffin, yet after two or three days to have reviv'd again, but whoever awakes out of this fit, whether it be of short or long continuance, does not for that reason fall into a Palsie, or half Palsie of one side, as those for the most part do, who are distemper'd with the *Apoplexy*.[102]

Willis's assistant, Richard Lower, wrote (in a letter to Boyle), how they ligatured the carotid arteries of a dog when they were studying the intracranial circulation.

> ... this week we took a young spaniel, and tied both carotid arteries in the neck very fast and close with silk, and the dog was not at all altered by it, but continued very lively and brisk, and was so far from taking unkindly what was done to him, that within a quarter of an hour after, he got loose and followed the doctor into the town, as he visited his patients. In this pleasant humour he continued two or three days, and then we opened his head, and found all the vessels of the brain as full of blood as usually they are in other dogs, who did not suffer the same experiment. But this I might have told you in a shorter time; for if one artery be syringed with any tincted liquor, all the parts of the brain will equally be filled with it at the same time, as several times we have tried ...[103]

Sydenham may have been a better clinician than Willis[104] but his approach was narrower. To Sydenham anatomy was unimportant and Harvey's discovery unimpressive,[105, 106] while his pathology was 'in all respects inferior to Willis's.[107] In his approach to the problem of the blood supply to the brain Willis demonstrated his versatility.

Psychiatric disorders. The word *Psychologia* was said to have been used for the first time by Rudolf Goeckel in 1590.[108] Willis used it in *De anima brutorum* and Pordage usually translated it as the 'doctrine of the soul'. But, as pointed out by Cranefield,[109] at least on one occasion Pordage used the English word 'psycheology' and this may be the first use of the word in that language.

The importance of Willis in the history of neuropsychiatry was emphasized in 1928 by Vinchon and Vie[110] of Paris, working in the department of Professor Laignel-Lavastine. The latter, a distinguished historian in this field, once told the author that this aspect of Willis's work had gone quite unappreciated in England. This was in 1947 at a meeting in Paris of British and French neurologists. It was only in 1961, on reading

Cranefield's important paper, that I began to appreciate the truth of Laignel-Lavastine's comment. Cranefield said that he had only been able to discover one published survey of *De anima brutorum*, that by Vinchon and Vie. When I came to read their paper I discovered that they worked in Laignel-Lavastine's department at that time.

Although Willis is often credited with one of the first descriptions of dementia paralytica,[111, 112] his chapters on psychiatric disturbances in general are more important. The lines which are usually quoted as descriptive of dementia paralytica come from the chapter on the palsy. Hare[113] was unable to discover who first drew attention to the relevant passages, which are as follows:

I have observed in many that when, the Brain being first indisposed, they have been distemper'd with a dullness of mind and forgetfulness, and afterwards with a stupidity and foolishness, after that have fallen into a Palsie, which I oft did predict; to wit, the Morbifick matter being by degrees fallen down, and at length being heaped up some where within the Medullar Trunk (where the Marrowy Tracts are more straitned than in the Streaked Body) to a stopping fulness. For according as the places obstructed are more or less large, so either a universal Palsie, or an half Palsie of one side, or else some partial resolutions of members happen . . .[114]

The oppilative or Stopping Particles being fallen down from the Brain and carried forward into the oblong Marrow, enter into the Nerves destinated to the Muscles of some parts of the Face, and by obstructing the ways of the Spirits in them, bring forth the Palsie in the Tongue, and sometimes a loosening of these or those Muscles of the Eyes, Eyelids, Lips and other parts.[115]

From the general context of Willis's discussion of cases of cerebral impairment with palsy, associated or following each other in different ways, it is difficult to detect the emergence of a recognizable picture of dementia paralytica. I agree with Hare who concluded that the patients Willis described could equally well be showing symptoms of cerebral arterio-sclerosis. Others (with 'Colick') may have had lead encephalopathy or neuritis, and those (who recovered), encephalitis. In the passages in which he described 'narcolepsy' and 'myasthenia gravis', on the other hand, we see much clearer justification for the designation of originality. Pages of general clinical observation and comment, however much they may hint at the truth, may be quite inadequate when compared to the obvious identification contained in just one clear case history.

Another much quoted statement is that Willis noted that fever might cure mental disturbance. When this is added to the claim we have been considering it sounds most impressive. In discussing Stupidity and Foolishness he wrote,

Sometimes a Feavour has cured some Fools, and stupid, and render'd them more acute . . . We our selves have known a certain man of a very blunt, Boeotick or dull wit, who talked idly in a Feavour, most suddenly brought forth most acute speeches, and seasoned with a great deal of salt or ingenious wit. Further, we before spoke of a generous old Gentleman, who having lost his memory, and so the use of discourse, received great help by the distemper of a Feavour happening afterwards; the reason of which seems to be, because the feavourish burning sometimes rarifies and dispels the darkness covering the Brain.[116]

Again, no really profitable discussion can be based on such observations, despite their acknowledged interest. We can only say that they do give us some indication, if we needed it, of Willis's sharp clinical astuteness and desire to understand. But the beneficial effects of fever was an ancient belief; Hippocrates found it helpful in convulsions and Galen in mental illness.[117]

Hysteria. The word 'Hysterical' ('belonging to the womb or mother, or troubled with the disease called the mother') appears in the index compiled by Pordage for his translation of *Cerebri anatome* – but not the word 'Hysteria'. Lord Brain[118] said that the earliest reference to hysteria so far discovered was in William Cullen's Clinical Lectures in 1766. In considering convulsions Willis wrote of 'the Passions commonly called Hysterical or Fits of the Mother'. He did not think they were uterine in origin.

... The hysterical passion is of so ill-fame, among the diseases belonging to women, that like one half damn'd, it bears the faults of many other Distempers; For when at any time, a sickness happens in a woman's body, of an unusual manner, or more occult original, so that its Cause lies hid, and the Curatory indication is altogether uncertain, presently we accuse the evill influence of the womb (which for the most part is innocent) and in every unusual Symptom, we declare it to be something hysterical, and so to this Scope, which oftentimes is only the subterfuge of Ignorance, and medical Intentions, and use of Remedies are directed.'[119]

But, like others, Willis noted that hysterical symptoms sometimes occurred in men; and that autopsies of hysterical women often revealed a normal womb.

... Women of every age, and condition, are obnoxious to these kind of Distempers ... yea, sometimes the same kind of Passions infest Men ... I have opened some women dead of other Diseases, though while they were sick, very obnoxious to Hysterical passions, in whom the Womb being very well, I have found in the hinder part of the head, the beginnings of the nerves, moistened and wholly drowned with a sharp serum ...

Willis makes it clear, nevertheless, that convulsions could be excited by disorders of the womb, as of other viscera. But, as with epilepsy, the cause nearly always arose in the brain. The general run of hysterical symptoms he describes as follows:

The most Common, and which commonly are said to constitute the formal Reason of the hysterical distemper, are these, viz. A motion in the bottom of the belly, and an ascension of the same, as it were a certain round thing, then a belching, or a striving to vomit, a distention, and murmur of the hypochondria, with a breaking forth of blasts of winde, an unequall breathing, and a very much hindred, a choaking in the throat, a vertigo, an inversion, a rolling about the eyes, oftentimes laughing, or weeping, absurd talking, sometimes want of speech, and motionless, with an obscure or no pulse, a deadish aspect, sometimes Convulsive motions, in the face and limbs, and sometimes in the whole body are excited; But universal Convulsions rarely happen ...[120]

Willis could not conceive of a 'wandering womb', writing:

... for that the body of the womb is of so small bulk in virgins, and widdows, and is so strictly tyed by the neighbouring parts round about, that it cannot of itself be moved, or ascend from its place, nor could its motion be felt, if there were any.[121]

Concluding that hysterical symptoms arose in the brain he thought they derived from disturbance, not in 'the middle of the brain', as in epilepsy, but in 'hinder parts', where he found 'the beginning of the nerves within the head'. These nerves, such as the vagi and intercostals (sympathetic), were distributed to the viscera of the thorax and abdomen, where hysterical symptoms were experienced.

Willis's hysterical symptomatology largely consisted of spasms, fits, and convulsions of varying kinds. Although he clearly saw the significance of the emotions in the causation of bodily ills his concept of hysteria was focused on the episodes he describes. He had not progressed to the view that hysteria was but one manifestation of that broad group of illnesses which we now call the neuroses.

Melancholia and madness.[122] In these chapters Willis shows he appreciates that depression and agitation are related symptoms, frequently following one upon the other.

Melancholy . . . is a complicated Distemper of the Brain and Heart . . . [it] passes oftentimes into Stupidity or Foolishness, and sometimes also into Madness. . . . Further, there is scarce any better thing to be expected from them who lying sick with only imaginary Diseases, take all Remedies, and require still more, and of diverse kinds to be given them . . . the Evident cause of this Disease, if any noted thing went before, should be inquired into . . .

Therefore, for the healing of the Spirits, first of all it is to be procured that the Soul should be withdrawn from all troublesome and restraining passion, viz. from mad Love, Jealousie, Sorrow, Pity, Hatred, Fear and the like, and composed to cheerfulness and joy; pleasant talk, or Jesting, Singing, Musick, Pictures, Dancing, Hunting, Fishing and other pleasant Exercises are to be used. They who are not for Sports or Pleasures (for to some Melancholicks they are always ingrateful) are to be roused up by imploying them in more light business; sometimes Mathematical or Chymical Studies, also Travelling, do very much help; moreover, it is often expedient to change the place of habitation, in their native soil. Those who stay at home are to be warned, that they take care of their Household affairs. . . .

Willis pointed to three characteristic features of the depressed patient:

1. [The patient was] continually busied in thinking, their Phantasie is scarce ever idle or at quiet.

2. They comprehend in their mind fewer things than before they were wont, that oftentimes they roll about in their mind day and night the same thing, never thinking of other things that are sometimes of far greater moment.

3. The *Ideas* of objects or conceptions appear often deformed . . . so that all small things seem to them great and difficult.

Sometimes the patient recovered from depression but there was always a danger of further symptoms. 'After Melancholy, Madness is next to be treated of, both which are so much akin, that these Distempers often change, and pass from one into the other. . . .'

As in depression Willis stressed three typical features of agitation:

1. Their Phantasies or Imaginations are perpetually busied with a storm of impetuous thoughts.

2. Their Notions or conceptions are either incongruous, or represented to them under a false or erroneous image.

3. To their delirium is most often joyned Audaciousness and Fury, contrary to Melancholicks, who are always infected with fear and sadness.

Stupidity or foolishness.[123] In Chapter XIII of Part 2 of *De anima brutorum* Willis discusses these two topics; their aetiology, recognition, differences, pathology, prognosis, and treatment. When one contemplates the significance of the chapter as a whole admiration for Willis grows anew. The obscurity of the rendering of the English translation of the book, with its rather murky title *Two discourses of the soul of brutes* has probably not encouraged its study, but nevertheless, it is difficult to appreciate why it was neglected for so long. Cranefield[124] remedied this by reprinting the entire chapter in his paper, and by analysing its content in detail. He came to the conclusion that it was 'a treasury of clinical astuteness'.

Willis begins by saying that these two afflictions are 'not improperly reckoned among the Diseases of the Head or Brain'. They arise 'when there is a failure of the Imagination and Memory ... forthwith the eye of the Intellect, as if covered with a vail, is wont to be very much dulled, or wholly darkened'. Stupidity was a term Willis applied to both amentia and dementia; it arose either from lesions of the brain or from lack of the animal spirits. In other words Willis recognized that the responsible brain disorder may or may not be recognized at autopsy. Foolishness also might be congenital or acquired but he saw an important clinical difference.

Many differences of this Disease are to be met with; and first, there is commonly wont to be a distinction between *Stupidity* and *Foolishness*, for those affected with this latter, apprehend simple things well enough, dextrously and swiftly, and retain them firm in their memory, but by reason of a defect of judgment, they compose or divide their notions evilly, and very badly infer one thing from another; moreover, by their folly, and acting sinistrously and ridiculously, they move laughter in the by standers.

On the contrary, those who are Stupid, by reason of the defect of the Imagination and Memory, as well as of the Judgment, do neither apprehend well, or quickly, nor argue well; besides they behave themselves not as the others by toying and gesticulation, but sottishly, foolishly, or like a dull Ass; so the *simplicity* of these is the more miserable, who shew so the Disease in their countenance and behaviour.

Thus, in foolishness we find the patient is in touch with his surroundings (apprehends), possesses a good memory, but has poor judgement and he moves and behaves in a way which amuses others. In stupidity, however, the patient has lack of apprehension, of memory, and of judgement and in consequence he is dull, simple, and readily recognizable. Cranefield thought this description of foolishness, with its 'by reason of a defect of judgment, they compose or divide their notions evilly, and very badly infer one thing from another', refers to schizophrenic thought disorder. If so it is probably the first such description of simple schizophrenia in psychiatric literature. Certainly we have here a much stronger argument in favour of the claim than in the case of dementia paralytica.

In the rest of this chapter Willis has much of interest to say of subnormality and the growth and decline of intellect. He had seen promising children turn out 'dull and heavy', and others who were originally 'unapt to learn, and wholly unfit for literature, and seeming of an ill favour'd countenance, when they have become young men, or have put off their childhood, have had both an excellent wit, and become beautiful'. He also had some thoughts which would have interested nineteenth-century anthropologists and phrenologists.

> The wit and ingenuity doth depend somewhat on the magnitude and figure of the Head, and consequently on its Brain ...
>
> Those who have a flat head, or too sharp, or otherways improportionate, are effected for the most part with some noted fault of the Animal Function.
>
> The evil conformation of the Brain, as to its pores and passages ... it sometimes happens that these are defective or perverted, and so brings on a dulness of mind, or Foolishness.

In *Cerebri anatome* he had referred to two autopsies of patients with congenital subnormality. In the legend to Fig. IV of that volume we read;

> The Effigies of an humane Brain of a certain Youth that was foolish from his birth, and of that sort which are commonly called Changelings; the bulk of whose Brain, as it was thinner and lesser than is usual, its border could be farther lifted up and turned back, that all the more interior parts might be more deeply beheld together.

In Chapter XXVI (p. 162), he mentioned the second case; 'we could find no defect or fault in the Brain less it was that its substance or bulk was very small'.

Willis recognized four 'Degrees of Stupidity': (1) 'Some being wholly fools in the learning of letters or the liberal Sciences, are yet able enough for *Mechanical Arts*.' (2) 'Others of either of these incapable, yet easily comprehend *Agriculture*, or Husbandry and Country busness.' (3) 'Others unfit almost for all affairs, are only able to learn what belongs to eating or the common means of living.' (4) 'Others mere *Dolts* or drivling Fools, scarce understand any thing at all, or do any thing knowingly.'

Subnormality could be hereditary or sporadic. Thus 'Fools [could] beget Fools' but so also could 'wise men and highly ingenious'. Bookish parents might have a stupid child. 'To be born of Parents who *have a sound mind in a sound body*, is far beyond a large patrimony.' Epilepsy when 'long continued', injuries to the head, alcohol, opiates, convulsions, and palsy may be followed by loss of intellect. But senile dementia may occur without any evident predisposition or cause. Trepanning is advocated in some cases but in the usual run of congenital subnormality it is the combination of physician and teacher which is most likely to help. 'Wherefore it must be the work both of a *Physician* and a *Teacher*, that the wit of such that are so affected, may be somewhat trimmed, and they being at least brought to the use of reason in a little measure, may be accounted out of the number of Brutes.'

Professor Alfred Meyer concluded that in these pages of Willis, in which he conceived that mental disorder could arise either from anatomical lesions of the white matter or by disintegration of the animal spirits, Willis had offered 'a very early anticipation of the division between organic and functional psychoses'.[125]

Willis was forty-three years of age when he published *Cerebri anatome*. He had then been in practice in Oxford for eighteen years, and for the last four he had also been Professor of Natural Philosophy. He could have learned little anatomy there as a student – or indeed of any form of science except that of Aristotle and Galen. In England the study of anatomy still lagged behind that on the Continent. The two scholarly humanists – Thomas Linacre (1460–1524) of Oxford, founder and first President of the College of Physicians, and John Caius (1510–73) of Cambridge – were both graduates of Padua. Linacre spent twelve years in Italy and his polished translations of Galen from Greek into Latin were no doubt very influential. Caius, although a lecturer in anatomy for many years, merely edited some of Galen's works and 'added nothing to anatomical knowledge'.[126] He did arrange for lectures and dissections in Cambridge, but their Vesalian content was probably slight.[127]

Harvey began his anatomical lectures in London in 1616. (There are recent translations of the *Prelectiones*.[128,129]) At that time he was reluctant to criticize Galenical teaching and Keynes[130] concluded that the lectures reveal how little Harvey then knew of the circulation rather than how much. Harvey spoke of the 'divine banquet of the brain', describing its general topography, the ventricles, the meninges, and the venous sinuses in a satisfactory but limited manner.[128] He thought the brain 'is cold that it may temper the spirits from the heart' and that 'sometimes it is swollen in full moon' (p. 217). He noted that 'the brain (draws in) external air through the nostrils' (p. 219); that the 'sutures (act) as breathing devices for the cerebrum' (p. 210); that the brain is always convoluted 'but of what I do not know . . . wherefore, it does not seem as in Erasistratus that (it is) for the sake of intelligence' (p. 216). He mentions the *rete mirabile* as if he thought it existed in man. He confessed he did not know 'which is the principal part [of the brain], whether the ventricle or the substance' (p. 217). He noticed that coughing caused the brain to swell and that all movements of the brain were derived from arterial pulsation (p. 210). He quoted Fallopius's observation that he had never been able to see the brain move in the way Galen had described.

Harvey commented on the confusion concerning the number of cranial nerves, whether seven, eight, or nine, and said that the optic nerves were arranged in the form of a cross so that double vision was eliminated (p. 225). Concerning nerve transmission he said 'I believe that the spirit does not advance by way of the nerves but occurs like a ray of light or an impulse, wherefore sensation and motion [are] as light in the air; perhaps [as] in the flux and reflux of the sea' (p. 224).

Hunter and Macalpine[131] examined Harvey's scattered neurological notes and concluded that he did in fact foreshadow the distinction between motor and sensory nerves, and the differentiation of irritability from sensibility and contractility. His observation that a servant in the College of Physicians had hands which were strong, but analgesic (probably syringomyelic), suggests that its functional significance was not lost upon him.

We do not know whether the ageing Harvey met the youthful Willis at Oxford in the years 1642–46 but Keynes thinks they must have been well acquainted.[132] Willis did not actually receive his medical degree until 1646 but he was busy observing and recording the fevers. Harvey's four years at Oxford must have directed the attention of physicians there toward the new physiology. Certainly Willis caught the message – unlike Sydenham – and was destined to become the 'Harvey of the Nervous System'.[133] 'Our most Famous Harvey', Willis said, 'hath laid, the Circulation of the Blood, as a new foundation in Medicine'.[134]

Willis's contributions to knowledge of the anatomy of the brain have been well established. He gave us new terms such as hemisphere, lobe, pyramid, corpus striatum, and peduncle. He identified structures such as the spinal accessory nerve, the anterior commissure, the olives (quoting Fallopius), and improved the descriptions of others. He made the olfactory the first cranial nerve, and the trochlear and abducens our fourth and sixth; he named the ophthalmic division of the trigeminal nerve; his description of the glossopharyngeal nerve, however, is confusing. Willis's list of ten pairs of cranial nerves was in general use until Soemmerring in 1778 introduced the present system of twelve pairs. Finally, of course, Willis demonstrated the structure and function of the arterial circle at the base of the brain.

Meyer and Hierons, [135–139] in a series of detailed studies, have examined Willis's anatomical and physiological contributions in a scholarly fashion, clarifying certain points, correcting others, and evaluating his writings in a way not previously attempted. Then, there are the excellent new translations of Willis, which are more valuable to the reader than Pordage's text, in Clark and O'Malley's indispensable *The human brain and spinal cord*.[140]

The first, and only, monograph on Willis was published in German in 1965 by Isler,[141] a Zurich neurologist. He furnished an English edition in 1968. No other publication has provided such a view of Willis as a whole.

The modern reader is now in a position to accept an invitation to the 'divine banquet of the brain', to study the menu and wine list, and tackle everything. Here I wish only to select a few topics of general interest to convey the manner in which Willis developed his conception of the function of the nervous system.

THE STRUCTURE AND FUNCTION OF THE BRAIN

Willis realized that it was the brain itself, its stuff and substance, and not the hollows within it, that really mattered. The doctrine of the ventricles could not survive.

> ... there yet remains that we speak of its Ventricles; But since they are only a vacuity resulting from the folding up of its exterior border, I see no reason we have to discourse much of their office, no more than Astronomers are wont of the empty space contained within the vacuity of the Sphere.[142]

In Clarke and O'Malley's translation[143] of this passage, with their wording that the ventricles were 'an empty space resulting from the folding of the exterior of the brain', the meaning is clearer.

Willis proceeded to say that the Ancients had so magnified the importance of the ventricles that they had neglected the brain itself. Some anatomists had come to regard the ventricles as 'mere sinks', discharging the end-products of brain metabolism The 'ventricles are often seen in the dead to be filled with water' and 'serous humours' accumulated there 'in men dying of Cephalick diseases' so that excretion through the infundibulum of the third ventricle seemed a reasonable possibility. But there were 'no manifest apertures or openings' in the 'wedged-shaped bone' (sphenoid) or the 'sieve-like bone' (cribriform plate of the ethmoid). Nevertheless, Willis did not entirely reject the old idea of excretion. Humours could easily pass 'through places that seem impervious and unpassable', so 'why in like manner may we not suppose the serous humours falling down from the ventricles of the brain into the pituitary glandula and the mamillary processes to be carried away through the nerves and membranes passing through here or there?'[144] He quoted the two patients with possible cerebrospinal rhinorrhoea, referred to on page 64, in support of this notion.

It is not clear whether he considered that the ventricular fluid was a *normal* constituent, but he surely must have noted that at times it was clear, and at others, turbid. He did not think that the animal spirits were formed in the ventricles, and in discussing the choroid plexuses he seems to have conceived the idea that they were the source of the ventricular fluid.

He thought that the vessels of the choroid plexuses 'instill nothing to the substance of the brain' but that in diseases of the brain, when 'the ventricles

FIG. 27 (*below left*). Willis did not slice the brain *in situ* like Vesalius but removed it as did Varolius (1543–75). He began with the base. Figure V from *Cerebri anatome* 'shews the interior Basis of an humane skull; where is shewn after what manner the Vessels of every kind cut off from the Brain, and about to go out of the skull, are hid or laid up under the *dura Mater*'. Olfactory nerves, C; optic, D; oculomotor, G; trochlear, H; trigeminal, I; abducens, K; facial and auditory, L (seventh pair); glossopharyngeal, vagus, and accessory, M (eighth pair); spinal accessory, N; hypoglossal, O (ninth pair); Willis's tenth pair, P, 'tending downward with the vertebral artery' was made up of upper cervical rootlets. The pituitary gland, E; the carotid arteries, F.

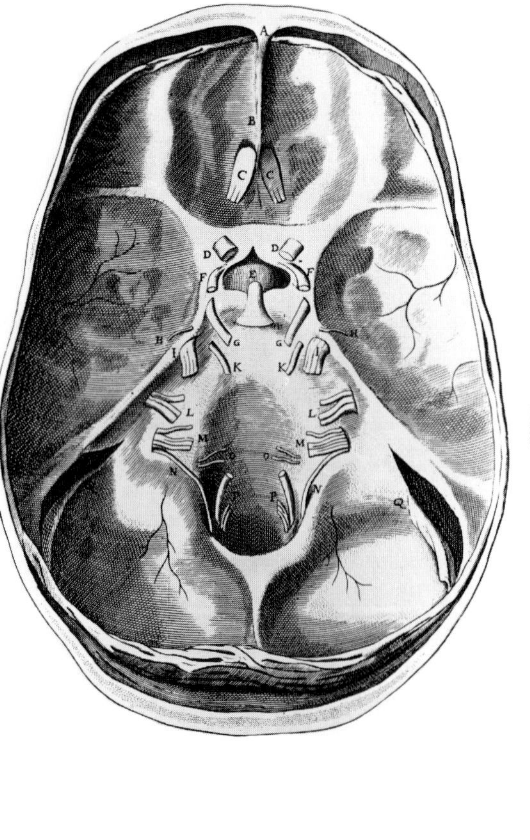

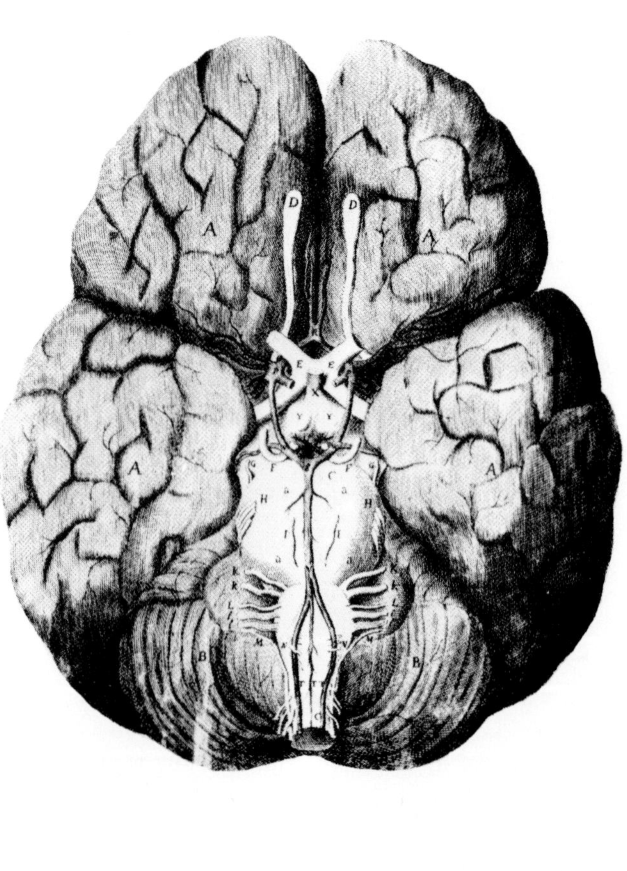

are filled with water . . . the continuity of the infolding [the choroid plexus] is dissolved by too much moisture'.

It was possible, he said, 'that the more watery part of the blood destined for the brain may be sent off into its [the plexus] vessels'. Moreover, he had examined the vascular 'choroeidal infoldings' carefully, possibly with a microscope, and noted that they were 'beset with many lesser glandula's or kernels, and every where interwoven with them, which imbibe the serum secreted from the blood, in the smaller vessels'.[145] He thought that 'when the vessels of that infolding, carrying too watry blood, lay aside more serum than the glandula's are able to receive or contain', they discharge the superfluous fluid into the ventricles.

This concept, admittedly not clearly stated, of a fluid being produced by the choroid plexuses was, nevertheless, some two hundred years before Luschka's suggestion of its role in the formation of the cerebrospinal fluid.

The brain itself was composed of 'double hemisphere' and 'double substance'. There were two 'lobes' to each hemisphere, the anterior and posterior, demarcated by the middle cerebral artery 'like a Bounding river to both, distinguishing them as it were into two provinces'. Such 'partitioning' of the brain ensured that its function might continue when one hemisphere or lobe was injured or diseased. 'So the Brain, like a Castle, divided into many Towers or places of Defence, is thereby made the stronger and harder to take.'[146] The hemispheres were joined together in several places 'either by a contiguity, or by processes setforth', so that 'every impression coming this

FIG. 28 (*facing*). Figure I from *Cerebri anatome* 'shews the Basis of an humane brain taken out from the skull with the roots of the vessels cut off'. A, 'the anterior and posterior lobes of the brain quadripartite or divided into four parts'. B, 'the cerebel'. C, 'the long marrow or pith'. D–O, the ten cranial pairs of nerves. P–S, the carotid artery with branches, the posterior 'meeting with the vertebral trunk'. T, 'the vertebral arteries and their branches ascending'. V, 'the vertebral growing together into one Trunk'. W, 'the place designed where the Vertebrals and the Carotides are united', X, 'the tunnel', (infundibum). Y, 'the two glandula's or Kernels placed behind the tunnel' (corpora quadrigemina). a, 'the annulary Protuberance (pons), which being sent from the Cerebel, embraces the stock of the long Marrow' (medulla oblongata).

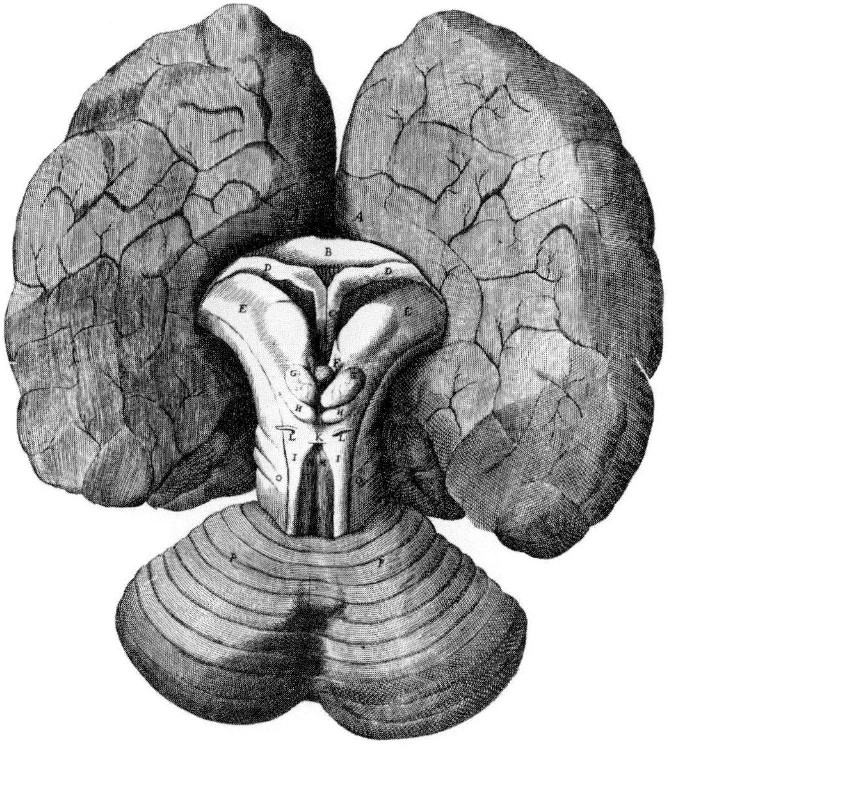

FIG. 29. Figure III from *Cerebri anatome* with the 'border of the brain being loosened . . . elevated and turned outward' to show 'the shanks of the oblong Marrow, the Fornix or arched Vault, the Nates and Testes (corpora quadrigemina), with the Pineal Kernel, and other Processes . . .'. A, the 'border of the brain'. B, 'the callous body' (corpus callosum). C, the fornix. D, 'the arms of the fornix'. E, 'the shanks of the oblong Marrow'. F, 'the pineal glandula'. G, 'the orbicular protuberances, Nates' (superior corpora quadrigemina). H, 'the lesser protuberances, Testes,' (Inferior corpora quadrigemina). I, 'the medullary processes which ascend obliquely from the testes into the cerebel' (superior cerebellar peduncle). K, 'a transverse process'. L, 'the pathetick nerves' (trochlear). M, 'the oblong marrow' (medulla oblongata). N, 'the hole of the ventricle or cavity'. O, 'a portion of the annulary protuberance sent from the Cerebel, and embracing the oblong Marrow' (inferior cerebellar peduncle).

or that way, becomes still one and the same'. In this respect he referred to the corpus callosum, the corpus striatum, and the optic decussation. Within the brain substance

may be observed many white parallel lines, which cut the partition of the brain in right angles, as if they were certain tracts or footsteps, in which the animal Spirits, travel from one hemisphere of the brain to the other, and return back again.[147]

The 'double substance' was the grey and white matter, the 'cortical and medullary'. The former comprised the 'crust', 'shell', or 'rind' of the brain, cerebral and cerebellar. It was more richly vascularized than the white matter. Within the brain there were symmetrical masses of grey matter. The external surface was 'rendered uneven and twisted by gyri and convolutions, almost like those of the small intestine'; a haphazard arrangement but one which protected the surface vessels in the sulci and which also considerably enlarged the surface area of the grey cortex. The gyri were more numerous and larger in man than in any other animal 'because of the variety and number of acts of the higher faculties'.

At this point it is essential that the reader appreciates that certain of the anatomical terms Willis used do not conform to their present usage. This applies particularly to the corpus callosum, the medulla oblongata, and the cerebellum. Thus the corpus callosum comprised all the cerebral white matter; the term did not refer only to the commissure we know today. Then the medulla oblongata was very extensive. It was Y-shaped 'like Parnassus',† that is, bifurcate, reaching up into the brain 'like a trunk', as far as the corpus callosum. 'Where the callous Body is thought to end, the oblong Marrow begins.' It thus took in all the brain stem, and each limb comprised thalamus, basal ganglia, internal capsule, a lateral ventricle, together with all the deep grey and white matter.

... The Tract of the oblong marrow, which as it were the King's High-way, leads from the Brain, as the Metropolis, into many Provinces of the nervous stock, by private recesses and cross-ways; it follows now that we view the other city of the animal Kingdom.[148]

That 'other city' was the cerebellum, but it included the lower part of the brain stem. Both the pons (annular protuberance) and the corpora quadrigemina (orbicular prominences) are several times referred to as 'processes' or 'appendices' of the cerebellum, 'with one part proportionate to the magnitude of the other'.[149] Through them, the three cerebellar peduncles, and the hemispheres of the cerebellum 'reciprocal commerces' were facilitated 'between the brain and Organs of involuntary functions.'[150] The cerebellum possessed 'a different structure' from the cerebrum, and had 'certain Privileges and a peculiar Jurisdiction'. Its anatomy and physiology, in other words, were different. Unlike the random' 'intestinal' foldings of the cerebral cortex, the cerebellar convolutions were parallel, disposed in a certain orderly series in 'thin lappets, or little rings or circles'. Within, the white matter connected the two lobes to the brain stem by 'three distinct medullary processes', the cerebellar peduncles.

Although the brain stem was 'made unequal by prominences and

† Mount Parnassus rises out of the Boeotian plain in central Greece. The Boeotians were derided by Athenians as dull and backward. Willis refers to the Boeotians in Chapter 13, 'Of Stupidity or Foolishness,' in *De anima brutorum*, in connection with the possible effects of environment on intelligence.

processes', its surface was not 'garnished with any turnings about' (not convoluted) and its cortex was not grey like the hemispheres. When sectioned he observed it to be 'marrowy and white' and 'much darkened with fibres and hairs . . . figured in various places . . . direct or stretched out at length, and in other places again circular'. He realized that there were major and minor pathways, 'ascending and descending', and interspersed with areas of grey matter. The corpus striatum was the only area which was 'streaked like ivory'. Eight years later, in *De anima brutorum* he recorded that he and his colleagues had a new method of examining the central matter. By gently scraping away the soft darker matter they were better able to see the white substance and they judged it was fibrous. But from the beginning, this had been conjectured.

Like Harvey before him, Willis studied the brains of different animals. Figure II in *Cerebri anatome* is an illustration of the base of a sheep's brain, placed opposite that of the celebrated representation of the base of the human brain for comparison. The legend refers to 'Two Hemispheres of the Brain without lobes, different from that in a Man'. The fifth and sixth figures show the interior of the base of the skull of man and calf, respectively. Figures VII and VIII are also of sheep brain; dissected and 'unfolded' in the former to illustrate the general arrangement of the white matter; in the latter, to display the corpus striatum, midbrain, medulla, and cerebellum. In Chapter VIII of *Cerebri anatome*, devoted to comparison of the manner in which the carotid and vertebral arteries enter the skull in different animals, he provides illustrations from a horse and a calf, as well as from man. He compared and discussed the significance of the arterial siphons and he thought that if the *rete mirabile* was actually encountered in man it would only be 'in those sort of men being of a slender wit' (mentally subnormal). He also devoted a chapter to describing the 'Brains of Fowls and Fishes'. In *De anima brutorum*, he described the brain of the lobster, the oyster, and even the humble earthworm.

He noted that not only were the convolutions more developed in man but that there was considerable variation in the size and shape of certain structures, such as the corpus callosum, the corpus striatum, the thalamus, pons, and corpora quadrigemina. Man had the largest pons; but the dog and cat had larger pons than the calf and sheep. There was an inverse relationship between pons and the corpora quadrigemina; in man the latter were small and in the calf and sheep they were large. The cerebellum, on the other hand, was singularly uniform in appearance, another indication that it had some function common to man and other animals. He also observed that 'the vertebral Arteries, different from the *Carotides*, are found alike in all without any great difference.'[151] But like the carotids and the cerebral cortex they supplied the cerebellar cortex in a rich manner. Observing and contemplating these similarities and differences in the brains of animals provided one way of approaching the study of function. 'A compared Anatomy', he said, 'may yield us a more full and exact Physiology of the Use of the Parts.'[152]

These anatomical observations led him to a concept of general nervous function. The animal spirits were 'procreated only in the brain and cerebellum'. Moreover, because of the vascularity of the grey cortex, and the fibrous nature of the underlying white matter, he judged that their functions were different. He considered that the animal spirits were generated in the cortex and transmitted through the fibres threading their way through the white matter of the brain stem, spinal cord, and nerves. The passage downward and upward of the spirits provided the basis of motion and sensation. The central masses of grey matter were subsidiary centres for the storage and generation of the spirits.

The blood ... is carried by the fourfold Chariot of the Arteries to four distinct regions of the Head ... nigh the cortical substance of either, out of which the Spirits are distilled ... which presently flowing from the Cortical substance into the medullary, there exercise the gifts of the animal Function ... In the meantime, the oblong marrow and its various processes and protuberances are either retreating places, or high roads for the animal Spirits ... [and so] irradiate the nervous *System* ... Wherefore, it is observed, that all parts of the whole body, by which motion and sense are performed do not only swell up with the animal Spirit.[153]

The nerves themselves were not hollow but under a lens or microscope they resembled the porous nature of 'sugar-cane'. They served both sensory and motor functions. The 'proper organ of feeling' was not skin, muscle, or membrane, but the nervous fibres implanted in them. There was no particular specificity in nerve structure or function but there were probably different types of sensory modalities.

Which Fibres, tho' everywhere of the same conformation; yet exhibit various Species, according to the various approaches of tangible things.
... the Fibres, tho' of the same nature or frame, enter into divers ways of Contraction or wrinklings ... the Fibres which are the Instruments of Touching, are affected after a different manner, by the various impulse of Tangible things. For it seems, that these are irritated or provoked one way with heat, and another way with cold, and so from the rest of the Qualities, after a manifold manner.[154]

Sensations were transmitted to the brain and received in the corpus striatum, the 'First' or 'Common Sensory', which was also concerned with voluntary motor function. The corpus striatum

receives the strokes of all sensible things dilated from the Nerves of every Organ, and so causes the perception of every sense.[155]

A sensory impulse might travel further into the brain; in the corpus callosum it became imagination, and if it reached the cortex it was stored as a memory.

If that this impression, being carried farther, passes through the *callous Body*, Imagination follows the Sense; Then if the same fluctuation of Spirits is struck against the *Cortex* of the Brain, as its outmost banks, it impresses on it the image or character of the sensible Object, which, when it is afterwards reflected or bent back, raises up the Memory of the same thing.[156]

Concerning the faculty of memory and his choice of the cerebral cortex for its location, Willis reminded his readers that 'For as often as we endeavour to remember objects long since past, we rub the Temples and forepart of the Head.' He does not seem to have had any cogent reasons for placing memory in the cortex, where, it will be recalled, he also said began the process of sleep. He simply affirmed that he had shown that 'phantasie and imagination' took place in the brain, and that 'Memory depends so upon the Imagination'.

The curious mixture of sharp clinical observation and fanciful conjecture so characteristic of Willis's writings is exemplified in a passage about sensation in which he seems to indicate his appreciation of stereognosis – and also his belief in ghosts!

> For since that the Sensible Qualities so called, are manifold and divers, to wit, Heat and Cold, Moisture and Dryness, Hardness and Softness, and other Modifications of Bodies, their Make, Motions, Influences and Types, or Figures of Appearance ... the greatest part of them by much are the proper Objects of Feeling, and are discerned only by its Judgment. ...[157]

But although common touch seemed to be a rather crude faculty.

> [It] gives notes of Judgment to all the other Senses concerning uncertain Objects; for when the Sight cannot distinguish a Ghost or Spectre, from a solid Body, by the tryal of Feeling, presently the thing is put out of doubt.[157]

The two oval-shaped corpora striata, strategically placed 'between the cerebrum and cerebellum and the whole nervous appendix [brain stem and spinal cord]', whose 'streaks have a double aspect or tendency', suggested ascending and descending tracts. The corpus striatum was therefore likely to possess two functions. One, as we have said, was sensory; the other was motor. 'These bodies, as they receive the forces of all the Senses, so also the first instinct of spontaneous local motions ... For here, as in a most famous Mart, the animal Spirits, preparing for the performance of the thing willed, are directed into appropriate nerves.' Willis wrote that in patients 'who dyed of a long Palsie, and most grievous resolution of the Nerves, I always found these bodies less firm than others in the Brain, discoloured like filth or dirt, and many chamferings [streaks] obliterated.'[158] Lesions at these sites caused paralysis. Further, in new born pups the normal appearance of the striatum was undeveloped.

> Further, in Whelps newly littered, that want their sight, and hardly perform the other faculties of motion and sense, these streaks or chamferings, being scarce wholly formed, appear only rude.[158]

Here we have an illustration of the modern method of clinico pathological correlation in the study of function. What is more, although we now know that it is the adjacent thalamus which is the 'first Sensory', and that the cortex and not the corpus striatum contains the motor centres, we are reading in Willis's pages one of the earliest indications of the localization of cerebral function. Another two hundred years were to pass before these centres were identified.

Another step forward was his recognition that motion could be voluntary or involuntary; the former was determined by the corpus striatum and the latter by the cerebellum (again, we should remember how he used the term cerebellum).

When some time past I diligently and seriously meditated on the Office of the Cerebel, and revolved in my mind several things concerning it, at length, from the analogy and frequent Ratiocination, this (as I think), true and genuine use of it occurred; to wit, that the Cerebel is a peculiar fountain of animal spirits designed for some works, and wholly distinct from the Brain ... by which all the spontaneous motions, to wit, of which we are knowing and will, are performed. But the office of the Cerebel seems to be for the animal Spirits to supply some Nerves, by which involuntary actions (such as are the beating of the Heart, easie Respiration, the Concoction of the Aliment, the protrusion of the Chyle, and many others) which are made after a constant manner unknown to us, or whether we will or no, are performed.[159]

He explains that he came to this opinion because (1) of the simple unvarying structure of the cerebellum in all animals; (2) the nerves derived from it were largely distributed to the viscera; (3) the actions of the heart, lungs, and gastrointestinal tract continued automatically; (4) autopsy experience showed that lesions in the cerebellum 'or nigh its confines' were often associated with 'crule and horrid Symptoms' in the 'Praecordia' and 'Belly'.

When Sherrington[160] came to define the cerebellum as 'The head ganglion of the proprioceptive system' he pointed out that 'its size from animal species strikingly accords with the range and complexity of the habitual movements of the species'.

Willis devoted three chapters (XV, XVI and XVII) of *Cerebri anatome* to a discussion of the cerebellum and involuntary movements. When they are examined together with his accounts of the 'eighth pair' (the vagus) and the 'intercostal' (the sympathetic) we have some of the earliest expressions of the concepts of reflex action and of the autonomic nervous system.

Willis's famous contemporary, Thomas Sydenham (1624–89), did not believe that studies such as these would ever disclose the workings of the human brain. He wrote

The brain is the source of sense and motion. It is the storehouse of thought and memory as well. Yet no diligent contemplation of its structure will tell us how so coarse a substance (a mere pulp, and that not over-nicely wrought) should subserve so noble an end. No one, either, can determine from the nature and structure of its parts, whether this or that faculty would be exerted.[161]

Sydenham's attitude is not uncommon in the history of medicine. Neurological history abounds in examples of men, distinguished and learned, who have inveighed against some development which ultimately proves sound. The authoritarian quality of medical teaching in the past rather encouraged the adoption of pronouncements 'from the bedside' – as if it was only there that wisdom resided.

REFLEX ACTION

In devising his system of neurophysiology Willis was influenced by the writings of Galen, Descartes (1596–1650), and Gassendi (1592–1655), all of whom he mentioned. Here were the animal spirits, the mechanistic interpretations, and the chemical concepts which he took up in turn, developing analogies such as rivulets and flowing streams, beams of light rays or guiding reins, and fermentation and chemical explosion. At times there appears to be cohesion and synthesis, at others only a jumble of obscure notions. He obviously possessed a powerful, vivid imagination and, impelled by his desire to devise satisfactory explanations, he gave it free rein. 'We have resolved to undertake the task of the Doctrine of the Nerves', because without it 'the Doctrine of the Brain ... would be left wholly lame and imperfect'.

All down the centuries the existence of voluntary and involuntary motion had been recognized. Hippocrates, Galen, and their successors had used the terms to distinguish between 'willed' muscular action and 'vital' movements such as those of the heart, thorax, and alimentary tract. There were also references to the blinking of eyes, the reactions of pupils, to grimacing, and to movements during sleep and in decapitated animals. Then, also, there was the ancient philosophical concept of 'Sympathy', which implied the existence of 'consent' or 'sympathy' between different parts of the body. A lesion in one part might affect another. Galen envisaged several types of sympathy in which communication between the parts was effected by humours or by irritation of nervous pathways. But the idea of reflex action did not emerge until the seventeenth century, with the work of Descartes and Willis. Descartes continued to speculate like those before him, but Willis also endeavoured to provide an anatomical basis for his ideas on the subject.

Willis believed that muscular contraction was basically a chemical process resulting from the 'explosive' interaction of 'arterial juice' brought to muscle in the blood stream, and 'nervous juice' transmitted by the nerves. Not content with the analogy of explosion in a trail of gunpowder he also said that the conjunction of the two juices '... being married together, are as it were the male and female seed, which being mingled in a fruitful womb'[162] created muscle contraction. Although Willis knew that nerves were not hollow and that when 'Nerves being cut asunder, it [the juice] is not perceived to flow out' and that 'Nerves being also bound, they do not swell above the ligature, as Arteries and Veins',[163] he, nevertheless, like Galen, found explanations to deploy. The juice was 'very subtil and spirituous' which could readily 'evaporate and be blown away or dispersed unperceivably' when a nerve was cut. And in new-born pups, nerves did swell above a ligature. He also believed that a muscle did swell when it contracted.

The concept of the essential irritability of muscle tissue had yet to be established but Willis had noted apparently spontaneous movements in voluntary and involuntary muscle, although the histological distinction between them was also unknown. He mentioned the 'trembling' of limb muscles in a skinned animal just after death and the 'contraction and relaxation' of the muscles of the heart, thorax, and diaphragm in living animals. He was also aware of the significance of associated movements, citing the example of the action of the diaphragm during animal activities such as running and flying. That was why the phrenic nerve was attached to the plexus of nerves supplying the shoulders and forelimbs. This was an instance of 'consent' or 'sympathy', and he suggested that intercommunication between nerves could take place peripherally, as well as in the brain.

> ... when many Nerves together are required to some motion of a Muscle equally, all these by reason of the commerce mutually had between themselves, might conspire in the same action; hence in some motions of the members, as in the striking of a Harp or Lute and other complicated actions, many muscles cooperate with admirable celerity, so that, although many may be employed at once, they perform their task severally without confusion. Besides, there is need for the Nerves to communicate mutually among themselves, because of the Sympathetical motions of the members and of some of the parts ...[164]

Galen and others, of course, believed that animal spirits could flow from one nerve to another wherever there was anatomical communication. The optic decussation was often quoted in this context.

In his essay 'De motu musculari', Willis speaks of 'our Myology or Doctrine of the Muscles', stressing that various, apparently spontaneous, movements were commonly encountered, but that normally

> The Instincts of Motions, to be obeyed by the Muscles, so delivered by the Nerves, are, being sent either from the Brain, performed at the command, and with the knowledge of the Appetite; or from the Cerebel, according to the Laws of Nature, for the most part unknown to us.[165]

Willis's favourite analogy when discussing the transmission of messages was that of light rays and their reflection and refraction about which Descartes had written. Willis spoke of 'dioptric mirrors' and 'whitened walls' when writing of the function of the corpus striatum and the conversion of sensory into motor impulses. A passage in which the term 'reflection' occurs may be quoted;

> Further, when the Tangible Impression [sensory stimulus] arrives first and immediately at the Streaked Bodies [corpus striatum], if the same be light, it is there terminated, and the sensible Species [Image] presently vanishes; but if the Impulse of the Object be somewhat stronger, it passes further to the Callous Body [corpus callosum], and oftentimes to the Shell of the Brain [the cortex] ... [but there may also take place] ... a divergency or bending down of the Spirits, from thence is reflected into the same Nerve, or others related to it, so it stirs up local Motions. These sort of Effects are sufficiently known by the Common Proverb, *Where the Pain is, there the Finger will be*; for it is implanted by Nature in every Animal, to rub or press the place with its finger or foot, where any sense of Trouble or Pain is.[166]

The process of reflection is mentioned three times in the passages in which he describes the successive steps of perception, imagination, and memory taking place in the brain.

> ... which, when it is afterwards reflected or bent back, raises up the Memory of the same thing.[167]

> ... so in sleep (the Appetite knowing nothing of it) when pain troubles, presently we rub the place, moving the hand to it; but more often after that the sensible Species, having past from the common Sensory to the *callous Body*, hath stirred up the Imagination, the Spirits, reflecting from thence, and flowing back towards the nervous Appendix, raise up the Appetite and Local Motions, the Executors or Performers of the same.[167]

Wherefore whilst the chief reflection of the Brain and Spirits is celebrated, sleep, or an Eclipse of the animal Spirits happens.[167]

Although Willis envisaged a cerebello-medullary mecanism controlling the involuntary functions of the body and mediating reflex activity he stressed that certain parts of this 'Dominion, are compelled to obey the beck and call of the government of the Brain', so that 'we are able also in a measure to alter the motions and actions of the *Praecordia* and *Viscera* at the will or command of the appetite'.

In all this it is possible to see not only the stirrings of the concept and mechanism of reflex action, with its varying degree of complexity, but also the prospect, as it were, of higher and lower levels of activity in the nervous system. Reflex action was still a vague notion with the brain playing the essential part, but with peripheral nervous intercommunication providing a suggestion of more elementary activity. There is no real hint of Willis identifying the spinal cord as a key structure, although Brazier (1959) thought that he may have viewed it as a centre for communication between nerves.[168] That was achieved by Whytt (1714–66) in the next century.

The contributions of Descartes and Willis to this chapter of neurological history have been discussed by many authorities, and one gains the impression that Willis's place is now more firmly established than it was earlier in this century.

In 1901 Willis's arch critic, Foster, wrote that Willis's views were 'indeed to a large extent the views of Descartes, modified by more exact anatomical knowledge, occasionally by sound physiological deductions', but although Descartes' anatomy was 'fantastic and unreal', his account, with 'very little change in the details ... and some of that hardly more than a change in terminology would convert that exposition into a statement of modern views'.[169] Willis, on the other hand, according to Foster, 'in no case dwells on Descartes' main thesis' (that the human body was a machine) and he only 'dimly laid hold of the modern doctrine of reflex action'.[170]

Foster's pupil, Sherrington, in *The integrative action of the nervous system* (1906) did not mention Willis, but Descartes is frequently quoted and stands at the head of his list of bibliographical references. Later, however, in *Man on his nature* (1941) and in *The endeavour of Jean Fernel* (1946) Sherrington had this to say of Willis and reflex action:

As to the term itself, Descartes in describing his automata did not say 'reflex', or rather he scarcely did so. It is to be found once, and then not in substantial form. It was Willis, Professor of Medicine at Oxford, who writing, rather later, on the nervous system gave numerous instances of automatic acts, where stimulus was promptly followed by movement without conscious participation of the 'will'. He spoke of this action as being 'reflex'.[171]

But this thesis that the body is the mainspring of its own motions was slow in getting across – even to the physician as a physician. In the latter part of the eighteenth century, Haller's full treatise on physiology – seven volumes – makes no mention of 'reflex action', that part of motor behaviour mediated according to Descartes by nerves not actuated by 'reason' or 'will', and called 'reflex'. The notion of reflex action is traceable to Descartes, but the term hardly so. The term is traced more clearly to Thomas Willis.[172]

We may note, in passing, that Foster's own *Textbook of physiology*†, used by Sherrington when a student, only contained 'a mere 5¾ pages' on 'Reflex Action' in 1879.[173] But Sherrington, and in turn Meyer and Hierons,[174] were incorrect when they said that Willis did not mention Descartes. He referred to him as 'the Famous *Cartes*' when he was discussing the pineal gland (A.B. p. 64).

In *Reflex action, a study in the history of physiological psychology*, Fearing[175] considered that Willis's account was 'more precise, anatomically speaking, than that of Descartes' and he thought that Willis's preoccupation with animal spirits 'should not obscure the importance of his attempt to account for integrated and co-ordinated muscle action'.

A similar growth in the appreciation of Willis's contribution in this field can be detected in Fulton's writings. In the historical section of his book, *Muscular contraction and reflex control* (1926), he said Willis 'had little of the originality of scientific insight possessed by his contemporaries',[176] making no reference to Willis's ideas of reflex action, and his only quotation is one of Foster's translated passages concerning the flow of animal spirits into muscle. In his *Selected readings in the history of physiology* (1930) Fulton depicted the growth of the concept of reflex action in the works of Fernel, Descartes, and Whytt, omitting Willis entirely.[177] He also neglected him, when recounting the history of the reflex, in his *Physiology of the nervous system* (1938),[178] but mentioned him in connection with the thalamus, basal ganglia, the autonomic nervous system, and the cerebellum. In 1953, when writing of the 'Forerunners of the Reflex', in an essay on 'The Historical Contribution of Physiology to Neurology' Fulton described Willis as 'an Oxford Physician who restricted his practice almost entirely to neurology ... who dissected the cranial nerves, recognising all twelve pairs' and who decided that the cerebellum presided over involuntary and the cerebrum over voluntary movements, because he 'studied the effects of ablating the cerebellum' and noted that 'animals suffered paralysis when the forebrain was injured or removed'.[179] Here, Fulton was indicating that Willis was one of the early investigators who used the experimental approach to the study of the nervous system. But his summary is not really satisfactory, or even accurate.

In their study, *The early history of the reflex*, Hoff and Kellaway[180] stated that Willis was the first to suggest that all intercommunication between nerves need not take place in the brain. Descartes' view of a sensory stimulus evoking, in a mechanical fashion, a response in the brain through the medium of nerve threads certainly did not imply any particular function for the spinal cord. It served to further the notion that the cord was but a bundle of nerve fibres. Descartes' nerve fibres all terminated in the ventricles. Willis's view of reflex action was clearly more physiological than Descartes'; a travelling spirit was nearer the truth than a cord which rang a bell, an analogy Descartes employed in the legend to his famous diagram of the reflex response to fire.

Liddell's[181] *The discovery of reflexes* contains little about Willis although he is credited with being the first to use the word 'reflexion'. Elsewhere there

† It was in this book that Sherrington subsequently introduced the word 'synapse' (see Ref. 178, p. 55).

is only mention of the arterial circle, the *sensorium commune*, and the suggested function of the cerebellum in relation to involuntary movements.

In all these studies there is no explanation of what Willis meant when he used the word 'cerebellum' and one gains the impression that Foster's initial appraisal was too readily accepted by the English school of physiology.

Indeed, the stoutest protagonist of Willis in this particular field of neurophysiology is a Frenchman – Dr Georges Canguilhem.[182] His monograph *La formation du concept de reflexe aux XVII et XVIII siècles*, published in 1955, deserves to be better known in this country, judging by the few libraries which possess a copy. It is an admirable study in which the author devotes an entire chapter of twenty-two pages to Willis. He analyses Willis's use of the words 'motus reflexus' and points out that they served to indicate a particular kind of movement, one example of which Willis often cited, namely, the scratch reflex. 'Here,' Canguilhem said, 'we are in the presence of a concept.'

> In summary, concerning the reflex, we find in Willis, the thing, the word and the idea. The thing, in the form of an original observation, a cutaneous reflex of the nervous system, the scratch reflex: the word, which passed into classical use both as an adjective and a noun; the idea, initially a question of discernment or classification, finally being interpreted as a principle (p. 68).

Canghuilhem concluded that Willis did not just adopt the views of Descartes as has often been suggested. He made original and notable advances. He conceived of a class of movement that was involuntary; one that was not initiated in the brain, but that depended on a free flow of spirits – centrifugally and centripetally, 'the birth certificate of reflex action' (p. 77).

THE AUTONOMIC NERVOUS SYSTEM

Sheehan's[183] memorable paper entitled 'Discovery of the Autonomic Nervous System' proved to be an important step in the renewal of Willis's reputation in this century. We have seen how Galen described the sympathetic nerve trunks and their ganglia but without clearly distinguishing them from the vagi, and how he thought they arose from the brain. Vesalius made the same errors but Meyer and Hierons[184] credit him with providing the first illustration of the sympathetic nerve and point out that Eustachius (1520–74) and Willis were the only anatomists of this period who provided clear illustrations of the two separate vagus and sympathetic nerves. They both also, apparently independently, gave the sympathetic a cerebral origin, Eustachius deriving it from the VI nerve, and Willis from the V and VI nerves.

Willis's illustration (Table IX; *Cerebri anatome*) is shown in Fig. 30. It is rather schematic but it is accompanied by two pages of detailed legend and shows the relation of the vagus and sympathetic nerve trunks, with their ganglia, plexuses, and their branches to the heart, and great vessels, the trachea and oesophagus. The three cervical sympathetic ganglia are demonstrated, with the cardiac plexus, the branches 'binding' the axillary

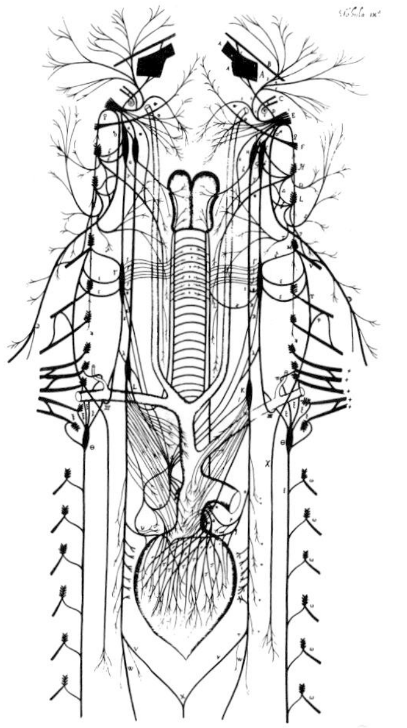

FIG. 30. Table IX from *Cerebri anatome* showing 'the fifth and sixth pair of nerves . . . the Intercostal Nerve (Sympathetic) and the wandring Pair (Vagus) and the Accessory Nerve'. In this schematic representation are seen the three sympathetic ganglia, the visceral plexuses, and the recurrent laryngeal and phrenic nerves. The intracranial portion of the sympathetic is depicted arising from the fifth and sixth cranial pairs.

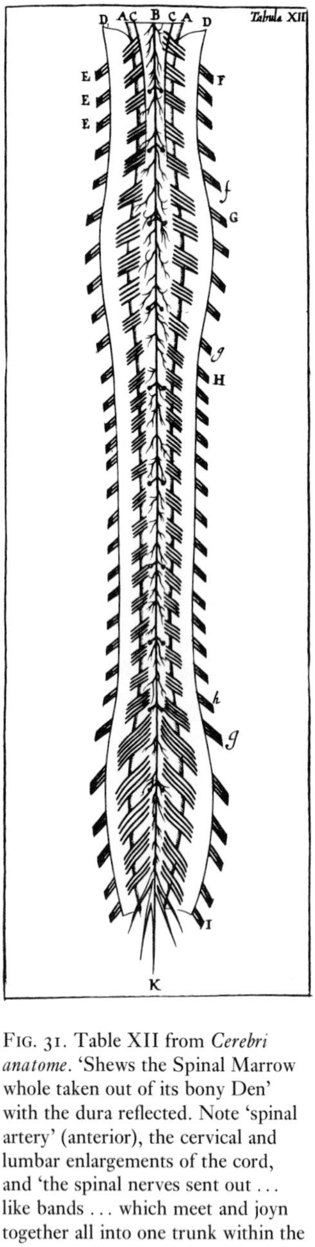

FIG. 31. Table XII from *Cerebri anatome*. 'Shews the Spinal Marrow whole taken out of its bony Den' with the dura reflected. Note 'spinal artery' (anterior), the cervical and lumbar enlargements of the cord, and 'the spinal nerves sent out . . . like bands . . . which meet and joyn together all into one trunk within the junctures of the vertebrae . . . and carried to their respective Provinces'.

and vertebral arteries, the rami communicantes, and the communications between vagal and sympathetic ganglia and nerves. Finally this splendid plate also illustrates the glossopharyngeal, the spinal accessory, the recurrent laryngeal, and the phrenic nerves. In Table X, Willis shows the same structures in an animal, with the union of the cervical portion of the sympathetic trunk and the vagus nerve. In many animals the cardiac nerves were largely vagal; there was little sympathetic supply.

All this, wrote Sheehan, 'represents an important milestone along the road to knowledge of the autonomic nervous system'.

The vagus nerves[185]

Willis's text on the eighth or 'wandring Pair' (the Vagus) and the 'Intercostal Pair' (the Sympathetic) takes up some twenty-seven pages of *Cerebri anatome*. Their peculiar origins, distribution, complexity, and their ganglia or 'infoldings' like 'knots in the stem of a tree', clearly intrigued him and he sensed they possessed special functions.

The vagus nerve had a 'large province' and many other nerves temporarily united with it in various parts of its course. They 'are accounted part of it, although they have distinct beginnings . . . going away again' from it, in a strange manner. Links with the sympathetic nerves were less in man than in animals and the latter had larger vagus nerves. Ganglia were situated where there was rich branching but some nerves were more in the nature of 'companions' using the 'same coat'. A branch in the cervical area was distributed to 'the sphincter of the throat', another formed an anastomosis with the recurrent laryngeal nerve, others 'compass about the trunk' of the carotid artery, or 'are inserted into its coats'. There were two cardiac 'infoldings', both with communicating sympathetic supply, which 'compassed' the arch of the aorta, the pulmonary artery, and the heart itself. In the lungs the vagal branches 'in their passage step by step they follow the pipes of the *Bronchia*, both the Arteries and the Veins . . . and compass about these Vessels'.

Willis discussed the physiological significance of this distribution of the vagus nerves in the following chapter (XXIV). The vagi 'serve almost only to the involuntary Function . . . stirred up either by the instinct of Nature, or by the force of the Passions, the animal in the meantime scarce knowing it'. Communicating nerves assisted this activity 'in divers parts', facilitating 'a certain Sympathy and consent in their actions'.

The laryngeal nerves ensured that in times of excitement, the tracheal rings and the vocal cords would respond in 'double motion' (breathing and voice) to the requirements and expression of flight, anger, fear, or joy. Of the nerve supply to the heart, he wrote

Truly this copious distribution of the nerves doth effect the pulsifick force in the little ears of the Heart and in the Arteries, or at least seems to excite it; . . . that they may be able to sustain an undiscontinued reciprocation of *Systole* and *Diastole*. Moreover, that the thick fibres and shoots of the nerves are inserted both into the Veins and Arteries, and bind both those kind of Vessels, and variously compass them about, we may lawfully suppose, that these nerves, as it were Reins put upon these blood-carrying vessels, do sometimes dilate, and sometimes bind them hard together for the determining the motion of the Blood according to the various force of the Passions, or to deduce it here and there after a manifold manner; for by this means it comes to pass, that in fear the excursion of the blood is hindred, and in other Affections its motion is respectively altered.[186]

In addition there is further comment that these cardiac nerves about the aorta and pulmonary artery control the rate and rhythm of the heart beat and that disturbance of the vagi may cause 'inordinate tremblings and shakings of the heart, which are manifestly different from its natural pulse'. Normally, these nerves 'compose themselves to the requisite analogies and proportions of the Pulses'. These observations must be among the earliest explanations of the basis for nervous regulation of the heart.

Then follows the famous account of the ligation and subsequent section of the vagus nerves in a dog.

The skin about the throat being cut long-ways and the Trunk of both the wandring pair being separated apart, we made a very strict Ligature; which being done, the Dog was presently silent, and seemed stunned, and suffered about the Hypochondria convulsive motions with a great trembling of the Heart. But this affection quickly ceasing, afterwards he lay without any strength or lively aspect, as if dying, slow and impotent to any motion, and vomiting up any food that was given him; nevertheless his life as yet continued, neither was it presently extinguished after those nerves were wholly cut asunder; but this Animal lived for many days, and so long, till through long fasting, his strength and spirits being worn out, he died. The carcass being opened, the blood within the Ventricles of the Heart, and the Vessels on every side reaching from thence, to wit, both the Veins and Arteries, being greatly coagulated, was gathered into clotters; to wit, for this cause, because the blood, though for the sustaining of life, it was in some measure circulated, yet for the most part it stagnated both in the Heart, and in the Vessels. The cause of which stagnation I can assign to no other thing, than that the *Praecordia*, the influence of the animal spirits being hindred, wanted its usual motions.[187]

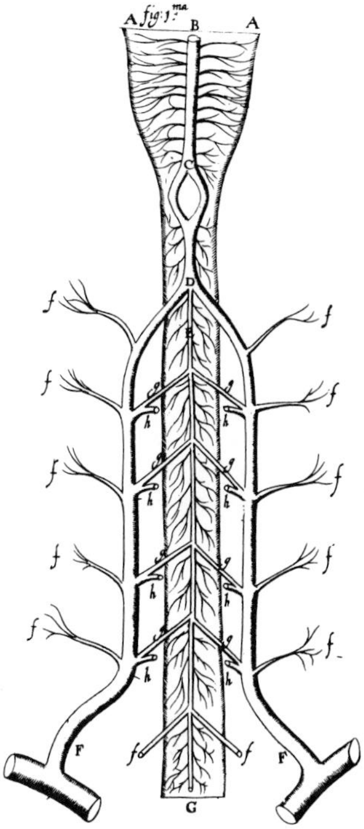

FIG. 32. From Table XIII of *Cerebri anatome, Fig. 1*. The vertebral arteries (F), the spinal cord (G), the anterior spinal artery (E), the basilar artery (B), and the radicular arteries (g and h). C is the 'double coalition' of the vertebral arteries seen in some animals. In Fig. 3 of this Table is shown the anastomotic chain of arteries formed on the spinal cord.

Willis did not actually state that the pulse was slowed but he did aver that 'the vigour and elastick force of the Heart was suppressed, so that the Pulse being by degrees weakened, life is by little and little extinguished'. He concluded that in noting 'the tenour of the Pulse' the physician might be able to decide whether there was 'alteration of the spirits' or a 'fault of the blood'.

The pulmonary vagal branches were an indication that the lungs did not just move passively as a result of contraction of the muscles of the thorax and diaphragm.

And so when Nerves of a twofold kind, to wit, some from the spine being inserted into the muscles of the *Diaphragma* and the *Thorax*, and others from the wandring pair distributed into the lungs, actuate the Organs of Respiration, of itself unforced and involuntary, may be at our pleasure somewhat restrained, interrupted, and diversly altered.[188]

Normal function depended on reflex activity in somatic and autonomic innervation, but there was also cerebral control. In coughing and laughter 'all the organs of respiration intimately conspire'. In asthma, 'a spasmodick

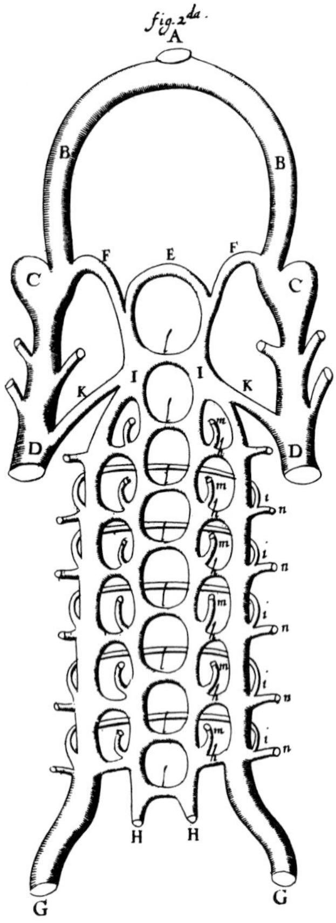

FIG. 33. From Table XIII of *Cerebri anatome, Fig. 2*. The venous channels 'which are Companions' to the vertebral arteries. B, lateral sinus; C, jugular bulb; D, jugular vein; G, vertebral vein.

Affection' which 'afflicted the pneumonick nerves ... the *bronchia* themselves were pulled together ... so that they cannot take in and send forth the air after its due manner'. Disorders of breathing of this kind may also occur in patients with lesions of the brain – and also in hysteria.

Willis ends his account of the vagus nerves by describing how the two trunks unite in the epigastrium, sending only 'little bands of spirits' lower in the abdomen. This did not surprise him because 'it seems an unworthy thing, that the same path which leads to the chief office of nutrition and to the Palaces of life itself, should lye open to the more vile intestines also, and the sink of the whole body'. He was never at a loss for an explanation.

The sympathetic nerves[189]

Willis called these nerves the 'Intercostal' nerves 'because that going near the roots of the ribs, it receives in every one of their interstices a branch from the spinal marrow' (the rami communicantes). Many thought, he said, it was but a branch of the vagus nerve, probably because of the manner in which 'conjugation' took place between them. 'In its whole descent through the thorax ... it sends forth from itself not a shoot.' In the upper abdomen the solar plexus, 'the greatest infolding of all stands like the Sun in the midst of the planets'. The sympathetic nerve ended in the sacral plexus.

It had a common origin with the vagus; there were three ganglia in the neck and the numerous communications with the vagal and spinal nerves ensured 'a more mutual commerce together'. (The spinal links also provided some protection in the sympathetic's 'long journey' and also an additional avenue of excretion of humours from the spinal cord.)

The sympathetic nerves had two principal functions. They provided the means by which the brain influenced the viscera and they served as a network of nervous communication between the different parts of the body.

The upper reaches of the sympathetic were concerned with the functions of the throat and heart.

> This nerve in the sphincter of the Throat corresponds with others akin ... and is helpful to them in the business of chewing ... whereby the throat being opened, the chewed meats may be thrust forward into its passage.[190]

'A sense of choaking in the throat' could arise from a lesion 'anywhere in any nerve of the wandring or intercostal pair'. It was common in 'hysterick distempers' and in Hypochondria.

The sympathetic nerve had a special function in man; it 'serves in the place of a special *Internuncius* before the cloister of the breast, which bears the mutual senses of the brain and heart this way and that way ...'. The heart beat, the motion of the blood, and respiration, were all under the influence of this nerve. There were 'reciprocal affections of the heart and brain'. The cardiac nerves were of 'either family', vagal and sympathetic. Their 'joynt action' could be seen in the expressions and colour of the face during excitement; the blood flows more swiftly, the heart's action increases, the lungs are raised up when 'the heart desires to rejoice'. That was why the ancients 'placed wisdom in the heart'.

The lower group of sympathetic nerves were distributed to the viscera of the abdomen and pelvis. The intestinal supply was concerned with the 'culinary work of nutrition', and 'the peristaltick motion of the vermiculation'. The muscular contractions of the gut were different from those of voluntary muscles; the muscular fibres were varied in their arrangement, some straight, others circular or oblique. The woof was of a finer texture and the movements spiral or screw-like. The processes of digestion, absorption, and excretion quietly maintained themselves, even in sleep; 'whilst the organs of other faculties are at rest, there is no quiet granted to these'. All was involuntary, 'For the nerves knowing best the wants of either part, warn them both of their mutual duty, and as occasion serves, stir them into action'.[191]

The sphincter of the anus was served with many nerves of a diverse kind, spinal, vagal, and sympathetic. This ensured co-ordinated action, whether reflexly or at will.

At times, when he was describing the ramifications and 'uses' of the vagi and sympathetics, Willis frequently adopted analogies of a mechanical kind, in the fashion of Descartes, mentioning cords, ropes, reins, bridles, and even a 'windlace' (windlass). The way in which he mixed these and interchanged them with those of a natural or chemical nature is one of the most characteristic features of his writings.

Eleven years later, in *Pharmaceutice rationalis*, writing of the 'vast number of nerves and nervous fibres [which] did embrace and encompass the trunks of the arteries in many places, and especially about the bottom of the heart' Willis modified his view that the nerves acted in a mechanical manner. 'They did onely convey fresh supplies of spirits and instincts' and did not 'draw or streighten the parts one jot.' The motions of the heart and vessels were actually performed by their 'fleshy' muscle fibres: 'Those arteries contract and extend themselves by their own strength.'[192]

Despite his excessive use of analogies and his fanciful 'speculation' (a word he used), one can nevertheless see how hard he strove to unify his observations and come to some coherent idea of the nature of this strange portion of the nervous system. The body and soul, the brain and heart, the instincts and emotions, the vital and natural, the voluntary and involuntary were all subjects of his meditation. In the brain stem he sensed there were pathways from the hemispheres through the corpora quadrigemina and the cerebellar peduncles to the cerebellum, the seat of involuntary function. From the pons emerged motor fibres which served the viscera of the thorax and abdomen, and also the expressive muscles of the eyes and face. The importance of the brain stem in this self-regulating system was beginning to emerge.

If we read between the lines, as Foster encouraged us to do when writing of Descartes and reflex action, altering the terminology and so on, Willis's account of the vagus and sympathetic nerves carries quite a modern ring. Meyer and Hierons[193] have indeed said 'If one substitutes the medulla for the cerebellum (of which it was thought to be a part) and the hypothalamus for the corpora quadrigemina, the error would indeed be small and we would be very close to our modern ideas of the cerebral control of the autonomic nervous system.'

I do not think Willis would be at all surprised to learn that we regard this system as a homeostatic mechanism whose head ganglion is the hypothalamus. Neither would he be surprised with our concept of psychosomatic medicine, for was there not a wonderful commerce between heart and brain?

THE CONCEPT OF INTERNAL SECRETIONS

There are statements in Willis's writings which require assessment of the role he played in the origin of the concept of internal secretion. The problem has recently been admirably analysed by Simmer (1974).[194] Although it is not primarily a neurological one the question is of great interest and arises out of certain passages in which he was discussing the gonads and the pituitary gland.

The gonads

In his first treatises on fevers and fermentation in 1659, Willis referred to the effects of 'fermentation' from the womb and the testes on the health and appearance of the individual. The female who lacks ferment is pale and languid; in the male the ferment provides strength, a manly voice, and beard. Male castrates lacked these features. But it was the following passage from convulsive diseases that led Adams[195] to suggest that Willis was the first to express the concept of an internal secretion of the testes. (Simmer incorrectly attributes this to Rolleston.[196]) Willis was commenting that in some epileptic children convulsions tended to cease at puberty.

> About the time of ripe age, as the Blood pours forth something before destinated for the brain through the spermatic arteries to the genitals, so also it receives as a recompense a certain ferment from those parts through the veins to wit, certain particles imbued with a seminal tincture, are carried back into the bloody mass, which makes it vigorous, and inspire into it a new and lively virtue; wherefore at the time the gifts both of the body and mind chiefly show themselves; hairs break out, the voice becomes greater, the courses of women flow, and other accidents happen, whereby it is plain, that both the blood and nervous juyce, are impregnated with a certain fresh ferment.[197]

Miller[198] referred to this passage describing the development of secondary sexual characteristics and thought it 'clearly hints at internal secretion' but Rolleston[199] did not mention it. In 1936, however, Rolleston[200] wrote that the passage 'may be interpreted as a conception of internal secretion', an opinion supported by Symonds,[201–2] Feindel,[203–4] and Isler.[205] Hierons[206] noted the suggestion, but expressed no opinion.

Another relevant passage, which I have not seen quoted, occurs in Part I of *De anima brutorum*.

> The genital humour is not, as Hippocrates formerly taught, and as now commonly believed, carried from the brain into the spermatick vessels . . . the genital humour is not from the brain but the blood . . . loss of seed disturbs the brain and nerves . . . there is wonderful commerce of brain with genital members . . .[207]

Simmer examined the origin of Willis's concept of a gonadal ferment. He pointed out that Willis did not specifically mention the ovaries ('the female testes'; ovarian function was then not understood) when writing of the ferment from the womb. But concerning the testes Willis was probably influenced by the writings of Van Helmont on ferments and Glisson and Wharton on glandular secretion, all of whom he mentioned in his writings. Willis postulated that the testes released a secretion, a ferment, into the venous blood which exerted effects on various organs of the body. Isler[208] indicated that in the preface to *Cerebri anatome*, Willis used the Greek word for hormones which Pordage translated as 'the rushings on or impressions' when he was speaking of the invisible animal spirits in the brain and nerves. Isler thought that the concept of substances thus distilled from the blood and influencing the body 'is very near to our concept of hormones'. But I feel, with Simmer, that Willis was not there referring to gonadal secretion. Willis's affirmation that we come into being, live, and die by the properties of ferments was correctly stressed by Isler as being a fundamental conviction which pervades all his work. Simmer concluded that 'in proposing the release by the testes of a substance into the blood and assigning a specific action to this material, Willis apparently was the first to forecast internal secretion in all regards'.[209]

The pituitary

The arterial circle in man (which he often referred to as the *rete mirabile*), the *rete mirabile* of animals, and the pituitary gland all fascinated Willis. Their unusual anatomy and close proximity suggested important functions. 'Each of these deserve consideration, the more, for that in divers animals they are after a different manner.' The pituitary gland 'is found in all perfect creatures ... from whence we may conclude it to have some necessary uses in the brain'.[210] Its size and the degree to which it is enclosed in its 'cell or stall' varied in different animals. It consisted of two parts. Although it looked 'but one and undivided, in truth, it is made up of a substance which is of a twofold nature or kind'. Its size seemed to be related to that of the brain and of the carotid arteries, sometimes to 'both these together, or only to one'.

Willis said that

> for if an inky liquor be squirted into the carotids with a syringe, the exterior part of the glandula, that is interwoven with the blood-carrying vessels, will be very much dyed with a black colour. Wherefore without doubt, it may be thought, that this glandula doth receive into itself the humors, to wit, flowing into it from the Tunnel [infundibulum] in all kind of living creatures, and in some from the branches of the carotides.[211]

He accepted Schneider's demonstration that there was no discharge from the pituitary through the sphenoid into the nasopharynx. He injected ink into the 'great hole' of the sphenoid bone in a calf and found it emerged in the jugular veins.

On another page (A.B. p. 85) Willis writes that the function of the vessels entering the pituitary gland was to 'separate the serosities of the too watry blood, and to lay them up in to that glandula, whereby the rest of the bloody *Latex*, to be carried to the brain, becomes more pure and free from dregs'.[212]

Again, he wrote

... the serous humors ... do all slide down ... into the steep opening of the Tunnel ... and pituitary glandula. Further, it is manifest that this glandula, in some animals, is charged with a double office; to wit, as it receives the serosities sent from above from the brain, so also it separates the humors from the blood brought to the same from the wonderful net by the arteries, and prepossessing them, imbibes them before their ingress to the brain. Wherefore this part is furnished with a substance of a double kind; viz. one reddish, more thin, and interwoven with blood-carrying vessels, which constitutes either side of it; and the other more white placed in the middle, to which the tunnel is inserted.[213]

But having shewn, that this Glandula receives the humors so brought by a double Tribute, we did diligently enquire concerning the ways and means whereby they are at length carried away from thence; and as it appears by an Experiment, that there is a passage open from this Glandula into the Vessels lying underneath the bone, and from thence into the Jugular veins, we affirmed, that 'twas most likely, that the humors to be carried away from this glandula, (after the manner of others) may be reduced at last into the bloody mass.[214]

Thus we see Willis visualizing the pituitary gland as an organ for the purification of blood on its way to the brain, and also as an excretory organ for the products of brain metabolism. He cannot be said to have actually identified the anterior and posterior lobes of the gland.

Why, then, did Cushing, in 1930, write that Willis's views on pituitary function contained 'the kernel of the modern conception of an internal secretion'?[215] Cushing was referring, not to any of the passages quoted above, but to another in which Willis was giving his reasons for the vascular arrangements at the base of the brain; viz. the carotid siphons to reduce the force of entry of blood into the cranium, the pituitary branches so that jblood could be first purified, and the circle which reduced the possible consequences of arterial obstruction. With regard to the second point Willis wrote,

The divarication of the *Carotides* into net-like infoldings, hath another use of no less moment, to wit, that the more watry blood being (as it is its temperament in most beasts, and especially in those who are fed with herbage) before it be poured upon the brain, might carry away some part of the superfluous Serum to the pituitary Glandula, and instil the other part into the branches or shoots of the Veins to be returned towards the Heart.[216]

The answer is provided by Simmer. He explains that Cushing did not use Pordage's translation from Willis's Latin text, but his own. And by just using '*to*' instead of '*of*', the above passage might be taken to mean that the blood took some part of the superfluous serum *of* the pituitary gland. It is clear that Cushing's interpretation is not correct if the previous passages on the pituitary gland are also taken into account. So the claim of Rolleston that here we had 'the germ of the conception of an internal secretion' cannot be justified.

Cushing and Simmer agree, however, about the outcome of Willis's views in this field of internal secretion. Cushing said 'the idea was stillborn'; Simmer, that 'a major conceptual contribution of seventeenth-century English medicine was long forgotten. Why it was so ill fated needs further study.'[217]

WILLIS IN HISTORY

An historical reputation is a fragile thing and in Willis particularly we have an example of how it may flourish and wane and rise again. Even now one doubts whether it has been securely established and widely appreciated, in the sense, for example, of that of his contemporary Thomas Sydenham.

Sir Charles Symonds, more than anyone, has succeeded in proving the slanderous nature of some of the writings about him, with their baleful influence on subsequent interpretations. But there was also, from the first, criticism of an entirely objective nature, the most memorable being launched only a year after the publication of *Cerebri anatome*.

The tragic life and scientific contributions (on glands, the lymphatic system, the muscles, the heart, the foetus, the brain, and on geology) of the Dane, Niels Stensen (Nicolaus Steno; 1638–86), are well known.[218] An English translation of his famous *Discours sur l'anatomie du cerveau*, delivered in Paris in 1665, and published there in 1669, is contained in Scherz's commemorative symposium volume of 1965.[219]

The lecture, of some thirty-three pages, was delivered when Stensen was only twenty-seven years of age, after studies in Copenhagen, Amsterdam, and Leiden. Anatomy had been his main interest during these years and he had not actually practised medicine. The lecture began with the strange words that 'I confess sincerely and publicly here that I know nothing about it'. Nevertheless his lecture has been universally acclaimed.

He said that terminology and methods of dissection were both far from satisfactory. Willis's technique, for example, of removing the brain from the skull was liable to result in injury to soft and delicate structures at the base. Slicing, unfolding, and separating grey from white matter were, in themselves, incomplete; they should be used in combination, and sections in transverse and longitudinal planes should be examined. But 'we should not delude ourselves' for the only valuable form of dissection 'would be one following the nerve filaments through the substance of the brain to see where they come to an end'. And that at present was impossible. Nevertheless, if the white matter did prove to be fibrous, the arrangement of its pattern was doubtless concerned with the functions of motion and sensation. This 'pregnant passage' so impressed Foster[220] that he said that if Stensen had not deserted his study of the brain the story of neurophysiology would have been very different!

Stensen found minor faults in Willis's representations of certain structures in his diagrams, notably the details of the pineal gland, the white matter of the cerebellum, the pons, the corpus striatum, the anterior roots of the fornix, the origin of the trochlear nerve, and the slant of the oculomotor nerve. But Willis's diagrams were the best to date. He agreed with Willis

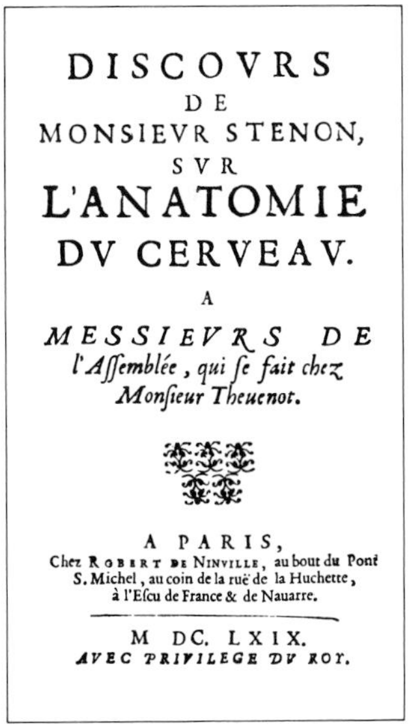
DISCOVRS
DE
MONSIEVR STENON,
SVR
L'ANATOMIE
DV CERVEAV.
A
MESSIEVRS DE l'Assemblée, qui se fait chez Monsieur Theuenot.

A PARIS,
Chez ROBERT DE NINVILLE, au bout du Pont S. Michel, au coin de la ruë de la Huchette, à l'Escu de France & de Nauarre.

M DC. LXIX.
AVEC PRIVILEGE DV ROY.

FIG. 34. Title page of Stensen's (Steno's) *Discourse on the anatomy of the brain*, published in Paris in 1669. The lecture, in which Willis was criticized, was delivered in 1665.

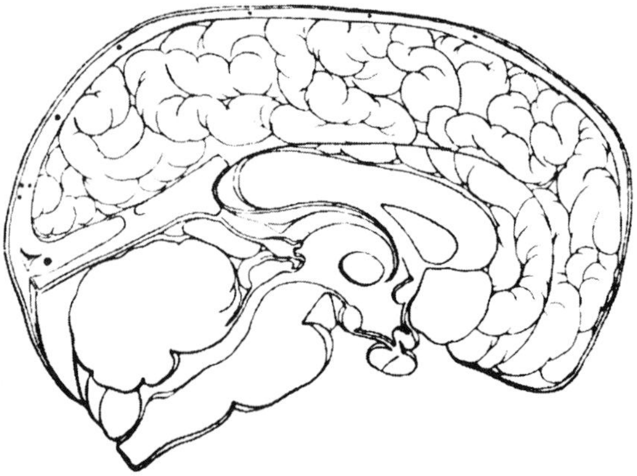

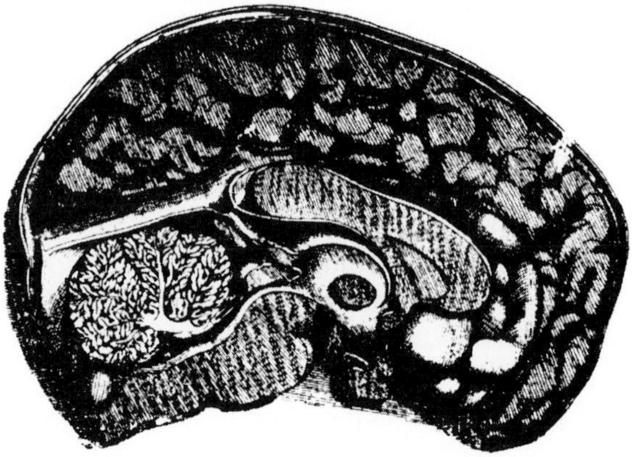

FIG. 35 (*left*). Sagittal section of brain in Stensen's *Discourse*. The convolutions are poorly shown; the interventricular foramina and the posterior commissure are not depicted.

FIG. 36 (*centre*). Coronal section of brain in Stensen's *Discourse*, posterior to corpora mamillaria, showing clear outline of the cortex. The internal capsule is schematically indicated but the grey matter of the basal ganglia is not shown.

FIG. 37 (*right*). Coronal sections of brain in Stensen's *Discourse*. In the upper diagram are the thalami with commissure, a rather big fornix, and poorly defined basal ganglia. The choroid plexus in the ventricles is not shown. In the lower diagram, through the brain stem, we see indications of the vermis and fourth ventricle. These diagrams of Stensen did not carry legends but they represent some of the earliest illustrations of coronal and sagittal sections of the brain.

that there was nothing in the ancient notion of ventricular function but he castigated him for erecting such 'fantastic interpretations' of cerebral function.

M. Willis gives us a quite extraordinary system. He houses common sense in the *corpus striatum*, imagination in the *corpus callosum* and memory in the *cortex* ...

He describes for us the *corpus striatum* as if it had two types of *striae*, one rising the other descending, and yet if you separate the grey matter from the white, you see that these striae are all of one type ...

What assurance can we have then that would be credible to us, that these three operations exist in the three bodies to which he assigns them?. Who can say whether the nerve fibres begin in the *corpus striatum*, or pass through the *corpus callosum* as far as the *cortex* or grey substance?

He even thought there was little reason for giving a name to that part of the white substance termed the *corpus callosum*. He was rather petulant and over-critical.

Stensen ends his discourse by stressing that physicians and surgeons usually have insufficient time to criticize anatomical research; academics 'when they have demonstrated clearly what is in their notes and their students have understood it, both think themselves satisfied with the

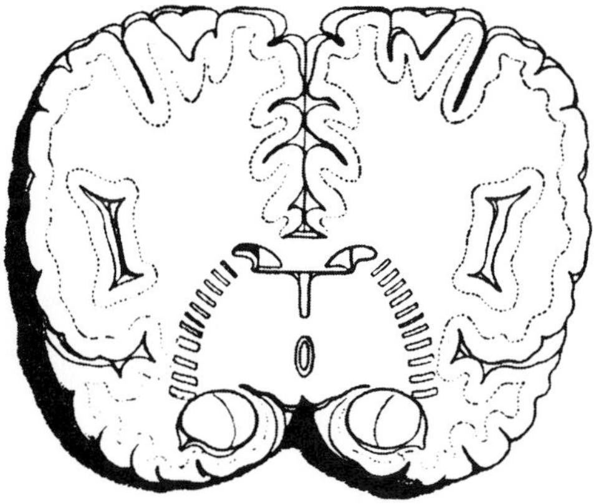

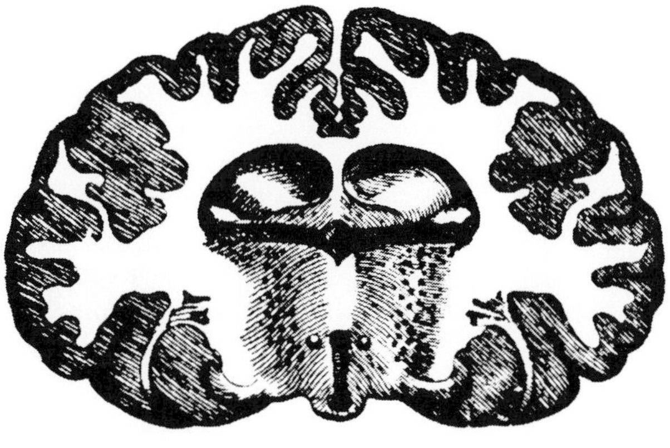

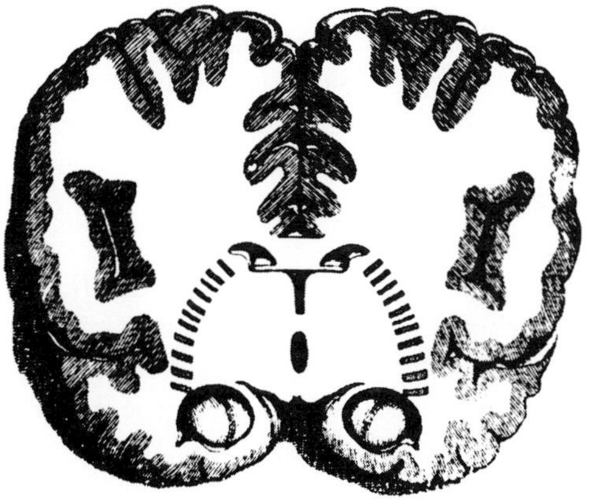

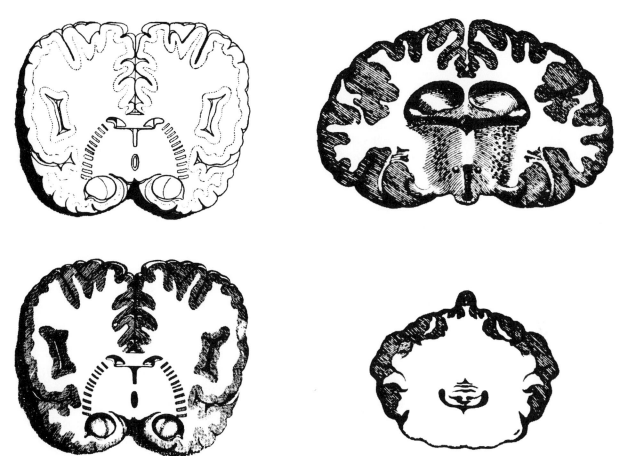

exercise'. Research, he said, 'requires a dedicated man'. He advocated more care in brain dissection; scrutiny and note-taking should always precede cutting or moving, lest unknowingly 'you change the interior' and 'the attachment of parts'. Removal of the skull cap could be improved; 'a circular saw might be made', trepanning used, or a liquid devised which would soften or dissolve bone. Comparative anatomical studies were essential; 'in the foetus of animals one sees how the brain develops'. Vivisection of animals should be encouraged; intravenous injections might affect the brain, and indeed, applying drugs to the brain surface or injecting them into the ventricles might help to determine if they possessed specific properties.

Stensen warned that standards of research should be improved. 'We shall always be miserably ignorant if we are satisfied by the scraps of information that are left us.'

Willis, no less dedicated, had actually begun what Stensen was advocating although he had marred his image by retaining so much of Galen and speculating too widely. The value of Stensen's lecture was that it introduced a new type of rigorous, scientific criticism and at the same time made proposals for further studies. A reader of today will find that it carries quite a modern ring. Nevertheless, Stensen did underestimate the significance of Willis's suggestions concerning the localization of brain function. He may have been in error anatomically – but not conceptually.

Another major critic was the celebrated John Mayow (1645–79) whose studies of the physiology of muscle and respiration made him famous. He thought Willis's views on muscle action were unsound. 'The theory of the learned author is certainly very ingenious, but I am not sure that it is in the same degree in accordance with truth.'[221] Mayow did not think contraction of a muscle caused it to swell, but only to harden. Willis's contributions to muscle physiology were not of lasting importance, according to Hierons and Meyer.[222] But Mayow also criticized Willis's use of the analogies of 'flame' and 'light' in connection with nervous physiology.

> ... I ask how it comes about that the light which is supposed to illumine the whole brain and all the nerves can never be seen by the eye? Assuredly Fires of this kind and New Lights no less in Anatomy than in Religion appear to me things wholly vain and fanatic.[223]

Had Willis possessed more of this faculty of critical analysis and less of the faculty of imagination, his recognition by physiologists would perhaps not have been so delayed. What one misses in his writings are passages in which the analysis of an idea is followed by its rejection. He was a great promoter of ideas, some sound, others absurd.

Willis wrote in Latin. Twenty years after his death in 1675, the first monograph on neuroanatomy in the English language was published. It was entitled *The anatomy of the brain* and its author was Humphry Ridley[224] (1653–1708) of London. His copperplate engraving of the base of the brain (Fig. 38) shows 'the ten pairs of nerves belonging to the brain', the 'blood-vessels injected with wax', and the spinal dura reflected on the right side. He indicated the siphons of the vertebral arteries, the basilar ('cervical') artery and its two branches, the superior cerebellar and the posterior cerebral arteries (with the emerging third nerve between them), and the posterior communicating artery. Not shown is the anterior cerebral branch of the divided internal carotids. He studied venous drainage of the corpus striatum and the intercavernous sinuses[225] and introduced the term restiform body for the inferior cerebellar peduncle of Willis.[226] He noted that the infundibulum, which was thought to drain the brain effluvia, was actually solid in its lower part. He did not think the branches of the internal carotid artery had been correctly described, by some anatomists; they were 'taking it on trust from Wepfer'.[227] He agreed with Willis that the arterial communication at the base of the brain 'was of great use and benefit to the brain' in the case of obstruction of one of the carotid or vertebral arteries.[228]

But the expression 'contrary to what Willis says' is not infrequently encountered. He said 'I have never found this *rete* wanting' in man[229] and of Willis's idea that the cerebrum controlled voluntary and the cerebellum involuntary motion, he said 'I am apt to think that Learned Person too soon fell in love with his first thought ...'[230]

In the eighteenth century Willis gained notice in the first English history of medicine – John Freind's (1675–1728) *The history of physick*.[231] Freind, a London physician, a Harveian orator, and friend of Dr Mead, planned his

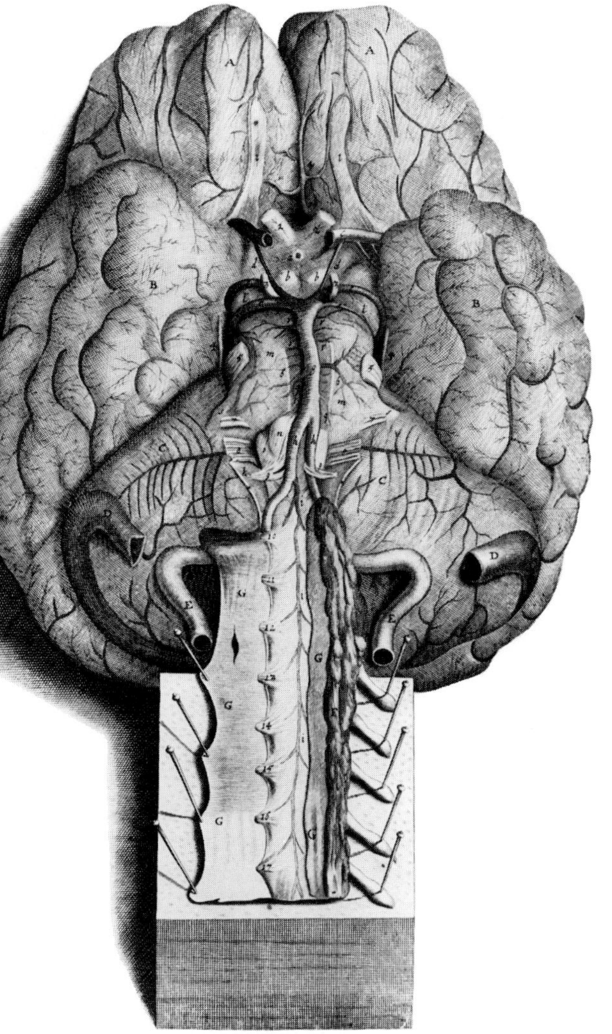

FIG. 38. After Ridley (1653–1708) of London, author of the first book in the English language on neuroanatomy.[224] The legend to this plate states that the blood vessels were injected with wax. D, lateral sinus; E, vertebral arteries; G, basilar ('cervical') artery; C, carotid artery; D, posterior communicating artery ('communicant branches'); E, posterior cerebral artery. And an odd-shaped pons.

book in the three months he spent in the Tower of London in 1722 on a charge of high treason.[232] He was a member of the Tory opposition after the Hanoverian succession and Mead engineered his release by refusing to treat the Prime Minister, Sir Robert Walpole, for his renal calculi, before Freind was released. At a celebratory dinner Mead gave Freind five hundred guineas which represented fees he received from Freind's patients during the doctor's spell in the Tower.[233]

In discussing the question of voluntary and involuntary motion Freind (Vol. 2, p. 315) said 'I take notice of this, because it is exactly the notion of the famous Dr. Willis, the first inventor of the nervous system'. But the respective roles of cerebrum and cerebellum he did not accept. 'But this notion is entirely overthrown . . . by what one may observe of the nerves. . . .' Freind was also puzzled by 'the medulla oblongata, which by him is reckon'd to belong to the cerebellum'. And in the treatment of palpitation he said 'I have often wondered that our countryman, Dr Willis, mentions none

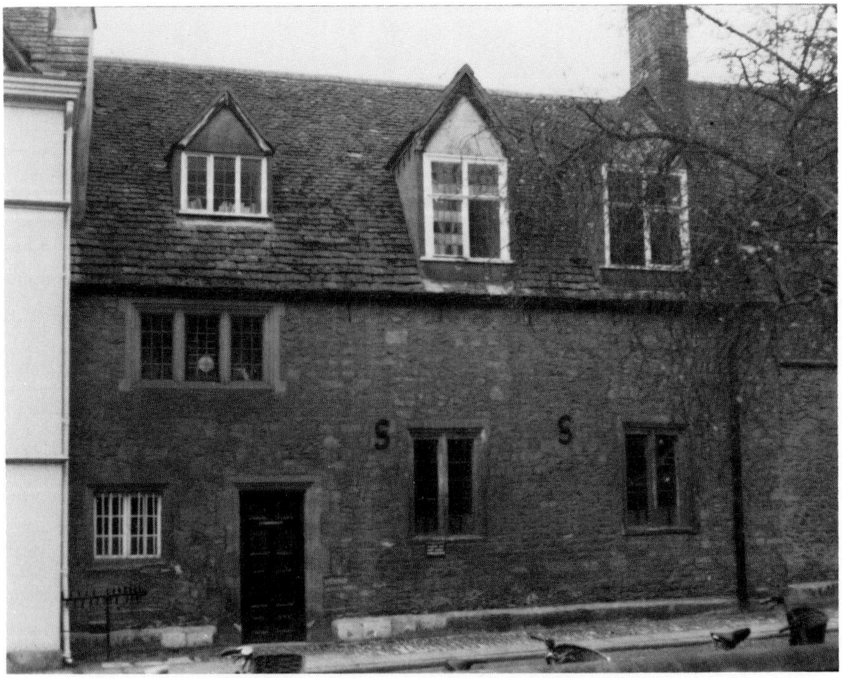

FIG. 39. Willis's Oxford home, Beam Hall, opposite Merton College. (Photograph by the author, 1977.)

of these [bleeding and purging] in his method of curing this distemper.'

At the end of the century Benjamin Hutchinson[234] in his two-volume *Biographia medica* (1799) devoted four pages to Willis. He said that Willis 'had refused the honour of knighthood' and that 'his table was the resort of most of the great men in London'. But he thought Willis 'hath founded a body of physic, chiefly on hypotheses of his own framing [quoting Wood]; but it will not be agreed that this foundation will be lasting'. He goes on to say that

> ... the truth is, nothing could be more unfortunate than this method of proceeding of Dr. Willis; who, instead of deducing real knowledge from observation and experiment, exercised himself in framing theories. Hence it is, that, while his books show the greatest ingenuity and learning, very little knowledge is to be drawn from them, very little use to be made of them. And perhaps no writings, which are so admirably executed, and prove such uncommon talents to have been in the writer, were ever so soon laid aside and neglected, as the works of Dr Willis.[234]

But he admitted that there were 'many curious things to be found in the works of this ingenious and able physician' and he quotes a Dr Wotton who considered that Willis had shown 'not only the brain was demonstrably proved to be the fountain of sense and motion, but also, by the course of the nerves ... that sense ... and motion were caused by nerves going into every one of those parts, which are all struck together'. He also quoted Vieussens as having corrected some of Willis's anatomical errors.

Perhaps the decline in the prestige of Willis is best demonstrated by the neglect he suffered at the hands of John Cooke (1756–1838). He was a physician to the London Hospital and wrote a book, *Treatise on nervous diseases* (1820–23) which McHenry,[235] considers to be 'the first separate work in neurology' and 'the most significant single contribution to neurology for its time'. The bulk of the book concerns the three diseases of apoplexy, paralysis, and epilepsy but its value is enhanced by the historical approach which McHenry says is 'the first history of neurological thought from the ancients to the turn of the nineteenth century'. It is a fascinating book to which I shall return (p. 167) and its author was clearly a classical scholar and widely read, so his treatment of Willis, in contrast to those of Hippocrates, Galen, Vesalius, Descartes, Whytt, and others, is all the more disappointing and revealing. He could not have thought Willis an important historical figure.

Another nineteenth-century indication of Willis's decline may be gauged from Pettigrew's[236] *Biographical memoirs of the most celebrated physicians and surgeons*. Pettigrew was senior surgeon to Charing Cross Hospital, London, and FRS, and in the preface to his four-volume compendium, he wrote 'None will be admitted into this Portrait Gallery who have not promoted the advancement of Medical Science.' Forty-seven qualified, of whom thirty-seven were English; Vesalius was there but not Willis. Not even the illustrations in *Cerebri anatome* won Willis a mention in that classic work of Choulant[237] on the *History and bibliography of anatomic illustration*.

Munk's *Roll of the Royal College of Physicians* (1878, 2nd edn, p. 341) simply quoted Hutchinson's indictment already mentioned. But redemption was in sight. Medical historians began to disclose that Willis could no longer be thus neglected.

Described as 'one of the finest short works on medical history'[238] Withington's *Medical history from the earliest times*[239] had this to say. After pointing out the significance of Willis's explanation of fermentation, and commenting that it was 'what we now call "metabolism" ', Withington said

> ... Willis and his writings hardly received the attention they deserved, for the countrymen of Harvey and Newton were less attracted by chemical theories than by the rival doctrines of the so-called mathematical or mechanical school (p. 313).

Across the English Channel two illustrious medical historians, Max Neuburger (1868–1955) of Vienna and Jules Soury (1842–1915) of Paris, were starting the process of the re-examination of Willis and evaluating his worth.

Neuburger's book was entitled *The historical development of experimental physiology of the brain and spinal cord prior to Flourens*.[240] In it he convincingly portrays Willis as a scientist of vision who inaugurated 'a new era in the physiology of the brain' (p. 2). He said there were three distinct phases in this field between the middle of the seventeenth and nineteenth centuries. The first, initiated by Willis, brought the concept of localization of cerebral function. The second was the period of Haller (1708–77) and his development of Glisson's concept of irritability, with his rejection of Willis. The third period comprised the years after Haller, ending with the memorable labours of Flourens (1794–1867) who was one of the first to ascribe different functions to different parts of the brain. Each of these periods had its own characteristics; in the Hegelian concept of history they portrayed the negation of the first period by the second, with, in the third period, the negation of the second and the reaffirmation of the first. Willis may have been incorrect in many of his conclusions but he showed that the nervous control of the vital functions probably lay in the brain stem, and he provided experimentalists with a basis for their investigations. He was the first to define precisely the relationship between the central nervous system and the vital organs of the body (p. 7).

Neuburger concluded that the great merit of Willis's work was that it led indirectly to two important developments, which are a feature of modern science. They were the testing of hypotheses in the light of fresh knowledge, and the introduction of new standards in the conduct and interpretation of experiments.[241]

Soury's[242] massive tome of 1899, *The central nervous system; structure and functions; a critical history of theories and doctrines*, is one of those untranslated classics of medicine. Soury devoted fourteen pages to Willis, quoting from the three books *Cerebri anatome*, *Pathologiae cerebri*, and *De anima brutorum*. He praised the manner in which Willis had based his ideas on observations of human anatomy, comparative anatomy, embryology, pathology, experiment, and clinical practice. He was impressed by the demonstration of the sensitivity of the dura and the insensitivity of the brain; by the clear separation of grey and white matter, their distribution and obviously different roles; the importance of the cerebellum and brain stem and the explanation of voluntary and involuntary motion. The anastomotic nature of the vascular supply to the brain was well portrayed ('contre Duret et Charcot'). As for reflex action, both 'the thing and the name, have been clearly observed and described by Willis'.[243] His 'explosion' theory of the epileptic convulsion reminded him of the modern concept of 'nervous discharge'.

Willis, he said,

> ... presents a comprehensive account of the phenomena of life, and the anatomy, physiology and pathology of the nervous system, with the ardour of an artist and with penetrating genius. Whether one considers the structure, the functions, or the diseases of the brain, especially those important disorders of epilepsy and hysteria, there is no point of fact or of theory where one cannot detect the influence of Willis today, and one can readily see, on re-reading the works of the old master, that the living force of his genius is not yet exhausted.[244]

A year later these opinions were not at all shared by a distinguished English professor lecturing in San Francisco. He was Sir Michael Foster FRS, Professor of Physiology at Cambridge University, a founder of the Physiological Society (1875) and the *Journal of Physiology* (1878), a former President of the British Association, a Secretary of the Royal Society for twenty-two years, one of the inaugurators of the first International Congress of Physiology (1889), and author of a textbook of physiology (1876) which with 'its rolling prose, authoritative scholarship, and good sense made it a textbook unexampled among English books'.[245] Moreover he was a classical scholar and antiquarian, although Professor O'Malley has pointed out that all Foster's historical books 'have been criticised for lack of proper historical scholarship.'[246]

When Foster published his *Lectures on the history of physiology* in 1901 he actually confessed in the preface that there were 'many mistakes' but he pleaded 'in excuse that historical research, perhaps above all other kinds of research, demands ample leisure' of which he had little. But surely sufficient to get a couple of Willis dates correct? *Cerebri anatome* was not published in 1659 and Willis did not die in 1666. A modern reader would be excused a wry smile on hearing that a Cambridge professor of that era, after twenty years in his chair, writing on the history of his own subject, should say that 'his little work has been snatched from a life broken into bits by many and varied duties'. But in all fairness it probably was. Foster was an eminent organizer and administrator who sat on many commissions of one kind or another, and he eventually became a member of parliament for the University of London. The Royal Society obituary said 'Foster's active additions to our knowledge by way of research are small and not of great importance. He was a discoverer of men rather than of facts.'[247] There is little doubt that he would have relished the opportunities which the State now offers to such men.

Yet his 'little work' is unique and immensely readable, as generations of students have learned. Foster was able to offer his own eloquent translations of Vesalius, Servetus, Columbus, Fabricius, Harvey, Descartes, Borelli, Malpighi, Stensen, van Helmont, Franciscus Sylvius, De Graaf, Mayow, Lower, von Haller, Stahl, Lavoisier, and Willis. Despite all that has been discovered since it was written it still presents a perspective invaluable to the modern student of physiology. But on Willis he erred; and inexcusably. I am inclined to agree with Sir Charles Symonds who, in telling the story of Foster's account of old Oxford calumnies about Willis, wrote that 'In this I scent something of the odour in which the physiologist held the successful practitioner 50 years ago.'[248]

In the preface to his lectures Foster said that he included some biographical data not only to add to the human interest of the tale 'but also and even more so because, in most cases at least, the fruitfulness of the labours of an inquirer is largely dependent on the inquirer's character and belongings' (presumably intellectual). Willis, he said, quoting Wood, wore himself out 'mostly for lucre sake', and was 'helped or rather instructed' by Lower. The latter, Foster reminded the reader, was 'a real man of science, with a clear penetrating mind, with a genuine love of truth for truth's sake'. But, Foster continued,

> Willis was of a different type; love of truth was in him less potent than love of fame. Mixing with and indeed in daily intercourse with the band of exact inquirers, who at Oxford and in London were striving to establish the new philosophy and advance by experiment natural knowledge, Willis caught up their phrases and thinking himself one of them, attempted to expound in their fashion the physiology of the nervous system . . . Willis's mind was of the rhetorical sort, he loved words as words, looked upon an illustration as an argument, and when he had discovered an analogy thought he had found a proof. Hence when we come to examine the views which he put forward, we find that while they are expounded with a certain philosophical air which perhaps goes far to explain the influence which they had in their time, they do not of themselves form any real solid contribution to knowledge.[249]

Foster did not question that *Cerebri anatome* 'became a classic work' but added that 'The value of the book is indeed much above the worth of the author.' He also considered that in trying to explain the transmission of the nervous impulse, '... Willis may be regarded as dimly striving to explain nervous phenomena on the hypothesis of a specific nervous fluid, possessed of peculiar properties, a kind of foreshadowing of an electric fluid.'[250] Also, as we have said, 'he had dimly laid hold of the modern doctrine of reflex action', and he had 'many sound physiological views'.

But, aside from Foster's poor estimate of Willis's character and scientific talent, what we do not read in his account is any indication that he appreciated how widely Willis had cast his net. Foster's quotations are almost all from sections dealing with Willis's ideas and it is generally agreed that some of them did not make much sense. He does not mention how Willis focused attention on the cortex, how he deduced that in the white matter there were pathways that provided communication between different parts of the nervous system, nor how he demonstrated by dissection, injection, and clinicopathological observation the significance of the arterial circle. There is no record of how he used his studies in comparative anatomy to develop his ideas of cerebral localization, nor any word of the autonomic nervous system. Neither does Foster mention Willis's suggestion that nervous intercommunication might take place in the periphery. With its hint that not all ingoing and outgoing fibres travelled to and from the brain, there was here a glimmer of what Foster so stressed in his textbook – the segmental organization of the spinal cord.

Foster specifically names only *Cerebri anatome* among Willis's books, adding that one other 'special treatise' was devoted to proving 'that the blood is aflame, is burning, that a flame exists in the blood'. Willis's 'great discovery was simply this, that the part of the soul residing in the blood was of the nature of "flame", and the part residing in the brain and nervous system was of the nature of "light"'[251] Naturally, Willis the clinician was not discussed.

It is not surprising, therefore, that anyone reading Foster at the turn of the century should have a very distorted view of the 'Harvey of the Nervous System'. But Foster was an 'impulsive' man, who 'quickly judged a character and – never relinquished it'.[252] His judgement on Willis, seemingly authoritative and indisputable, must have exerted a wide influence in the medical world.

But there were other voices to be heard, less authoritative, perhaps but one at least who emphasized the wide range of Willis's enquiries. Sir Benjamin Ward Richardson (1828–96),[253] one of the ardent social reformers of the nineteenth century, physician,† man of science and letters, has left us his estimate of Willis in his *Disciples of Aesculapius* (published posthumously). In it he said 'The works of Thomas Willis in the physiological department of medical learning are more original and remarkable than the anatomical. They display a genius of the highest order.'[254] Richardson referred to all eleven treatises and concluded, in regard to *De anima brutorum*, that 'two souls was not a bad working hypothesis for one who lived

† He was the first to note the effects of inhaling amyl nitrite, and of spraying the skin with ether.

when belief in witchcraft and cure by Royal Touch were accepted as real truth. ... In reality he ranks among the great decemvirate of physic and is not second to any one of that immortal band.' A glimpse of the extent of Richardson's own vision of things may be caught in the title of a book he had planned to write with Cardinal Manning – *The physiology of sin*!

During the twentieth century, as we have seen, there has been a searching examination and reassessment of Willis's works, crowned by the reprinting of *Cerebri anatome* and the publication of the first monograph on Willis in 1965. In the introduction to the English edition of Isler's monograph in 1968, the eminent Zurich historian of medicine, Professor Erwin H. Ackerknecht, wrote that the book presented a view of 'Willis's work as a whole and not as an agglomeration of discoveries'. He continued,

> In the case of British medical history of the seventeenth century, for decades the interest of medical historians has been concentrated on William Harvey and Thomas Sydenham, and numerous other outstanding figures of that most brilliant period have not been considered. Probably the greatest of these forgotten men is Thomas Willis.[255]

Now, fortunately, we can understand why that celebrated German scientist, Karl Friedrich Burdach (1776–1847)[256] said, a hundred and sixty years ago, that 'England with Willis is in the front line'.[257] Now, too, we can echo the words of Sherrington that Willis 'put the brain and nervous system on their modern footing'.[258] Today, Sigerist's[259] *The great doctors* and D'Arcy Power's[260] *British masters of medicine* would have to include Willis; and if another symposium with the title 'The history and philosophy of the brain and its functions' was to be held, Willis would assuredly receive more than the passing consideration dispensed only twenty years ago.[261]

Some have thought that Willis was no scientist. But Sir Peter Medawar[262] has explained that you cannot formally separate the creative and the critical components of scientific thinking – 'Though imaginative thought and criticism are equally necessary to a scientist, they are often very unequally developed in any one man.' What Willis's writings do disclose is his 'imaginative grasp of *what might be true*',[263] and he adopted all the means at his disposal to ascertain the truth. To wit, as the old master would say, 'To unlock the secret places of Man's mind'.

Willis in history recalls the words of the historian G. M. Trevelyan[264] in his essay on 'Bias in History'. 'All history is a matter of opinion based on facts, of opinion guided and limited by facts that have been scientifically discovered. But the opinion, or bias, cannot itself be scientific. It must be philosophic.'

Analogies are often superficial but one cannot resist commenting that Willis's star declined like Haydn's, as those of Mozart and Beethoven rose, only to glitter again in recent years.

PART II

The eighteenth century

CHAPTER 4

AN AGE OF TRANSITION: PHILOSOPHY TO SCIENCE

Whether or not is there in the brain any principal part, in which resides the origin of all motion, the end of all the sensations, and where the soul has its seat?

The nervous liquor then, which is the instrument of sense and motion, must be exceedingly moveable, so as to carry the impressions of sense, or the commands of the will, to the places of their destination, without any remarkable delay.

But concerning the nature of this nervous fluid, there are many doubts. Many of the moderns will have it to be extremely elastic, of an etherial or of an electrical matter.

Albrecht von Haller in *First Lines of Physiology*, 1767, 3rd edn.

INTRODUCTION

The medical landscape of the eighteenth century is not one that is universally attractive. The picture of the fashionable physician or quack which has come down to us in portraits, caricatures, and writings, with his periwig, gilt-buttoned satin coat, breeches, silver-buckled shoes, and gold-headed cane, is certainly not one to inspire respect. Then, too, there was the intellectual atmosphere of the times which, despite the growth of humanism, was still deeply charged with philosophy, much of it tiresome and hindering the emancipation of science. Newton said 'I have long since determined to concern myself no further about the promotion of philosophy.'[1a] One might have expected, after Harvey, a great burst of discoveries, but it was only toward the end of the century that things livened up with Lavoisier's (1743–94) discovery of the gaseous exchange in respiration and Galvani's (1737–98) electrophysiology. In addition, there were the too ambitious schemes of the classifiers and systematists, not to mention the cults of mesmerism, homeopathy, and magnetism.[1b]

Robert Frost said of the system-makers

> I love to toy with the Platonic notion
> That wisdom need not be of Athens Attic,
> But well may be laconic, even Boeotian.
> At least I will not have it systematic.[2]

The years 1700 to 1750 have recently been called 'The lost half-century in English Medicine' by one medical historian.[3] Of course, the educated man had much to assimilate and think about. There was an unprecedented spread of knowledge, with new institutions, encyclopaedias, and periodicals, and the replacement of Latin by the vernacular. William Cullen's (1712–90) lectures in Glasgow in 1757 were among the first to be given in the English language. The sensational discoveries of Galileo, Kepler, and Newton had led to concepts of the Universe and Nature freed of any spiritual order. There were fresh ways of investigating the structure and function of the human body with the advent of physics, chemistry, embryology, and comparative anatomy. There were new instruments that measured time, temperature, and pressure, and there was the microscope. But the most important influence of all must have been the lesson of Harvey's discovery, namely, the value of physiological experiment when combined with accurate observation and correct inference. Yet theorizing remained more popular than experimentation and the new instruments were only really developed and exploited in the nineteenth century.

The halting nature of medical progress may even be exemplified in the case of two outstanding developments of the century, Boerhaave's (1668–1738) method of bedside teaching in Leyden and Morgagni's (1682–1771) method of clinicopathological correlation. After the death of Boerhaave bedside teaching in Leyden lapsed for forty years,[4] while, despite the pioneering work of Malpighi (1628–94), his compatriot Morgagni wholly neglected the microscope, as also did Bichat (1771–1802) who is rightly honoured as the founder of histology. Had he not died so young Bichat would surely have taken up the microscope in the course of his study of tissues. But Morgagni had enjoyed ample time, living as he did to the ripe old age of ninety.

Nevertheless the eighteenth century saw the change from speculative systems to pathological and clinical concepts, and the rise of nosology. And throughout the century the conflict between animism and mechanism was a persistent theme in medical thought.[5] The forces thought to be at work in the nervous system, traditionally immaterial or humoral, were now also envisaged in mechanical forms.[6] At the end of the century they were replaced by electrical forces, and for a time the notion of an electric fluid in nerves was thereby extended. But the way was now open to the discovery of 'the universal currency of the nervous system' – the nerve impulse.

GENERAL CONCEPTS OF NERVOUS FUNCTION

We have seen that by the eighteenth century the humoral neurophysiology of Galen was largely, but not wholly, discredited. But what was to replace it? What was known of the composition of the gross structures of the nervous system – the brain, the spinal cord, and the nerves – and the interrelation of their parts was quite elementary, while the mode of transmission within the system remained wholly mysterious.

Descartes' purely mechanistic views and Willis's chemical ones were to be overtaken, largely through the influence of Newtonian physics. The significance of the ideas of force and motion in the universe came to be appreciated by those investigating the function of the human body. Newton himself suggested that sensation and motion might be transmitted by the vibrations of a 'spirit' which might be 'electric' or 'elastic'. The pursuit of this spirit and its passage through the nerve fibre was a dominant theme throughout the century, and, with the continuing search for the sensorium commune, marks the final years of the long history of these concepts.

There was a general acceptance of the notion that within the brain there was a common centre or zone – the sensorium commune – where all forms of sensation were correlated. It was sought for no longer in the ventricles or in the vicinity of the pineal gland, but in the solid parts of the brain itself. Vieussens (1641–1715) preferred to locate it in the centrum ovale, rather than in Willis's corpus striatum; Haller (1708–77) chose the medullary white matter, others the corpora quadrigemina, the thalamus, and even the spinal cord. Prochaska[7] (1749–1820) excluded only the hemispheres of the cerebrum and cerebellum and wrote that 'the sensorium commune reflects sensorial into motor impressions'. The century ended with Soemmerring (1755–1830), apparently impressed by the way in which most of the cranial nerves originated in the walls of the ventricles where they were bathed in the cerebrospinal fluid, concluded that the fluid, as of yore, must contain the seat of the soul and the sensorium commune. It was an extraordinary quixotic judgement to come from the leading anatomist of his day, but the sensorium commune was still being sought by Rolando (1773–1821) who placed it in the medulla oblongata.[8]

With regard to transmission in nerves, the ancient view that they were hollow still persisted in many quarters and what flowed through them was thought to be a very 'subtle' fluid or vapour. The idea of circulation in the nervous system was probably sustained to some extent by Harvey's success in proving that there was one in the cardiovascular system. Some, like Willis, thought that nerves or their fibres were porous, but Haller and Boerhaave both favoured the concept of hollow threads or fibres. The fluid, some argued, might be invisible, like air. Nerve ligation, though it produced motor and sensory paralysis, did not cause the nerve to swell above the ligature from arrest of flow, and few saw any juice escape from the cut end. But that 'something' was stopped in its path seemed to be a reasonable inference, and observation of artefacts, minute vascular channels, and imagination did the rest. At the end of the century hollow nerve fibres became a dying concept, with the coming of electrophysiology, but they were not finally banished until 1883 when Remak demonstrated the solid nature of the axon – the true nerve fibre.[9]

In the eighteenth century Rather[10] has suggested that the 'fibre' occupied a position in physiology that was taken up by the 'cell' in the nineteenth century. To Boerhaave, Haller, and others the 'fibre' represented a fundamental unit in structure and function, and, to a considerable extent, also in their notions of pathology. 'What was being searched for by these investigators', Rather writes, 'was an ultimate structural and functional unit of life.' Their answer was the 'fibre'. To Morgagni the anatomical elements were 'apparently nothing else than the fibrils arranged in different ways'[11] so it is astonishing that he should have so wholly rejected the microscope.

NEUROANATOMY

Just as the inadequacy of the early microscopes extended the belief in the hollow nerve doctrine, so also did it retard the examination of the internal structure of the brain and spinal cord. Stensen (p. 99) had warned anatomists of the difficulties and limitations of brain dissection, and in advocating his method of tracing fibre pathways he said that 'it is so full of difficulties that I do not know whether one may hope ever to complete the task *without very special preparations*' (my italics).[12] Eighteenth-century anatomists employed all the methods discussed by Stensen and macroscopic tracing of fibre tracts was pursued until the early decades of the nineteenth century. Reil's (1759–1813) technique of hardening the brain in alcohol came only at the end of the century and particularly simplified the task of unravelling the ramifications of the white matter in the hemispheres and brain stem. Willis had advocated the study of comparative neuroanatomy and Steno had emphasized the potential value of studying the growth of nervous tissue. But little had been done in these directions until the nineteenth century, when Stensen's 'very special preparations' proved to be the techniques of fixation, staining, and the application of the processes of Wallerian degeneration and myelogenesis to this field of neuro-anatomy.

Despite the crude nature of the microscopes Malpighi, two years after the publication of Willis's *Anatomy of the brain*, in which he had read of Willis's observations on the grey matter of the cortex, reported that it resembled the structure of a pomegranate and was composed of tiny 'glands'. Malpighi prepared his brains by boiling them, stripping away the three meningeal membranes, and pouring ink over the convolutions before examining them.

> I have discovered in the brain of the higher sanguinous animals that the cortex is formed from a mass of very minute glands. These are found in the cerebral gyri which are like tiny intestines and in which the white roots of the nerves terminate or, if you prefer, from which they originate.[13]

In 1684 Leeuwenhoek (1632–1723) thought that the cortex of a turkey's brain was full of 'globules'. Neither of these findings about the cortex was confirmed by Ruysch (1638–1731) who asserted (in 1699) that it was composed of nothing more than a mass of tiny blood vessels. Ruysch was the subject of one of the many medical biographies written by Dr Samuel Johnson who described the evolution of Ruysch's technique, with the use of de Graaf's 'new species of syringe' and Swammerdam's 'warm substance' which solidified on cooling and was 'retained in the vessels'. This was wax and it enabled one to see vessels 'as slender as the threads of a spider's web', even 'without the assistance of a microscope'. Ruysch's corpses were thus made to 'glow with the striking lustre and bloom of youth.'[14] 'In short, the mummies of Mr. Ruysch were so many prolongations of life; whereas those of the ancient Egyptians were only so many continuations of death.'[15]

Dr Johnson even commented on Ruysch's finding that 'the cortical substance of the brain was not glandular, as was commonly thought, but consisted of vessels infinitely ramified'. Ruysch indeed came to believe that tissues were but vascular networks variously arranged, so completely did his injected vessels mask any parenchymatous elements.

Clarke and Bearn,[16] adopting Malpighi's techniques and using a seventeenth-century microscope to scrutinize specimens of cerebral cortex, came to the conclusion that his 'glands' were not neurones, but artefacts, areas of brain tissue outlined by the ink-stained capillaries of the grey matter.

But the inference of these early investigators of the cortical grey matter was that it probably secreted a substance which was transmitted to the white matter and thence to the rest of the nervous system. There was general acceptance of this view and it conformed to the traditional concept of neuro-humoral activity. Meyer[17] suggests that Malpighi's observations may have even influenced Soemmerring in deciding the location of the sensorium commune.

Microscopists fared better when it came to the nerves. The findings of Leeuwenhoek, Monro II (1733–1817), and Fontana (1730–1805) are generally regarded as the most significant. Leeuwenhoek sectioned nerves and spinal cord and thought that nerve fibres were composed of a series of globules. He looked for canals, failed to find them, but later thought they were actually there, tending to disappear like the globules, when his specimens dried up. One of his illustrations is thought to be the first

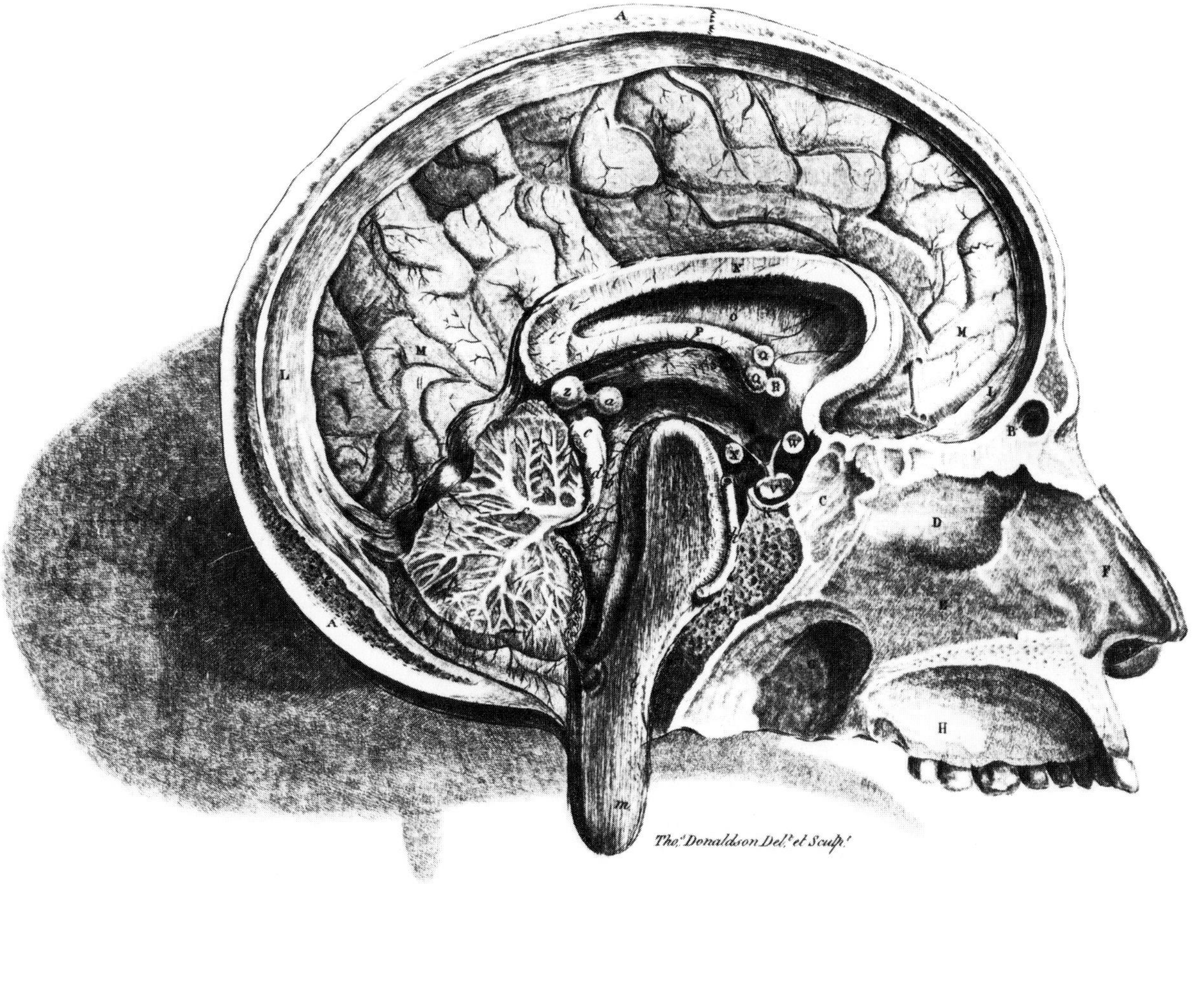

FIG. 40. Sagittal section of the head; the interventricular foramen (S) behind the anterior crura of the fornix (QQ); the anterior commissure (R); the posterior commissure (a) anterior to the pineal gland (Z); the valve of Vieussens (e); Note the closed lower end of the fourth ventricle 'shut by the vascular or choroid plexus and pia mater'. (After Monro II.[32])

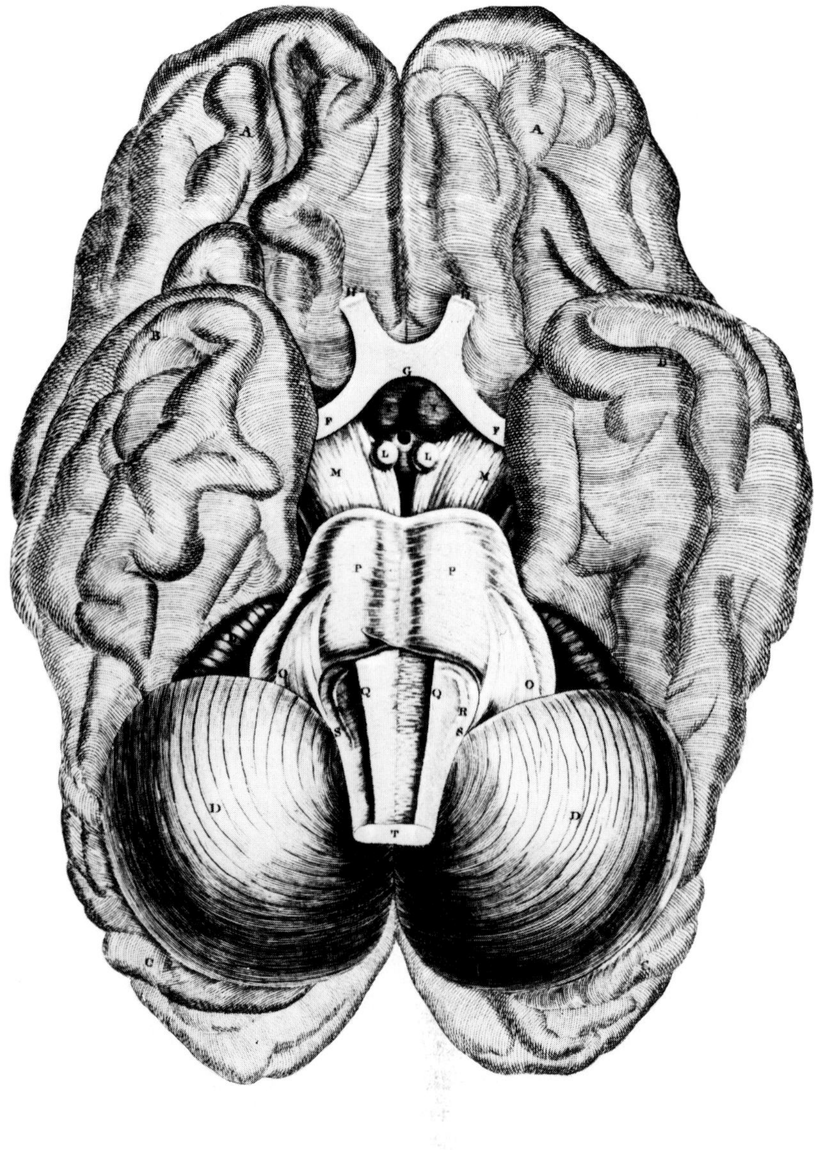

FIG. 41. Base of brain, without the cranial nerves, to show 'the general direction of the medullary fibres' in cerebral peduncles (M), the cerebellar peduncles (O), the pons (P), and the pyramids (Q). On the surface of the latter are 'fibres disposed transversely'; in the fissure between the pyramids are 'decussating bundles'. In the original plate, lines of decussation can be seen in the optic chiasm. 'But unless I am much deceived I have seen in man an intermixture and partial decussation of the cords which compose the optic nerves' (p. 43). (After Monro II.[32])

representation of a cross-section of a nerve.[18] Whether he actually observed axons and myelin sheath is uncertain. Monro I (1697–1767) wrote in 1746 that 'the nerves are composed of a great many threads lying parallel to each other' and that of the 'minimum visible it is demonstrated that each fibre of the retina, or expanded optic nerve, cannot exceed the size of the 32 400th part of a hair'.[19] He was one of those who found no sign of a nerve fluid in the course of ligation experiments. His son (Monro II) used a microscope to study nerve fibres but was troubled by artefacts and did not pursue the matter. However, it is thought that his work stimulated Fontana who provided the best descriptions of nerves in the eighteenth century. He identified the fibre as the essential element of the nerve, naming it the 'primitive axis cylinder' and he noted the presence of an outer sheath. Authorities are not sure whether he was describing actual axis cylinders with their myelin sheaths, or only fibres and endoneurium.[20, 21]

Naked eye dissection of the brain, especially in the second half of the century, continued to provide many valuable descriptions and illustrations of the various structures and regions of the brain. Even Gall (1758–1828) and Spurzheim (1776–1832), near the turn of the century, found that in tracing fibre tracts the scraping technique used by Willis was preferable to the microscope. Their skill and success were renowned. Reil (1759–1813) wrote that 'In Gall's anatomic demonstrations of the brain I have seen more than I thought possible for one man to discover in the course of a long lifetime.'[22] Mention has been made (p. 18) of Gennari's discovery of the lamination of the cortex in 1776, independently confirmed by Vicq d'Azyr in 1786 and by Soemmerring in 1788. Gennari's frozen brain also contained 'in their ventricles, water converted into minute icicles' presumably Cotugno's (1736–1822) cerebrospinal fluid which he described in 1761.[23]

The internal structure of the brain attracted more attention than the convolutions and sulci, few of which were identified or named by 1900. Vicq d'Azyr began to draw attention to them, illustrating the fissure of Sylvius, the central sulcus, the occipito-parietal and calcaine fissures, and the pre- and post-central convolutions.[24, 25] The varying size, shape, colour, and relationships of the internal masses of grey matter were described and illustrated in the atlases of the day. Among the most renowned were those of Ruysch (1724), Winslow (1733), Santorini (1775), Haller (1781), Vicq d'Azyr (1786), and Soemmerring (1788). The identification and naming of anatomical structures is a complex process and the importance of the historical perspective in neuroanatomy has been emphasized by Meyer.[26] Nomenclature was a considerable problem; even now, for example, there is no general agreement as to what exactly comprise the 'basal ganglia'.

Willis's corpus striatum was gradually subdivided into what we now call the lentiform and caudate nuclei, the former with an outer putamen and an inner, paler, globus pallidus. Santorini's name is associated with the red nucleus, and Soemmerring's with the substantia nigra. The characteristic shapes of the caudate nucleus, the fornix, and the thalamus were increasingly defined. The term 'medulla oblongata' came to be restricted to that portion of the brain stem below the cerebral peduncles (named by Winslow) and the pons. Winslow renamed the 'intercostal nerve', calling it the 'grand sympathetic'.

Illustrations of the base of the brain were more detailed and accurate; those of Vicq d'Azyr and Soemmerring were renowned. Soemmerring, 'Herr Neurologue' to his professor (Wrisberg, 1739–1808), is now best remembered for his classification of the cranial nerves into twelve pairs. Previously the ninth, tenth, and eleventh nerves were grouped together as one pair because of their common exit from the skull.

The cerebellum

The distinctive appearance of the cerebellum with its rather flat lobes and

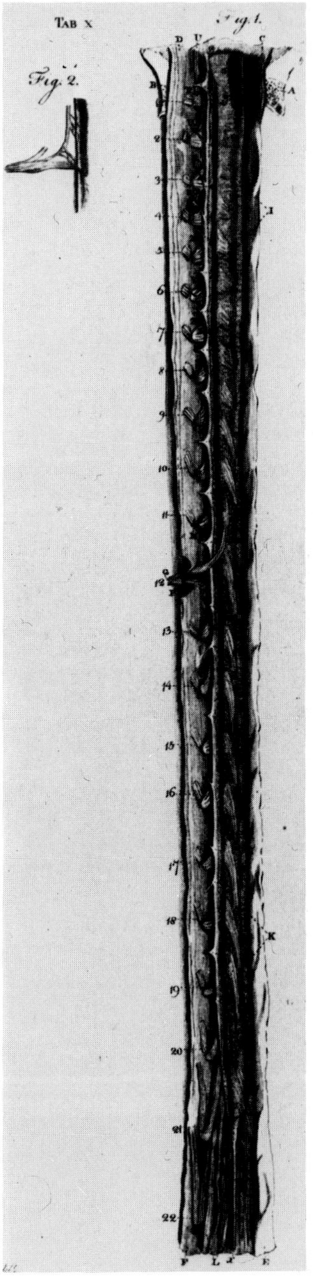

FIG. 42. Anterior view of spinal cord, with meninges reflected on right, and anterior roots sectioned. At (12), the fifth dorsal roots, a ganglion is depicted (P). Monro noted the septum which separated the anterior and posterior root bundles in the dural foramen. *Fig. 2* illustrates the accessory nerve connection to the cord and spinal nerve. (After Monro II.[32])

thin, uniform convolutions, continued to intrigue anatomists and invite comment. Galen's notion of a valvular function for the vermis was replaced by Vieussen's interpretation of a similar role for the anterior medullary velum. Stretching between the superior cerebellar peduncles, across the roof of the fourth ventricle, he viewed it as a mechanism which effectively closed off the upper end of the fourth ventricle. He was among the first to note the tree-like branching of the cerebellar white matter; he confirmed Willis's description of the three cerebellar peduncles, and noted a rhomboid-shaped mass of central grey matter in each hemisphere which was later to be named the dentate necleus by Vicq d'Azyr. In 1776, the first monograph devoted to the cerebellum was published by the Italian surgeon and anatomist, Malacarne.[27] It was not illustrated but he discussed the grouping of the convolutions into lobes and gave us the terms tonsil, uvula, and lingula. He also wrote on anomalies of the nervous system and on comparative anatomy.

The spinal cord

Neither Vesalius nor Willis had focused much attention on the spinal cord although Coiter (1534–76) and Blasius (1626?–92) had both noted the anterior and posterior spinal nerve roots and the grey and white matter of the cord itself (Fig. 43).[28,29] But by the end of the eighteenth century, the two Edinburgh medical students, Charles Bell (1774–1842) and Marshall Hall (1790–1857) who subsequently made outstanding contributions to

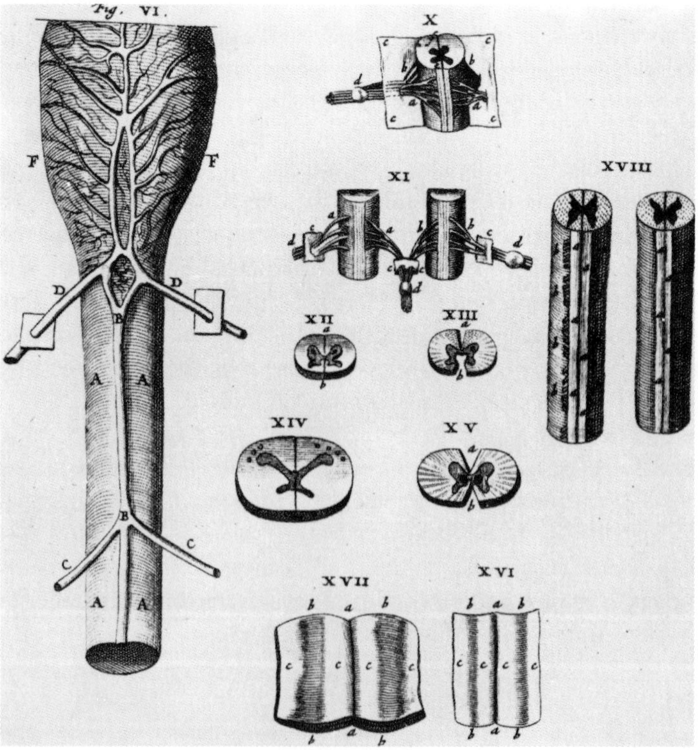

FIG. 43. After Blasius (1626?–92) of Amsterdam, author of the first important book on the spinal cord.[20] He illustrated the shape of the grey matter within the cord, the separate origin of the spinal roots, the dorsal root ganglion, the anterior spinal and vertebral arteries, and a double basilar artery. Blasius edited an *Opera omnia* of Thomas Willis in 1682.

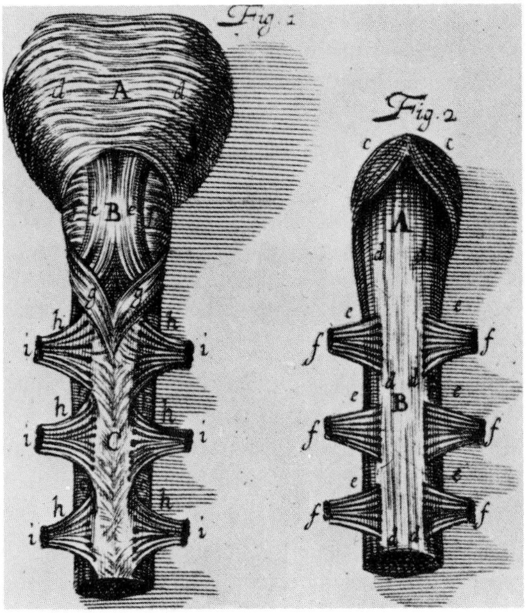

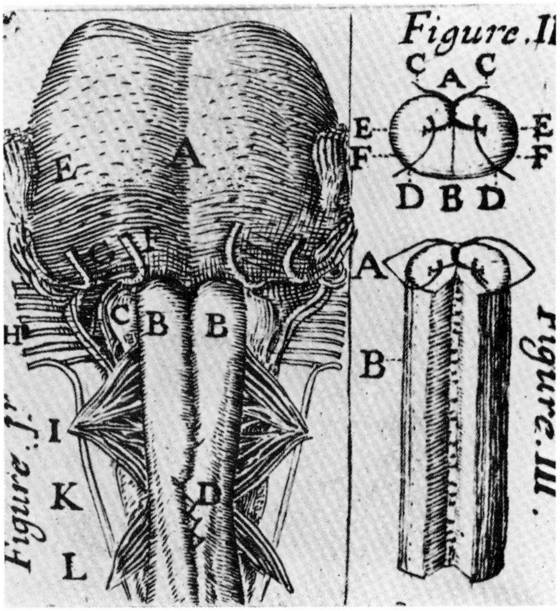

FIG. 44 (*left*). *Fig. 1* shows decussating external fibres in the brain stem at *g*. *Fig. 2* shows them at *c*. In another illustration he showed the outward rotation of a hemiplegic leg. (After Mistichelli (1675–1715). *Tratto dell'apoplessia*. Rome (1709).) A microfilm copy of this very rare document may be seen at the Wellcome Institute for the History of Medicine, London.

FIG. 45 (*right*). The legend for *Fig. I* reads 'It represents the change of the medullary fibres (*D*) from one side to the other.' For *Fig. II*, 'The spinal cord cut across'; *E*, transverse fibres; *F*, 'dark lines from the transverse fibres to posterior part.' For *Fig. III*, A section of cord to show at *A*, 'the junction of anterior and posterior nerves', and at *B*, the transverse fibres 'in the depth of the posterior longitudinal division' of the cord. (After Pourfour du Petit (1664–1741). *Lettres d'un medecin* (1710).) A copy of the book may be seen in the British Museum.

knowledge of the spinal cord, could have learned little about it from their books and lectures. The 'double' nature, or symmetry, of the cord, with its shallow posterior and deep anterior median sulci and transverse commissural fibres, was noted by many anatomists and during the century it was increasingly appreciated that the cord was composed of two substances. There was the H-shaped arrangement of the grey matter as it appeared in cross section, and the columnar distribution of the fibrous white matter. But the vital question of the decussation of the pyramidal motor pathways was still unresolved at the end of the century.

The ancients had known that an injury to one side of the head might cause contralateral epilepsy or hemiplegia, and autopsies by Wepfer, Willis, Morgagni, and others had revealed the hemisphere lesions. But it was not yet appreciated that the hemisphere lesion was *always* contralateral. The crossed paralysis was thought merely to disclose that each side of the body received nervous energy from both sides of the brain, one of Nature's arrangements which ensured that unilateral brain damage would not *always* result in hemiparesis. The apparently 'double' nature of the spinal cord seemed to support this explanation.

But decussation of pathways in the brain stem had actually been described and illustrated by Mistichelli (1675–1715) in 1709 and by Pourfour du Petit (1664–1741) in 1710. Both works are very rare but Thomas[30] in 1910 was able to study them, and it appears that Mistichelli's famous illustration (Fig. 44) depicts the crossing of the fibres of the meningeal membranes of the medulla, from which he thought that nerves arose. On the other hand, Pourfour du Petit described and illustrated the actual decussation of the pyramids (Fig. 45) in explanation of the clinical effects of hemisphere lesions he had seen in patients or produced experimentally in dogs. Nevertheless, for most of the century, the generally accepted view was that of the 'double' nature of the spinal cord, and there were various accounts of the connections between the two halves. Haller saw them as part of the system of commissures which included the corpus callosum and other cerebral and cerebellar cross-connections.

Moreover, by this contrivance, nature seems to have provided, that, in whatever part of the brain any injury may happen, the nerve that arises from thence is, by this means, not always deprived of its use. For if the said nerve receives its fibres by communicating bundles, as well from the opposite as from its own hemisphere of the brain, its office may in some measure be continued entire by the fibres which it receives from the opposite side, even after those of its own side are destroyed.[31]

Vicq d'Azyr had similar views. Monro II was less impressed by the extent of the commissural fibres and did not describe or illustrate the decussation in 1783.[32] It was left to Gall and Spurzheim to definitely establish the decussation of the pyramids, rediscovering, as it were, the works of Mistichelli and Pourfour du Petit, and making clear the distinction from the transverse medullary and spinal connections.

The sensory pathways of the spinal cord were not elucidated until the nineteenth century.

'Animated anatomy' was how Haller regarded physiology, and his neurophysiology was based on an anatomy in which he accepted that injection studies had shown that the cerebral cortex was essentially vascular, that 'much the greater part of it consists of mere vessels'[33]; that 'the fibres of the brain are continuous with those of the nerves, so as to form one extended and open continuation'[34]; and in which the nerves themselves were composed of fibres that were hollow, although 'not visible by any microscope'.[35] If they had been solid, he argued, to transmit sensation and motion, they would have to be hard, tense, or elastic; and they were not.

The cerebrospinal fluid

The ventricular system, with its disputed communicating channels, and its contents, was another area to be explored. The wetness of the brain and the occurrence of hydrocephalus were known since ancient times; moist or watery humours were an accepted feature, but whether there was any difference between the living and the dead remained unknown. Willis had suggested that the choroid plexuses had something to do with the ventricular contents but the fluid's excretory role continued to be discussed well into the eighteenth century. The concept of a circulation of the fluid depended on knowledge of the foramina of Monro (first described by Galen, see p. 18), which he described in 1783, although he failed to find any exit foramina in the fourth ventricle. Magendie's and Luschka's findings were published in 1828 and 1855, respectively. As for the communication between the third and fourth ventricles, which Galen sought but seemingly did not discover (see p. 19), it is generally agreed that it was Franciscus Sylvius (1614–72) who established that the aqueduct passed through the substance of the mid-brain.[36]

There was confusion, however, about the origin and destination of the cerebral fluid, whether it was a normal or abnormal constituent, and whether it began as a vapour or not. It was a mysterious substance and Willis's observations and conjectures about it were disputed. Indeed, Ridley (1695) doubted its existence and failed to find any in the third and fourth ventricles 'in subjects free from those diseases incident to that part'. They both considered the fourth ventricle to be too small to serve as a reservoir. No one had established that it was one and the same fluid which was found in the ventricles and basal cisterns, and which covered the hemispheres. And it was certainly not known that it also bathed the spinal cord.

Here the story of the role played by Swedenborg (1688–1772), mystic and theologian, is an extraordinary one.[37,38] A native of Stockholm, he graduated from the University of Uppsala in 1709, mathematics, mineralogy, and geology being his initial interests and mining his occupation until middle life. Then, he took up the study of biology, anatomy, and physiology, spending several years studying and dissecting (and apparently experimenting) in various European medical schools. His biological writings, which included some on the brain, were published between 1740 and 1744, but a treatise on *The brain* was left in manuscript form when he abruptly turned to considerations of the soul, an exercise that occupied him for the rest of his life. He died in poverty in London in 1772. Maudsley[39] considered that Swedenborg suffered from episodes of insanity, an opinion hotly contested by Tafel, a member of the New Church of America, a denomination that grew up around Swedenborg's teachings. In 1868 Tafel discovered unpublished manuscripts of Swedenborg in the Library of the Academy of Sciences in Stockholm. He translated them into English and they were published by the Swedenborg Society in London, in two volumes, in 1882 and 1887, entitled *The brain considered anatomically, physiologically and philosophically*.[40] Further translations of other Swedenborg manuscripts on the brain were published in 1938 and 1940.[41]

The cerebrospinal fluid, Swedenborg said, was formed in the cerebrum and cerebellum, and the choroid plexuses of the lateral and fourth ventricles took part in its formation.

> This most refined lymph of the cerebellum is soon joined by a lymph, endowed with a fresh spirit from the choroid plexus which lines both sides of the ventricle. This plexus serves to show that the same kind of lymph is distilled into this cistern, as into the lateral ventricles . . .[42]

Swedenborg also said that the fourth ventricle 'hands it [the cerebrospinal fluid] over for distribution to the medulla oblongata, and especially over the spinal marrow'.[43] 'It seems also to express this liquid through a cleft in its ceiling, between the pia and dura mater, and thence into the spinal cord' where it filled the subarachnoid space, bathing the cord and its nerve roots.[44]

But the fluid in the lateral and third ventricles was confined there by Vieussen's valve; it was a coarser substance of an excretory nature. The liquid which bathed the surface of the brain was probably a product of the pia mater or the surface arterioles. It collected at the base of the brain and around the medulla, and

Thither it flows from both brains, and thither it is conveyed from the whole circumference of the medulla oblongata, and thence, through the foramen magnum of the occiput, it descends toward the posterior surface of the cord.[45]

How fascinated Magendie would have been. He had retrieved Cotugno's neglected contribution, buried as it was in his account of sciatica, and republished it with his own work. Magendie found his foramen 'at the base of the fourth ventricle opposite to the calamus scriptorius'. Swedenborg had written, nearly a hundred years earlier,

Whether there are still other channels for the discharge of the lymph, namely, whether such a channel opens immediately from the calamus scriptorius into the medullary portion of the spinal marrow, to my knowledge has not yet been discovered.[46]

In the meantime, Haller had emphasized the physical properties of the fluid and its vaporous origin from the arteries in the form of a 'sweat' or 'exhalation', and its absorption by the veins. He also suggested that it flowed out 'through the bottom of the skull, and from thence into the spinal medulla'. But he thought the fluid lay between the dura and the arachnoid.

When the renowned Haller was writing these words in Bern, after seventeen years in Göttingen, young Cotugno (1736–1822), in Naples, was busy examining 'this large and capital cavity of the spine', so neglected 'by many famous men'. 'I have no doubt', he concluded, 'that the great Physician Haller's opinion is founded on fact'. Cotugno was seeking the cause of sciatica† and had recognized that there was a 'nervous' and an 'arthritic' type; it was the former which puzzled him, especially the 'posterior' variety. He concluded, without ever seeing an autopsy on such a case, that the responsible lesion lay in the sciatic nerve.

If the patient will but point out with his finger the track of the pain from the sacrum to the foot, we shall find him, like a skilful anatomist, tracing out the precise progress of the sciatic nerve ... In this nerve the pain is felt, in this nerve we should search for the cause of lameness, and from its affection the origin of the paresis and wasting.[47]

Cotugno referred to the Eustachius plates which depicted the course of the nerve and recommended blisters at certain points. The nerve, he thought, was irritated by some 'acrid matter' which might be derived from the cerebrospinal fluid, 'as they [the nerves] are full of a humour which they receive from the brain'. He noted that the sheaths of the spinal nerves ended at the ganglia and that fluid could not flow beyond them. Only when forced†† would air or quicksilver pass peripherally, but 'dropsy' of the nerve, he considered, was a likely lesion in sciatica, and so he was led to look further into 'this collection of water about the brain, and in the spine'. Anatomists had missed it, he said, 'owing to the preposterous method of dissecting, for when they are about to examine the brain, they commonly cut off the head from the neck ... all the water flows out ... and is foolishly lost'.

He dissected the 'dural tube' of the spine in twenty human autopsies and, seeking to learn whether the cerebrospinal fluid was present in living animals, he carried out vivisections in fishes, fowl, dogs, and the 'sea-

† The Boston neurologist and medical historian, H. R. Viets, writing about Cotugno in 1935 (*Bull. Hist. Med.* 3, 701), made the curious statement that sciatica was 'now a rare disease' thanks to 'modern therapeusis with the removal of foci of infection in teeth, tonsils, sinuses, appendix, prostate and gall bladder, and less exposure to damp and faulty working conditions'. The classic paper of Mixter and Barr, also of Boston, proving the role of the intervertebral disc, had appeared in the *New England Journal of Medicine* in 1934).

†† The author regretfully remembers the treatment of sciatica by pumping oxygen into the buttock.

tortoise of about fifteen pounds weight'. He concluded that 'all that space, therefore, which is around the spinal marrow, is filled with water naturally, and in this respect, a dead body varies little or nothing from a living one'.

He noted that the brain and spinal cord shrank in old people and consumptives, so that water accumulated around them. In the erect position when the brain of a corpse is exposed and the dura punctured, water may flow out; if the brain is then lifted up gently more water will be seen at its base; if the brain is removed by cutting through the medulla 'the tube of the dura mater will be found to be exactly full of this water all around the spinal marrow'; on spinal transection in the lumbar region 'you will find a limpid stream flow out . . .'.

Lastly, he wrote of the erect corpse, 'If you open the vertebrae of the loins before the head is touched, and cut the enclosed tube of the dura mater, a great quantity of water will burst out . . .'.

His watery fluid was clear, occasionally a little yellow, and in adults he usually succeeded in drawing off five or six ounces. But it was red and opaque 'in foetuses strangled in difficult labour'. Unlike Haller, who said that cerebrospinal fluid coagulated on heating, Cotugno's merely steamed away and left no residue.

The cerebrospinal fluid of Cotugno, then, was a liquid and not a vapour.

> Those waters which the ventricle of the *Cerebellum* received, either from the greater ventricles of the brain, by the Lacunae, or Sylvius's aqueduct, or the proper exhaling arteries, were afterwards mixed with those of the spine; as here, their perpendicular position, and the free passage that is about the cavity of the spine, sufficiently prove to us that there is a defluxion of humours to the spine.[48]

All this at the age of twenty-eight years.

ALBRECHT VON HALLER (1708–1777) AND NEUROPHYSIOLOGY

There were major advances in two fields of neurophysiology in the eighteenth century. These were the elaboration of the concept of reflex action and the discovery of the role played by the spinal cord, and the introduction of electrophysiology. Progress was also made in the doctrine of the localization of cerebral function. As it happened, the foremost physiologist of the century, that phenomenal scholar and tireless experimenter, Haller, subscribed little to these developments, and indeed, through his authority and the multitude of his scientific publications (said to have been over 1300), one could argue that he actually retarded the approach to the concepts of reflex action and cortical supremacy initiated by Willis in the previous century. He is certainly not deserving of the title 'The Harvey of the Nervous System', bestowed on him by the German medical historian, Baas.[49] Haller's fame in neurophysiology rests on his contributions to different concepts – those of 'irritability' and 'sensitivity' – which dominated physiological thought for a century.†[51–56]

An extraordinarily indefatigable man, poet, botanist, classicist, philosopher, he was a pupil of Boerhaave, and for seventeen years Professor of Medicine in the newly-founded University of Göttingen. A Fellow of the

† Claude Bernard was to say that Haller's 'physiology is reduced to an irritable fibre and a sensitive fibre'. (*Introduction to the study of experimental medicine*. Dover, New York (1957). p. 106.)

Royal Society of London, he was created a Baron by George II and appointed his consultant physician, but he declined an invitation to the Chair of Medicine at Oxford. His *First lines of physiology* (1747) was translated into English and has recently been reprinted[57] but his monumental, eight-volume *elementa physiologiae* (1757–66) remains in its original Latin. He also published a treatise on anatomy and he may be regarded as the founder of medical bibliography. In his four volumes on the bibliography of botany, anatomy, surgery, and medicine he classified more than 52 000 publications providing annotations and reviews. It is sad to read that his funeral in his native city of Bern was a humble affair, without ceremony or oration, or even a permanent memorial to mark his grave. Robert Whytt (1714–66) of Edinburgh, Haller's doughty opponent, fared better in this respect, with a public funeral, 'the Principal and Professors of the University, attired in their gowns and preceded by the mace attended his remains to the grave, while the whole body of the College of physicians joined in the procession'.[58] A Latin-inscribed tombstone marks his grave in Greyfriars Churchyard.

In his classic paper of 1753, 'A Dissertation on *the* Sensible and Irritable Parts of Animals,'[59] Haller explained that 'irritability' was a biological property first discovered and named by Glisson (1597–1667). But Temkin[60] has shown that the notion of 'irritation' can be traced back to Galen, just as we have seen in the case of the term 'tonus'. Irritation in Galenic physiology meant an attempt by an organ or tissue to eliminate disturbing material, a faculty possessed by every living part. To Glisson, irritation indicated the existence of perception, which required the presence of nerves. Sensation or feeling may or may not attend perception and reaction.

For many years Haller brooded and wrote on the problems of irritability and sensibility, undertaking hundreds of animal experiments, 'a species of cruelty for which I felt such a reluctance', and finally concluding that animal tissues could be divided according to their possession of these properties.

> I call that part of the human body irritable, which becomes shorter on being touched . . . I call that a sensible part of the human body, which upon being touched transmits the impression of it to the soul [the brain] . . .[16]

> I took living animals of different kinds, and different ages, and after laying bare that part which I wanted to examine, I waited till the animal ceased to struggle or complain; after which I irritated the part, by blowing, heat, spirit of wine, the scalpel, *lapis infinalis*, oil of vitriol, and butter of antimony. I examined attentively, whether upon touching, cutting, burning, or lacerating the part, the animal seemed disquieted, made a noise, struggled, or pulled back the wounded limb, if the part was convulsed, or if nothing of all this happened.[62]

He found that the sensitive tissues were the skin, muscles, nerves, and mucous membranes. The subcutaneous tissues, tendons, joint capsules, ligaments, periosteum, and external membranes covering the brain, lungs, heart, and viscera were insensitive. The pain of gout and pleurisy could not therefore arise in joint capsule or pleura. Headache could not arise from the dura. He was not sure about bone and blood vessels, and in general attributed insensitivity to lack of nerve fibres.

The irritable parts of the body were the muscular parts, whose fibres could still contract when rendered nerveless. The heart was the most irritable organ, capable of movement, 'even after death, for four and twenty, or thirty hours, or longer'. He suspected the 'thin' auricles were the most irritable portion of the heart, 'but if you ask me whence proceeds the greater irritability of the heart than of the other muscles, I shall find it very difficult to answer the question'. 'It lay concealed in the very structure of the heart itself', he said, thereby laying the foundation of the myogenic theory of the heart beat. He was not sure whether the blood vessels possessed irritability.

Irritability was not proportional to sensitivity. 'The most irritable parts are not all sensible, and vice versa, the most sensible are not irritable.' The nerves, the organs of sensation, were not irritable. When stimulated they conveyed motion only to the muscles to which they were distributed, and 'whatever irritation I gave to a muscle, it never communicated the least motion to the nerve'. Mechanical forms of nerve transmission, oscillations and the like, were thus improbable. Cutting the nerve supply to a muscle deprived it of sensitivity but not irritaility.

Lastly, in small animals I have tied the trunk of the nerves which go to the extremities, and thereby rendered the limbs insensible and paralytic. Afterwards I have irritated the muscles, and seen them contract the same as before, though they were no longer subject to the command of the will.

From all these experiments collected together it appears, that there is nothing irritable in the animal body but the muscular fibre . . . From the same experiments it likewise follows, that the vital parts are the most irritable . . . the diaphragm . . . the stomach and intestines . . . and lastly the heart.[64]

But the complete independence of sensitivity and irritability sounded unlikely to many, and clinicians held other views about the sensitivity of tissues such as the pleura, peritoneum, tendons, and periosteum. De Haen (1704–76) criticized Haller's experiments and 'fictitious reasoning' although he felt that Haller's reputation was such that 'I will be censured for questioning authority and gentlemen may make reprisals . . .'[65] Robert Whytt realized that Haller's views did not take into account the phenomena of 'sympathy' and the 'reflex act'. One can see how Haller failed to lay hold of the idea of reflex action when he referred to those who 'are obliged to introduce an insensible sensation, and involuntary acts of the will, that is to say, to admit contradictory propositions'.[66] Yet he knew that the pithed frog cannot be stirred into motion. By the end of the century, the term 'irritability' was no longer used in the restricted sense of Haller, meaning only contractility of muscle, and in the years that followed it was replaced by the term 'excitability' of tissues.

Haller considered that the sensibility of a nerve resided in its 'medullary part, which is a product of the internal substance of the brain.'[67] All nerves were mixed; he did not conceive of separate sensory and motor nerves. When he exposed the brain of an animal, he noticed the movements that accompanied respiration, but he considered these were a consequence of removing the calvarium. However, 'Upon touching the brain, in whatever manner I did it, the animal was instantly seized with violent convulsions, which bended its body to one side in the form of a bow.'[68] But he did not interpret this as indicating cortical motor activity for, elsewhere, he wrote that although the cortex must feel, no movement results when it is irritated.[69] In his experiments on the brain he deduced that movements meant that sensation had been excited. The central parts of the brain were where external impressions were appreciated and where movements were initiated.

> Nor in the cortex of the brain alone is the seat of sensation or the full origin of the cause of muscular movement; each of these lies also in the medulla of the cerebrum and of the cerebellum.[70]

With regard to Willis's suggestion of the possible localization of function within the brain, experimental and pathological observations led Haller to reject the notion. He did not think the corpus striatum was the seat of sensation and the source of movement. The cerebellum was not essential to vital activity.[71] 'Imagination', 'sensation', and 'memory' could not be assigned any actual location, such hypotheses were 'feeble, fleeting, and of a short life'. Experiment seemed to be everything to him, the greatest source of error was 'substituting analogy instead of them', a trait he no doubt noted in Willis. Nevertheless, Haller did ask the question 'Whether or not there is in the brain any principal part, in which resides the origin of all motion, the end of all the sensations, and where the soul has its seat?'[72] He thought the latter 'lies not in the cortex, but in the medulla'. 'The seat of the mind must be where the nerve first begins its formation or origin.'[73] This was the *sensorium commune*, where sensations arrived and motions were initiated.

In muscles, then, there was the inherent force, the *vis insita*, which could cause contraction of the fibres without the aid of the nervous system. In the nerves there was another force, the *vis nervosa*, sent down from the 'soft' centres of the brain to promote willed motion. The absence of irritability in nerves suggested that a mechanical form of transmission in solid fibres was unlikely, and although Haller had found no hollows in nerves a fluid medium seemed, as it had to Boerhaave, more probable. But he said he would not speculate on the nature of a substance 'known to us only by its effects'. Stensen would have reiterated his words that spirits, humours, vapours, and juices 'are mere words, meaning nothing'. 'An electrical matter', said Haller, 'is, indeed very powerful, and fit for motion, but then it is not confinable within the nerves . . . and a ligature on the nerve takes away sense and motion, but cannot stop the motion of a torrent of electrical matter.'[74] Insulation and transmission of an electrical impulse in nerve seemed altogether too chimerical for one who vowed never to 'go beyond the testimony of our senses'. But his views changed.

Haller seems to have been a difficult colleague, rigid in his ideas, oversensitive to criticism, and devoid of humour.[75] When he left Göttingen, which he said was 'the grave of his wives' (he had three), and returned to

Bern, he spent the remaining twenty-five years of his life in bureaucratic and administrative posts. His great library, voluminous writings, and wide fame did not, it seems, provide much happiness. He lamented 'O my poor brain, which must return to dust; and all the knowledge and information which I have been collecting with such unwearied labour, will *fade away* like the dream of an infant.'[76]

One wonders whether Galen would have been surprised to learn that sixteen hundred years later, the foremost physiologist of the day reaffirmed one of his theories.† Surprised maybe, but delighted, most assuredly. Nowhere, however, in Haller's *First lines of physiology* nor in his *elementa* would Galen have encountered the new term 'reflex action'. This was a concept developed by a contemporary of Haller, of whom he said, 'He never mentions me but when he wants to criticise me, and has adopted several of my ideas, without mentioning whence he had them.'[77] Robert Whytt, no less.

ROBERT WHYTT (1714 – 1766) and REFLEX ACTION

Haller's Scottish adversary was also a former Leyden student, a Fellow of the Royal Society, and a Physician to George II. In 1763 he became President of the Royal College of Physicians of Edinburgh. A practising physician and a professor of medicine, he lectured in Latin, in which language he is said to have shone, and wrote in English, free (said a contemporary reviewer) 'from the least peculiarity of the Scottish idiom'.[79–82] A collection of his writings, *The works of Robert Whytt, M.D.*, was published by his son in 1768.[83] This included *An essay on the vital and other involuntary motions of animals* (1751);[84] *Observations on the sensibility and irritability of parts of men and other animals* (1755);[85] *Observations on the nature, causes, and cure of those disorders which are commonly called nervous, hypochondriac or histeric* (1764);[86] and, published for the first time, *Observations on the dropsy of the brain*.[87] These were his four principal treatises.

The first of these, his *Essay* of 1751, begun in 1744, comprises 208 quarto pages, divided into fourteen chapters. He considers the motions of the heart and respiration, the motions of the blood vessels, the gastrointestinal tract, the urinary bladder, the pupil, and the inner ear. He discusses the effects of sleep and the role of the mind in these activities, and the problem of the contraction of muscles, during life, after death, or after excision from the animal body. It is remarkably general in its scope and one cannot but admire the lucid way in which he marshalls his data, observational and experimental, and develops his theme. 'Landmark' is an historical title sometimes inaptly bestowed upon a work – but assuredly not in this case.

In the preface Whytt said that his interest in the subject arose from his dissatisfaction with the 'common theories of respiration and the heart's motion'. He thought that the function of respiration was to cool the blood and assist its circulation; he did not accept the new notion that air contained something that was absorbed into the blood from the lungs. Nor did he

† The German medical historian, J. H. Baas,[78] said Haller had dealt a 'death blow to the doctrine of the vital spirits'.

agree with Boerhaave's explanation for the alternating movements of inflation and contraction of the lungs, and the systole and diastole of the heart. Boerhaave taught that the former arose as a consequence of temporary compression of thoracic nerves (with transient paralysis) by the expanded lungs. Similarly, intermittent compression of the cardiac nerves at the junction of heart and great vessels intercepted the flow of spirit. Such mechanistic explanations were too abject for the pious Whytt. He preferred to conceive and nourish the notion that in man there was 'one sentient and intelligent principle, which is equally the source of life, sense and motion, as of reason'. All his neurophysiology was built around this conjecture, although, ultimately, what actually emerged was the idea of reflex action, its nature, purpose, and anatomical basis. The mechanistic element in an axon reflex would have astonished him.

He begins his first *Essay* by stating 'a certain power or influence' in the nervous system is essential for muscle contraction. This explains why stimulation of the medulla of nerves, spinal cord, brain stem, or cerebral hemispheres causes movements or convulsions, and why compression causes paralysis. He cites Galen's experiments on the recurrent laryngeal and peripheral nerves. Muscle action does not depend on blood supply although the latter provides nourishment. Muscle contraction is due to shortening of fibres and normally there is always some 'state of tension', sphincter muscles being 'always contracted'. This state of 'natural contraction' is maintained by the nerves, in a 'constant and equable' manner, but may be increased by the action of the will. 'Voluntary contraction' may be controlled in terms of force and duration. A third type of contraction he termed 'involuntary', that which arises from a stimulus. This cannot be influenced by the will.

'Numberless experiments and observations' show that not only 'pricking' a muscle causes it to contract, but that 'whatever stretches the fibres of any muscle, so as to extend them beyond their usual length, excites them into contraction'[88] – Sherrington's stretch reflex. Because isolated pieces of skeletal or visceral muscle may be seen to twitch after death, or may be stimulated to do so, this did not necessarily mean that the nerve supply was not normally essential. Contraction varies with the strength of the stimulus, 'but the effects of different stimuli depend very much upon the peculiar constitution of the nerves and fibres of the muscles to which they are applied'.[89] A stimulus which provokes a strong reaction in one part of the body may have no effect in another. Examples were the effect of cold water, 'agreeable to the nerves of the stomach', yet which 'excites violent coughing ... in the windpipe'. And 'Light, which by irritating the *retina* occasions the contraction of the pupil, does not act, sensibly, as a *stimulus* on any other part of the body.'[90] Such observations have been rightly regarded as among the earliest to indicate what later, after Muller (1801–58), came to be called the doctrine of specific energies of the nerves or senses.

In the two following quotations concerning direct stimulation of exposed muscle we see a reference to Sherrington's refractory period.

An irritated muscle does not remain in a contracted state, although the stimulating cause continues to act upon it; but is alternately contracted and relaxed.[91]

It might perhaps be imagined, that a muscle ought to remain contracted as long as the *stimulus* or cause of its contraction continues to act upon it; but the fact we see is otherwise; ... [it may continue] for some time after it is removed, although these motions become gradually weaker, and are repeated more slowly.[92]

Later, he develops the view that the purpose of reflex action is essentially protective, that all voluntary muscles may act involuntarily, and that even the memory or sight of a stimulus may serve to repeat the initial response. 'Thus the sight, or even the recalled idea of grateful food, causes the saliva to flow ...'.[93] 'The idea of a stimulus has, in many cases, almost the same effect as the thing itself.'[94] Pavlow's conditioned reflex.

The motions of the pupil

Whytt recognized that the eye would be 'ill-fitted' for its function if there were no mechanisms which enabled it to operate in various intensities of light and to adjust to near or distant vision. He studied the movements of the pupil to light and on accommodation, in animals and man, and in his patients.

He described the constrictor and dilator fibres of the iris, quoting Winslow and Ruysch, noting their anatomical arrangement and mode of action. He said the circular fibres 'may properly be called the *sphincter pupillae*'. He mentioned the various shapes of the pupils in different animals and their significance. Both pupils constrict when light falls only on one eye, but it is more marked in the exposed eye. He quoted Galen's observation (see p. 10) that closing one eye led to pupillary dilatation in the other, and he mentioned others who had noted the constrictor effect of strong light. In syncope, apoplexy, or at the moment of death, the pupil dilates. A lesion of an eye such as a corneal opacity or a cataract which 'intercepts the rays of light', or one of the retina which renders it 'insensible', or of the iris itself, will impair the pupillary reaction to light.

Light rays do not exert a local effect on the muscles of the iris. When a normal eye is covered the opposite pupil dilates so that direct action is impossible. When an eye is closed 'its pupil must be widened by the natural contraction of the stronger longitudinal fibres of that membrane (the uvea)' and the other pupil dilates 'as the mind has, from the time of birth, been always accustomed to contract the pupils of both eyes at the same time.'[95]

In unilateral blindness, on closure of the good eye the pupil of the blind one remains inactive to light; but the pupil of the blind eye will constrict when a bright light is shone on the good eye. The iris of the blind eye is not, therefore, paralysed. This consensual reaction 'can only arise from the sympathy between the two pupils' normally present. It is possibly lost when there is 'a perfect amaurosis' on one side.

In blindness the pupils were usually dilated but he had a patient 'almost totally blind of both eyes', without opacities, in whom the pupil of the completely blind eye (right) was normal in size but wholly inactive. In the other eye there was light perception only, the pupil was dilated but responded feebly to light. He concluded that on the right side both the retina and the iris were affected whereas on the left side both were still capable of some response.

He described the case of a boy of five years who went into a coma.[96] The pupils were at first dilated and inactive. Later they appeared normal. When the boy was roused they dilated but remained inactive to light; when he relapsed they contracted. At autopsy there was internal hydrocephalus. Whytt concluded that the initial pupillary dilatation was due to 'compression of the *thalami nervorum opticorum* ... which rendered the retina insensible to the *stimulus* of light'. Later, pressure 'on the origins of the nerves of the *uvea*' led to paresis of the pupillary dilator fibres and some shrinking of the pupils. These compressive lesions were asymmetrical. Since, on rousing, the pupils, remained inactive to light, he concluded that the optic nerves were more compressed than those to the iris. That Whytt did not know the actual innervation of the constrictor and dilator fibres of the iris nor of the pupillary effects of tentorial herniation makes this analysis all the more interesting.

He observed the pupillary response in a cat whose head was submerged in water; the pupils 'immediately dilated though exposed to the sun-beams'.[97] This could not be explained if light rays exerted their effect directly upon the fibres of the iris. Alternatively, light rays under water suffer less refraction on entering the eye and do not focus so sharply on the retina, so the response is less than in air. This confirmed his belief that the response was determined by reflex action.

When he comes to consider the pupillary movements on accommodation-convergence, he describes the changing shape of the lens effected through the ciliary muscles, and, like Descartes before him, he noted the dilatation on near vision and the contraction on distant vision.

> Thus if one with his back to the windows of a room, brings a small printed book so near his eyes, that he cannot, without straining, distinguish the letters; upon turning his face quickly to the light, he will be able to read with little difficulty; because, by the action of the stronger light on the *retina*, the pupil is immediately lessened; and therefore its power, to prevent the dissipation of the rays, and consequently indistinct vision, is increased. Hence neither the single effort of the mind to avoid indistinct vision, nor a vivid light alone, can contract the pupil to its least size, that is, not so much as when both these causes of its contraction are united.[98]

But whereas the light reaction is a muscle response like that occurring in hiccup, sneezing, or ejaculation, the accommodation response is different. The latter is voluntary, 'though often not attended with consciousness of volition', and 'can be restrained if we please'. Combining with the lens adjustment and 'the uniform motion of the eyes in looking at objects' it facilitates vision. Descartes believed that whereas the 'desire' to look at an object caused the pupil to adjust, merely 'thinking' about it was not effective. Whytt considered that 'habit' was responsible for the way in which lens and iris combined without conscious effort or awareness. It was acquired after birth (the infant's retina was not fully sensitive so the pupil remained dilated, and accommodation had yet to develop) and was often impaired in old age. Iritis could also affect accommodation by 'leaving a rigidity' in the fibres of the iris. Whytt mentions the case of a seaman whose sight failed at night 'owing to the pupil's not being dilated'; by day he saw well, but his pupils were 'always pretty narrow' and responded little to light. He did not say whether they reacted on accommodation but his patient may well have had Argyll-Robertson pupils.

In these discussions of pupillary responses Whytt does not mention the word 'accommodation'. This is curious, because, in the next section of the same chapter, when he discusses the movements of the muscles of the internal ear, he says that they adjust the tension of the membranes of the tympanum and oval window, 'and so accommodated to almost all possible sounds'.

From these observations he draws the conclusion that a central reflex mechanism is responsible for pupillary movements.

Since the optic nerves and those of the *uvea* arise from different parts of the brain, and have no communication with each other in their course to the eye, it seems evident, that light affecting the *retina* cannot excite the *sphincter* of the pupil into contraction by any immediate mechanical change which it produces, either in the muscle itself, or in the nerves which actuate it; but the uneasy sensation occasioned in the *retina* by the admission of too much light into the eye, may so affect the sentient principle, which is present and ready to act where-ever the nerves have their origin, as to excite it to contract the orbicular muscle of the *uvea*, in order to lessen the pupil, and exclude the offending cause ...[99]

The alternate motions of respiration were those of the chest, not the lungs, and he thought they showed 'a remarkable analogy' with those of the pupils. Constriction of the pupil and inspiration resulted from muscular contraction; both were followed by relaxation. But 'respiration differed from most of the other spontaneous movements, in being subject to the power of the will'. Yet it is not voluntary as it continues during sleep. He described periodic apnoea in 'acute diseases, where the head is much affected' and in a case of laudanum poisoning.[100]

Muscular contraction[101]

This arises 'either from an effort of the will, or a stimulus of some kind or another'. The former is voluntary and the latter is vital or spontaneous. He rejects the notions that contraction arises because of some 'elastic' property; an elastic body 'is no more than a piece of dead matter, without any power of generating motion'. Neither is there any good evidence that contraction depends on 'any effervescence, explosion, ethereal oscillation, or electrical power excited in its fibres or membranes'. 'It makes no odds whether the stimulating substances be electrics *per se* or non-electrics.' 'Every kind of irritation, excites muscles' and the stimulus may be remote from the muscle itself.[102]

If a spark from the fire, or a drop of boiling water falls upon one's foot, the leg is instantly drawn in towards the body; but as the muscles employed in this action are those which run along the thigh, and are inserted about the head of the *tibia*, it is manifest that this *stimulus* cannot excite those muscles into contraction in consequence of any mechanical action upon them; and if the sympathy of the nerves, or continuation of membranes, shall be assigned as the cause of this motion, it may be justly asked, why the muscles which run along the leg, and are inserted into the foot, are not more moved than those of the thigh, since they have a nearer connection with that part to which the stimulus is applied; or why the extensors of the leg are not brought equally into action with its flexors?[103]

Clearly 'there is some intervention of the mind' in such phenomena. This should not surprise us as 'many remarkable changes and involuntary motions are suddenly produced in the body by affections of the mind'. He cites the examples of fear causing urination, sounds occasioning tremor, fright producing pallor and palpitation, and so on. Even 'the sound of a bagpipe has been said to give some people an inclination to make water'.

Involuntary contraction may be continuous or intermittent according to the purpose of the movement. Peristalsis is intermittent, contraction of the urinary bladder is sustained during urination, and in the penis, it is maintained in erection, but spasmodic in ejaculation.

Whytt saw movements as voluntary, involuntary, or mixed, the second and third being spontaneous. Sneezing, coughing, or hiccupping were purely involuntary. The heartbeat was a form of 'vital' involuntary movement, while that of respiration was mixed, as it could be influenced by the will. The stimulus to movement could arise in the mind, in the nerve, or in the muscle itself, but the unconscious sentient principle was an agent in each case. In an involuntary movement it is not that there is unawareness of the stimulus or of the ensuing muscular contraction but that there is no consciousness of anything interposed between the two, as in the example he quotes of the drops of hot water falling on a foot. Equally 'some voluntary motions are performed while we are insensible of the power of the will' as in walking. Or again, seeing a kettle about to boil over, the foot can be withdrawn. In both withdrawals there is consciousness of an initial impression but in the conscious withdrawal there is also awareness of a voluntary act. So although mind plays a part in involuntary motion its involvement is predetermined ('the mind is not a free but a necessary agent') and the whole process becomes as automatic as the mechanical concept of Descartes. But Whytt did not see it this way and derided Descartes' view that we were but 'machines formed entirely of matter, and, as it were, so many pieces of clock-work wound up and set agoing'.[104] And whereas Descartes considered that 'reflection' took place in the ventricles and Willis suggested it might occur in peripheral nerve connections, it was Whytt's achievement to show that it took place mainly in the spinal cord.

In the concluding pages of this essay on vital motions, when he is discussing the matter of sympathy between parts and its possible central location, he said that he wished it to be understood that he includes the spinal cord in his considerations for it 'does not seem altogether derived from the brain and cerebellum, but probably prepares a fluid itself; whence it is enabled to keep up the vital and other motions for several months, in a tortoise, after the head is cut off'. He referred to the persistence of movements after decapitation in a frog, cock, viper, and tortoise; in a frog 'divided into two'; and in a tortoise whose brain was completely extracted.

He observed that the duration of life after decapitation was influenced by the size of the brain, relative to the spinal cord. 'Those animals who have a small *brain* and large spinal *marrow*, live long after decollation, man, and most quadrupeds, which have a large brain, survive the loss of it only for a few moments.'[105] His attention was also drawn to reports of anencephaly and the like in which movements both spontaneous and reflex occurred. The spinal cord clearly required consideration.

The spinal cord

He investigated this question in his next book of physiological essays, published four years later, in 1755, *Observations on sensibility and irritability*. It is here that he published the famous words from his friend Stephen Hales (1677–1761) about the effect of pithing a frog.

> The late Reverend and learned Dr. Hales informed me, that having many years since, tied a ligature about the neck of a frog, to prevent any effusion of blood, he cut off its head, and thirty hours after, observed the blood circulating freely in the web of the foot; the frog also at this time moved its body when stimulated; but that, on thrusting a needle down the spinal marrow, the animal was strongly convulsed and immediately after became motionless.[106]

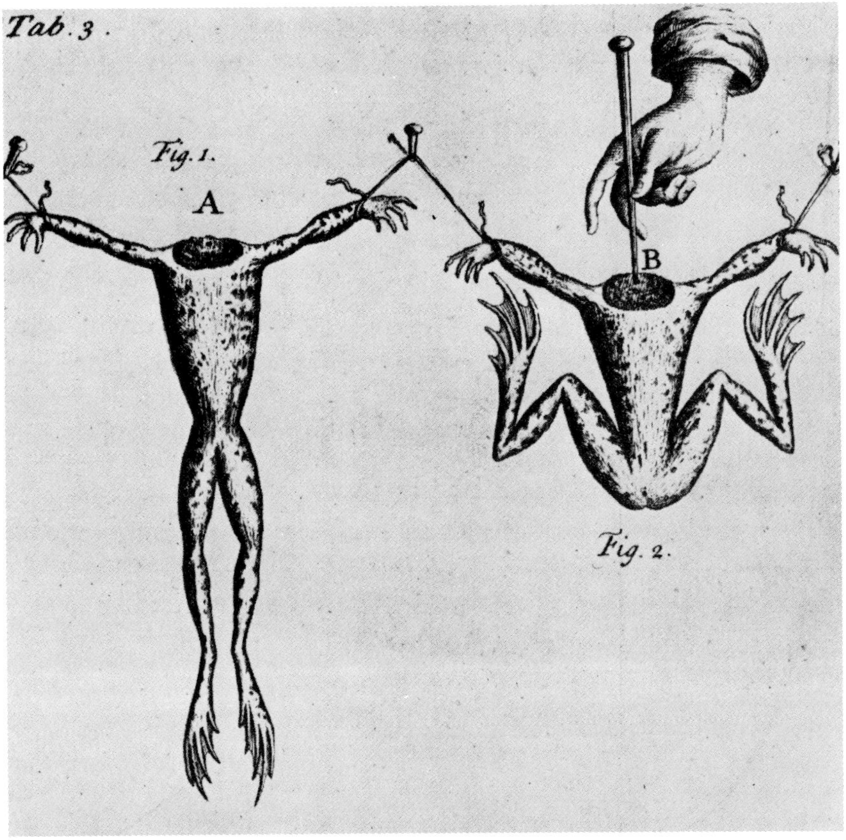

FIG. 46. Illustration of the effect of pithing a frog. (After Stuart.[108]) *Fig. 1*. Suspended decapitated frog hangs limp and motionless. *Fig. 2*. Flexion of legs on inserting a probe into the spinal canal. He found that if the probe destroyed the spinal cord, the movements ceased. His interpretation was that the reflex movements were produced by compression of the cord and forcing nerve-fluid into the nerves. We have it on Whytt's sole authority that this experiment was first performed by Stephen Hales (1677–1761) at some unknown date. But Leonardo da Vinci (1452–1519) had made a similar observation.

Others, before Hales, had noted this consequence of pithing a decapitated frog. Leonardo da Vinci appended the following note to a drawing of the spinal cord, in which, incidentally it is shown reaching to the sacral region of the vertebral column. 'The frog retains life for some hours when deprived of its head, heart and all the intestines. And if you prick the said nerve [spinal medulla] it suddenly twitches and dies.'[107] In 1739, Alexander Stuart (1673–1742) illustrated the phenomenon in one of his lectures on muscular motion (Fig. 46).[108] Haller, and no doubt other physiologists, knew that movements occurred in the decapitated frog, but so far as I have been able to discover he did not demonstrate that they ceased when the spinal cord was then destroyed. Liddell's quotation,[109] attributed to Haller, is certainly to be found in Whytt, where it runs as follows.

> But further, it ought to be observed, that when after decollation, a frog's spinal marrow is destroyed with a red-hot wire, no visible motion is produced in its limbs, or body, by pricking, cutting, or otherwise hurting them . . .[110]

Whytt took the matter further. Removing the skin from the thighs of a decapitated, pithed frog, and stimulating the muscles directly, he obtained only weak tremulous movements. He reasoned that these resulted from 'the influence of power of their nerves, which still remain entire'. He also noticed that 'there was no sympathy between the different muscles, or other parts of the body, as was observed when the spinal marrow was entire'. He concluded that nerves had no communication 'but at their termination in the spinal marrow; and to this, perhaps alone, is owing the consent and sympathy between them'.[111]

It is generally agreed that these observations by Whytt established that reflex activity depended on an intact spinal cord. But in 1751 he had already written that 'when the body of a frog is divided in two, both the anterior and posterior extremities preserve the life and power of motion for a considerable time'.[112] In turn, these words have been understood to mean that Whytt had shown that only a portion of the cord is necessary, but as French[113] has pointed out, Whytt did not specifically indicate that the lower limbs of the frog responded to irritation. A segment of spinal cord was clearly capable of originating movements but this experiment did not actually prove that it was also sufficient to maintain reflex response to irritation. French observed that Whytt makes it clear, a few pages further on in this *essay*, that both spontaneous and stimulated movements were abolished when the spinal cord was destroyed. For Sherrington this was the fundamental experiment of reflex physiology; 'Whytt was the first to show that the integrity of even a fraction of the length of the spinal cord suffices to enable reflex reactions to occur in response to skin stimuli, and therefore that reflex function does not depend on the integrity of the cord as a whole. Legallois extended similar observations to the mammalian cord.'[114]

The immediate effect of decapitation in a frog was one of immobility; responses could not at first be obtained.[115] A hundred years later this phenomenon Marshall Hall (1790–1857) called 'spinal shock'.

In arguing his thesis Whytt did not know of the specificity of the sensory and motor nerves, nor in what way central connections were arranged but he seems to have conjectured, as did Haller, that nerve fibres were unbranched from their origin in the brain or spinal cord to their termination. The nerves 'appear to be no more than continuations of the medullary substance of the parts whence they proceed ... without any communications between their branches ...' unlike the arterial system.[116]

every individual nerve appears to be quite distinct from every other, not only in its rise from the medullary substance of the brain or spinal marrow, but also in its progress to that part where it terminates. ...[117]

He thought that peripheral anastomoses would only cause 'confusion' of incoming sensations; our wires would be crossed.[118] Hence he thought Willis's conjecture was wrong but he agreed that he was responsible for the concept that sympathy was a function of nerves. Of course, like Willis and others, his clinical examples in this field included symptoms such as referred pain, trismus, the body manifestations of anxiety, and a variety of phenomena which today we would not include under the heading of reflex action. A 'large draught of very cold water in winter' causing a painful sensation in 'that part of the forehead immediately above the nose' may well be the equivalent of 'ice-cream headache' as suggested by Hoff and Kellaway,[119] but that 'pain in the head is sometimes the consequence of wearing strait shoes'[120] is scarcely a reflex phenomenon.

As for the term itself, Whytt, although using the words 'stimulus' and 'response', spoke of the 'reflex act' and 'reflex consciousness' in a way bearing no resemblance to the simple sensori-motor responses of modern neurophysiology.[119]

Why may not a muscle, whose nerve is tied or cut, continue for some little time, sensible and irritable? Its sensibility will not indeed be attended with what is called *consciousness*, as distinguished from simple sensation; because this reflex act, by which a person knows his thoughts or sensations to be his own, is a faculty of the soul exercised in the brain only, with which all communication is now cut off.[121]

... the soul is equally present in the extremities of the nerves through the whole body as in the brain. In those it is only capable of feeling or simple sensation; but in this, it exercises the powers of reflex consciousness and reason.[122]

Though he rejected Willis's idea of 'reflection' in the periphery, and Descartes' 'reflection' in the brain, Whytt was not able to offer a satisfactory explanation of reflex action, one that was wholly scientific. He had to fall back, again and again, on his 'sentient principle' but he sensed his dilemma when, referring to the anatomical basis of nervous sympathy, he said 'It would be vain to enquire into this matter, unless we knew the minute structure and connections of the several parts of the brain ...'.[123]

A decade after Whytt's death, Unzer (1727–99) echoed Whytt's words when he said, writing of the motor and sensory pathways, 'neither anatomy or experiment can determine the question; for it is so microscopically minute, as to escape the cognisance of our senses'.[124] Nevertheless, he deduced that there must be 'afferent' and 'efferent' pathways; 'I meditated on certain phenomena and found that it was absolutely impossible to explain them, except by assuming that afferent and efferent fibrils do exist.' The Göttingen reviewer of his book (probably Haller, according to Laycock, Unzer's translator) thought that there was no evidence for this conjecture. In the next decade Prochaska (1749–99) wrote that 'reflexion follows according to certain laws, writ, as it were, by nature on the medullary pulp of the sensorium, which laws we are able to know from their effects only . . .'.[125]

Both of these physiologists supported Whytt in his view that the contractility of muscles depended on the nerves, which was one of the major issues in his celebrated dispute with Haller.

The controversy with Haller

This has been admirably analysed by French,[126] and although the arguments became somewhat metaphysical and the issues obsolete it was a classical encounter in the history of neurology and still deserves reference.

Haller had been writing for some years on the irritability and sensibility of tissues, and when Whytt's first *Essay*, on vital motions, appeared in 1751, Haller criticized it, and in his own 'Dissertation' in the following year he extended his criticism. The subtitle to Whytt's *Observations on sensibility and irritability*, in 1755, was *Occasioned by the celebrated M. de Haller's late treatise on those subjects*. The debate continued for more than a decade, Haller maintaining his views in his *Elementa physiologiae*, the last volume of which was published in 1766, the year of Whytt's death. The Scottish medical historian, Comrie, writing in 1925, thought 'Whether he convinced Haller or not, Whytt, in the opinion of his contemporaries, seems to have got the better of him in the dispute.'[127] But it was a dispute which only succeeding generations could correctly judge, when new knowledge made possible a better appreciation of his views.

Whytt's criticism of Haller's views on the absolute distinction between sensibility and irritability were made on practical, as well as theoretical grounds. As a clinician, with colleagues such as the Monros and Cullen, his experience taught him that tendons, joints, and ligaments were sensitive to the knife and that an inflamed pleura or dura mater was very painful. As an experimenter he realized that an animal could not communicate its pain except by crying out or struggling and that 'shock' and pain itself might inhibit these. He quoted the Hippocratic aphorism that a greater pain obscures the lesser, 'Of two pains occurring together, not in the same part of the body, the stronger weakens the other.'[128] Whereas Haller asserted that membranes and tendons could not be sensitive because no one had found nerves in them (which was not true), to Whytt sensibility meant that nerves must be there. Sympathy depended on 'feeling'.

Similarly, for Whytt, irritability was a property only of muscle. Here he agreed with Haller but was opposed to the idea that it was inherent in muscle and unrelated to sensibility, Haller's insistence meant that he had closed his mind to the notions developing in Whytt's, namely, that sensori-motor mechanisms helped explain the nature of involuntary movements and sympathy. Canghuilhem[129] has pointed out that Haller also frequently cited Willis with reference to his ideas of involuntary movement but nevertheless he remained indifferent to the term and the idea of reflex action as developed by both these men. To the modern reader it would appear that Haller was literally obsessed with the 'irritability' of muscle.

It is interesting to note that Foster,[130] who regarded Haller's 'Dissertation' as his 'chief work' and 'a remarkable advancement of knowledge', made no mention of the entire absence from it of any reference to reflex action; nor indeed to Robert Whytt. Do we see here, as in the case of Willis (p. 106), a physiologist's prejudice against the physician who dabbled in experimental physiology? Haller boasted that he had done many more experiments than Whytt. But Whytt thought that this was to some extent just 'to overpower the incredulous by their number'.

The conflicting views of Haller, Whytt, and others were noted by Fontana (1730–1805). In his 'Laws of Irritability' he said, 'Hallerian Irritability had caused many disagreements' and was sometimes referred to as '*an irritation to all Italy*'. 'Irritability now seems to reign in universal Philosophy much as Attraction does in Celestial Physics.' 'The reward of my effort on this problem has been to read the animal Spirits out of office, forever, by sound logic and new reasoning . . .'.[131]

Fontana stated that contraction of a muscle fibre required a stimulus; 'when the blood is drawn from either ventricle of the heart of larger animals, the movement immediately ceases' as claimed by Haller and Whytt. Secondly, there was 'the definite interval of time' so that, 'new action of the stimulus is necessary for all single contractions of a muscle'. This temporary diminution of irritability came to be termed the 'refractory period' by Marey (1830–1904). Fontana stressed Whytt's contribution to this phenomenon. Whytt had shown that heart muscle went on contracting and relaxing in the presence of a continuous stimulus. Thirdly, Fontana found that fatigue was a state within the muscle fibre itself; the nervous system could *excite* a muscle to contract but did not actually cause the contraction, otherwise 'muscles would never grow quiet, never remain motionless . . .'. Thus, the paralysed muscles of a patient contract 'under the influence of the electric spark . . .'. 'Paralyses can therefore occur through defects of the muscle alone, particularly in certain parts, without involvement of the nervous fluid.' Vigorous exertion reduced muscular irritability; the muscle fatigued. The responses in the legs of a decapitated frog were much reduced if the legs were first kept contracted for some time by applying an electric current to the spinal cord.

Fontana's fourth law referred to the harmful effects on muscular contractility of overstretching or compression. He observed the former when he dilated the urinary bladder in animals, causing retention, and immobility of the exposed organ. His fifth law concerned the weakening effects of disuse and atrophy.

In venturing to differ from Haller, to whom he dedicated one volume of his publications on this subject, Fontana assured him that 'love for the truth will serve as the centre for the union of our spirits in our diversity of opinion'. No such sentiments characterized the disputations of Haller and Whytt.

The clinician

Whytt's book on nervous disorders is a rambling one, rather repetitious, but full of clinical observations. The first chapter is devoted to the doctrine of sympathy, the role of involuntary movements, and his ideas of reflex action. In his preface he wished 'to wipe off the reproach' that physicians were using the term 'nervous' merely to cloak their ignorance. In one sense, all disorders were nervous 'because in almost every disease the nerves are more or less hurt'. 'There are few disorders which may not in a large sense be called nervous.' He agreed with Sydenham that 'the shapes of Proteus, or the colour of the chameleon, are not more numerous and inconstant than the variations of the hypochondriac or hysteric disease'. There are many lively case summaries. He described a case of 'collapse' after a bee sting,[132] and 'uneasiness relieved by getting out of bed',[133] and the waning of anxiety when tuberculosis spread to the lungs.[134] He would have been interested to learn that a radiograph may show unilateral paresis in cervical zoster; 'why should not the diaphragm be disturbed in its motions when the second and third cervical nerves are irritated by blisters etc.?'[135] Brandy reduced tremor of the hands.[136] One cannot say he actually recognized anorexia nervosa but he did mention that in 'nervous atrophy' there is a 'sensible wasting of the body' and that the patient 'may suddenly start eating'.[137]

Some patients were affected by 'undue sensibility' in general; in others only 'certain organs' were affected. 'Faults may arise in the coats, the medullary substance or in the fluid of the nerves.'[138]

Reading these pages of Whytt leaves one in no doubt of his appreciation of the role of emotional factors in illness. His successor in the Chair of Medicine, William Cullen (1710–90), held similar views on the importance of general 'sympathy' and inherent power in nerves, and one of his disease types he termed the 'Neuroses'.

But as a clinician Whytt is best remembered for his admirable account of tuberculous meningitis. This appeared in the collected works published in 1768, in an essay of seventeen pages entitled 'Observations on the Most Frequent Species of the Hydrocephalous Internus, viz. the Dropsy of the Ventricles of the Brain'.

That fluid could accumulate inside the head and cause its enlargement in children had been known since Hippocratic times. Fluid over the surface of the brain, compressing it, was often noted during the ensuing centuries, but cases in which the fluid remained confined to the ventricles were rarely observed. Vesalius described one example. Whytt used the term internal hydrocephalus when the fluid collected in the ventricles or between the brain and the skull. The term external hydrocephalus indicated that the fluid lay external to the cranium. Although internal hydrocephalus was known to physicians of the day, such as Boerhaave and Haller, little was known of its clinical manifestations. Whytt remedied this on the basis of his study of twenty cases, with ten autopsies.

Osler's reference in his textbook to the three stages of 'acute hydrocephalus' which Whytt described, on the basis of the pulse changes, served to enhance Whytt's reputation which had sadly declined during the nineteenth century.

The illness affected children and was invariably fatal in four to six weeks. In the first stage there was anorexia, thirst, constipation, lassitude, increasing headache, photophobia, and vomiting. The child was pale, with a high temperature and a rapid pulse (100 to 140). With the second stage the pulse became slower (often down to about 60) and irregular. There was drowsiness, difficulty in sitting up, and squinting. In the final stage, the patient lapsed into coma, there was paralysis of one or both eyelids, the pupils dilated, and convulsive movements occurred. Respiration was impaired and the pulse became rapid again and progressively feebler. He did not record head retraction or neck stiffness.

At autopsy there was dilation of the lateral ventricles from which he was able to remove two to five ounces of fluid. The third and fourth ventricles also frequently contained an excess of fluid. But he observed no accumulation between the dura and the brain, nor between the hemispheres. Like Cotugno he found that the fluid did not coagulate on heat, as did serum, lymph, or that from the pericardium or on abdominal paracentesis.

Whytt did not suggest that the illness was tuberculous. Dropsical remedies were not really indicated and surgery was considered impossible.

In seeking to differentiate these cases from other forms of fever, coma, or infestation with worms, Whytt stressed the falling of the pulse in the second stage, with the onset of restlessness and cranial nerve palsies. He thought the dropsy was a result of an imbalance between the 'exhalant' arteries and the absorbing 'bibulous' veins. The clinical features were a consequence of the compression of the brain.

Seventeen years later, William Withering (1741–99) referred to Whytt's account of hydrocephalus, in 'An Account of the Foxglove.'[139] He thought that the fluid was a consequence and not a cause of the illness, 'which I believe originates in inflammation'. Although Whytt's clinical description was accurate, Withering thought that the sequence of events could vary, and that the pulse changes were not invariable. He did not suggest where the inflammation originated nor that the illness might be tuberculous. Of phthisis, he said 'it is certainly infectious'.

EMANUEL SWEDENBORG (1688–1772) and CEREBRAL LOCALIZATION

Although we do not know how much practical experience of dissection and experiment Swedenborg actually acquired, on opening his volumes on the brain[40, 41] it soon becomes evident that he had studied extensively. He knew exactly what anatomists had described, and he quotes extensively and in detail from their works. Indeed, in his pages a modern student would find quite a good introduction to the neuroanatomical writings of such men as Eustachius, Malpighi, Ruysch, Willis, Leeuwenhoek, Vieussens, Ridley, Morgagni, and others. Each chapter begins with a summary of existing knowledge of the topic under discussion – the membranes, the sinuses, the ventricles, the inner structures and so on – and is followed by an 'Analysis'.

He freely admits that his data are largely derived from well known authorities, and he makes an introductory comment which modern researchers and their sponsors would not contradict.

Indeed there are some that are born for experimental observation ... and others again who enjoy a natural faculty for contemplating facts already discovered, and eliciting their causes. Both are peculiar gifts and are seldom united in the same person.

It becomes apparent that his interest in the detailed structure of the brain was solely so that he could construct a hypothesis of its function. He is often long-winded and repetitious and prone to the use of fanciful analogies after the manner of Willis. Indeed, many of them are similar. He was convinced that there was motion in the brain, and also indeed in the medulla oblongata, the spinal cord, and the pituitary gland, which was of a respiratory and pulsatile character. Fluids moved from the brain to the cord and nerves. Yet he achieved an extraordinary insight into the integrative functions of the nervous system, its hierarchical construction, and the likely function of particular parts of the brain, such as the frontal lobes, the motor cortex, the corpora quadrigemina, the pituitary gland, and the medulla oblongata and spinal cord. But these deductions lay hidden for one hundred and forty years so they had no influence on neurological thought, and few books on the history of medicine or neurology mention them. McHenry's[141] and Rasmussen's[142] volumes are among the exceptions. Perhaps if Neuburger[143] had not called Swedenborg 'The Swedish Aristotle' his writings would have won a place in the modern literature of neurology which they are gaining in that of science.[144–146]

Swedenborg's deductions about the brain were based on considerations of its anatomy, the effects of injury and disease, and upon experiment. It was the organ of consciousness, the intellect, and of power and sensation.

The cortex

This was the most important substance in the brain.

The cortical substance is the unit of the whole brain; in this unit or substance, then, we ought to find that superior power of which we are in quest. Therefore in this, and not in any ulterior unit ... we ought to find the soul's faculty of understanding, thinking, judging, willing.[147]

He had studied the microscopic descriptions of the cortex by Malpighi and deduced that sensory impulses arrived there, and motor impulses were initiated there. The glandulae or spherulae and their fibres formed the anatomical basis for these activities.

The abundant supply of these spherules is so great that they can not be counted by units, but by myriads, especially in the human brain which exceeds all others in size. The greater their number, the greater the skill by which they are distributed and connected; and the more perfect they are by nature, the more do they exceed in power ...[148]

This noble substance [the cortex] is the centre and, as it were, the meeting place of all contingencies ... the seat wherein sensation finally ceases.[149]

The fact that Malpighi's 'glands' and 'ducts' were not actually nerve cells and fibres does not really detract from Swedenborg's conception of the supremacy of the cortex but it can scarcely be claimed that it represented the introduction of the neurone theory. It is not correct to say that the 'glands' were 'probably Betz cells'[145] or that 'larger, pyramidal cells had also been differentiated'.[146] Swedenborg was writing in the seventeen-forties, a century before nerve cells and their axons were seen and their vital continuity was being established. Betz did not describe his cells until 1874.

Cortical localization

Swedenborg spoke of 'areas', 'regions', 'centres', 'courts', and 'provinces' of the brain as well as hemispheres, lobes, and convolutions. Intellect was represented in the frontal lobes.

These fibres of the cerebrum proceed from its anterior province, which is divided into lobes – a highest, a middle, and a lowest. ... These lobes are marked out and encompassed by the carotid artery. ... If this portion of the cerebrum therefore is wounded, then the internal senses – imagination, memory, thought – suffer; the very will is weakened, and the power of its determination blunted. ... This is not the case if the injury is in the back part of the cerebrum.[150]

The highest court of the cerebrum is among the topmost protuberances, or in the crown, where the highest lobe is. The middle court, which is adjoined to the former is the middle lobe; and the lowest is the third lobe. Thither all sensations aspire ...[151]

Where the faculty of perception resides, there also is that of volition and determination ... even in such a manner that the muscles and actions which are the ultimates in the body or in the soles of the feet depend more immediately upon the highest parts; upon the middle lobe the muscles which belong to the abdomen and thorax; and upon the third lobe those which belong to the face and head; for they seem to correspond to one another in an inverse ratio.[152]

Ramstrom enquires 'Whence did Swedenborg derive all this information?'[144] Retzius[153] thought that experiments must have been the basis of such precise statements but it is quite possible that critical analysis of the facts of anatomy and pathology, combined with 'an imaginative grasp of what might be true', may have sufficed. Swedenborg did also discuss Ridley's and Baglivi's cerebral experiments and noted that cortical injury caused convulsive movements, so he may have deduced that there was a motor cortex. And Ramstrom pointed out that Vieussens had already described upper, middle, and lower regions of the white matter of the brain tracing them to differently positioned tracts in the medulla oblongata and the spinal cord.

The corpora striata

Swedenborg was prompted to conclude from studies of 'petrified brains, as well as acephalous and hydrocephalous heads' that subcortical centres played a role in voluntary and involuntary motion.

the corpora striata are vicarious cerebra and that they succeed in the place of the cerebrum whenever it is deprived of its power of acting. ... These carry out into action whatever the cerebrum decrees; the cerebrum without the auxillary forces of these medullae being unable to operate anything whatever in the human body. . . . [Always there is] the mediation of the medulla oblongata and the spinal marrow . . . [these] may act from themselves, without consulting the cerebrum, when the latter relaxes and loosens its fibres. In this case the striated bodies can initiate motions which at first originated with the cerebrum and were voluntary; for it is a well known fact that voluntary acts by daily habit become spontaneous, or that habit is like second nature.[154]

The medulla and spinal cord

He saw in these structures and their connections further indications that there were higher and lower activities within the nervous system.

The fibres of the cerebrum, as well as those of the cerebellum . . . flow together . . . in the medulla oblongata, where they are also joined by new or recent fibres born from the caudex [medulla oblongata] itself.[155]

The fibrous medulla oblongata arises from the coalescence of this three-fold progeny [cerebral, cerebellar and medullary], and thus constitutes a common forum and halting place. . . .[156]

The medulla oblongata does not start anything of its own accord, but is compelled to act with the two brains [cerebrum and cerebellum].[157]

The medulla oblongata is the medium, uniting the determinations of the cerebrum with those of the cerebellum . . . the cerebrum acts from the will; the cerebellum, from nature.[158]

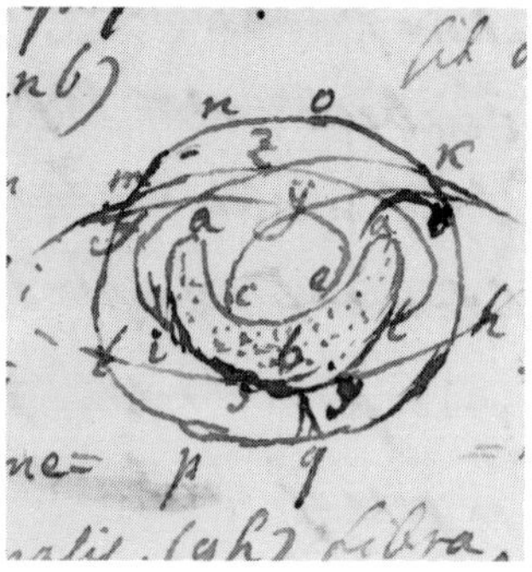

FIG. 47. Drawing of transverse section of spinal cord in one of Swedenborg's manuscripts. In the accompanying text he explains that the central 'ashy axis' varies in size and shape in different animals; in man it is 'orbicular' in the neck' with 'a hollowed-out pit'. Here, it resembles 'a horse's hoof' but 'spread open' to show the 'fluxions of the fibres'. Nerves emerge 'almost horizontal' in the cervical region and increasingly oblique toward the 'cauda equina'. In the white matter, fibres from the cerebrum descend anteriorly; those from the cerebellum posteriorly in the cord. 'The two principles go out from the medullary stalk always like comrades and companions.' (Courtesy of the Royal Swedish Academy of Sciences.)

In speaking of the conduction of motor and sensory impulses through the medulla he suggested that fibres did not run, without interruption, from cortex to periphery and vice versa. There were 'halts' and 'infinite anastomoses'. Spinal fibres originated not only in the hemispheres of the cerebrum and cerebellum, but also in the medulla oblongata and in the grey matter of the cord itself. He was aware of the decussation of the pyramidal fibres, which '. . . little by little come to the central axis, and there, by oblique decussations, they pass over to the fibres of the other side. . .'.[159]

He wondered about their origin and destination as 'the facts of experience are in twilight as it were'. He also made this extraordinary statement about the spinal nerve roots.

. . . the anterior roots of the spinal nerves receive fibres from the anterior part of the grey matter. The posterior roots, on the other hand, are furnished with fibres from the front and back parts of the grey matter, but always from the opposite side, so that there is a decussation of fibres.[160]

His manuscript contains a drawing to illustrate his idea of what a transverse section of the spinal cord would reveal (Fig. 47).

The corpora quadrigemina

Swedenborg often referred to the brain as 'A Chymical Laboratory' and he pictured within that laboratory various 'illustrious' pieces of 'apparatus'. Certain 'active little bodies' were the 'anterior and posterior tubercles of the corpora quadrigemina'. They had connections with the cerebellum, the optic thalamus, and the eyeball.

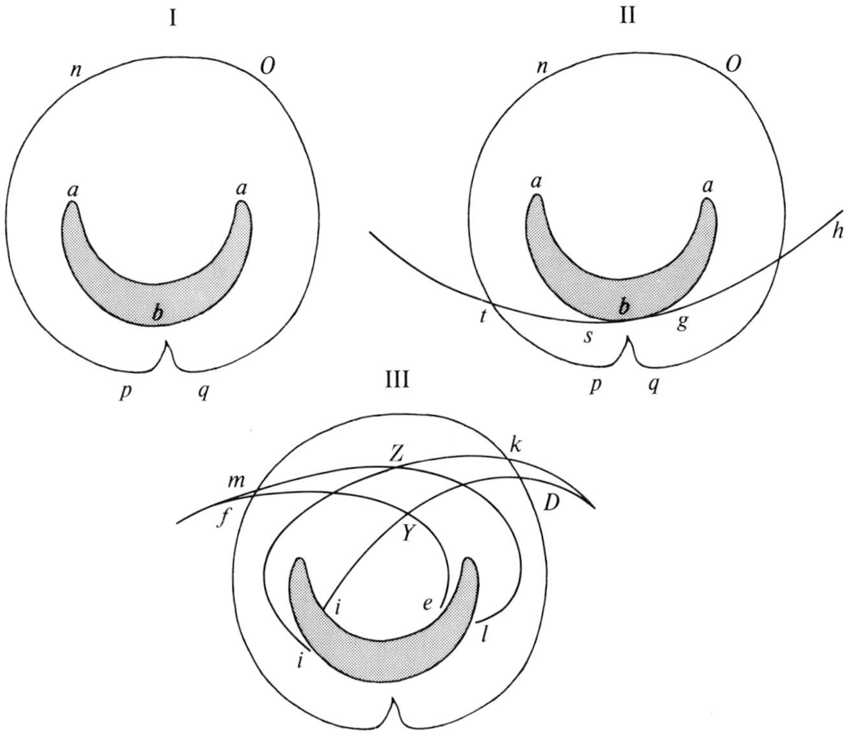

FIG. 48. Three diagrams to show how Swedenborg constructed his drawing in Fig. 47. I. The cord circumference – n, O, q, p, The grey matter – a, b, a. II. The anterior fibres – g, h, and s, t – 'which flow from the convex face to the anterior principle'. III. The posterior crossing fibres – l, m, and i, k – from the convex surface; e, f, and i, d from the concave surface. Decussation at Z and Y. (I am indebted to the Curator of Swedenborgiana Library, Bryn Athyn, Pennsylvania, Lennart O. Alfelt, for sending me Dr Iungerich's translation of the Latin text of the pages, referring to this drawing by Swedenborg.)

By this way these fibres [from the cerebellum] tend upwards into the surface or into the delicate membrane of the optic thalami, and at the same time more deeply into them, and thence, in conjunction with the fibres of the cerebrum, they direct their ways towards the bulb, the coatings, the humours, the iris and the pupil of the eye; that is, chiefly towards those parts of the eye which are being adjusted to the state of the objects at the time, and indeed, spontaneously, and without any previous will of the cerebrum . . . the region of the corpora quadrigemina, is subjected both to the cerebrum and the cerebellum.[161]

It was not until the eighteen-twenties that Flourens (1794–1867) showed that the corpora quadrigemina were centres of coordination between retinal impressions and movements of the iris. This led to the discovery of the role of the superior body in the reflex movements of the head which occur in response to visual stimuli.

The pituitary gland

This was 'the only undivided organ belonging to both hemispheres'. Swedenborg devoted twenty pages to summarizing its anatomy as described by Willis and others, and he spent thirty further pages in analysing its function. He concluded that it was 'the arch-gland' because

. . . it receives the whole spirit of the brain and communicates it to the blood, to which it thereby imparts a special quality, upon which quality compared with its quantity, depends the life of the whole of its kingdom.[162]

If, therefore, the brain ... concentrates in this one gland, as in a certain terminus of its work, it must needs be that it has in view, and carries out here, some sublime and grand work which concerns the whole animal kingdom, and on which its welfare depends. On this account the pituitary gland may deservedly be styled the gland of life, or the arch-gland.[163]

This gland expends all its action, both within itself and without, on the receiving, the transmitting, and, to some extent, the simultaneous secreting of liquids ...[164]

When we recall that at the turn of the present century all that was virtually known about the pituitary gland was that it was enlarged in acromegaly, these conjectures of Swedenborg were remarkable.

Throughout his writings on the brain it is clear that Swedenborg had grasped the importance of the function of integration in the nervous system.

In order that these essential parts of the cerebrum or of the cortical substance may be properly coordinated, and at the same time subordinated ... the whole of it is bipartite; again, there are lobes in it; further, convolutions and gyres; there are also particular clusters and individual substances. In order that the particular and individual parts may act freely in their own sphere according to their own nature, they are divided from one another by intervals ... each part thus has its own sensation and motion ... all conspire together unanimously in the production of general and specific effects.[165]

When reading Swedenborg, on the one hand, you feel you are in the presence of a man inspired, a man thinking and feeling in images, like a poet whose lines come from unconscious depths of creativity. On the other hand, so strange and bizarre are some of his thoughts, there is the suspicion, all the time, that his contact with reality is a frail one. Maudsley[39] did, in fact, find evidence of an episode of 'acute insanity' in Swedenborg's London diary of 1744. There was mention of hallucinations and delusions.† Although Maudsley thought that 'because a man's mind is unsound all of which he says is not therefore folly', he nevertheless concluded that Swedenborg was 'scientifically as sound as sounding brass or a tinkling cymbal'.

'Not many notices and reviews' of the 1882 volume on the brain appeared, complained Tafel, but the review in the journal *Brain* was 'fair and considerate'. It was indeed, all ten pages of it.[166] The reviewer thought it was 'one of the most remarkable books we have seen'. There were 'hopelessly unintelligible parts' but Swedenborg had clearly 'anticipated modern discoveries' in the localization of cerebral function, in which field two of *Brain*'s editors – Ferrier and Hughlings Jackson – had laboured so well.

One London medical school returned a presentation copy of Volume I, saying that 'the work was undesirable for their library', provoking Tafel to reply that such a spirit 'reminds one more of the bigoted ages of the past'.

In 1910, to celebrate the hundredth anniversary of the Swedenborg Society, an international congress was held in London, with four hundred representatives. I do not know whether Hughlings Jackson, Ferrier, or Sherrington attended any of the scientific sections of the meeting, but they might have read about it. I feel sure, however, that the men who charted the concepts of levels in the nervous system, of cortical localization, and of

† In the *Journals and letters of Caroline Fox*, there is an entry (7 April 1847) that Swedenborg was eating in a Bishopsgate Inn, in 1785, when he thought he saw in the corner of the room a vision of Jesus Christ, who said to him 'Eat slower.' 'This was the beginning of all his visions and mysterious communications'.

integration, would have been intrigued by the uncanny anticipations which this strange genius forecast over two hundred years ago. Contrast them, for example, with the tentative expressions of opinion by such as Unzer in 1771 and Prochaska in 1784, whose two books on the nervous system were widely acclaimed.[167, 168]

Unzer (1727–99) wrote,

The whole brain is not immediately necessary to thought since large portions of it may be lost or defective, or be compressed or ossified, or its function otherwise interrupted, without any perceptible influence on the mental powers, which, as to the cortical substance at least, is not remarkable, because it is not the seat of the mind. ... It is not known, whether there be one point only in the whole brain appropriated to consciousness and the conceptive force, and which can be termed the seat of the mind.[169]

Although Unzer was unimpressed by the importance of the cortex, which he said was 'almost wholly a tissue of tubes', he nevertheless admitted that old age or head injury could impair one faculty and not another, as they 'are scattered about the brain'.

Prochaska (1749–1820), at the end of his dissertation, asked the question 'Do each of the divisions of the intellect occupy a separate portion of the brain?'. Since the brain was 'composed of many parts, variously figured' he thought it quite likely that they did.

It is, therefore, by no means improbable, that each division of the intellect has its allotted organ in the brain, so that there is one for the perceptions, another for the understanding, probably others also for the will, and imagination, and memory, which act wonderfully in concert and mutually excite each other to action.[170]

But such statements do not take us further than did those of Willis, a century before, with Unzer, in fact, not accepting Willis's suggestion of cortical supremacy.

*

Looking back, one can see how little was known of the functions of the brain and spinal cord at the end of the century. There were, it is true, a few hints of a segmental arrangement in the spinal cord, and of regional differences within the brain, but the whole problem of nervous conduction was still wrapped in mystery. Progress demanded the discovery of a new phenomenon, or the forging of a new doctrine. This came about as a consequence of the work of Galvani.

LUIGI GALVANI (1737 – 1798) AND THE BIRTH OF ELECTROPHYSIOLOGY

It is not without interest that although the general outline of the story of Galvani is well known[171–174] and not in dispute, an English translation of his celebrated *De viribus electricitatis in motu musculari commentarius* of 1791 was not made until 1953. German and French translations were published in 1793 and 1939, respectively. Curiously, in 1953, two English translations were published, both by Americans.

'The affair began at first as follows' said Galvani.

I dissected and prepared a frog, as in Fig. 2, Tab. I, and placed it on a table, on which was an electrical machine, Fig. 1, Tab. 1 widely removed from its conductor and separated by no brief interval. When by chance one of those who were assisting me gently touched the point of a scalpel to the medial crural nerves, DD, of this frog, immediately all the muscles of the limbs seemed to be so contracted that they appeared to have fallen into violent tonic convulsions. But another of the assistants, who was on hand when I did electrical experiments, seemed to observe that the same thing occurred whenever a spark was discharged from the conductor of the machine (Fig. 1, B).[177]

Galvani, then 54 years of age and a professor in the medical faculty of the University of Bologna, had been studying 'animal electricity' since 1780. It was a popular scientific topic of the day. Although much of his work had ultimately to be rejected it did serve as a powerful stimulus, exerting a great influence on the development both of physiology and physics. This indirect achievement, Galvani hoped for, when he said, in the opening page of his Commentary, 'if we cannot attain the truth, at least a new approach thereto may be opened'. The new approach was to the age-old problem of nervous transmission.

It is not important whether we conclude, with Hoff,[171] that 'electrophysiology began almost a half century before Galvani with the discovery of the Leyden Jar', or whether, with Brazier,[178] that 'The birthday of electrophysiology falls on September 20th 1786', when Galvani watched the twitching of some frog legs on his terrace. Neither is it important that there was an element of chance in the discoveries in Leyden and Bologna. But it

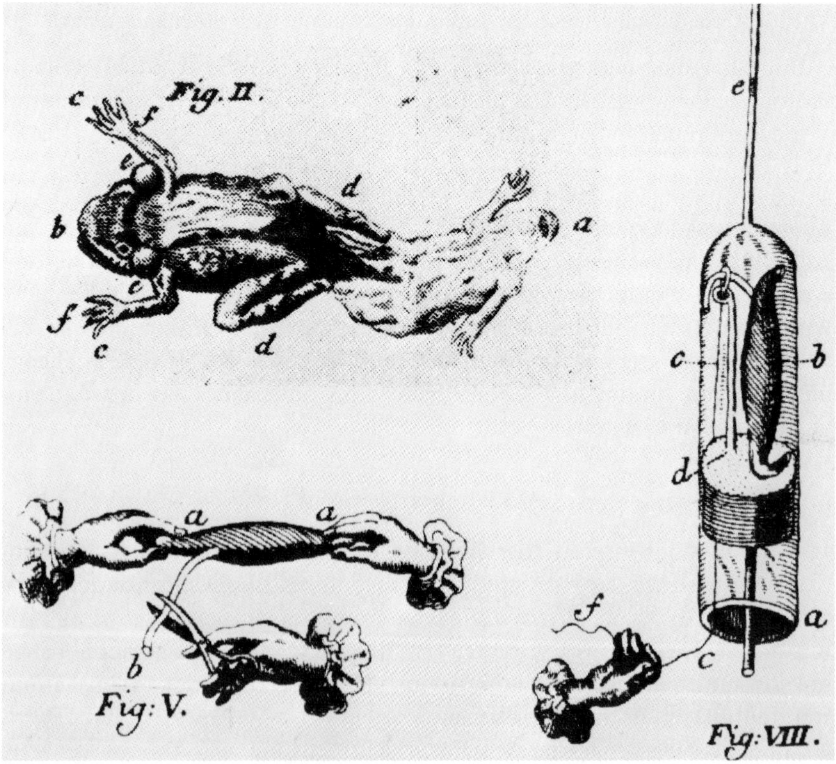

FIG. 49 Illustrations of use of frog nerve-muscle preparations (1665–67). *Fig. V.* The muscle *aa*, contracts when the nerve *b* is stimulated. *Fig. VIII.* The muscle-nerve preparation is enclosed in a glass tube and a drop of water is trapped at *e* in a narrow tube. The muscle *b* contracts when the silver wire *c* is pulled. As the drop of water did not move, he concluded that the muscle had not swelled when it contracted. As the silver wire *c* is threaded through a loop in the copper wire *d*, some have thought that the stimulus was not mechanical but electrical. But this is very unlikely. (After Swammerdam[206].)

was important that in each case the initial perception was a vivid one and that it was followed by an energetic search. Physicist and physiologist each 'grasped the skirt of happy chance' and the sciences of electricity and physiology came together – and each took a great leap forward.

Electricity

In the ancient world phenomena such as lightning, the thunderbolts of Jove, haloes and flames around human heads, and beams of light from warriors' eyes were familiar in life or legend. So also were the effects of friction on amber and the shock-producing power of certain fish. Although Gilbert (p. 54) may have 'made a philosophy from a lodestone' only the static form of electricity was known until the end of the eighteenth century. Gilbert's 'Electric Force' was gradually differentiated from those other 'imponderable' forces of nature – heat, light, magnetism and chemical action, not to mention 'phlogiston' and 'aether'. If friction could produce both fire and electricity it is not difficult to understand how they could be confused.

In 1768, Joseph Priestley (1733–1804) said a spark 'has not only the appearance of fire, but is capable of actually setting fire to various substances'. His *The history and present state of electricity, with original experiments* (1767),[179] had proved too 'difficult' for his readers, so a year later he wrote *A familiar introduction to the study of electricity*.[180] In these books he summarized and explained what was known of electricity and, concerning the history of his subject, he said that he was 'peculiarly fortunate' as 'the materials were neither too few, nor too many to make a history'. The ancient Greeks had imagined amber was 'animated'. Gilbert thought that friction 'excited the virtue' of electric bodies by 'alteration of cohesion'. To Boyle, electrics 'emitted a glutinous effluvium which laid hold of small bodies'. The phenomena of attraction and repulsion, Priestley wrote, were first shown by Otto von Guericke (1602–86), Burgomaster of Magdebourg, with his 'globe of sulphur'.

Priestley described the various types of electrical machines then available, explaining that their 'principal part was a globe or cylinder of glass with a machine to give it friction'. He explained the terms 'positive' and 'negative', 'charging' and 'discharging', and 'battery' ('a number of jars'). With his own new machine which he offered for sale he presented a copy of his second book, for 'philosophical purposes ... and entertainment'.

The popularity of the new medium had been heralded by Stephen Gray (?–1736), 'a pensioner at Charter House' who succeeded in electrifying 'a boy of eight or nine years'. Gray's report to the Royal Society of London in 1731 was one of a series of publications in the *Philosophical Transactions* on the phenomena of electricity. Gray said he had begun his experience in 1729 and found that 'the Electrick Vertue of a glass tube may be conveyed to any other Bodies, so as to give them the same Property of attracting and repelling'.[181] He found that the 'Electrical Effluvia will be carried in a circle and be communicated from one circle to another'. The famous experiment with the suspended boy was performed several times in April 1730.

Upon the tube's being rubbed and held near his feet, without touching them, the leaf-Brass was attracted by the boy's face with much vigour ...[181]

By these experiments we see that Animals receive a greater quantity of Electrical Effluvia, and that they may be conveyed from them several ways at the same time to considerable distances ...

'Hithertoo', said Priestley, 'the spirit of electricity seems to have been confined to England', but the Frenchman Du Fay (1698–1739), on learning of Gray's experiments, repeated and extended them, and succeeded in showing the difference between conductors and insulators (metals and electrics). Du Fay thought there were probably two kinds of electrical fluid, which were separated by friction; he conceived the idea of something 'flowing'. Benjamin Franklin (1706–90), who showed that lightning was electric in 1752, argued that there was only one fluid which flowed.

It had always been amusing to see a spark jump a gap, or to hear a crackle of discharge, but when conduction through the human body could be so dramatically demonstrated by the Abbé Nollet that, holding hands, 180 Royal guards at Versailles, or a mile-long line of monks in a monastery, were seen to jump with the passage of the new medium,[171] it is not surprising that doctors and quacks should choose it as a form of therapy.[182] Priestley said there were reports of 'great cures' of paralysis from Italy and Germany, but he had known a person with epilepsy made worse by electrical treatment. Whytt wrote

A man aged 25, who, from a palsy of twelve years continuance, had lost all power of motion in his left arm, after trying other remedies in vain, at last had recourse to electricity; by every shock of which the muscles of this arm were made to contract; and the member itself, which was very much withered, after having been electrified for some weeks, became plumper.[183]

A weapon which could 'beatify' with a halo, and cure paralytics was clearly one of Nature's wonders. Could it also be the *vis nervosa* which would, in Fontana's words, 'read the animal spirits out of office'? There were some who argued; others experimented. What helped to formulate the concept of 'innate', as opposed to 'communicated', electricity were the investigations upon electric fish.

Electric fish

Kellaway,[184] in his fine study of ancient views on these animals, said that 'Undoubtedly the first bio-electric phenomenon of which man became aware was the electric discharge of certain types of fish.' The numbing or paralysing effect of these species of fish, eel, or ray (torpedo, viz. torpor-inducing) was well known in classical antiquity. It was also appreciated that the shock came from certain parts of the fish, and that it could pass through the length of a line or trident. The fish could be safely eaten. As early as the twelfth century, Averroes, the last of the great Arabic physicians, actually suggested that the force exerted by the electric fish was analogous to that exerted by the lodestone on iron. But it was not until the third quarter of the eighteenth century that the electrical nature of the shock was revealed.

In July 1772, from La Rochelle, on the Atlantic coast of France, came the first of a series of letters from John Walsh (1725–95) to Benjamin Franklin, requesting him to lay before the Royal Society of London, the observations he had made 'On the Electrical Property of *the* Torpedo.'

> The effect of the Torpedo appears to be absolutely electrical . . . we have discovered the back and breast of the animal to be in different states of electricity . . . [we were able] to direct his shocks through a circuit of four persons . . . the conductors are the same in the torpedo as in the Leyden jar . . . we have not observed any spark to accompany the shock . . .[185]

In his second letter, from the adjacent Ile de Ré, Walsh wrote,

> The effect of the Torpedo appears to arise from a compressed elastic fluid, restoring itself to its equilibrium in the same way, and by the same medium, as the elastic fluid in charged glass.[185]

Walsh's account included drawings of the electric organs which showed they had a 'hexagonal arrangement' resembling 'a honeycomb in miniature'. Electricity, he said 'wings the formidable bolt of the atmosphere . . . and . . . in the deep it speeds an humbler bolt, silent and invisible'. In the following year came a second paper from Walsh, 'Of Torpedos found on the Coast of England.'[186] Caught in Torbay and Brixham, 'This wonderful guest' was much bigger, and would surely 'felicitate our invalids'. Walsh referred to its reputation in ancient Greece and Rome for curing Headache and gout; the patient stood barefoot on the animal until its power was exhausted. Walsh won the Copley Medal of the Royal Society for his work but what puzzled everyone was that the discharge of electricity came from a muscle which was itself a conductor of electrical fluid.

John Hunter (1728–93) dissected a torpedo furnished by Walsh and found that the two electric organs lay on each side of the cranium and gills, each about five inches in length, 'consisting wholly of perpendicular columns, reaching from the upper to the under surface of the body . . . each column is divided by horizontal partitions . . . 470 columns in each organ'.[187] Hunter noted that the nerves inserted into each organ arose from three 'extraordinary' large trunks coming from the posterior part of the animal's brain. He surmised that they must be for the 'formation, collection or management of the electric fluid', and he wondered how this could be related to an explanation of nervous function.

Henry Cavendish (1731–1810) noted that 'a shock may be perceived when the fish is held under water . . . and where the electrical effluvia hath a much readier passage than thro the person's body'.[188] He devised an artificial torpedo.

Electric nerve fluid

In the mid-eighteenth century physicians such as Boerhaave and Haller were forced to speculate about the nature of the fluid which they believed responsible for nerve conduction. Boerhaave had seen 'drops of dew' at the cut ends of nerves, and wrote that nerve-fluid must be 'the most subtle of the whole body! . . . [and the] . . . 'swiftest'.[189] Under the influence of the will it could speed in and out of muscles in a moment. Haller held similar views. In an annotation by Wrisberg (1739–1808) in an edition of Haller's *First lines of physiology*, we read

The doctrine of the nervous fluid, or animal spirits is confirmed by many arguments drawn from anatomy; but is fully refuted by as many, if not more, of a similar nature. But ocular demonstration of the nerves, proves, that such a fluid . . . does not exist. . . . Since 1766, I have been inclined to think, that it perhaps resembles the electric and magnetical fluids; . . . We may expect that this obscurity will be greatly removed by the very celebrated anatomists Drs. Monro and Prochaska, who have extended and directed their study to the physiology of the nerves.[190]

Wrisberg was referring to Monro II, but the first Alexander Monro, a pupil of Boerhaave, had also written on 'The Anatomy of the Human Nerves,' in 1732. His essay is to be found in *The works of Alexander Monro*, published by his son in 1781.[191] A cautious observer, who 'personally attended the opening of every body' at post-mortem, he was uncertain about the nerve-fluid hypothesis. He saw no 'dew' emerge from the cut end of a nerve, nor any swelling above a ligature. But these observations 'did not prove the absence of liquor'.[192] He found that compression of the phrenic nerve in a living animal paralysed the diaphragm on that side. (Haller had found that it caused the diaphragm to move.) Then, 'milking' the nerve below the compression, he noted a transient return of movement. He concluded that this was because some nerve fluid had remained in the nerve below the compression. The following oft-quoted passage is taken from *The works* (p. 333).

We are not sufficiently acquainted with the properties of an *aether* or *electrical effluvia* pervading everything, to apply them justly in the animal oeconomy; and it is difficult to conceive how they should be retained or conducted in a long nervous cord.[193]

But this apparently cannot be taken to be the first known reference to the idea of electrical conduction in nerve. Clarke and O'Malley[194] have pointed out that the words 'electrical effluvia' and 'conducted' were additions which appeared in editions after 1746. Published with his 'Osteology' and other essays, his book was translated into most European languages and went through eight editions in Monro's lifetime (1697–1767).[195]

The first person to speculate that nerve conduction might be electrical was none other than that curious cleric Stephen Hales (1677–1761).[196] In 1732 he wrote that some stronger form of circulation than that of the blood was needed to enter a muscle and force it to contract. Muscular contraction

. . . must therefore be owing to some more vigorous and active Energy, whose Force is regulated by the Nerves; But whether it be confined in Canals within the Nerves, or acts along their Surfaces like electrical Powers, is not easy to determine.[197]

Whytt however felt that no known form of energy could satisfactorily explain nerve conduction and muscular contraction. Electricity was being used 'to explain almost every hidden operation in nature':[198]

Gravity, magnetism, and electricity are all regular and uniform in their operations; they bespeak nothing of feeling or life in the bodies which are endowed with them . . .[199]

In 1767, Fontana had little to say about electricity in 'The laws of irritability' but in 1781, his famous *Traite sur le venin de la vipère*, etc. included a lecture he gave in London in 1779 on the structure of nerves. He said that a 'nerve is made up of a large number of transparent cylinders, homogeneous, uniform, and very simple'.[200] He did not think his primitive nerve cylinders contained a swiftly moving fluid. Some other principle should be considered.

If not ordinary electricity, then something at least strongly analogous to it. The electrical eel and ray, if not actually making it probable at least suggest such a possibility.[201]

He suggested that the laws governing electricity might determine the nature of nerve conduction and muscular contraction.

During the fifty years that Monro II (1733–1817) occupied the Chair of Anatomy at Edinburgh he published three books on the nervous system: *Observations on the structure and functions of the nervous system* (1783),[202] *Experiments on the nervous system . . . with a view of determining the nature and effects of animal electricity* (1793),[203] and *Three treatises; On the brain, the eye and the ear* (1797).[204] The last book does not concern us here as it is a description of fifteen cases of internal hydrocephalus, with a repetition of his original account, thirty-three years previously, of the interventricular foramina.† The first book appeared nearly a decade before Galvani's *De viribus electricitatis*; the second book, two years after Galvani's.

In Chapter 22 of the first book (p. 67) he recounts his experience of using a compound microscope to examine the structure and size of nerve fibres. He estimated that optic nerve fibres measured 1/9000th of an inch, but he found the appearances generally 'deceptive' and 'misleading'. He commented (p. 74) on Haller's estimate of the velocity of nerve fluid at 9000 feet a minute and was not convinced. As for the electric torpedo and eel, all he felt we could conclude was that 'the nerves enable this machinery to perform its proper office of collecting the electrical fluid, but without directly furnishing to it any of that fluid'. He did not think the evidence warranted the conclusion 'that the nerves operate by the medium of an electrical fluid'. Neither did he think that there was a '*vis insita* different from *vis nervea*' (p. 94). Galvani's claims, therefore, must have caused a great stir in Edinburgh and Monro II was quick to study this new animal electricity and in his second book he concluded that the nervous and electrical fluids were not identical.

Lastly, we should recall that in this pre-Galvanic era of neurophysiology, Prochaska thought in much the same way as the Monros, Haller, and Whytt in regarding electricity as only a new form of stimulus that could excite neuromuscular action.

A stimulus is necessary to the action of the *vis nervosa* . . . as the spark is latent in the steel or flint, and is not elicited, unless there be friction between the flint and the steel, so the *vis nervosa* is latent, nor excites action of the nervous system until excited by an applied stimulus. ... I have conjectured however that there is an analogy between the *vis nervosa* and electricity ...[205]

The paths to Bologna

In the city of Whytt and the Monros, 1745 was the year of 'The Rising'; in Boerhaave's it was the year of 'The Leyden Jar'. This first useful condenser or capacitor not only enabled quacks and doctors to employ their electrostatic machines more freely, but it also provided the physiologist with a valuable tool. Haller, in his experimental onslaught on those unfortunate 190 animals, used all manner of torture, even burning out a womb. Why he never used electrical stimulation is a mystery; the only mention of it in his 'Dissertation' of 1753 is in reference to its use in a patient with paralysed limbs. Perhaps if he had not given up his work at Göttingen and returned to Berne he might have taken it up.

Physiologists now turned increasingly to *Rana Temporaria* – the common European frog – evolving the humble nerve-muscle preparation which has played a classical role in experimental physiology.† With the nineteenth-century smoked drum it became a familiar sight in laboratories throughout the world. Doubtless, tickling frogs' legs and noting the response to different stimuli have interested man through the ages. Izaak Walton (1593–1683) described in *The Compleat Angler* how he used the frog as bait when fishing for pike. Judging from his account of keeping a frog for six months, hooked up through mouth and gills, with a leg tied up to the arming-wire, it would not be surprising if he had noted an occasional bimetallically-induced twitch. Stensen's friend, Swammerdam (1637–80),[206] left splendid drawings of the use of frog nerve-muscle preparations (Fig. 49). He showed that mechanical stimulation of a nerve induced contraction, but not swelling, of the muscle. In one experiment his employment of silver and copper wires in his preparation led to the suggestion that the stimulus may have been electrical. There is disagreement on this point; some, such as Liddell[207] and Schulte and Endtz,[208] favour the probability of a closed circuit; others, such as Licht[209] and Brazier,[210] find it improbable. Swammerdam's work was not published until 1738, but in the meantime, in 1700, it was a professor of anatomy in Paris, Du Verney, who is authoritatively reported to have been the first to publicly demonstrate that irritation of a nerve in a frog preparation caused contraction of the muscle.[211] Contrary to Licht's[209] claim there is nothing in the account, admittedly an abridged translation, to suggest that there was any electrical stimulus.

It is clear, however, that the most popular experimental preparation in the history of physiology was first used over two hundred years ago.

By the middle of the eighteenth century electrical stimulation of animal tissues was an accepted mode of investigation in physiology. Means of measurement were lacking and Priestley said 'I cannot help wishing the experiments were resumed with some more accurate measure of conducting power than hath yet been contrived.'[213] He had been comparing the

† 'The Job of physiology.' (Claude Bernard in *An introduction to the study of experimental medicine*. Dover, New York (1957). p. 115.)

conducting powers of 'spinal marrow' and 'muscle tissue' in 'an ox and other animals'.

Galvani's predecessor in the Chair of Anatomy at Bologna, Leopoldo Caldani (1725–1813), used frog nerve-muscle preparations for a lecture there, in 1756.[171] It was to Caldani that Haller had turned during his controversy with Whytt, when he read of the latter's discovery of 'spinal shock'. He asked Caldani to study the effects of decapitation of a frog and he confirmed Whytt's observations.[214] Galvani was a student in Bologna at the time of Caldani's lecture, graduating in 1759. So, when he began his own researches in about 1780, it was not with a new technique, but he was the first to use it to demonstrate that electric fishes were not the only animals possessing the 'vertue'.

Galvani's experiments

Galvani's *Commentarius* of 1791, in the English translation[175] on which this account is based, is some 24,000 words in length. The original Latin sentences were clearly long and often tortuous; their meaning is sometimes obscure. This writer will forever remain puzzled by Professor O'Malley's comment that the following lines merely represent a 'stylistic conceit'.[215] 'The peculiar and not previously recognised nature of this seems to be that it (animal electricity) flows from muscles to nerves, or rather from the latter to the former' (p. 60). When Galvani refers to his four illustrative plates the reader must be patient and prepared to use a magnifying glass. Each plate is used to demonstrate a number of different experiments. But the reader will soon appreciate that Galvani did not publish his experience in the manner of a modern scientist, on a well-constructed plan, with an introduction, a review of the literature, the reasons for the research, and a summary of his results and conclusions. Instead he chose to present his 'discoveries and findings in the order and relation in which partly chance and fortune presented and partly diligence and industry revealed them to me' (p. 1). It becomes an account in which, step by step, the reader is invited to share Galvani's puzzlement and witness the manner of his endeavour, over a period of at least ten years. It is a very personal, and at times, even a homely, document, as when he mentions that he was burned with wax in one experiment (p. 46), and when he names and identifies friends who assisted him in another when they were 'rusticating in a villa' (p. 41).

But this approach, though interesting, deprives the reader of an opportunity of judging how much Galvani knew of the experience of others in this and relevant fields. For he mentions only four scientists; Volta, when he used his electrometer (p. 31); Cotugno, in reference to sciatica (p. 73); Bartholinus,† on the term 'animal electricity'; and Gardiner,‡ whom he mentions when discussing the subjects of the influence of weather on health (p. 78) and lightning on plant growth (p. 81). There is frequent reference to 'physicists' and 'learned' men but nowhere is there a summary about the current state of relevant knowledge. As already mentioned, however, the evidence makes it very unlikely that he was unacquainted with it, and the familiar note he often strikes supports this impression.

† Bartholinus; Abbé Pierre Bertholot (1742–1800), author of *De l'électricité des vegetaux* (Lyons, 1783).

‡ Gardiner, J. (1738?–90?), author of *Observations on the animal oeconomy, and on the causes and cures of diseases* (Edinburgh, 1784), in which he said (p. 42), 'When old men are unfortunately addicted to venereal pleasures, they consult their passions, rather than their ability . . . it is true they seldom die in action . . . but after palsies'.

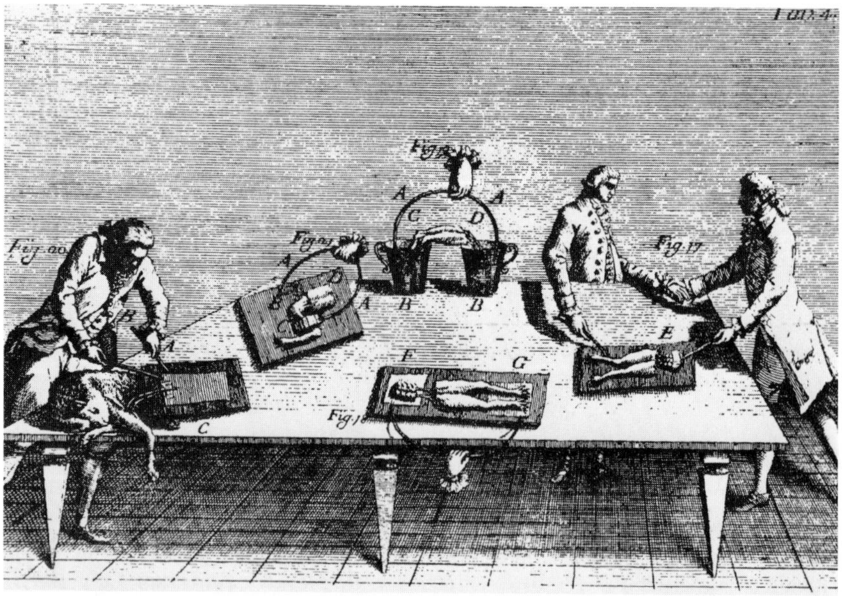

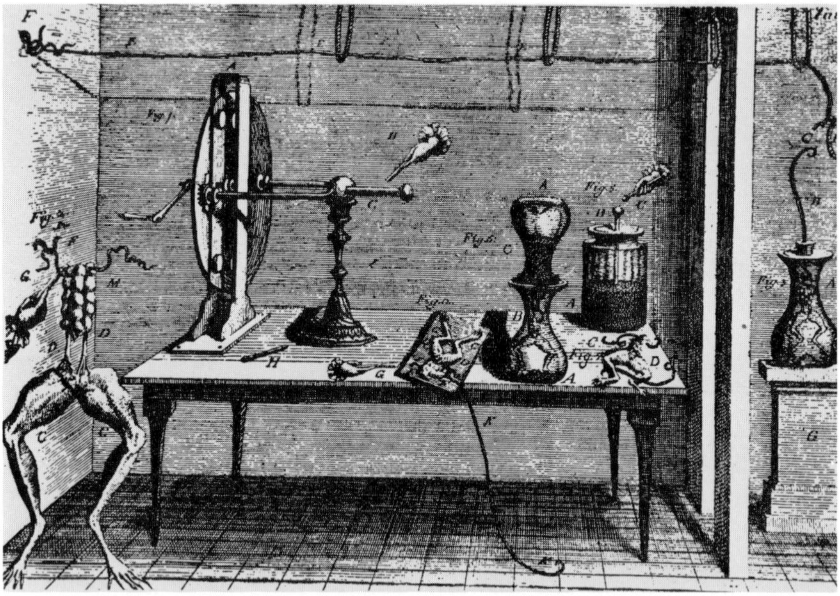

FIG. 50. On the left a live sheep with its thigh nerves removed and armatured with tin foil to a plate. On the right two assistants complete an arc. Centre (rear); the frog preparation lies in two jars of water, feet on left, spine and nerves on right. Centre (front); the preparation rests on two unconnected surfaces; F. silver; G, copper foil. Centre (left); an armatured preparation of a chick.

FIG. 51. On the table, to the left, stands an 'electrical machine', of the revolving plate type. A Leyden jar containing lead shot stands on the right. Between them is Galvani's 'little machine', two glass jars, one inverted on the other. The upper contains lead shot, and the lower a frog preparation and more lead shot. He used it in experiments designed to exclude the possibility of electricity reaching the preparation from the frictional machine. In front of the Leyden jar is a frog preparation with a conductor attached to the spinal stump and another to the legs. A second preparation lies on a plate, wired to the ground. On the left of the table is the customary preparation Galvani employed; only the nerves connect the legs to spine. Metal wire is threaded through the spine and connects with an iron hook on the wall. From the ceiling, slung on silk threads, is an iron wire 150 feet in length, running to an adjoining room. It connects with another wire attached to a frog preparation in a glass jar. The muscles contracted when the electrical machine sparked.

The majority of his experiments were performed in his home, on dead animals, usually frogs and turtles, but he also used living animals, dissecting out the sciatic nerve in the thigh and applying his electric conductor to it. He used cold-blooded and warm-blooded animals (birds, chicks, hens, and sheep). One of his plates shows a sheep (Fig. 50). Muscular responses were more readily obtained in dead, cold-blooded animals. He worked outdoors and indoors, in different weathers and seasons, because he was concerned to learn the source of animal electricity. He employed glass, resin, wood, and marble as insulating surfaces, and iron and bronze wires and hooks as

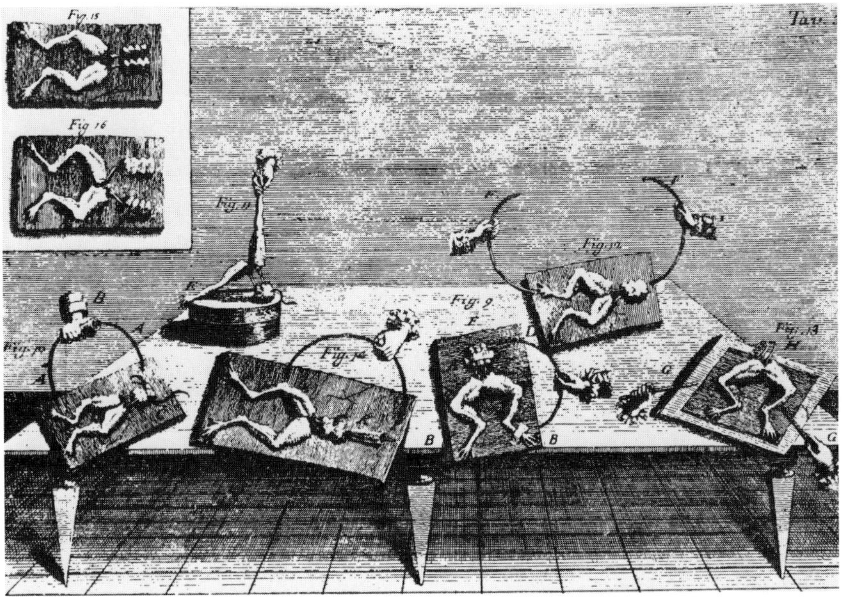

FIG. 52. A series of demonstrations. There are two wall plates, *Figs. 15* and *16*. In the upper the legs are divided in the pelvis and separated. Only the leg connected to the spinal stump would twitch. In the lower, the spinal stump is split and separated, the legs are rejoined, and the result is the same. To the right of the wall plates (*Fig. 8*) is the experiment of the 'electric pendulum' (p. 157), with the preparation held by one foot over the silver box. The remaining figures illustrate various hand-held arcs, insulated and non-insulated, and one made of two separate halves. Note tin foil on leg and spinal stump in *Fig. 9*. On far right, *Fig. 13*, the preparation lies on a 'magic square' with the ends of an arc touching its two surfaces and the nerves (H) arranged to make contact with its lower surface.

conductors. He normally used his frog preparations on a table, but sometimes he enclosed them in glass jars, or submerged them in water, or oil, before applying the electric stimulus. The latter was obtained from a frictional machine of the revolving disc type, or a Leyden jar, and he mentions 'magic squares' – glass plate condensers covered on each side with metal foil. Taking a hint from the physicists who used tin foil in their magic squares and Leyden jars, he found that if he covered his nerves with tin foil, the responses were augmented. He was able to obtain them even in a tadpole. Galvani had previously failed to obtain any response when he applied his conductors to the brain, but 'if the denuded cerebrum and denuded spinal cord are covered in some part with the same metal foil, when the arc was applied according to custom, contractions both vigorous and prompt then began to appear' (pp. 47 and 71). His arcs were curved iron or copper rods held in the hand.

In his customary frog preparation he completely removed the thighs so that the lower end of the vertebral column, with its enclosed spinal cord, was connected to the legs only through the sciatic nerves. In some experiments he divided the pelvis sagittally and separated the legs, joining them 'in some artificial way' when required (Figs. 51 and 52). One end of the arc was applied to the spinal cord or sciatic nerve and the other to the foot.

He divided his commentary into four chapters, dealing successively with 'artificial', 'atmospheric', and 'animal' electricity. The fourth chapter was entitled 'Conjectures and Conclusions' wherein he considered in what way his observations might have relevance to human physiology. The cramps of sciatica, the spasms of tetanus, the convulsions of epilepsy, and the paralysis of apoplexy and other diseases of the nervous system would, he hoped, be better understood. But his concept of a 'neuro-electric fluid' that was distilled in the brain and flowed throughout the spinal cord and nerves into the muscles provided no new basis for consideration of aetiology. He could only suggest that lesions might develop as a consequence of 'accumulation' or 'contamination' of this fluid. He also reasoned that in epilepsy, animal electricity might do what he had shown artifical electricity could do in his animals 'rushing into ... and ... stimulating and injuring the brain' (p. 75).

He was wary of the therapeutic use of electricity in paralysis 'for it is difficult to diagnosticate whether a disease arises from damaged and impaired structure of nerves or brain, or from insulating material blocking either the internal parts of a nerve, or others whereby we think that the circulation of electricity in us is performed' (p. 79).

The chance contact of the scalpel with the nerve led to a whole series of experiments. First, Galvani had to be certain that the stimulus was not just mechanical. He assured himself on this score when he found that movements only occurred when the machine was sparking and when he held the scalpel by its metal blade or when his fingers touched the iron nails in the bone handle; no movements occurred when he only touched the bone of the handle. 'To place the matter beyond all doubt' he next touched the nerve with a slender glass, then an iron cylinder, and found that contractions only occurred with the latter. There was clearly an electrical element at work and he wrote that 'contact of a conducting body with the nerves is also required'. Then he found that a long wire 'would replace the lack of a man'. Further experiments produced similar results when he used a Leyden jar or electrophore instead of an electrical machine, and live animals instead of his preparations. He removed the machine to a distance, enclosed his frog in a glass jar, and was still able to produce muscular contractions.

The experiments were repeated 'in the fresh air, in a lofty part of the house' to see whether atmospheric electricity would have similar effects. Prepared legs of frogs and warm-blooded animals were attached by their

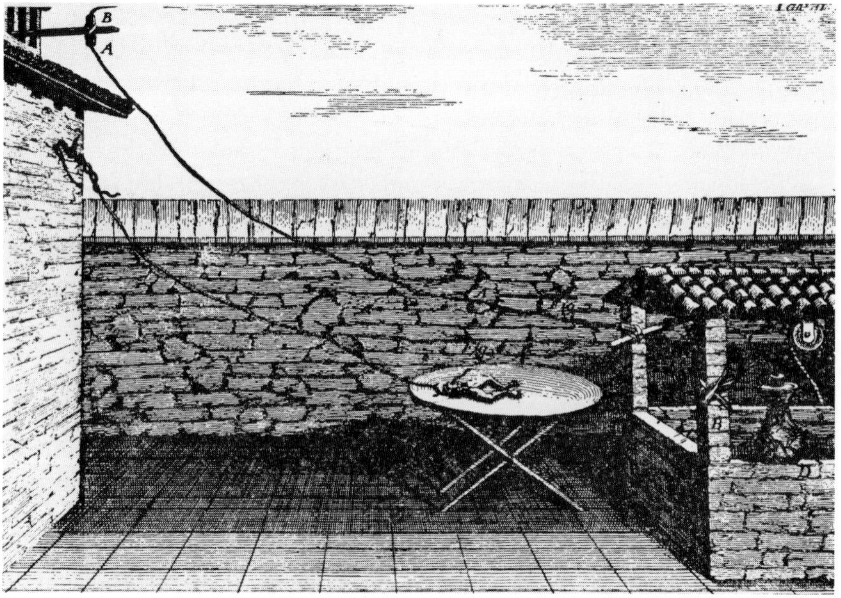

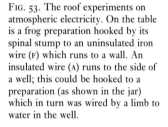

FIG. 53. The roof experiments on atmospheric electricity. On the table is a frog preparation hooked by its spinal stump to an uninsulated iron wire (F) which runs to a wall. An insulated wire (A) runs to the side of a well; this could be hooked to a preparation (as shown in the jar) which in turn was wired by a limb to water in the well.

nerves to long insulated iron wires, with the feet connected to another long wire, which dipped into the water of a roof well (Fig. 53). Not only did muscular contractions occur during lightning, 'preceding the thunders', but also when the sky was just 'stormy', when the conductors were not insulated or when they were placed 'on lower ground', and even when the preparation was enclosed in a jar or kept indoors. The same occurred with living animals.

In the third chapter Galvani began, 'my heart burned with desire to test the power of peaceful everyday electricity'. He had noticed that his preparations sometimes twitched as they hung on an iron trellis that surrounded 'a certain hanging garden of my house'. In his *Commentary* Galvani said the hooks by which the spinal columns were attached to the trellis were bronze, but Professor Pupilli[216] noted that in a manuscript Galvani first referred to iron hooks. He thought the twitching was the effect of atmospheric electricity so he watched them 'at different hours, for many days', when the weather was 'stormy' or 'serene'. Finally 'weary with vain expectation, I began to press the bronze hooks, against the iron gratings to see whether by this kind of device they excited muscular contractions'. They did, so he brought a preparation indoors, laid it on an iron plate, pressed the hook against the plate, and 'behold, the same contractions and the same motions!'

There were no contractions if glass, stone, or wooden plates were used. It appeared that the atmosphere was irrelevant and Galvani began to have 'some suspicion about inherent animal electricity itself'. He found that on a glass plate, movements were sometimes produced if he connected the bronze hook to a foot of the frog. If the connecting arc was made of a second metal, twitches were seen, but not when it was of the same metal, or made of nonconducting material.

'A casually observed phenomenon' particularly excited him, and led him to compare it to 'an electric pendulum'. He held up a prepared frog by one leg, with the bronze hook in the spinal column resting on a silver box. When the other leg touched the box it jumped up. The muscles relaxed when the circuit was broken. The leg could thus be made to rise and fall 'not without admiration and pleasure on the part of the beholder'.

As a result of his experiments, and notwithstanding how he noted the importance of contact between dissimilar metals, Galvani concluded that the phenomena proved the existence of animal electricity. As it transpired, Volta was to show that the frog's leg merely played the part of a sensitive electroscope, and he argued that *all* the electricity was artificial. But three years later, Galvani did succeed in demonstrating the truth of his original claim, when he held up a preparation by one foot and manipulated it so that the spinal stump and the sciatic nerve touched the muscles of the other leg. The muscles contracted, and also when the spinal column was allowed to fall on the thigh. Here there was no problem about metals or artificial electricity. We now know, of course, that this 'animal electricity' was the injury current of cut muscle.

Galvani continued to investigate animal electricity in his preparations, and also in the electric ray in Rimini and Senigallia on the Adriatic coast. He found no difference in them from his laboratory animals. But his last years were not happy ones. In addition to his dispute with Volta, there were family worries; he died in 1798.

When Volta wrote in 1793 to the Royal Society of London about Galvani's discoveries, he said that there was proof of 'the existence of a genuine animal electricity in all, or nearly all animals'.[217] But when he reported again, in 1800, his views had changed. He no longer believed that a muscle could be compared to the coating on a Leyden jar and he was able to show that an electrical discharge could stimulate sensory nerves as well as muscle fibres. 'In certain cases, conductors are also creators of electricity . . . [his] organ of artificial electricity [the Voltaic Pile or Crown of Cups] was fundamentally the same and structurally similar to the natural organ of the ray.'[218] He, too, was awarded the Copley Medal.

Monro II, in 1793, also published an account of the experiments he had undertaken 'with the view of determining the Nature and Effects of Animal Electricity'.[219] He used frogs, rabbits, and a pig, employing opium and 'metalline substances' and concluded that the 'nervous fluid' and the 'electrical fluid' were not identical. Nerve power was excited by mechanical or chemical stimuli, and abolished by opium, 'which cannot be imagined to act on the electrical fluid'. Galvani's notion that 'the nerve was electrified *plus* and the muscle *minus*, resembling the Leyden phial' was refuted. 'Muscles are convulsed when the only communication between muscles and metals, is by the nerve . . . a muscle forming 'no part of the circle' could contract. . . . His experiments showed that the 'nervous and electrical fluids were moving in opposite directions,' so they must be essentially different. Moreover, the electrical fluid was not arrested by ligature or section of a nerve. The new knowledge, he concluded, had merely shown that there was a new way of 'exciting the nervous fluid or energy'.

Galvani's nephew, Aldini (1762–1834), who had assisted in the Bologna series of experiments (and who may have been one of the two assistants who made the chance observations with the scalpel and the sparking machine) continued to experiment, and seemingly to exploit what came to be known as 'Galvanism'. He spoke of the 'animal pile', and experimented on decapitated criminals in Bologna. In 1803, on a visit to the Royal College of Surgeons in London, he carried out some worthless tests on 'the body of a malefactor executed at Newgate' by hanging, an hour previously.[220]

MORGAGNI (1682–1771) AND BAILLIE (1761–1823) AND THE PHENOMENA OF DISEASE

'In order to perform what I promised you, I will begin with the pain of the head.' So wrote Morgagni (1682–1771) as he began to write his *De sedibus, et causis morborum per anatomen indagatis libri quinque* which was published in 1761, when he was nearly eighty years of age. The only complete English translation of its five volumes was made by Benjamin Alexander in 1769,[221] selections from which, some two hundred pages, were published in *Medical*

Classics, in 1940.[222] Alexander's translation was reprinted in 1960.[223]

Although his university chair in Padua was in anatomy, following Malpighi and Valsalva, it is clear that in *De sedibus*, what he had 'promised' his friend, when he began the seventy letters concerning the seven hundred or so autopsies on which the work is based, was not, to quote Virchow, 'the furtherance of anatomy as a pure science but the development of it as a fundamental science of practical medicine'. *Ubi est morbus*? Where is the disease?, Morgagni enquired, as did Virchow.[224] But as a historian of pathology, Long wrote, although modern pathology properly began with Morgagni, the book itself 'is as much a clinical work, with anatomical explanations of disease symptoms'.[225] In his clinical histories you will often find the age, sex, and occupation of the patient, his build and habits, and perhaps some reference to intelligence or character. Jarcho[226] has pointed out that *De sedibus* represents only about two-fifths of Morgagni's published work. From the Parma manuscripts, in 1935, a volume was published, based on one hundred clinical consultations recorded by Morgagni.[227]

Volume I of *De sedibus*, 'Which Treats of Disorders of the Head', contains in its fourteen letters accounts of otitic cerebral abscess, infantile cerebral palsy, cerebral tumour, cerebral gumma, and hydrocephalus with adequate demonstration that hemisphere lesions caused contralateral paralysis. Of the latter, he confessed that, at first, 'I had never attended to it', but he excused himself in recalling that Wepfer, Valsalva 'and many others ... should have taken so little notice of it' though they had observed 'this contrast betwixt the injury of the brain, and the palsy of the body'.

Case 1 may have been an example of tuberculous meningitis. A boy of 13 years, whose brother and sister had died of tuberculosis, developed pain in the head, fever, lethargy, delirium, convulsions and died. At autopsy there were pulmonary tubercles, congested inflamed meninges, and basal exudate.

Case 4 may have been one of hepatic encephalopathy. An alcoholic man of forty suffered from recurrent bouts of abdominal pain and delirium and had a fatal apoplexy. His liver was cirrhotic but his brain was normal in appearance.

Case 10 was possibly a patient with a subdural haematoma or a meningioma. He was a beggar, 'silly', liable to headaches and confusion; at autopsy the brain was normal but the dura was thickened and adherent to the skull on one side and had 'degenerated into a middle state betwixt a bone and a ligament, and formed the figure of an ellipse'.

Morgagni's description – the first – of the Stokes-Adams syndrome, concerned Anastosio Poggi, aged 68, 'a grave and worthy priest ... moderately fat and of a florid complexion, when he was first seized with epilepsy which left behind it the greatest slowness of pulse ... the disorder often returned, but the slowness of the pulse still remained'. Concerning epilepsy he knew of 'its beginning, either from the side, the hand or the foot' and that 'if a tight bandage was timely thrown round the leg, the disease did not proceed'. He quoted Willis about these focal epilepsies but differed with him about their cerebral origin. He still held to the older view that they originated, not in the head, but in the extremities. 'For if it had its origin from the brain, why did it always go to that part first?'[228]

His cases of apoplexy are many and varied. He viewed them as serous or sanguinous, although he was undecided about the nature of the fluid-filled cavities in the brain substance, sometimes watery, sometimes bloody. He seems to have suspected that strokes were in some way related to the cerebral circulation, its vessels, or the state of its blood, and that the lesions he saw were a cause rather than a consequence of the strokes.

Morgagni's seed, Sir Clifford Allbutt contended, fell upon hard and sterile ground, 'Morgagni had to wait for Laennec and Bright'.[229] Matthew Baillie (1761–1823), in the preface to the first edition of his *Morbid anatomy of some of the most important parts of the body* (1794) did write that he was trying 'to judge more accurately how far the symptoms and the appearances agree with each other'.[230] He thought many of Morgagni's observations were 'too generally described' and that 'small collateral circumstances', which were frequently introduced, obscured the main issues. Baillie's book, nevertheless, was more of a systematic textbook of pathology. It was well written and concise, beautifully illustrated, but from the neurological point of view, his case histories are inadequate and he did not consider lesions of the spinal cord and nerves.

Adult paraplegia, he thought, had 'considerably increased in this country within the last 15 or 20 years'.[231] There was no 'obvious' spinal disease and he thought it 'most commonly depends, in a great measure, on disease affecting the brain itself'; 'Pressure on the brain' most likely. In two cases of adult paraplegia he wrote that in the hands 'I found the sense of touch considerably impaired, so that shillings and sixpences could not be distinguished from each other'.[232] He mentioned a case of a 'singular disease of muscles', giving no clinical account, in which 'many of the muscles were extremely altered from their natural appearance. They were converted in many places into a yellowish substance.'[233] Diseased appearances of the brain were described under captions such as inflammation (uncommon), scrofulous tumours, spongy tumours, ossifications, abscesses, softening, gangrene, hardening, serous collections, extravasations, and hydrocephalus. He observed parasellar 'cherry-sized aneurysms' on the internal carotid arteries and a 'gooseberry-sized tumour' at the optic decussation. The cranial nerves were 'rarely diseased'.

Baillie noted the diseased appearance of arteries in the brains of elderly persons and in patients who had suffered strokes. He spoke of 'bony or earthy matter being deposited in the coat of the arteries', especially the carotids and basilars.[234] He considered that it was in some way related to the haemorrhagic lesions in the substance of the brain which were usually in the 'medullary part' of a hemisphere, often near a ventricle.

In the preface to the second edition of his book (1797) Baillie again commented on the problems of clinico-pathological correlation. Symptoms might be the same when 'the pathologies' were so different, which was 'particularly exemplified in diseases of the brain'. And a clinical history could be 'easily wrong'. This is why he avoided 'minute detail' clinically. He

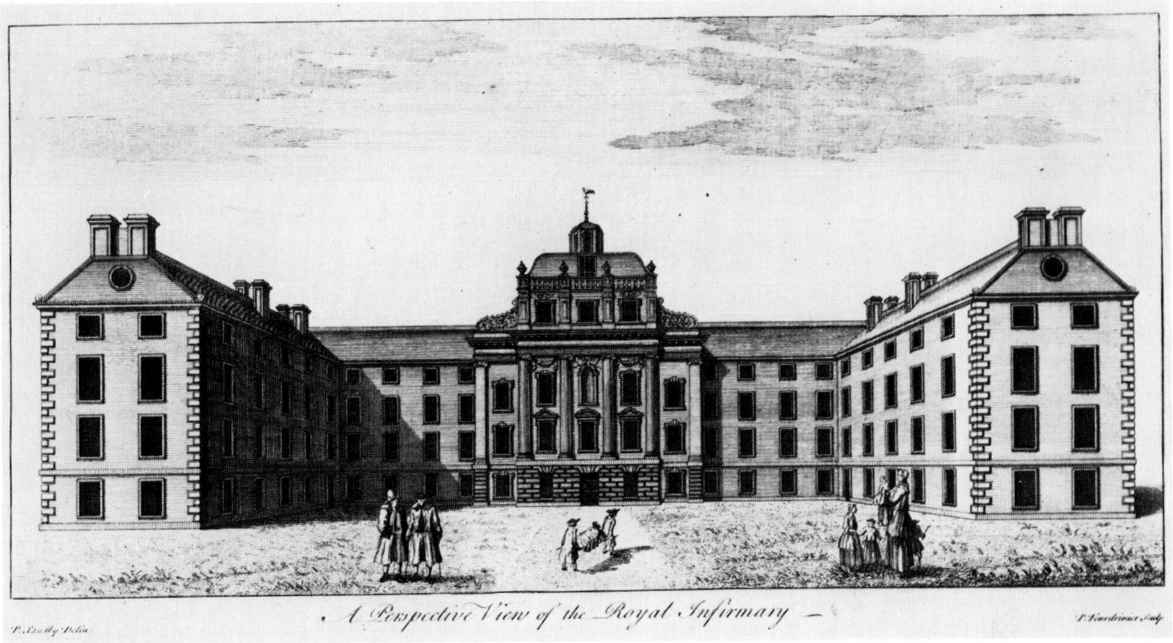

FIG. 54. The old Royal Infirmary of Edinburgh (engraver Sandby 1748). Robert Whytt was professor of medicine in Edinburgh from 1747 to 1766. (Courtesy of the Lothian Health Board, Edinburgh.)

concluded that there were many morbid appearances in which 'the symptoms are not known', 'too slight' to be mentioned, or 'so obvious' that their account would be 'superfluous'.

Despite Morgagni's errors and the rambling nature of many of his accounts, they are readable and lively, reflecting his knowledge of historical sources and of classical and contemporary authors. There is the feeling that he had a more scholarly comprehension of medicine.

WILLIAM CULLEN (1710–1790) AND NOSOGRAPHY

When Cullen published his *Synopsis nosologiae methodicae* in 1769, he was nearly sixty years of age and had been teaching in Glasgow and Edinburgh for some twenty-five years. He did not resign his Edinburgh professorship until he was seventy-nine, dying the following year.[235] His clinical experience over sixty years of practice must have been tremendous. His reputation was immense. Yet he adopted a system of classification of diseases that was soon forgotten. It was based solely on symptoms.

In the preface he said that there had been 'a certain affectation of learning' by many physicians and that before Sydenham 'there are hardly any full or accurately written histories of diseases'. To classify diseases it was essential to identify the essential symptoms 'the pathognomonics . . . the symptoms which are so peculiar to each disease'. 'If', he wrote, 'physicians actually can discriminate diseases from one another, they can likewise tell by what marks they do so.'[236] It was also necessary to recognize that the presence or absence of some symptoms often only indicated 'a variety' of a disease; 'species' of diseases included many varieties. In constructing his classification he

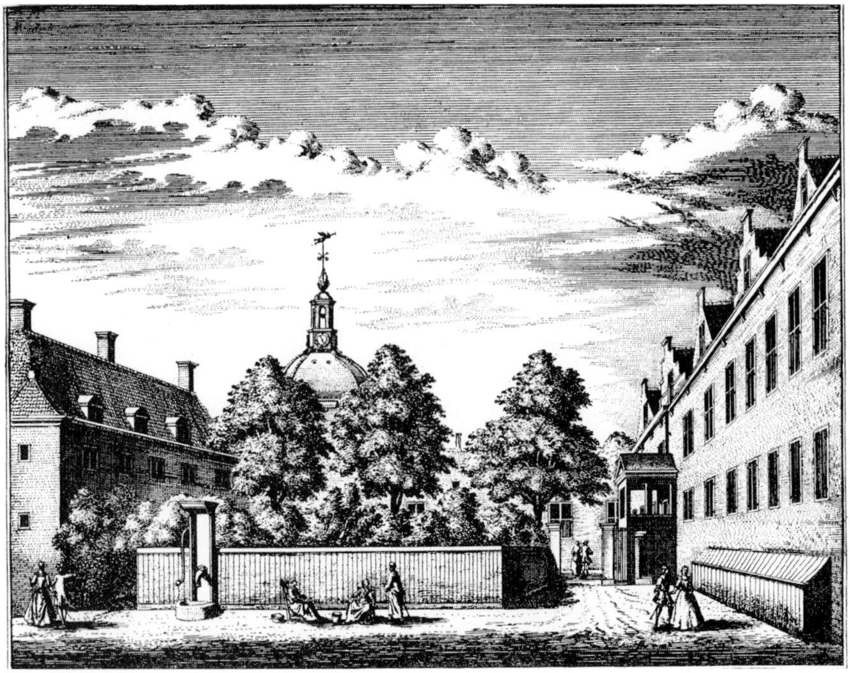

FIG. 55. The St. Caecilia Hospital courtyard, Leiden (engraver Rademaker c. 1730). Here, F. Sylvius made daily rounds and Boerhaave had twelve teaching beds at his disposal, 1714–38. The ward was on the first floor of the building on the right. (Courtesy of the Rijksmuseum voor de Geschiedenis der Naturwetenschappen, Leiden; Museum Boerhaare.)

'always selected those external marks which are easily observable by our senses . . . the never failing attendants of the disease'.

De sedibus had appeared eight years previously. Cullen's *Nosology* was written in Latin, appearing in the same year as Alexander's translation of Morgagni's work. But not only is there no hint then that Cullen had caught the message from Padua, there is none eight years later, when he published his *First lines on the practice of physic* (1777). 'The reader may peruse *Cullen*

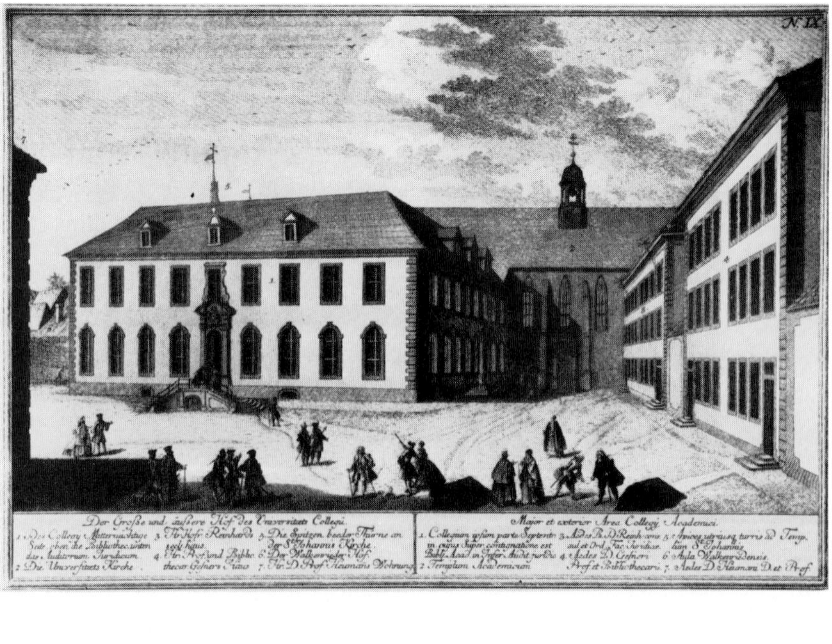

FIG. 56. Göttingen University (engraver Kaltenhofer c. 1765). On the left the library and auditorium; the University Church in the background; on the right, the professors' houses. Haller was professor of medicine at Göttingen from 1736 to 1753. (Courtesy of Gruber, G.B., Naturwissenschaftliche und Medizinische Einrichtungen der jungen Georg-August-Universität in Göttingen, 1955, Musterschmidt-Verlag, Göttingen.)

from cover to cover', wrote Allbutt,[237] 'and fail to find out that Morgagni had ever existed.' As is well known Cullen thought that all physiological and pathological processes were determined by the activity of some 'nervous power' in the brain. All diseases started there – and all drugs acted there.

Since the days of Willis, Cullen said, many diseases had been called 'nervous'. 'In my opinion, the generality of morbid affections so depend on the nervous system, that almost every disease might be called nervous.'[238] These words recall those of Whytt (p. 138). Cooke[239] quoted them in the opening sentence of his *Treatise on nervous diseases* (1820–3). Cullen's *Neuroses* were one of the four classes into which he divided all diseases. The other three were the *Pyrexiae*, *Cachexiae*, and *Locales* (diseases only affecting a particular part).

Cullen's *Neuroses* were affections of sense and motion, without fever, or local disease. They were divided into four orders; *Comata* (apoplexia, paralysis); *Adynamiae* (syncope, dyspepsia, hypochondriasis, chlorosis); *Spasmi* (convulsions, tetanus, chorea, hysteria, hydrophobia); and *Vesaniae* (impaired judgment, amentia, melancholia, mania). His *Nosology* brought him fame in the old world and the new. There were many translations of his small book; clearly the medical world yearned for some simple method of systematization. But Cullen's success must also have meant that the significance of Morgagni's work had yet to be grasped. In fifty years the *Nosology* was forgotten.

Yet, as Riese[240] has said, Cullen's nosography 'anticipated the anatomical and physiological discoveries of the nineteenth century, being a *classification of nervous disease according to a functional principle as to the leading one, related however to a structural principle, as to its corollary*'. When Romberg (1795–1873) came to write his epochal manual in the middle of the nineteenth century we shall see that he also adopted a physiological approach to the classification of nervous diseases. 'Neuroses of Motility' and 'Neuroses of Sensibility' were the basis of his scheme. Although the new knowledge of motor and sensory functions provided by Bell and Magendie was available, pathological grouping was neglected.

PART 3

The nineteenth century

CHAPTER 5

THE NERVOUS SYSTEM EXPLORED: MORPHOLOGY, PATHOLOGY, EXPERIMENT

It appears ... that to get any adequate comparison with the nineteenth century, we must take, not any preceding century or group of centuries, but rather the whole preceding epoch of human history.

Alfred Russel Wallace in *The Wonderful Century*, 1901.

INTRODUCTION

Where, we may now ask, have these centuries of endeavour and 'Capital Enquiries' brought us? What did a learned physician know of the nervous system – its structure, function, and disorders in the opening years of the nineteenth century. Fortunately, we are able to turn to a particularly illuminating and authoritative source, to the first book, in fact, devoted to clinical neurology. The author was John Cooke (1756–1838), physician to the London Hospital, and his book, published in two volumes in 1820 and 1824, when he was in his mid-sixties,† was entitled *A treatise on nervous diseases.*[1] Moreover, he was a classical scholar,[2] devoting seventy-four introductory pages to the history and philosophy of knowledge of the brain and its functions, which he entitled 'Of the Nature and Uses of the Nervous System'. He discusses and quotes the views of Aristotle, Socrates, Plato, Descartes, Locke, Hume, and Berkeley; of physicians such as Hippocrates, Galen, Vesalius, Whytt, Monro II, Haller, Prochaska, and men of his own times – John Hunter, Reil, Fontana, Galvani, Gall and Spurzheim, Bichat and Legallois. It is indeed, as McHenry[3] has said, 'The first history of neurological thought'. What, then, did Cooke say?

'The physiology of the nervous system', he concluded, 'remains involved in impenetrable obscurity.'

> The sensible qualities of the organs of the nervous system, the form, size, colour, relative situation, protuberances, cavities, and division of parts of the various substances contained within the cranium and spine, have been accurately described; but no satisfactory explanation has been given of the intimate nature, and of the manner in which they immediately act in producing sensation and motion. The most minute examination of the brain and nerves has thrown no light on this mystery ... we are utterly at a loss to form any rational conception, concerning the manner in which the mind acts, and is acted upon in sensation and motion.[4]

'Therefore,' he concluded, 'let us turn our attention to a subject better suited to our powers, namely the investigation of the diseases of the nervous system.'

But even here Cooke could only classify neurological illness into

† Cooke is not mentioned in Lord Brain's 'The Neurological Tradition of the London Hospital' (in *Doctors past and present*, Pitman (1964), p. 108) presumably because of the essay's subtitle, 'The Importance of Being Thirty.' Elsewhere in the same book (p. 10) Brain quoted Cooke's translation of a passage of Galen.

apoplexy, palsy, and epilepsy – as did Hippocrates and Galen. And in the field of therapy there were only the traditional rituals of purging, bleeding, cupping, and blistering and so on, whether the patient was a child with meningitis, a youth with paraplegia, or an adult with a stroke.

Yet, by the end of the century we shall have seen the successful removal of tumours from the brain and the spinal cord, the electrical nature of the nerve impulse will have been established, and we shall have the doctrine of the neuron and the principle of the integrative action of the nervous system. These major achievements were based on a wide variety of studies, with new instruments and techniques, which revealed the microstructure of the tissues of the nervous system and the regional manner in which its special functions were organized. All this against a background of increasingly competent clinical investigation and interpretation, and the growth of the science of pathology in all its forms.

JOHN COOKE'S TREATISE ON NERVOUS DISEASES

One of the interesting features of this work is that the author, who had been medically educated in London, Edinburgh, and Leyden, did actually achieve what he set out to do – 'to collect, to arrange and to communicate, in plain clear language, a variety of useful observations from the best authors, both ancient and modern, respecting the principal diseases of the nervous system'. He had retired from his position at the London Hospital in 1807, after serving for some twenty years, and by nature was studious and scholarly. He clearly devoted much time to preparing his book and was familiar with contemporary opinion.[2]

The first of the two volumes comprising this treatise was published in 1820 and entitled *On apoplexy*, but it contained, as I have mentioned, an excellent historical introduction, and also an essay on 'Apoplexia Hydrocephalica' (one of Cullen's many confusing terms) or acute internal hydrocephalus. This volume was based on his Croonian lectures at the Royal College of Physicians of London. The second volume, in 1824, was devoted to *Palsy and epilepsy*. My own copy is a one-volume American edition, of 432 pages, published in 1824,[1] and it is to that publication my references will apply.

Apoplexy

There are eight chapters in this volume, six of which are devoted to definition, pathology, aetiology, classification, diagnosis, and treatment. The seventh chapter deals with other 'soporose affections', and the eighth with acute hydrocephalus. It is worthy of note, and not unexpected, that whereas there are but eight pages of pathology, there are twenty-six on aetiology and forty on treatment.

He first considers the term 'apoplexy', commenting on the disagreements, ancient and modern, in definition and interpretation. Hippocrates used it and described the features of sudden loss of consciousness. Aretaeus and Galen, he inferred, thought that 'apoplexy is a general, and palsy a partial, abolition of sense and motion'. Modern nosologists used a great variety of definitions. Sauvages and Linnaeus stressed 'profound sleep and stertorous respiration', but Cullen thought that the latter was not always present. Cooke offered his own definition in the following words.

It is a disease in which the animal functions are suspended, while the vital and natural functions continue; respiration being generally laborious, and frequently attended with stertor (p. 78).

The cardinal features are described; the onset, though usually sudden, is often preceded by warning symptoms, referable to the head, the senses of vision, speech, hearing, balance, and so on. Avicenna had observed 'scotomia'. The pulse is usually normal or slow at first, but tends to weaken. Boerhaave measured the strength of the disease by the degree of stertor; Cheyne commented on the terminal periodic apnoea. Cooke said that few had commented on contraction of the pupils, but he found that it was an invariably fatal sign. *Sudden* death more commonly resulted from some affection of the heart, rather than the brain. 'Genuine apoplexy, I believe, seldom destroys life in less than one or two hours' (p. 83). Although Baillie had usually found that in hemiplegia the brain lesion was in the opposite hemisphere, 'however, he tells me that he has sometimes, although rarely, seen the effusion of blood on the same side as the paralysis' (p. 83).

Cooke found that the brain lesions had been 'imperfectly described'; 'even Morgagni's' accounts were inadequate. He pleaded for 'a comparison of symptoms, or a consideration of them, in connection with appearances on dissection' (p. 90). As it was, it was generally agreed that it was rare to find no abnormality in the brain and he recorded that haemorrhagic lesions were by far the commonest. Many other types of lesions – tumours, effusions, cysts, suppurations – were questionable causes of 'genuine apoplexy.' In the latter the commonest site was in the corpus striatum. In a careful search he said he could not find a single case in the Sepulchretum of Bonetus (Theophile Bonet; 1620–89) or in Morgagni's *De sedibus* 'in which organic lesion was observed in the brain unaccompanied with blood or serum' (p. 98). He thought all apoplexies were essentially 'sanguineous'; he questioned the existence of 'serous' apoplexy. The two eighteenth-century physicians – Heberden (1710–1801) and Fothergill (1712–80) – are quoted. The former thought serous apoplexy 'seems hardly ever looked for in practice'. Fothergill had thought that apoplexy in general arose when, in the head, there was 'more blood than ought to be there'.

Cooke was perplexed that in over twenty years at the London Hospital he had never seen there a single case of apoplexy, while colleagues at St. Thomas's and St. George's Hospitals had seen many. Cheyne (p. 176) had made a similar comment. Cooke thought it 'seldom occurs among the laborious poor, unless occasioned by drinking spirits to excess' (p. 96). He favoured Abercrombie's view that there was an 'interrupted circulation ... derangement of the relation betwixt the arteries and veins of the brains ... which diminish the capacity of the venous system ... or cause diminution of the impulse of the blood entering the head' (p. 108). As yet the idea of arterial occlusion causing softening of the brain had not crystallized. Hanging or strangling did not seem to result in death by apoplexy although constriction of the neck in soldiers 'obliged to wear their cravats too high' had been reported a likely agent. Fothergill had described the case of a man who had a stroke from twisting his neck too much while crossing the Thames in a boat; he had seen several similar such cases and advised his patients that giddiness provoked in this way could be avoided (p. 106). But the mechanism of neck stricture in all these types of case was thought to be venous, and not arterial compression.

'Temporary apoplexy' was how Cooke described a typical example of cough syncope (p. 98).

That cerebral arteries ruptured because they were diseased is nowhere actually suggested, despite Baillie's hint and the many old observations of arterial 'ossification'. The condition of hypertension, of course, was not known until the end of the century. Cooke thought that the commonest 'associated disease' in apoplexy was gout. He writes of 'gouty apoplexy,' citing the case of Malpighi who died of a stroke in 1604; Baglivi performed the autopsy and found ventricular haemorrhage 'with gravelly concretions' and blood vessels that were 'preternaturally distended' (p. 115). He did not think cerebral haemorrhage was invariably fatal because he recognized the signs of old lesions in fatal cases with known previous strokes.

In his account of acute internal hydrocephalus he discusses the differing views that it was a dropsy (Whytt, Monro, Fothergill), an apoplexy (Cullen), or an inflammation of the brain (Cheyne, Abercrombie, Rush). He favoured the latter. He mentions that it was primarily a disease of childhood, almost invariably fatal, and that early recognition of Whytt's first stage, although satisfying to the doctor, did not influence the outcome. At autopsy, in addition to the hydrocephalus, there were signs of 'inflammation of the brain and its membranes . . . tubercles, probably scrofulous, in the brain, on the surface of the liver, or in the lungs' (p. 190). He quotes Abercrombie's view that the effusion was a consequence of the inflammation and not a cause of the illness. He discusses the question of the brain being compressed by effusion and whether its presence can be recognized during life. Abercrombie thought that 'we have no certain mark which we can rely upon as indicating the presence of effusion in the brain' (p. 201). All the characteristic clinical features 'may exist without effusion'.

Palsy

There are seven chapters in this section. He divides palsy into three types; hemiplegia, paraplegia, and partial palsies. In all three the onset may be acute or gradual, and motor and sensory functions are usually both implicated. Sometimes there was pain. Affected limbs were usually colder and 'often become more soft and flaccid than natural; they waste and shrink, and sometimes appear oedematous'. In hemiplegia, speech is often affected; there is 'loss of the knowledge of language as well as of the power of speech' (p. 227). Intellect and emotional control may be affected in hemiplegia; 'the wisest men and the bravest soldiers [may] weep like children on the slightest occasions'. Recovery from hemiplegia usually began in the leg.

Hemiplegia. Hemiplegia usually resulted from an apoplectic fit; occasionally onset is 'intermittent' or 'gradual'. The unilateral distribution is a characteristic feature, applying not only to the limbs, but to the face, the tongue, the chest, and, in a case of Morgagni's, to the 'jaundice' the patient also suffered on the paralysed side, so that 'even the right part of the nose was yellow' (p. 231). Sensation was never completely lost. Cooke refers to several examples of what he termed 'anomalous hemiplegias'. They include cases of paralysis of an arm and leg on opposite sides; of paralysis of one leg with retained sensation but with the reverse in the other leg; loss of sensation without loss of motion; heightened sensation with loss of power; and what he termed 'double hemiplegia'.

Of particular interest in the pages on 'anomalous hemiplegias' are the two examples of physicians who described their own illnesses (p. 233). One was 'the celebrated De Saussure' who clearly had a 'thalamic syndrome'; the other was Vieusseux who had a lateral medullary infarction.

In the former case there was the characteristic unilateral hyperpathia and sensory loss with ataxia. Onset was sudden, with vertigo, and progressed 'by sudden accessions'. There is a vivid account of the difficulty encountered 'when he attempted to walk in a straight line' and in negotiating doorways (no hint that there may have been an hemianopia). The affected side was 'painful and agonising', with perversion of tactile sensation, dysaesthesiae – all 'extremely disagreeable'.

In Vieusseux's case there was acute onset of vertigo, loss of voice, dysphagia, and numbness of the right side of the body. There was episodic progression culminating in analgesia on the left side of the face and analgesia with thermanaesthesia on the right side of the body; also weakness of the left limbs with normally retained sensibility and ptosis of the left eyelid. Because of the 'depraved sensation' on the right side 'an etherised julep' and 'a new-laid egg' felt strangely different to his right hand; while in a bath 'it felt hot to the left side, and neither hot nor cold to the right'.[5]

The cerebral lesions in hemiplegia resembled those of apoplexy, but tumours, abscesses, cysts, and injuries had also to be considered. Willis, and Morgagni, had shown that the hemiplegic lesion was usually in the corpus striatum; in 'double hemiplegia' it might be in the pons (p. 279). The traditional explanation for the clinical effect was that the lesion caused 'pressure on the brain' but Serres, of Paris, had made extensive investigations which Cooke discusses at length. Serres usually failed to produce apoplexy or paralysis of limbs in animals by experimentally induced hemisphere lesions. Certainly, effusions thus caused did not seem to be responsible. Serres next endeavoured to correlate a history of apoplexy or hemiplegia with autopsy findings. He had examined the brains of some 370 hemiplegic patients from various Paris hospitals; in all, the lesions were in the opposite hemisphere. Of one hundred cases of apoplexy, seventy-nine were complicated by palsy. Effusions were common when there was no palsy; the brain was usually sound but the meninges were affected in varying degrees. On the other hand, in the palsied cases, there was invariably some destruction, recent or old, of the substance of a hemisphere. Serres concluded that hemiplegia was not caused by compression of the brain, but by destruction of some part of it – the cortex, the corpus striatum, or the thalamus, chiefly.

Cooke enquired of Abercrombie's views on Serres's findings. 'The subject', Abercrombie said, 'appears exceedingly obscure and difficult' but he was in general agreement that 'compression' of the brain was not a satisfactory explanation for palsy, which could be due to 'various and very different morbid conditions of the brain, some of them the very reverse of pressure' (p. 260).

Cooke's own view was that Serres had not 'overturned the doctrine of apoplexy and palsy from pressure', as he had claimed, although he admitted that 'meningeal' and 'cerebral' apoplexies might be considered an improvement on the old classification of 'serous' and 'sanguineous'. Much depended on the *degree* of pressure; 'In the generality of cases, apoplexy is produced by general, and palsy by partial compression.' An opinion, sound enough, but one that should not be taken to imply that we see here a hint of Monakow's (1853–1930) theory of 'diaschisis' or neural shock. In Cooke's day it was appreciated that the commonest lesion in apoplexy was in the corpus striatum, but that that reflected the existence of cerebral localization, was not inferred. Post-apoplectic hemiplegia was a matter of the severity of the lesion, rather than its locality.

Paraplegia. In paraplegia (p. 264) the lower limbs were much more frequently affected than the upper; motion and sensation were affected, but visceral function continued. Legallois (1770–1814) had shown that the respiratory centre was in the upper part of the medulla oblongata. In young children the onset was usually slower than in adults, and as they walked there was 'an involuntary crossing of the legs'. He pointed out that when the spine was curved 'Mr. Pott is not disposed to consider this as a paralytic affection', and that it differed from 'a nervous palsy'. Pott (1714–88), in his second paper of 1782, had written that 'the truth is that there is no dislocation, no unnatural pressure made on the spinal marrow, nor are the limbs by any means paralytic.'[6] Pott thought there was no 'true' paralysis in his cases, because the affected limb muscles were not 'soft, flabby, unresisting' but 'rigid' ... 'and always at least in a tonic state, by which the knees and ankles acquire a stiffness not very easy to overcome [so that] the legs are immediately and strongly drawn up ...'. But Cooke considered it a form of paraplegia due to a diseased spine – usually scrofulous. Paraplegic lesions were nearly always spinal in origin – injuries, inflammations, tumours of the vertebrae, or effusions and haemorrhages within the spinal canal. Baillie had occasionally found cerebral causes.

Partial palsies. These (p. 244) might arise from lesions of the brain, spinal cord, or nerves, particularly the latter. They were motor, sensory, or mixed.

Examples of sensory palsies were lesions of the nerves of smell, taste, vision, hearing, or touch. In the motor class, paralysis might be confined to a set of muscles, or to a single muscle. The part affected could be an eyelid, a lower lip, a sphincter, or even a single joint of a finger. Functions such as speech, swallowing, urination, or defecation might be singled out. One of the commonest causes of partial palsy was lead poisoning.

He sought the opinions of Abercrombie, Bell, and others. The former thought that isolated loss of speech could occur without any paralysis of tongue or larynx. In one such case visual and auditory understanding was 'entire', and the patient could write. 'What is it, then,' says Dr Abercrombie, 'that he has lost?' (p. 246). Lesions of the brain, no larger than a pea or bean, could cause focal palsies.

Tenderness over nerves, Bell said, was often a clue to the site of a partial palsy, citing the ulnar and 'fibular' nerves. Occupation, 'in a literary gentleman', was responsible for paralysis of thumb and forefinger of the right hand. 'Lifting a great weight' caused paralysis of the shoulder muscles in a young woman. But he did not mention the possibility of birth injury when the arm of an infant at the breast was paralysed 'among those wretched Irish women who apply as out-patients to our hospitals' (p. 269). The 'interruption of growth' of a paretic limb of a child perplexed Bell. 'Is it not owing to an affection of the nerves of the part?' (p. 269). A complete facial palsy, Bell had no hesitation in ascribing 'to lead palsy from a recently painted door of a bedroom' (p. 270).

Concluding his chapters on 'Palsy' Cooke takes up two questions which have 'a good deal engaged the attention of physiologists, ancient and modern'. These were the problems of motor and sensory functions, and the decussation of pathways.

He referred to Galen's notions of differing degrees of nervous power required for motor and sensory functions, and of the idea of mixed nerves. Cooke did not find much to help him from 'physiologists of the present day' but Bell informed him as follows.

> The nerves of sensation and motion are bound together in the same membranes, for the convenience of distribution, but there is reason to conclude that they are distinct through their whole course, and as distinct in their origin in the brain, as in their final distribution to the skin and muscles; why then should we suppose that they are similarly affected in diseases of the brain (p. 249).

The ulnar 'nerve for example', said Bell, 'has two roots, one connected with that part of the brain which receives sensation, and another with that which gives out the mandate of the will'. A partial lesion of the brain could 'cut off one root, and consequently one of its functions', but that, he thought, 'appears rather too mechanical an explanation'. He preferred to believe that 'the different functions of the brain are variously influenced by the same cause'. It is clear that when Bell used the term 'roots' he was not referring to the spinal nerve roots, but to the roots of origin of a nerve in the brain.

The site of decussation of motor pathways had been much debated. Lancisi thought it took place in the corpus callosum; Santorini, in the pyramids; Soemmerring, 'immediately below the lingual nerves'. Others preferred the spinal cord. The dissections of Gall and Spurzheim pointed to the medulla oblongata and had been confirmed by 'a committee of the French National Institute'. But, to Cooke, the 'minute structure of the brain' was still unknown; its 'fibrous structure . . . has not been satisfactorily proved' (p. 270).

Epilepsy

The picture of epilepsy portrayed in these pages of Cooke serves to remind one of how dreadfully it was still regarded. Demoniacal possession, the effects of celestial bodies, the violence of the convulsions, the uselessness of treatment, and the common outcome – 'idiocy or fatuity' – are all described and discussed. In a major convulsion there was 'prodigious force – terrifying the beholder – the eyes roll furiously – the foaming at the mouth – the gnashing of teeth, give to the countenance a horribly wild, and, as some fancy, supernatural expression, as if the wretched patient were possessed, or, in the language of the Scripture, *torn* by some malignant demon' (p. 330). Sometimes there was an aura – a feeling of oppression, a rising sensation, a change of mood, formication in a limb, 'flashes of light', 'disagreeable odours', or 'singing in the ears'. When the aura began in an extremity, it did not follow the path of a nerve, said Cullen, and a ligature sometimes aborted the general fit.

True, there were cases in which the fit was over in a few minutes, and tended to cease at puberty, on the appearance of the menses, or at marriage – but on the whole epilepsy was a formidable disability.

Cooke adopted Cullen's classification; idiopathic and symptomatic. The former included three species; the *cerebral*, in which the onset was sudden, without manifest cause; the *sympathetic*, in which there was an ascending aura; and the *occasional*, in which the fit resulted from a source of irritation which could be removed (a distorted toe; a lump on a nerve; worms, etc.). Constitution and heredity played their parts but there was no particular class of temperament of aetiological significance. Usually there was no known precipitating factor to a fit, but there was the case of a boy who reacted to the sound of a trumpet (p. 353) and a child to the sight of 'a vivid red colour' (p. 354). The tendency of some patients to react to odours was known to the ancients. Aretaeus remarked that purchasers of slaves would expose them to the odour of burning lapis gagates (jet), to test for susceptibility to epilepsy.

In the majority of cases no abnormality of the brain was found at autopsy. Depressed fractures, tumours, cysts, clots, abscesses were rarely found but 'congestion' and 'effusions' were fairly common. Cooke gives an interesting account (p. 338) of a Professor Wenzel's observations in Mayence. 'He instituted a society for the express purpose of assisting him in his investigation' of epilepsy, obtaining brains, and arranging new forms of treatment. He finally published his account of an examination of twenty brains from the idiopathic variety and found that the cerebellum, and not the cerebrum, was diseased. He also suspected there were pathological changes in the pineal gland.

Cooke also mentions Esquirol's (1772–1840) findings of 'diseased spinal marrow' in some cases.

The cause of epilepsy was not known. In some epileptic brains the lesions resembled those of apoplexy or palsy, but why similar lesions should have such different effects was a mystery. But occasionally an epileptic developed a palsy, or sustained a stroke, so they might have something in common.

Perhaps the different symptoms of these two diseases [apoplexy and epilepsy] arising from compression within the cranium, may, in some measure, depend upon the particular parts compressed (p. 350).

These lines contain the only hint of the possibility of cerebral localization. 'A derangement of the organisation of some part or parts of the brain' was opined by some physiologists, but more had to be learned of its 'exquisite structure'. Certainly you could have a gross brain lesion without epilepsy. The commonly found 'turgescence' of the brain might imply some degree of 'temporary superexcitement in the nervous structure of the parts', and this had been suggested. Another theory, proposed by a Mr Mansford, was that convulsions arose because of 'an accumulation of the electric matter in the brain'. 'The nervous and electric fluids are the same', wrote Mansford, and they were formed in the brain. Epilepsy arose when there was a loss of control over 'formation and expenditure'.

The treatment of apoplexy, palsy, and epilepsy

A physician of Cooke's day, called to see a patient with a stroke, a palsy, or a fit, would usually only have to decide *how much* to purge, bleed, cup, or blister. But he had an endless list of 'remedies' to hand and the section on treatment in this book takes up no less than a third of its content. One is struck by the zeal to treat; there is some suggestion that interference might at times be harmful, and the quotations from Heberden and Fothergill usually indicate reasonableness and moderation. There are long considerations of prescriptions, techniques, and regimes, with their now unfamiliar terminology. There are nervines, revellents, emmenagogues, sialogues, errhines, sternatories, cathartics, sinapisms, cataplasms, clysters, setons, and more. But at least the cordial for apoplexy prepared by the Dominican friars at Rouen – *Elixir Antapoplectique*, no less – could have done no harm. Indeed, for the disease 'lately described by Mr. Parkinson' (which Cooke summarizes, p. 317) it would have been better endured than the recommended treatment – 'blood should be taken from the upper part of the neck . . . vesicatories to the same part . . . sabine liniment . . . large issues to be kept open about the vertebrae . . . etc.'

THE PHYSICIAN-PATHOLOGISTS 1800–1850

Cullen's idea of the dominant role of the nervous system in general pathology lived on in Germany as a 'neural pathology'.[7] It was vigorously opposed by Virchow (1821–1902), whose 'cellular pathology' replaced it at mid-century. In revolutionary France, with its new medical schools and societies, Bichat (1771–1802), focusing on organs, tissues, and textures, led the way to the creation of the famous Parisian school of physician-pathologists, among whom, for neurologists, the most notable was Cruveilhier (1791–1873). In Britain, in the tradition of the Hunters and Baillie, there were also men who tackled the task of relating lesions to symptoms and signs. The most famous was Richard Bright (1789–1858).

The English School

John Cheyne (1777–1836). Two contributions of John Cheyne may be recalled. His *Essay on hydrocephalus acutus* appeared in 1808.[8] It was not illustrated but he stressed that his account 'may be implicitly relied on. These cases are not recollections ... they were invariably drawn up in the bed-chamber of the patient ...'. There were twenty-three cases but we can conclude that the six who recovered were not examples of tuberculous meningitis. He performed eight autopsies. He acknowledged Whytt's original description but he added that 'I am inclined to think he was directed to this disease by two articles in the Edinburgh Medical Essays.' Cheyne thought that Whytt had been 'too methodical in his arrangement of the history'. There were variations in its onset and course and he suggested a classification into acute, insidious, and abrupt. Fothergill (1712–80) had followed Whytt in regarding the disease as a dropsy of the brain, but it was a Dr Quin[9] 'who rectified the error'. The scrofulous aetiology was recognized; Cheyne mentioned one family in which eleven children died of acute hydrocephalus.

Cheyne's clinical descriptions are clear and vivid but one looks in vain to see whether he examined for neck rigidity, although he mentioned that the headache 'does not admit of the head being raised from the pillow'. Squinting was seen in all diseases of the brain. It arose from loss of sensibility falling first on the recti 'which are under the command of the will'. The obliques were not so influenced; they remained 'active ... and turned the eye'. The miliary lesions of the meninges, brain, lungs, liver, and mesenteric glands were commonly seen and the brunt of the disease was in 'the centre of the brain'. The most important differential diagnosis was from otitic cerebral abscess.

Following the publication of this *Essay*, which was one of several he wrote on diseases of children while he was practising in Edinburgh, Cheyne moved to Dublin in 1809 and remained there for twenty-two years. In 1812 there appeared his volume entitled *Cases of apoplexy and lethargy with observations upon the comatose diseases*.[10] A book of 224 pages it is sometimes omitted in historical accounts of stroke.[11, 12] Cheyne said that students rarely saw cases of apoplexy in hospital; he had seen only two or three in four years attendance at the Edinburgh Royal Infirmary. In five years military service, in England and Ireland, he had seen none.

There were various ways in which strokes presented. A patient, with or without any previous complaint, might just 'fall dead' or be 'found dead abed'. Loss of consciousness and hemiplegia were not inevitable. Speech was not always affected (no reference to laterality); convulsions sometimes occurred. Premonitory symptoms he listed were tinnitus, vertigo, headache, 'fits of blindness', 'flashes of light', 'restless nights', confusion, articulatory difficulties, 'spasms', numbness, and vomiting. Onset of apoplexy was sudden or gradual.

Physical examination recorded only the various degrees of loss of 'senses' and the extent of paralysis and convulsion. The quest for 'signs' had not begun.

Cheyne spoke of 'serous' and 'sanguineous' apoplexy but he was doubtful of the former entity, saying 'I know little of that species'. He quoted the opinions of Wepfer, Willis, Boerhaave, Cullen, and Morgagni, the latter's writings being 'rambling and parenthetical'. Cheyne did not think that the 'earthy or boney' appearance of the 'diseased' cerebral arteries was 'important'. Haemorrhage probably arose not from rupture of a single vessel, 'but from a number of smaller vessels' (p. 31). 'Rupture was not necessarily the consequence of the deposition of the gritty matter' in the arteries (p. 38). Haemorrhage was the result of 'a great and simultaneous action of the smaller arteries of a hemisphere, or of the whole brain ... (p. 39). He recounted twenty-three 'Cases and Dissections' but had never been able to trace extravasation to rupture of 'a considerable artery' (p. 41). (In Edinburgh he had assisted Charles Bell in autopsy studies.) The book contains five rather crude illustrations of apoplectic cerebral lesions from Bell's collection. They show congestion of the cortex, an intracerebral haemorrhage, an area of softening, a cyst, and, significantly, a basal haemorrhage. The latter, McHenry[13] considers to be the earliest illustration of a subarachnoid haemorrhage.

In his final commentary Cheyne wondered whether there was an increasing incidence of strokes and, not surprisingly, both 'indolence' and 'passion', gluttony, tobacco, and alcohol were apportioned their share of blame. He also mentioned a familial tendency, and the factors of 'temperament' and 'anxiety'.

This book does not contain his famous account of 'A Case of Apoplexy in Which the Fleshy Part of the Heart Was Converted into Fat' which contains his original description of periodic apnoea. This appeared in 1818.

> The only peculiarity in the last period of his illness, which lasted eight or nine days, was in the state of the respiration. For several days his breathing was irregular; it would entirely cease for a quarter of a minute, then it would become perceptible, though very low, then by degrees it became heaving and quick, and then it would gradually cease again. This revolution in the state of his breathing occupied about a minute, during which there were about thirty acts of respiration.[14]

His Dublin colleague, William Stokes (1804–78) referred to Cheyne's account when he published his own in 1854.[15]

Andrew Marshal (1742–1813). A book which Romberg (1795–1873) said aroused his interest in neurology was Marshal's *The morbid anatomy of the brain in mania and hydrophobia* (1815).[16] An Edinburgh graduate, Marshal had worked at the Windmill Street School of Anatomy, and taught at his own school in Thavies Inn from 1875 until 1800. The book deals largely with 'Mania' and 'Canine Madness', but there is a preliminary chapter on the physiology of the brain which contains a discussion of whether or not water is normally to be found in its ventricles. Marshal concluded that usually there was 'nothing more than a moist vapour in the ventricles'. In hydrophobia the brain was congested and showed various 'effusions'; in mania he had examined twenty-two brains (many from Bethlem Hospital) and usually there were similar findings. He also argued that as mania could be temporary and the patient recover, examination of the brain at autopsy might often reveal nothing abnormal.

He mentioned two cases of mania in which he would have expected negative findings. One was that of an Oxford don, who, 'fancying himself dead', retired to bed, but 'on hearing no bells toll', quickly repaired to the church and started tolling the bells himself. Upon which he was scolded by neighbours, and rather ashamed, he returned home 'mente sana'. His second case was of 'a servant girl' in the country, who, while making 'toast for tea' got it into her head to set fire to her master's barn – for which she was hanged.

Although his biographer, S. Sawrey, who provides a sketch of Marshal's life in this book, concluded that 'What he had was good', it is a curious work to have had such a significant influence. Young Romberg may have been romanticizing, or perhaps just indulging in a little flattery of the 'English' he subsequently quoted so lavishly.

Robert Hooper (1773–1835). There were no illustrations in Marshal's book but it was not long before neuropathology was to have its first atlas. This was Robert Hooper's *Morbid anatomy of the human brain*, printed in a series of loose sheets in 1826, and as a folio volume in 1828.[17] The work is notable for its fifteen splendid coloured illustrations using the new technique of lithography. A Londoner, Hooper was a physician to the St. Marylebone Infirmary, and practised from Savile Row. He had published books on botany, anatomy, epidemic diseases, and general medicine. His *Atlas*, he said, was based on over 4000 autopsies carried out over a period of thirty years, and he hoped it would 'enable the pathologist to distinguish organic diseases from one another, and thereby dispose them into classes, orders, genera, species, and varieties'. It was planned to be the first of a series covering all viscera, but only the second volume, on the uterus, was completed, before he died in 1835.

There are no clinical accounts of his cases, the text being confined to a description of the gross morbid appearances of the brain and its membranes, nerves, vessels, and the venous sinuses. 'Diseases states' of the brain are described in general terms such as 'softness' or 'pulpiness', 'hardness' or 'induration' and 'destruction of parts'. Not all were ante-mortem. Some areas of focal 'induration' may have been lesions of multiple sclerosis.

He recognized that there were acute and chronic forms of hydrocephalus, with varying degrees of compression of white matter and thinning of the cortex, but its obstructive nature was not appreciated. He noted the enlargement of the 'foramina of Monro' and the third ventricle – but not of the fourth. The idea of a circulating cerebrospinal fluid was not entertained.

The obvious morbid masses within the brain – tumours ('cephaloma', 'chondroma', 'osteoma', 'melanoma', etc.), – abscesses, aneurysms, and extravasations (haematomas and hygromas) – are described and illustrated. Tumours were 'circumscribed' or 'so blended with the surrounding cerebral substance, being lost imperceptibly in it, that their limits cannot be easily traced' (p. 11). They were 'soft' or 'hard'; 'solid' or 'cystic', and arose from the substance of the brain itself or its enveloping membranes. Gliomas and meningiomas may be recognized, as also yellowish tuberculomas, and black melanomas. Cystic masses, whether tumours or abscesses, might be multilocular or unilocular (Fig. 57).

Abscesses were classified as 'common', 'cellular', 'encysted', or 'scrofulous' but there is little to help one guess their origin or duration. Hooper does, however, speak of the encapsulating 'membrane' of an abscess, and sometimes refers to the degree of surrounding inflammation or swelling.

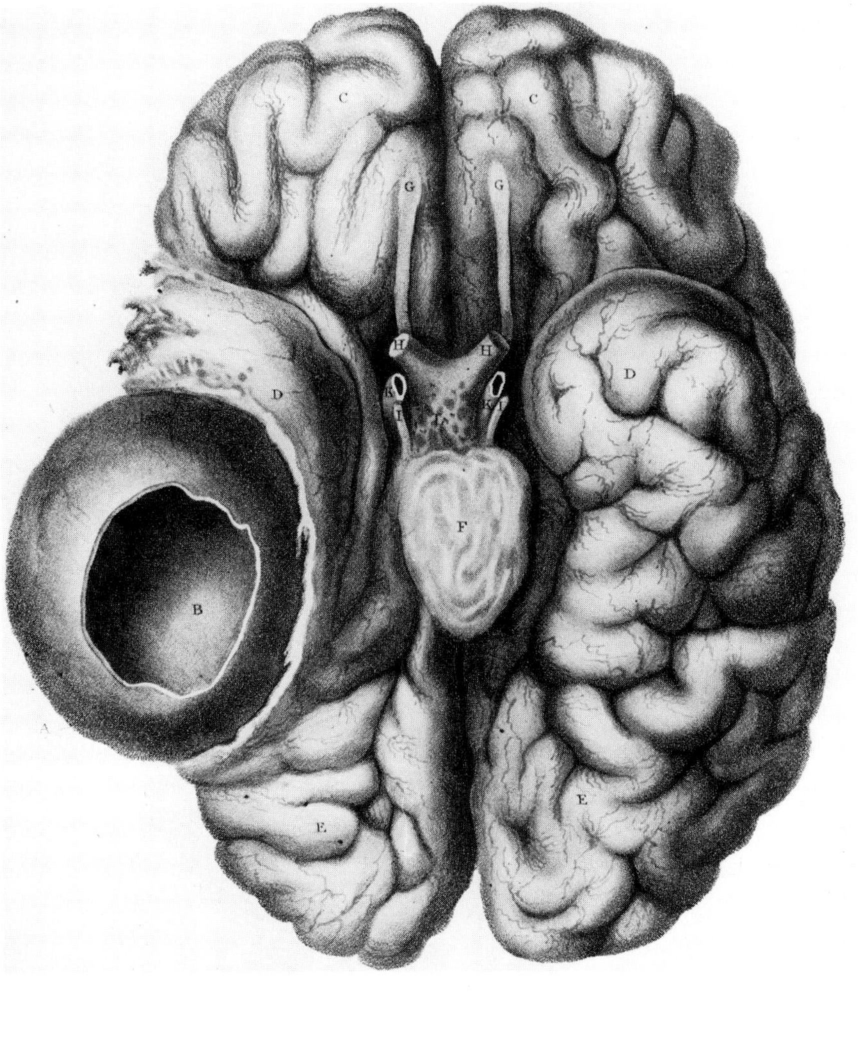

FIG. 57. Cyst; possibly abscess in view of the thick wall. F, pons sectioned; I, third cranial nerve; K, carotid artery. (After Hooper,[17] Plate XIII.)

Haemorrhages, massive and small, single and multiple, recent and old, are considered. They were usually found in the hemispheres but were also noted in the brain stem. The nature of the changes which took place in a clot, after a stroke, are described, with relevance to its consistency, colour and content, the developing 'membranous-like surface' around it, and the altered appearance of adjacent brain tissue.

'Ossification' of the cerebral arteries was associated with age, and with the aetiology of stroke. 'In most instances of apoplexy produced by the spontaneous rupture of a blood vessel in the brain, the arteries are found in this diseased state' (p. 22).

But it was in the field of suppurative lesions, Courville[18] stresses, that Hooper was so notable a pioneer. Figure 58 is an example of his depiction of acute basal meningitis. He recognized that involvement of the meninges might result from acute, subacute, or chronic inflammatory processes, and predominantly affect one or other of the three membranes. He described the varying types and location of exudates, the tendency to loculation, the

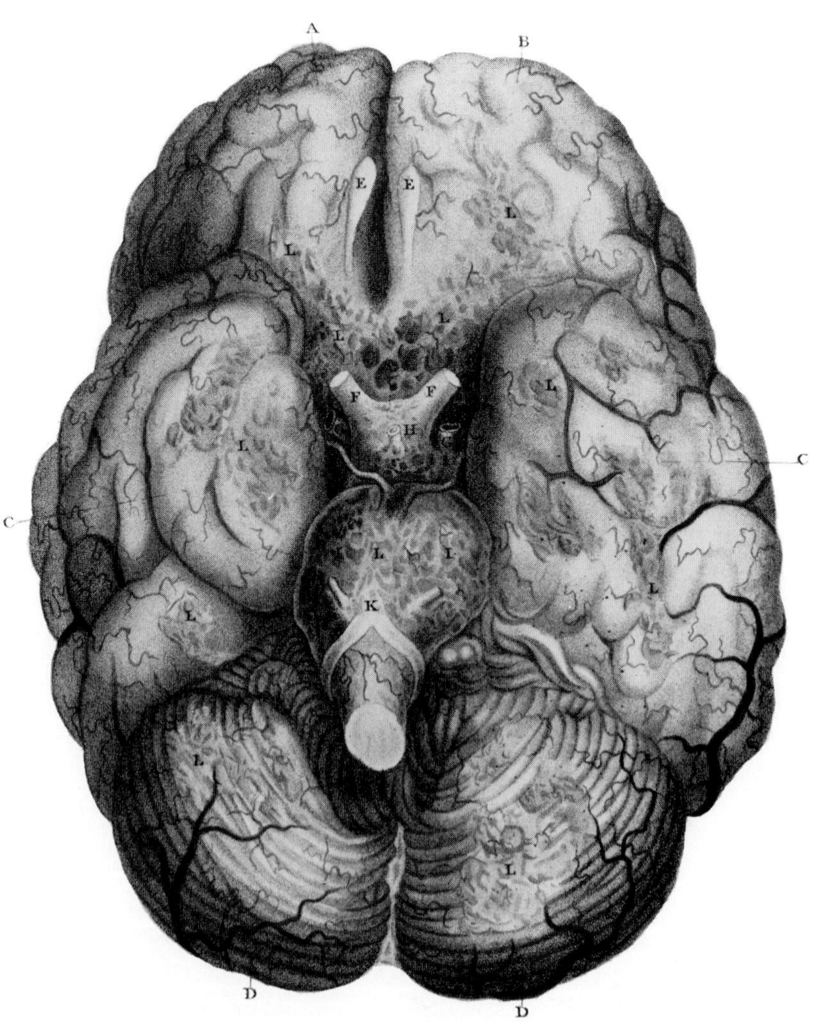

FIG. 58. Meningitis; the congested, opaque basal meninges, and the effusions, obscured the 'nerve origins, the infundibulum . . . and veins and arteries'. (After Hooper,[17] Plate IV.)

formation of abscesses, and the invasion of the venous sinuses. The lack of clinical data is particularly felt in this context.

John Abercrombie (1781–1844). This deficiency is not to be found in another publication of that year (1828) from Edinburgh. This was entitled *Pathological and practical researches on diseases of the brain and spinal cord*, by John Abercrombie.[19] If Hooper's book was the first atlas of neuropathology, this was the first textbook (476 pages, no illustrations). Abercrombie began by pointing out that there had come about 'a tacit but very general admission of the fallacy of medical hypotheses and the precarious nature of general principles in medicine ...'. He said he had 'no system to support, and no new doctrines to propose'. 'Every practitioner' should 'divest himself of system, and attend to what is passing before him ...'. Abercrombie offered him 'an extensive and accurate acquaintance with the pathology of disease' of the nervous system, with an analysis of 150 cases.

Clinical and pathological correlation was arranged in four parts; 'Inflammatory Affections', 'Apoplectic Affections', 'Organic Diseases of the Brain,' and 'Diseases of the Spinal Cord and Its Membranes'.

1 There was a great 'diversity of symptoms' resulting from intracranial *inflammation*. Most commonly the onset was characterized by what old writers called 'phrenitis'; there were fever, headache, photophobia, delirium, etc. On the other hand, the illness might be ushered in with a convulsion (sometimes one-sided). Presentation varied with the age of the patient. A child might rapidly become very ill, with vomiting, confusion, and disorientation, while an adult might just quietly retire to bed, 'unwilling to be disturbed'. The course of these illnesses also showed considerable variation, with 'deceitful appearances of amendment'. There were considerable difficulties in correlating the site and extent of the brain lesions with the clinical picture. Focal lesions could cause convulsive or paralytic symptoms, and only 'imperfect distinctions' could be made between superficial and deep lesions of the hemispheres, and between cerebral and cerebellar disease processes. Coma was common in many affections of the brain; effusions could be symptomless and were the result, not the cause, of the illness. Many febrile diseases could cause inflammation of the brain. In this first section he cited cases such as brain abscess with ear disease and erosion of the petrous temporal; brain abscess with ethmoid disease; and cerebellar abscess with a discharging ear. These were relationships not mentioned by Hooper. Other examples were of a subdural haematoma (p. 49) and a tuberculous abscess in the medulla oblongata (p. 108).

2 *Apoplexy* presented formidable problems of correlation because of the great variety of morbid conditions of the brain that might be encountered. Usually there was a haemorrhage or a serous effusion, but sometimes there was no apparent explanation. That was why, Abercrombie observed, men had speculated about 'suffocation' of animal spirits, 'relaxation' of nerves, or 'spasms' of the meninges, nerves, or vessels of the brain. In patients who recovered, the common sequels were hemiplegia and impairment of speech. There may or may not have been initial loss of consciousness. One patient

had suffered eight attacks of hemiparesis in thirteen years. Power suffered more than sensibility in affected limbs; it was rare to find sensory loss without motor loss; a paralysed limb was sometimes painful, and sensibility heightened or perverted. When speech was affected, 'there was a loss of memory for words' and the patient tended to replace one word with another, or even invent words. Yet the ability to read might be retained, although writing was not possible. He referred to Wepfer's case of right hemiplegia in which Latin speech was affected before German (p. 289).

Arteries which ruptured usually showed signs of disease. There was a patchy distribution of the 'earthy brittleness of Scarpa'; vessels, particularly the carotids, vertebrals, and basilars were 'ossified' or occluded. The vessels were large and their coats were thicker. Cerebral haemorrhage arose when there was 'an interruption between the arterial and venous systems' (p. 313). Any increase of pressure in one system must be at the expense of the other. The brain was protected from the effects of atmospheric pressure by its enclosure within the skull. The brain of an animal bled to death is not exsanguined, unless the skull is first trephined. These lines were 'conjectures on the circulation in the brain'.

3 *Organic diseases of the brain* took up only sixteen pages of Abercrombie's book. He wrote that

> When we endeavour to trace the leading symptoms with these various states of disease, we do not find any uniformity, by which particular symptoms can be distinctly referred to the various forms of the morbid affections; we can therefore attempt only a very general outline of the symptoms, which are connected with organic disease of the brain (p. 332).

Diseased states were usually 'permanent changes in the cerebral substance or new formations within the head'. He described the appearances already mentioned in Hooper's *Atlas* but he also tried to unravel the symptomatology. Masses within the head caused 'long-continued severe headache', which, nevertheless, could remit; it was often paroxysmal, accentuated by motion, or occurred in the early morning. Any of the special senses might be impaired, most commonly vision. Vomiting in cerebellar lesions might suggest a stomach disorder, but there was headache to consider. Convulsions in tumour might be the only symptom; they were sometimes unilateral. Hemiplegia from tumour was usually slow in development. 'All these diversities' Abercrombie wrote, 'do not depend on size or structure of tumours'. It was important to try and discover whether a tumour was 'of' and not just 'in' the brain.

4 *The spinal cord* is 'divided into four columns, the anterior of which take their origin from the crura cerebri, and the two posterior from the crura cerebelli'. There were two distinct spinal nerve roots, with 'recently shown diversity of function'. The central canal of the cord communicated with the fourth ventricle and might fill with fluid (no suggestion of recognizing syringomyelia). Extradural spinal effusions did not communicate intracranially because of the attachment of the dura mater to the anterior rim of

the foramen magnum. But subdural effusions did so, freely.

In trying to identify symptoms that would point to spinal, and not cerebral, lesions, Abercrombie felt he was on uncertain ground. There had been talk of convulsions, difficulty with speech, swallowing, trismus, and various respiratory difficulties. He doubted whether they 'proceed from the spinal cord'; paraplegia and sphincter troubles certainly did. He recognized girdle pains; 'a feeling of tightness or constriction along the margins of the ribs ... as if a tight band were passed across the stomach' (p. 401). He recognized tetraplegia from odontoid cord compression and thought that in caries of the spine 'the paralysis was not just due to the spinal deformity ... but to inflammation of the cord'.

In some cases of progressive paraplegia he found no explanation in the cord or brain. Some may have been examples of polyneuritis, but others suffered 'spasms', spinal pains, and loss of sphincter function. There were no cases of a remitting nature suggestive of multiple sclerosis nor any in which loss of motor and sensory function was distributed in a manner indicative of hemisection. Tumours, cysts, abscesses, and tuberculomas were noted to arise within the cord itself, or from the tissues enclosing it. Hence 'a minute examination of the spine' was necessary whenever there was a suggestion of spinal cord disease.

Although it was appreciated that spinal cord compression caused 'numbness' with paraplegia, actual examination of sensation is not mentioned.

At the end of his book, the author added a twenty-page appendix to 'Outline Diseases of Nerves'. Like the brain and the cord, lesions might be seen within the substance of a nerve, or in its membranes. There were segments of softening, discoloration, swelling, or shrinking; and nerves could be compressed by tumours. He referred to lesions of the fifth and seventh cranial nerves upon which Bell had been working. But 'the subject is entirely in its infancy'.

Abercrombie was educated in Aberdeen, Edinburgh, and in St. George's Hospital, London. He practised in Edinburgh, and became Lord-Rector of Marischal College, Aberdeen.

Richard Bright (1789–1858). Admittedly, in nervous tissue, changes could be 'so minute as to elude research ... minute particles are displaced ... fibres change their direction ...', but the study of such things should not be neglected. We would not expect 'the optician to neglect the transparency of his glass, or the machinist to despise the temper of his steel'. So wrote Richard Bright in the most celebrated text of its day on neuropathology. Under the unassuming title of *Reports of medical cases*, he had, in 1827, described his classical observations on dropsy, and diseases of the kidney. In the second volume, in 1831,[20] at the suggestion of his surgical colleague, Sir Astley Cooper (1768–1841), he confined his account 'to one particular organ' – the brain. Entitled *Diseases of the brain and nervous system*, it carried the subtitle, as it were, of the first volume; namely, *Selected with a view of illustrating the symptoms and cure of diseases by a reference to morbid anatomy.* An accomplished writer and artist, Bright's text on the brain was based on over two hundred autopsied cases, and includes many splendid illustrations, twenty-five in colour.

Bright commented on the difficulties presented in the case of the nervous system – 'a system the office and structure of which are so peculiar and so delicate, we may well conceive that trivial organic changes easily escaping observation – particularly if taking place over a large extent – might be capable of producing very important derangement and very marked symptoms' (p. 1). But there was no alternative but 'the careful comparison of symptoms with deviations from the natural structure and appearance discovered after death'.

The principal phenomena of cerebral disease could be ascribed to 'Inflammation, Interrupted Function, and Irritation', but he classified his material under four main headings; Inflammation, Pressure, Irritation, and Inanition. In the first category he listed the symptoms we now ascribe to meningitis and encephalitis. When pressure rose, there was paresis and coma. Irritation was marked by screaming, agitation, and convulsion. Inanition led to pallor, dull headache, tinnitus, indistinct vision, syncope, and coma. The morbid conditions responsible for these symptoms were usually 'blended together' and influenced by circulatory changes. It was not easy to say which was 'nervous' and which 'vascular' in origin, because 'we are unable to explain the action of the nerves on any known principle'.

Cerebral *inflammation* could follow head injury, fever, ear disease, and visceral diseases. *Pressure* within the head arose from arterial or venous 'derangements', from diseases of the heart and lungs, or from an impaired quality of the blood. Pressure effects also occurred when vessels ruptured, when the ventricles dilated, or when effusions collected. Masses forming within the skull were another source of pressure. Cerebral *irritation* originated in lesions within or without the skull. It often left no identifying mark in the brain and could then only be deduced from the clinical picture. This was usually characterized by 'paroxysms' – of mania, epilepsy, chorea, or neuralgia. Remote sources of cerebral irritation included diseases of the abdominal viscera, worms, teething, 'hysteria from uterine sympathy', tetanus, hydrophobia, and the effects of poisons such as mercury and strychnine.

One can sympathize with and admire Bright's endeavour to penetrate 'this obscure branch of pathology'. Clinical distinctions were still crude, and morbid anatomy still dependent on unaided vision.

The flavour of Bright's attractive and historical book on the brain is perhaps best captured by presenting examples in which a case history is accompanied by an illustration of the pathology.

1. *Case CXXV (p. 267). Ruptured cerebral aneurysm.* Bright was called to the home of a boy of 19 years and found him in bed unconscious; 'insensible ... throbbing carotid vessels ... active pupils'. He was told that 'while sitting upon a chamber utensil', he had suddenly cried out 'Oh, my head!' and was subsequently assisted to bed. He regained his senses and was

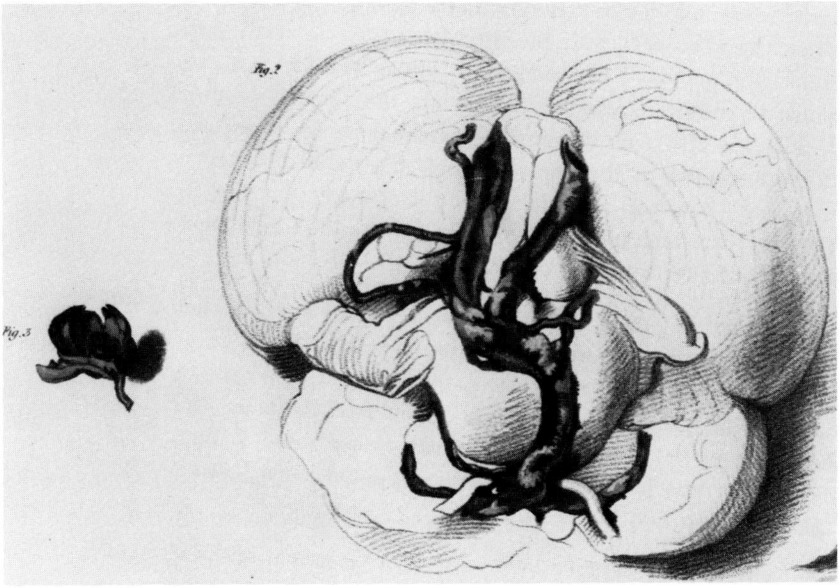

FIG. 59. 'Ossification' of vertebral and basilar arteries (Case CXXXV). *Fig. 3* shows the aneurysm which burst (Case CXXV). (After Bright,[20] Plate XIX.)

recovering, but nine days later, he had a second attack and died. At autopsy, amidst the intracranial clot, Bright found an aneurysm, the size of 'a large pea' on a branch of the left middle cerebral artery (see left-hand side of Fig. 59).

2. *Case CXXXV (p. 285). Apoplexy.* A 'stout man' of 61 years, with 'a short neck', was 'Aloft a ship' and fell. He was brought to hospital and found to have a left hemiplegia, dying three days later. His fall was judged to have been a consequence of the stroke. At autopsy his kidneys were 'granulated', his arteries diseased; there was a blood clot in the right hemisphere and the

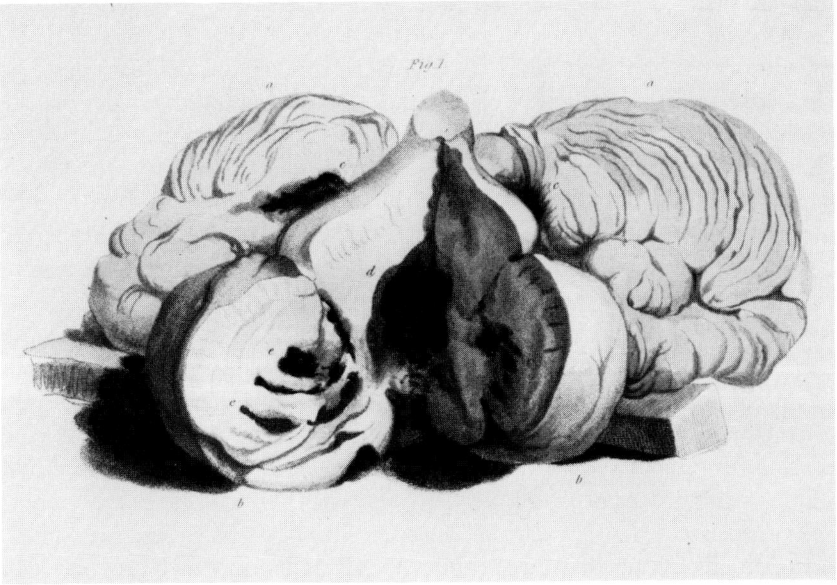

FIG. 60. Brain stem haemorrhages (Case CXXXII). (After Bright,[20] Plate XX.)

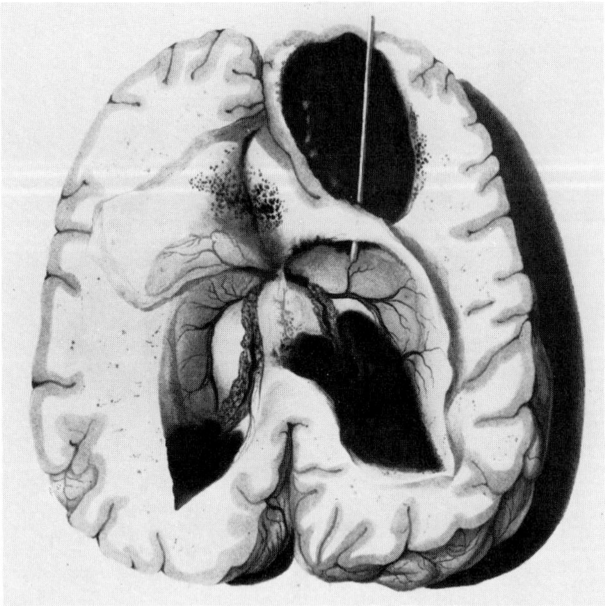

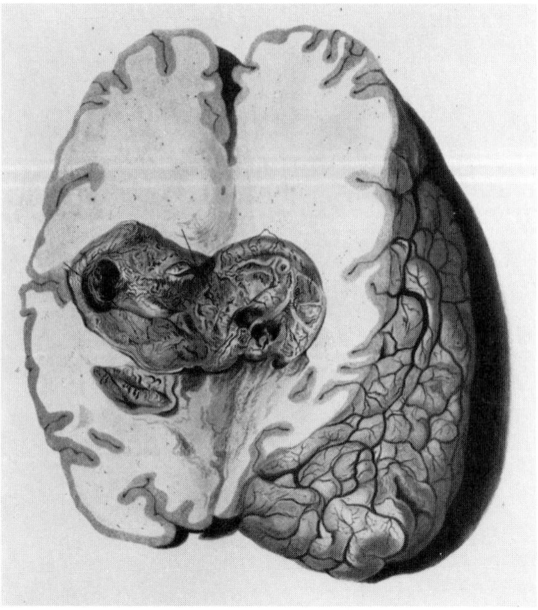

FIG. 61 (*left*). Right frontal lobe haemorrhage with rupture into lateral ventricle (Case CXXXVI). (After Bright,[20] Plate XXII.)

FIG. 62 (*right*). 'Cyst in Brain' with 'congeries of vessels' and fatal haemorrhage (Case CLXVI). Possibly an angioma. (After Bright,[20] Plate XXV.)

basal arteries were ossified, 'studded with numerous cartilaginous patches' (Fig. 59).

3. *Case CXXXII (p. 279). Apoplexy.* A 'stout ex-soldier' with 'a short neck', who had suffered from headaches for several years, fell unconscious in the street and was brought into hospital, dying the same day. At autopsy the arteries were hardened and the heart enlarged; haemorrhage in the left cerebral hemisphere, with rupture into the ventricles; haemorrhage in pons (Fig. 60).

4. *Case CXXXVI (p. 287). Apoplexy.* A woman, aged 55 years, was found unconscious on her kitchen floor, known to have lain there for at least half an hour. She died in hospital five days later, without regaining consciousness. 'The buccinators yielded in a powerless way to the air on expiration ... clenched right fist ... right arm flexed on her chest ... convulsive movements of the right hand.' Autopsy showed a haemorrhage in the right anterior lobe; a probe indicates where it ruptured into the ventricle (Fig. 61).

5. *Case CLXVI (p. 310). 'Cyst in Brain'.* Another stout, short-necked male; 44 years old, a street fruit-seller. Seventeen days before admission to hospital he noticed weakness of the left hand; it spread to the whole arm in four days, thence to the left leg and left side of his tongue. Died with a complete hemiplegia, with much headache, thirteen days after admission. Autopsy showed a large cystic lesion, and a smaller one, in the right hemisphere. The larger cyst was 'almost formed of a congeries of vessels'. No history of previous stroke, so Bright deduced there had been an 'effusion of blood into a vascular cyst ... the precise nature of this disease is not understood'. It was probably a cystic angioma (Fig. 62).

6. *Case CLXIV (p. 349). 'Tumour in Brain'.* A male, aged 45 years, complained of headache and numbness of his right arm which progressed to

a complete right hemiplegia, with loss of speech, over a period of eleven days. On command, he could open his mouth and protrude his tongue; he frequently raised his left hand to his head. He could say only 'Yes' and 'No'. He died 26 days after admission to hospital. At autopsy there was obvious swelling of the left cerebral hemisphere; horizontal section revealed the tumour (Fig. 63).

7. *Case CLXVII (p. 359). 'Scrofulous tubercles in the Brain'.* A boy aged 11 years. 'A fit' in school, five months previously. Gradually became 'dull' and 'helpless'. 'Leeched and blistered on the head'. On admission to hospital there was cough, he screamed with headache, his legs were 'stiff', 'spasms' affected his right arm, and he was incontinent. Increasing spasticity of right arm and left leg. He died eight days later (Fig. 64).

In the second part of his book, Bright offers a general discussion of the following topics: hysteria, chorea, palsy from mercury, neuralgia, epilepsy, tetanus, and hydrophobia.

Hysteria could 'imitate' many disorders, including inflammation and paralysis. Spasms of all kinds might occur, and sometimes there was 'mental affection' or 'delirium'. The uterus was still considered the source of trouble. 'This peculiar condition of the nerves seems to owe its origin, more or less directly, to the extensive sympathies of the uterus ... our first

FIG. 63 (a). Tumour in left hemisphere showing general swelling and posterior location (Case CLXIV). (After Bright,[20] Plate XXVII.) (b) Horizontal brain section of this case (Plate XXVIII).

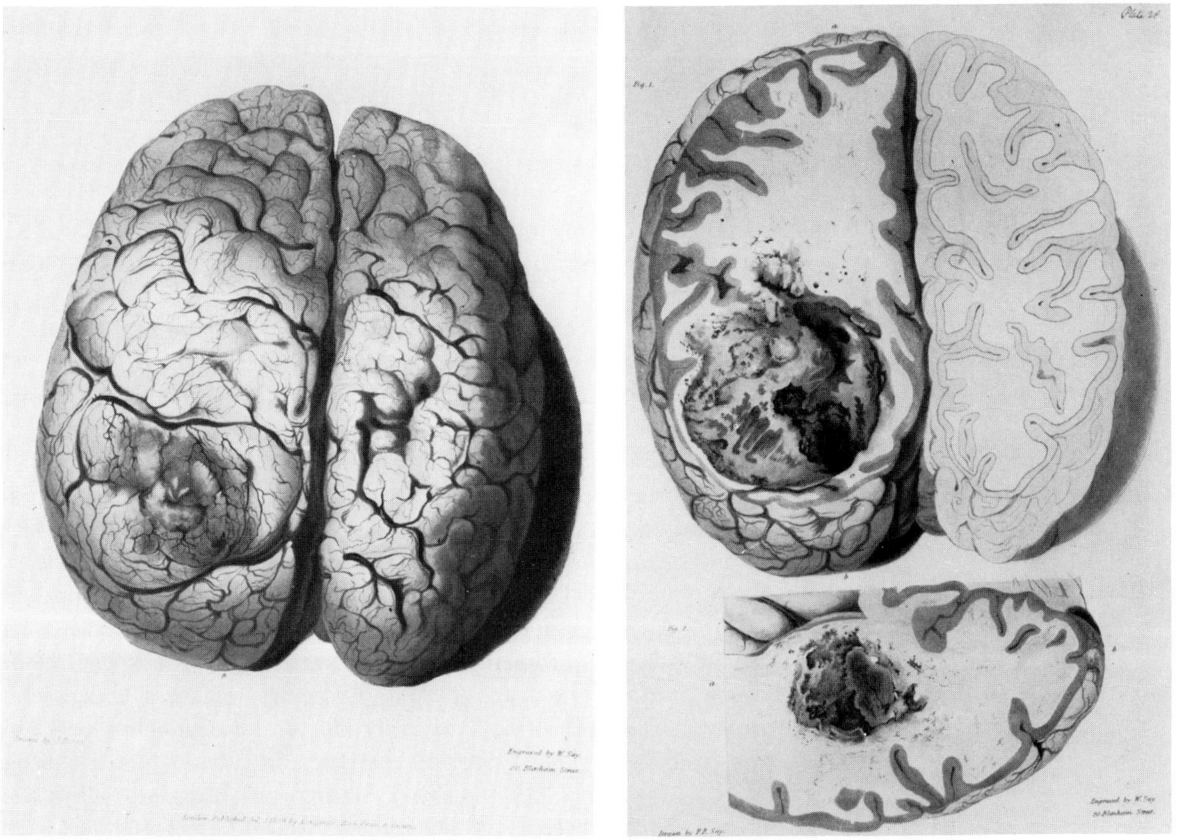

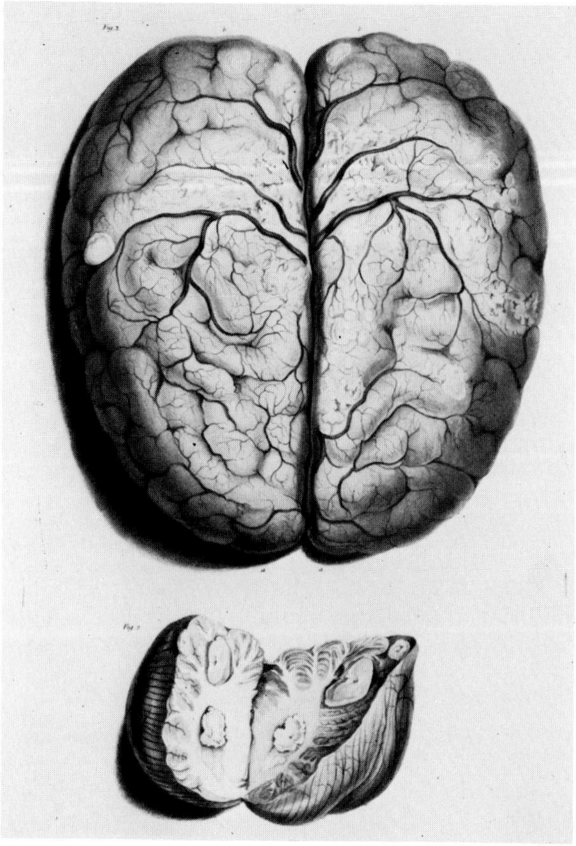

FIG. 64. Scrofulous tubercles in the brain; cerebellum below (Case CLXVII). (After Bright.[20] Plate XXIX.)

business is to seek out any indication of irregular uterine action . . .' (p. 466). We now know, of course, that many organic disorders of the nervous system can 'imitate' hysteria.

Chorea existed in acute and chronic forms. It was 'a general irritation which so strongly marks chorea'. The acute form primarily affected children, in which 'we have seen that rheumatism is so intimately connected . . . a peculiar connection' (p. 493). The chronic form was commoner in males and usually dated from childhood, 'attended with no danger but seldom admitting a cure'. Bright did not mention hemichorea, or its association with infantile hemiplegia, nor any hereditary form, or of cases which progressed to dementia.

Erethism, the clinical features of mercury poisoning, was encountered among people employed in silvering and gilding processes, and in venereal hospitals. In addition to stomatitis, salivation, and loss of teeth, speech itself could become unintelligible, and there were tremors, weakness, and general incoordination. Bright described a severely affected, emaciated husband and wife who lived in a single room, making their livelihood by 'procuring leathern bags in which quicksilver had been imported . . . and extracting the quicksilver which had been concealed in the pores', and selling it. They were persuaded to leave London, and recovered when the husband obtained employment in the country.

In the section on 'Neuralgia', Bright considered sciatica, 'an inflammatory affection of the investing membranes' of the nerve, post-herpetic neuralgia, hemicrania, and tic douloureux. The latter 'may attack any part . . . particularly the face'. When it affected a limb, division of a nerve had been tried, but it often failed. It was seen after amputation, when 'the common sensation of a limb' might also persist for years. Obviously the term tic douloureux was also used to describe paroxysmal pains of several kinds – including causalgia, and perhaps tabetic lightning pains. The phantom limb was known.

Epilepsy manifested itself, not only in major convulsions, but in attacks beginning in a hand or foot or 'a single finger', or remaining one-sided. Sometimes the attack consisted merely of 'a momentary absence of mind, the eye fixed as in thought, yet gazing vacantly' (p. 512). In other cases 'the head is drawn forcibly to one side'. 'Temporary paralysis' might follow a fit. One epileptic walked 'in a state of complete unconsciousness from Clapham Common to Shoreditch and was between four to five hours on the road.' The cause of epilepsy was 'nervous irritation' and when brain lesions were seen they were often on 'the surface'. He said that 'injury to the cineritious substance' (the grey matter) may be responsible. But usually there was little to observe in the brain at autopsy.

Tetanus 'originated in injury done to the extremities of nerves'. The trauma may have been forgotten and the wound healed, when the patient took ill. Treatment was usually to no avail. In a boy of fifteen years, on the tenth night, 'we contrived to get a pint of port-wine into his stomach, with the third of a pint of sheep's trotter jelly', but the boy died. Hydrophobia was also a lurking danger and invariably fatal.

In general, thought Bright, the brain was an organ that was exceptionally susceptible to 'excitements'. These were becoming 'unlimited . . . with every increase of luxury and civilisation' (p.652). But the wretched state of many of his patients can be inferred. 'Internal strife' could also agitate the brain and produce 'inflammation or congestion'. So there were psychological, as well as social, factors to be considered in aetiology.

He appreciated the importance of the cortical grey matter, citing Foville, mentioning its layers, and noting how in certain diseases it was shrunken, swollen, or discoloured. Cortical injury could cause epilepsy. As for the long white fibre tracts, those from the anterior portion of the spinal cord ascended through the corpora striata to the anterior lobes of the cerebrum; those from the posterior columns of the cord passed via the optic thalami *en route* to the posterior lobes of the brain. Bright thought lesions of the anterior lobes primarily affected the lower limbs; and lesions of the posterior lobes, the upper limbs.

Bright did not consider lesions of the spinal cord as such, but he recounted a case (CCCIII, p. 640) which may have been one of multiple sclerosis. A woman of 24 years, with a three-year history of weakness and numbness of the lower limbs, first on the right and then on the left, and with slight affection of her hands. She began to recover after two months in hospital, and eventually walked well. He also described three cases of disease of the upper cervical vertebrae, with 'slight paralysis of the arms' in two. Two had posterior pharyngeal abscesses; all three were probably tuberculous but there were no autopsies (p. 415).

Five years later, in the first volume of *Guy's Hospital Reports* (1836), Bright contributed his important paper on 'Diseased Arteries in the Brain'.[21]

Like the good man he was, Bright paid tribute to 'the sumptuous hospital to which I am attached' and from which there flowed such a splendid tradition in bedside and post-mortem observation.

Joseph Swan (1791–1874). 'There are few diseases so little understood as those of the nerves', wrote Joseph Swan in his *Treatise on diseases and injuries of the nerves* (1834).[22]

In his book, of 350 pages, he discussed the subjects of injury, inflammation, and tumours of nerves, the questions of pain, and repair, and he provided certain case histories and pathological findings.

FIG. 65. Injury to median nerve (*bb*) at the wrist which caused pain, weakness, contracture, and numbness for seven years. Hand amputated, median nerve swollen, no bony injury. (After Swan.[22])

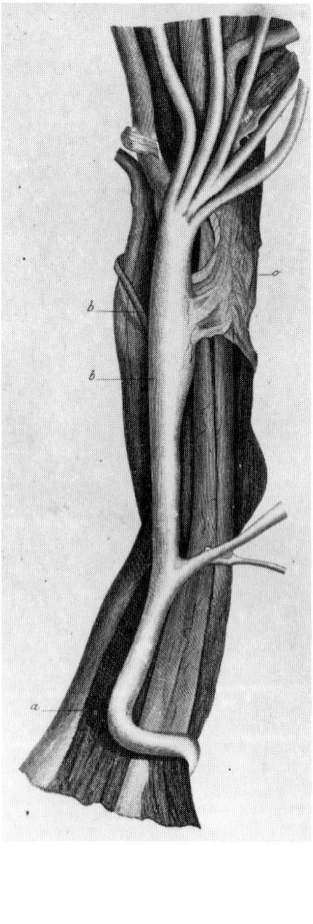

He first discussed pain as a symptom in 'general', and then in 'particular' nerves. 'Is pain only felt', he enquired, 'via the posterior spinal roots?' He thought that a muscle 'must be endowed with perceptibility, but not necessarily felt as a sensation by the mind' (p. 1). 'The same nerves can convey one impression to the muscular parts and another to the sentient' (p. 51). On a section of a nerve, if 'it retracts ... I conceive there must be contraction of the nerve itself'. Nerve function, like brain function, must depend on a blood supply; when it was cut off, nerve function was affected. Examples of referred pain were: (1) pain in the shoulder from disease of the liver – it must be distinguished from pain resulting from a lesion of the scapular nerve in the suprascapular notch; (2) pain in the bladder from a lesion of the penis; (3) pain in the sole of the foot from pelvic disease. Visceral pain was transmitted via the vagus and sympathetic nerves.

Common causes of injury were falls (from coach, carriage, shipmast, etc.), musket balls, and venesection. He described one case in which, for seven years, a man of twenty-two had suffered much pain, numbness, and weakness of one hand, as the result of injury to the median nerve at the wrist. A horse had suddenly jerked his arm, via a halter round his wrist. 'The hand was quite useless' and the patient could not extend the first three fingers, so Swan amputated the hand. There was no bony injury to the carpus, but the median nerve was 'enlarged' and the sheaths of the flexor tendons 'thickened' (Fig. 65). This illustration must be one of the earliest of this nature.

Partial injuries to nerves were more painful than complete ones. There was much more pain, with local 'quivering', 'sensitivity', and 'irritability' of an affected part when a nerve was incompletely divided. He wondered, as many have since done, whether 'constitution' was an influential factor in pain production. Some of the most troublesome cases were those in which the initial injury seemed slight. Particular care should be taken in venesection at the elbow. There is a sixteen-page account of the young wife of a Lincoln surgeon who suffered pains from 1805 to 1833, following a finger cut while peeling an orange. Amputation of the fingertip did not help, neither did amputation of the finger. The pains subsequently spread to the face and head.

Ligatures inexpertly applied were also a source of nerve injury. Swan quoted the case of an Army General who had to have an arm amputated following a gun-shot wound (p. 151). When a ligature was touched 'the pain was not in the stump itself, but referred to the finger, thumb, wrist and elbow of the lost arm'. The patient could trace the different course of the pains produced when the surgeon tweaked a ligature in various directions and was able to point out the track of the nerves in the surgeon's own arm. 'On one occasion I, with general astonishment, had the general neurology of my arm and fingers traced by him.'

What we now term 'causalgia' had already been described by Denmark[23] in 1813 in a soldier who sustained an arm wound in the storming of Badajoz in the Peninsular War. Amputation became necessary because of burning pain in the hand, thumb, and first and second fingers.

Swan studied the mode of repair of divided nerves in rabbits and dogs. He found that 'severed nerves do not set up anastomoses like arteries' but regeneration did take place. He illustrated (Fig. 66) this in a rabbit from which he removed one-half inch of sciatic nerve, and which he killed four months later.

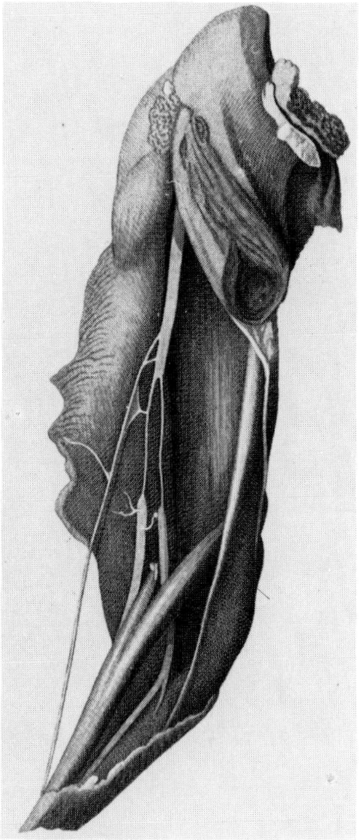

FIG. 66. Dissection of a rabbit leg, four months after half an inch of the sciatic nerve had been resected. Strands of nerve tissue now bridging the gap. (After Swan.[22])

In the chapter dealing with 'Diseases of the Nerves of the Senses' he included the eighth cranial nerve and discussed some aspects of deafness. He mentioned high- and low-tone loss, the various varieties of tinnitus, and how deafness resulted from lesions of the ear drum, the hearing apparatus, or the auditory nerve. In some types of deafness the patient might 'hear a conversation in a carriage in motion' (p. 279). He was also aware of sound conduction through the bones of the face or skull and wondered whether some form of instrument could be manufactured which would assist hearing. He thought some communication might exist between the facial and auditory nerves.

Swan also published a book entitled *A demonstration of the nerves of the human body* (1830),[24] an anatomical atlas containing twenty-five illustrative plates. Figure 67 depicts the brachial plexus.

Swan was a surgeon to the Lincoln County Hospital from 1814 to 1827, obtaining his FRCS in 1843. In London 'he never attained any practice but did much for the science of anatomy'.[25]

Robert Carswell (1793–1857). Whereas Hooper, Abercrombie, and Bright were experienced practising clinicians, Carswell (1793–1857), author of another historical atlas – *Illustrations of the elementary forms of disease* (1838)[26] – was primarily an artist-pathologist. Beginning in Glasgow and continuing his medical education in Edinburgh, London, and Paris, his career was an odd one, that included an appointment to the first chair in pathological anatomy in England, at University College, London, in 1828,

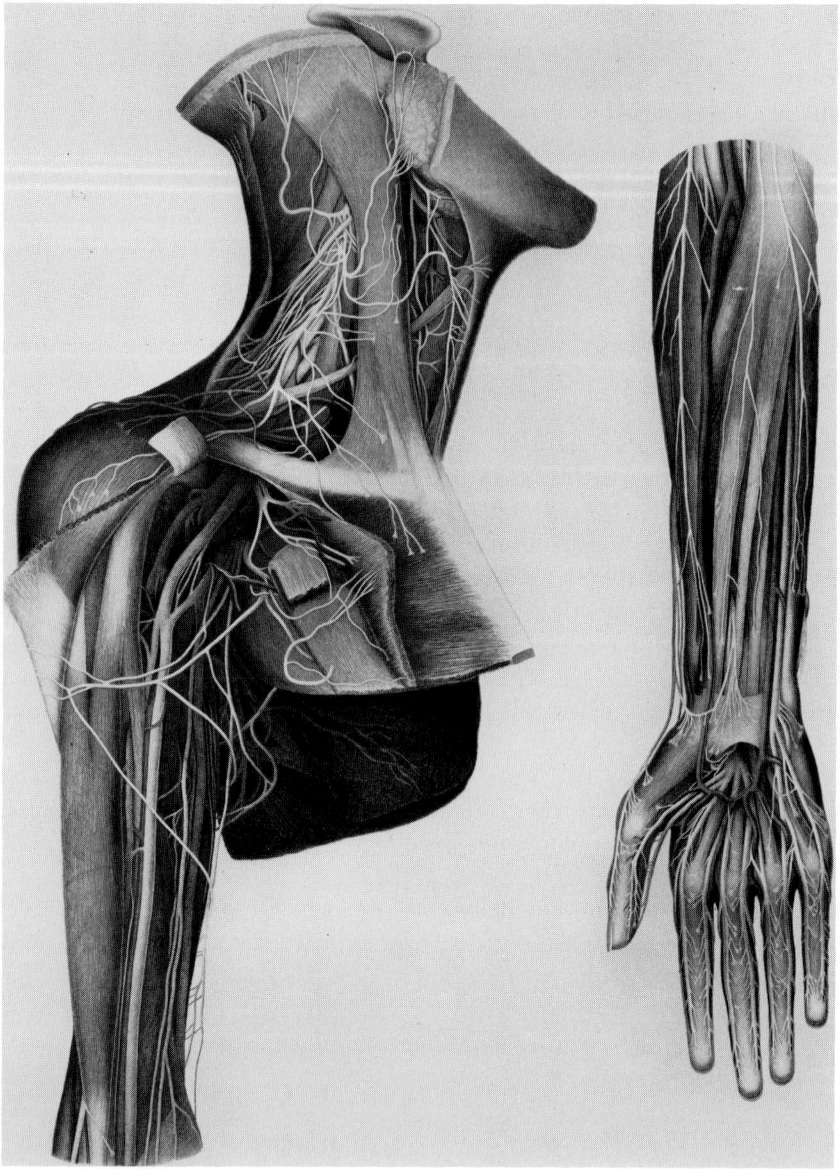

FIG. 67. Dissection of neck and cutaneous nerves of forearm. (After Swan,[24] Plate XXI.)

followed, in 1840, by that of personal physician to the King of the Belgians. He then resigned his professorship and lived in Belgium for the rest of his life. Knighted by Queen Victoria for his service to the exiled Louis-Philippe of France, of Entente cordiale fame, neither the *British Medical Journal* nor *The Lancet* published an obituary, although the latter promised one. His atlas has been described as representing 'the highest point which the science of morbid anatomy had reached before the introduction of the microscope'.[27]

It was based on two thousand water-colour drawings from which he produced his own lithographs – 'my coloured delineations'.† Carswell was primarily concerned with depicting the processes of disease in various

† Unfortunately with un-numbered pages.

organs – inflammation, atrophy, hypertrophy, haemorrhage, gangrene, softening, new growths, etc. – rather than with clinicopathological correlation. For neurologists, perhaps the three most interesting illustrations are from Plate IV of the atlas (see Fig. 68), in the section on 'Atrophy'.

Atrophy of the brain could be diffuse or focal, senile or pre-senile, cortical or subcortical. 'Ossification' of arteries such as the carotids and vertebrals caused atrophy by diminishing the blood supply. But softening itself was not necessarily ischaemic; it could result from inflammation or defective nutrition. Insanity was another condition in which there was cerebral atrophy, particularly when there was also 'a general paralysis', which he illustrated (Fig. 68, top right). In this disease the atrophy involved 'more especially the grey substance of the convolutions', and it could be focal or diffuse and bilateral. Fluid accumulated over the hemispheres and the meninges were 'opaque and thickened'. When the meninges were peeled away the convolutional atrophy and the 'irregular depressions or excavations, situated between', were disclosed. Carswell considered the cerebral atrophy as the cause of the insanity and general paralysis, and wondered whether it arose as a consequence of 'irritation or chronic inflammation' within the convolutions themselves, or as 'a consequence of compression, produced by the effusion and accumulation of this fluid between the convolutions, from a similar disease of the membranes'. In other words, whether there was primarily a cortical or a meningeal lesion. He favoured the latter.

He also appreciated that neural lesions could produce secondary atrophy. In convolutional atrophy he had noted a diminution in size of the corpus striatum and optic thalamus, on one or both sides, according to the extent of the cortical disease. 'Nor was the secondary occurrence of atrophy confined to those portions of the brain; it extended to the crura cerebri, pons Varolii, medulla oblongata, and spinal chord.' In his illustration (Fig. 68, bottom right) he indicates the ipsilateral distribution of this secondary atrophy, consequent on an apoplectic lesion in the corpus striatum, descending as far as the pyramids. He does not mention decussation or discuss the old problem of 'crossed paralysis'.

It was in this section of his atlas, on 'Atrophy', that we find the celebrated illustration of the lesions of multiple sclerosis (Fig. 68, top left). He called it 'a peculiar diseased state of the chord and pons Varollii, accompanied by atrophy of the discoloured portions'. He had seen two specimens showing these lesions, in Paris.

> One of the two patients was under the care of Mons. Louis in the hospital of La Pitié, the other under M. Chomel at La Charité, both of them affected with paralysis. I did not see either of the patients, but I could not ascertain that there was any thing in the character of the paralysis or the history of the cases, calculated to throw any light on the nature of the lesion found in the spinal chord.

In the case he illustrated, the pons was obviously affected; in the second case, the main lesions were in the spinal cord and medulla, with only 'smaller . . . distinct spots' in the pons.

Plate IV.

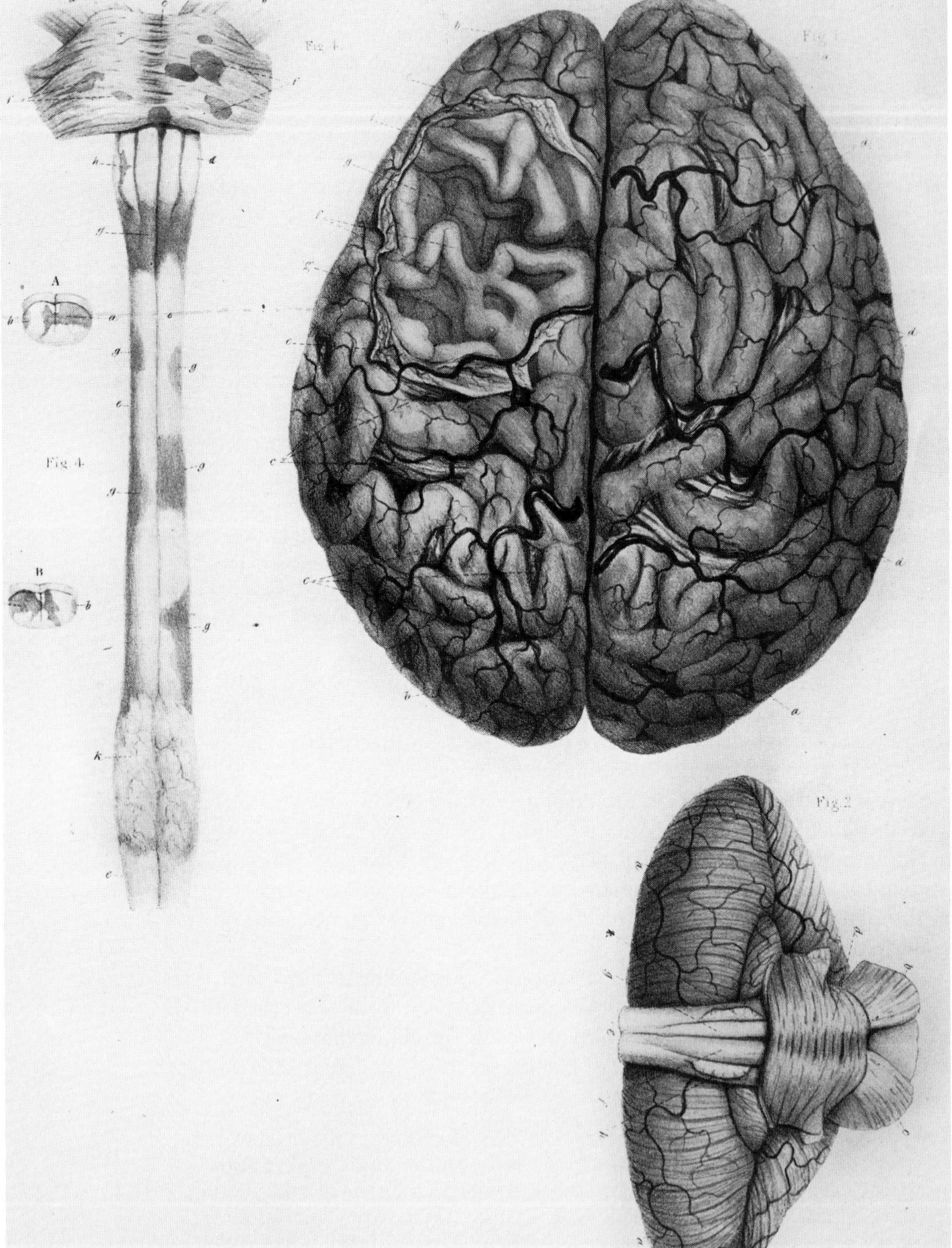

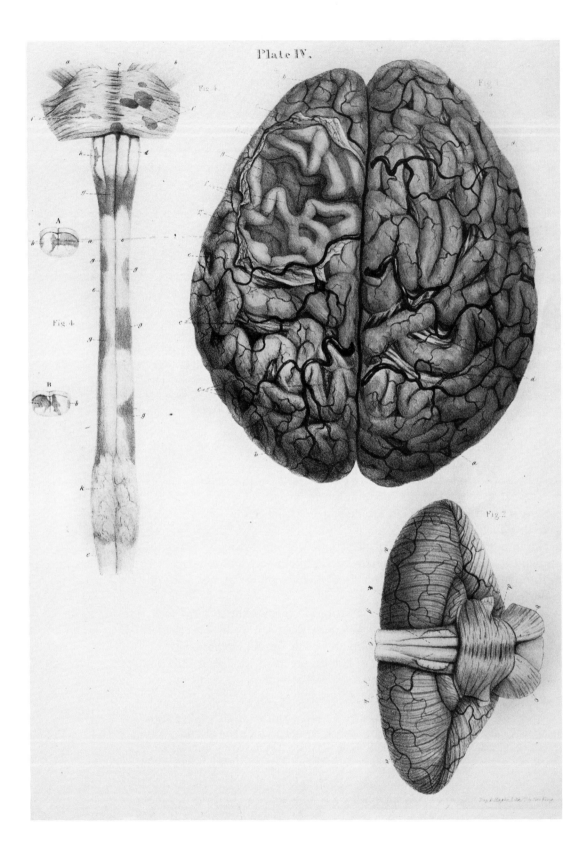

The anterior surface of the spinal cord presented a number of spots, from a quarter of an inch to half an inch in breadth, of an irregular form, of a yellowish-brown colour, smooth, glossy, without vascularity or any alteration in the colour or consistence of the surrounding medullary substance.

On dividing the spinal cord Carswell found that these discrete lesions were 'seen to penetrate as far as the grey substance'. They were unquestionably the plaques of multiple sclerosis, which Cruveilhier (1791–1874) was also observing in Paris at that time and which he also illustrated. But, in addition, Cruveilhier provided clinical histories.

Courville[28] concluded that other important contributions of Carswell were his illustrations of subdural haematoma, subdural abscess, metastatic melanoma, and traumatic petechial cerebral haemorrhages. In the section on tumours he did not include any examples of meningioma.

The Paris School

Bright's sentiment about his hospital was echoed by Cruveilhier (1791–1874), the first Professor of Pathological Anatomy of the Paris School of Medicine. The Salpêtrière, where he worked, had not, like Guy's, been built as a hospital, despite its name – 'Hôpital General' – but as a prison for female destitutes and incurables. Converted to an institution for sick, incurable, and insane women at the time of the Revolution, by 1822 it harboured 3900 incurables, 800 insane people, and 360 sick people.[29] It was still 'a grand asylum of human misery' in Charcot's day.[30] In the foreword to his atlas, *Anatomie pathologique du corps humain* (1829–42) Cruveilhier also spoke proudly of 'the hospital to which I am attached'. In the section on paraplegias he said that it was the remarkable concentration there of hemiplegias and paraplegias that afforded him such an opportunity to study 'cette classe si importante de maladies'.[31]

Cruveilhier's atlas was but one of a series of classical medical texts which reflected the glory of Paris medicine in the first half of the nineteenth century. After the Revolution, and with tremendous zeal, the state-owned hospitals were reorganized.[32] A new medical school was created, with twelve professorial chairs; proper professional recognition was given to surgeons and a system of competitive appointment of 'internes' and 'externes' was introduced.[29] These steps provided a setting in which the new Medicine was to flourish. This was based on a triad of precepts – the use of statistics, physical examination of the patient, and correlation with pathology. The introduction of the techniques of palpation, percussion and auscultation now ensured that correlation was not merely with symptoms, but also with signs. In the field of neurology this was vital, although it did not develop as rapidly as with diseases of the heart and lungs.

As early as 1806, Corvisart (1755–1821) had written that Morgagni's work 'has served more to adorn the works of other physicians than to advance the art of recognising organic diseases'.[33] To Laennec (1781–1826), pathological anatomy was 'le flambeau de la nosologie'.[34]

Ackerknecht[29] has given us a vivid and welcome picture of this unique epoch in the history of medicine. One reads of intense activity by teachers

FIG. 68 (*facing*). Plate IV from Carswell's *Pathological anatomy* (1838). *Fig. 1* (top right): 'Atrophy of the convolutions of the brain in general paralysis of the insane.' Anteriorly, on the left side, the pia has been resected to demonstrate the 'deep irregular hollows, in which the effused serosity was contained'. *Fig. 2* (bottom right): 'Atrophy of the left anterior pyramidal (*g*) and olivary (*k*) bodies, the left half of the pons (*d*), and crus (*b*) from extensive destruction of the left corpus striatum'. Secondary cortico-spinal atrophy. *Fig. 4* (top left): 'A peculiar diseased state of the chord and pons Varolii, accompanied by atrophy of the discoloured portions'. Multiple sclerosis: *ff* 'yellowish brown' lesions in pons; *ggg*, 'hard, semi-transparent, atrophied' 'patches' in spinal cord; *k*, 'softening of a portion of the chord'.

and students, with much illness and early deaths, specialization, the publication of hundreds of theses, monographs, and great dictionaries, atlases, and textbooks. Oliver Wendell Holmes (1809–94)[35] spent nearly two years in Paris as a medical student (1833–35), going on ward-rounds with the Barons Boyer, Larrey, and Dupuytren and Drs Lisfranc, Velpeau, and Chomel. He referred to 'that knotty-featured, savage old man', Broussais, then sixty-two, and to Andral, at thirty-seven, 'whose natural eloquence made it delightful to listen to him'. Pierre Louis, however, was 'the object of our reverence'. He was forty-seven.

Osler's *Alabama student* left an account of his fascination with the feverish activity in the Paris hospitals in 1835. He was at La Charité by 7 a.m., not leaving until 9 p.m., reading at home until midnight. 'There is not a solitary great man in France that is idle, for if he was, that moment he would be outstripped, it is a race. . . .'[36]

It was Pierre Louis (1787–1872) who appreciated the importance of studying large series of cases of particular diseases, thereby introducing the statistical approach. 'Systematic examinations, and systematic autopsies were systematically analysed through statistics.'[37] His books on phthisis and typhoid fever were landmarks. It was one of Louis' patients in whom Carswell found the lesions of multiple sclerosis (p. 193). The impetus given to pathological anatomy by Bichat (1771–1802) was tremendous; autopsies became almost routine in medical and surgical wards. Astley Cooper studied under Professor Desault (1744–95), 'the last great surgeon of the old school and the first great surgeon of the new',[38] and it was he who suggested to Bright the study of separate organs (p. 183).

But before Cruveilhier's great work, two other important monographs appeared from the Salpêtrière. The first was by Rostan (1790–1866) on softening of the brain (1820).[39] The second was by Lallemand (1790–1853) on brain pathology (1820–24).[40] From La Charité, in 1825, came two publications of Bouillaud (1796–1881), the first on inflammation of the brain,[41] and the second on impairment of speech in lesions of the anterior lobes.[42] And to the twenty-eight-year-old Paris physician, Ollivier d'Angers (1796–1845), belongs the credit of writing the first major treatise on diseases of the spinal cord in 1824.[34]

Professor Andral, who once said he had studied medicine three times[43] – first by way of pathological anatomy, then by physical methods of diagnosis, and finally through examination of the blood (introducing the term 'anaemia') – contributed sections on diseases of the nervous system in several of his treatises on medicine[44,45] and pathology.[46] He appreciated that one should not consider pathological anatomy 'comme une science definitivement arrêtée'. As well as the anatomist's scalpel, we needed the chemist's crucible, and the physician's microscope and electrometer. Chemistry had taught us there was iron in the blood, but what of the brain?

> Who knows, for example, if in cerebral diseases where careful anatomical investigation reveals nothing, who knows if there may not be an increase, reduction or alteration in the composition of the brain, in phosphorus, for example?[47]

But meanwhile, said Andral, there was encouraging progress to acknowledge in the investigation of diseases of the brain. 'Nous pourrions citer encore les belles recherches, faites en France et en Angleterre sur les maladies cérébrales . . .'.[48]

Concerning the 'doctrine of localisation' of function in the brain, Andral wrote, in this third decade of the century, that

On the one hand, it [the brain] is a great whole composed of a number of parts, each of which performs a special function; while on the one hand, these different parts are intimately connected with each other, in such a manner that they are mutually, jointly and severally responsible, if I can express it thus. Hence it follows that at the place where you discover a lesion there does not always reside the direct cause of the effects which are produced, and, according how it reacts on other sites, with specific functions, will depend the modification.[49]

Here, Andral seemed not merely to be saying that cerebral lesions exerted indirect as well as direct effects. He was also implying that there were difficulties to be faced in attempting to localize functions of certain areas of the brain, by observations of this kind. He pointed out that 'identical lesions could have variable effects', but he felt that if experience showed that particular lesions were consistently followed by the same effects one could not object to the 'doctrine of localisation'.

When discussing hemiplegia, Andral[50] was satisfied, in 1833, that he could refer to the crossed effects of cerebral lesions, as being 'a law', there were so few exceptions. The responsible lesion could be superficial or deep, and be no larger than 'a square-inch'. It might be found in the anterior, middle or posterior lobes of the hemispheres, in the thalamus, the corpus striatum, or the cerebral peduncle. There was some evidence to suggest that paralysis of the upper limbs was associated with lesions near the thalamus, and paralysis of the lower limbs with lesions near the corpus striatum. In seventy-five cases of hemiplegia there were forty in which upper and lower limbs were involved at the same time; twenty-one of them had lesions in the anterior lobes or corpus striatum and nineteen had lesions in the posterior lobes or thalami.

We cannot yet assign in the brain a distinct seat to the motions of the upper and lower limbs. No doubt such distinct seat exists, since each of these limbs may be paralysed separately, but we do not know it yet.[51]

*

With student audiences of over a thousand in the amphitheatre at l'École de Médicine, two-hundred and fifty in the surgical theatre at La Charité, fifty or more at every ward round, and, with a museum 'providing an inexhaustible magazine of materials composing the groundwork, substratum and apparatus of the healing art', Paris, to a visiting American doctor in 1828 was the 'Mecca of Medicine'.[52]

Rostan (1790–1866) *and Lallemand* (1790–1853). Rostan spent nine years collecting material for his monograph on softening of the brain – *Recherches sur le ramollisement du cerveau* (1820).[39] He was initially attracted to the problem when he saw a patient with an acute hemiplegia at the Salpêtrière, in whom a confident diagnosis of apoplexy had been made. 'A hundred students had seen the patient, more than fifty attended the autopsy.' The latter disclosed, not haemorrhage, but softening affecting one entire lobe, and he never forgot the case.

Not all his ninety-eight cases were examples of what we would now call cerebral infarction, but in the latter class the lesions varied from multiple bilateral 'ecchymoses', resembling 'une tache scorbutique', to massive hemispheral ones. Most commonly placed in the corpus striatum, thalamus, or central white matter, they were also found in the cortex, brain stem, and cerebellum. They were usually softer at the centre and displayed a range of discoloration, yellowish-green in old cases of apoplexy, rosé, chestnut, or reddish in recent cases. Some were frankly cystic, others rather indurated. Detection was not easy when the colour and firmness of the lesions were scarcely abnormal. There were no illustrations.

The clinical manifestions were described as occurring in two stages. In the first they were rather 'fugitive'; headache, giddiness, impairment of vision, tinnitus, difficulties with speech (slowness of response, 'brevity of language', or 'obstruction of the tongue') and numbness or clumsiness of a limb. But the patient did not consult a doctor. Sooner or later, in months or years, there followed the second stage, chiefly characterized by episodes of hemiplegia, resembling apoplectic haemorrhage and leading to coma and death. Indeed, 'ramollisement' appeared to be a fatal disease, unlike apoplexy. 'La marche de cette maladie est donc essentiellement continue et toujours croissante' (p. 21). In the hemiplegic patient the affected limbs did not usually convulse but they were often painful, hypersensitive to touch, and the seat of formication. The upper limbs developed flexion contractures.

Rostan considered that softening was the commonest lesion of the brain, commoner even than apoplexy (p. 457). Although, like others, he observed that it was most often found in old age, and in senility, and that it often surrounded or adjoined a haemorrhagic lesion, and that 'apoplexy' was the commonest 'complication' of softening, he did not, nevertheless, associate it with disturbance of the cerebral circulation. The significance of the arterial 'ossification', which was 'usually' present, escaped him. The general opinion of the day was that softening was a form of 'phlegmasia' or 'inflammation' of the brain ('encephalitis'), for there were the signs of 'congestion', 'redness', and 'exudation'. But Rostan did at least question this. Not all were inflammatory; some were definitely not so. 'Enfin, de toute autre nature inconnue' (p. 462), a contribution which although essentially negative was nevertheless significant.[12]

To Lallemand, however, things looked different. In a series of nine 'Lettres', in the manner of Morgagni, he respectfully admits, in three volumes (500 pages each), entitled *Recherches anatomico-pathologiques sur l'encephale et ses dépendences* (1820–24),[40] he sought to classify diseases of the brain on purely pathological grounds. As an intern at the Hôtel Dieu, he said in his preface, he had seen more cerebral disorders than any writer on the subject and he generally adopted a rather critical attitude to the work of others, which was usually full of 'préconceptions'. Cerebral pathology might be 'the despair of many' but he would attack the problem in a detached manner.

There were many difficulties to face when one came to interpretation. A fatal inflammation of the brain might leave little trace; a minor lesion might have gross consequences. Similar lesions might produce very different symptoms; similar symptoms may be produced by a variety of lesions. When the illness was acute, whatever the nature of the lesion, the clinical manifestations were much the same; similarly with chronic affections. Lastly, there were factors such as the age, temperament (and sex!) of the patient, and the location of the actual lesion within the brain. For all these reasons he thought it best to concentrate on the actual pathology.

The main changes comprised inflammation, induration, destruction, and atrophy. The processes of inflammation consisted of simple softening, suppuration, and encystment. In other words 'ramollisement' was inflammatory. Indurations were cerebral or meningeal, and some of them were tumours. Within the brain there were indurated areas of various shapes and sizes; thin, flat, radial, elongated, irregular, or cicatricial. Tumours were fibrous, fibrocartilaginous, cartilaginous, or osseous. Destruction, sometimes with ulceration, might be superficial or ventricular. Atrophy was usually localized. Case histories and autopsy studies, with comment, were provided under the separate headings – 1818 cases in all, but no illustrations.

But, as in Rostan's painstaking study, the true nature of the commonest cause of softening was not suspected. *Ramollisement* was merely that first stage of inflammation in which there was vascularity, infiltration, or effusion. Although he thought that there was some relationship, deserving study, between apoplexy and cardiac 'aneurysm' (enlargement), 'sans rétrécissement de l'orifice aortique' (p. xix), the idea that softening arose from arterial disease did not occur to him. Also meriting research was the influence of the liver on the brain (p. xix).

Thus, the earlier observations and suspicions of men such as Baillie and Hooper were not repeated, but in a few years, as we have seen, Abercrombie, and especially Bright, were directing attention to the arteries and the heart. Cardiac hypertrophy and the force of the pulse were being increasingly noted in relation to cerebral softening and haemorrhage. Andral wrote

> Thus then, from the state of hypertrophy of the heart, there may result with respect to the brain, (1) first, a degree of congestion, announced merely by pain in the head, vertigo and dizziness; (2) a second degree of this congestion violent enough to produce a total loss of consciousness and all the symptoms of cerebral haemorrhage; (3) this haemorrhage itself.[53]

> Increase in the force of the heart's impulse, whether entirely nervous, or owing to hypertrophy of this organ, has been a real influence in the production of cerebral congestion.[54]

But it was in Vienna and Berlin that the next vital steps took place. Rokitansky (1804–78), bringing together these observations on the heart, the arteries, and the brain, suggested that 'ossification' resulted from a process of deposition on the walls of the arteries, from the blood. And Virchow (1821–1902) proposed the concepts of 'thrombosis' and 'embolism' which led to 'infarction'.

Ollivier d'Angers (1796–1845). Introducing his monograph on the spinal cord – *De la moelle épinière et de ses maladies* (1824)[34] – Ollivier said that it was only an 'outline' but that study of the spinal cord had been neglected and that at autopsy it was too often not examined. Nevertheless, it presents a splendid 'l'ébauche', with its four hundred pages, in which he discusses, without the aid of a microscope, the anatomy, physiology, and pathology of an organ whose similarity to nerve he said had been much exaggerated. There are sixty-five case reports, not all his own, with two illustrative plates of his own drawings (Figs. 69 and 70). He was not entirely satisfied with the general arrangement he had adopted but publication had to be hastened. This perhaps explains why the autopsied case of syringomyelia is not placed in the chapter dealing with cavitation within the cord, in the section on congenital abnormalities, but is to be found in Chapter six (p. 275) devoted to spinal effusions. He devoted sixty pages to anatomy, twenty to physiology, and the rest to disorders of the cord.

In the first section he considers the development of the spinal cord in the embryo and foetus, noting the relative growths of the cord and spine during pregnancy, the communication between the central canal (which he did not think persisted after birth) and the fourth ventricle, and he compares the pyramidal tract in man with that in reptiles, birds, and fishes. The vexed question of its decussation (denied by Haller, Vicq d'Azyr, and 'Monro'?), he concluded, had been finally settled by Gall. The spinal canal varied in shape and size at different levels; triangular in the cervical region, oval in the dorsal, and becoming triangular again, inferiorly. The cord ended opposite the bodies of the first or second lumbar vertebrae. The arterial supply is described, and he wondered whether stasis occurred in the valveless venous network. The remarkable symmetrical nature of the internal structure of the cord clearly implied that its functions were intricate and vital. What was the significance of the curious configuration of the grey matter so well developed in man, and united across the middle? It had been variously described as resembling the hyoid bone (Huber), a tetragon (Haller), or a cross (Monro). The increase in size of the anterior and posterior horns in the cervical and lumbar enlargement was observed, and also the different size of the anterior and posterior spinal nerve roots at all levels. The disposition of the white columnar matter seems to have been determined by arrangement of the grey matter.

The main problem concerning the physiology of the spinal cord, said Ollivier, was to what extent it was independent of the brain. But he did not refer to Whytt. Its vital role in respect of the functions of respiration had been shown by Legallois, but Haller erred concerning its influence on the heartbeat. The anterior white columns proceeded to the cerebrum and the posterior to the cerebellum. The fibres composing the anterior and posterior nerve roots could be traced to the respective horns of the grey matter. The

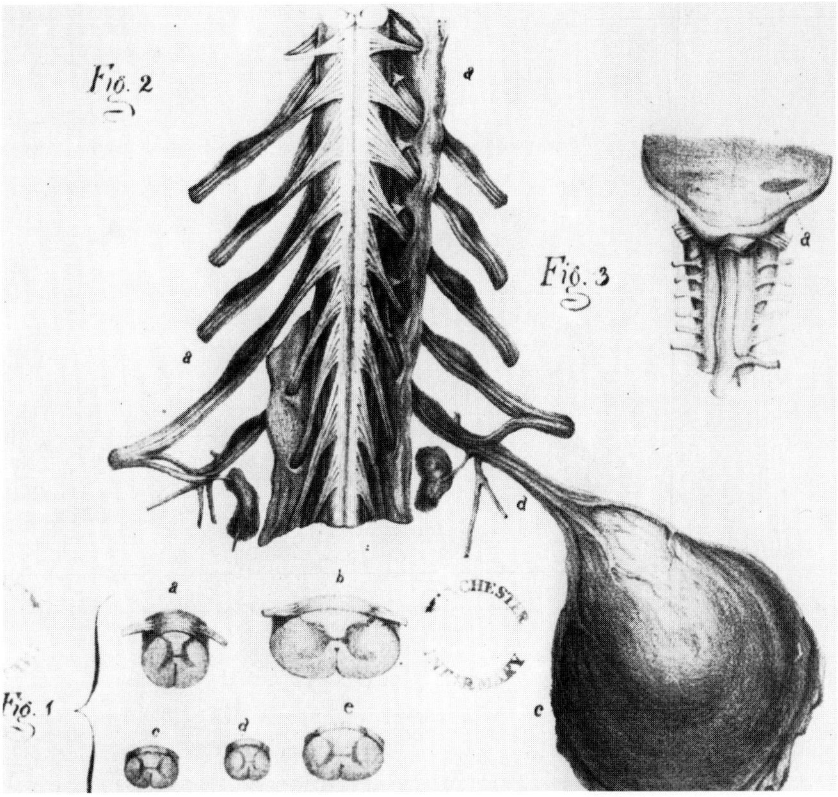

FIG. 69. Plate II of Ollivier d'Angers.[34] *Fig. 1, a, b.* Transverse sections of spinal cord of a horse, dorsal and lumbar, *c, d, e,* human. *Fig. 2. a, a.* Anterior view of human spinal cord, C.3 to D.4; meninges resected on right. *d,* Case 28. Tumour arising from first dorsal nerve (L) which caused severe pains for two years culminating in patient's suicide. Tumour was soft, solid, and showed a concentric arrangement of its fibres on section. Sheath continuous with neurilemma of thickened nerve. *Fig. 3.* Case 36. Anterior view of brain stem in old hemiplegia; scarring in pons on left.

former fibres were smaller, and to this difference in structure Bell and Magendie had added a difference in function. They had shown that the anterior roots were concerned with motion, and the posterior with sensation. But not exclusively so. The subsequent pathways for the transmission of these functions were not known but clinico-pathological studies had a part to play. Traumatic lesions of the anterior portion of the cord tended to primarily affect the motor functions; posterior lesions caused loss of sensation. Unilateral lesions caused ipsilateral paralysis of limbs. But the secret of these things would be found in the grey matter. '... la substance grise est le siège spécial où réside le principe d'action de la moelle rachidienne' (p. 73).

Disorders of the spinal cord were reviewed under the following headings; congenital malformations, atrophy, injuries, compression, commotion, effusions, inflammation, softening, induration, and tumours ('tissus morbides développés').

The section on congenital malformations (50 pp.) is remarkable for its originality. He clearly envisaged that only a thorough understanding of the embryonic development of the nervous system would enable one to decide whether there had been arrested development ('un retard dans leur développement') or some other pathological lesion ('consécutive à une altération particulière', p. 95). He describes the association of hydrociphalus with spina bifida, the various degrees of the latter with its external and

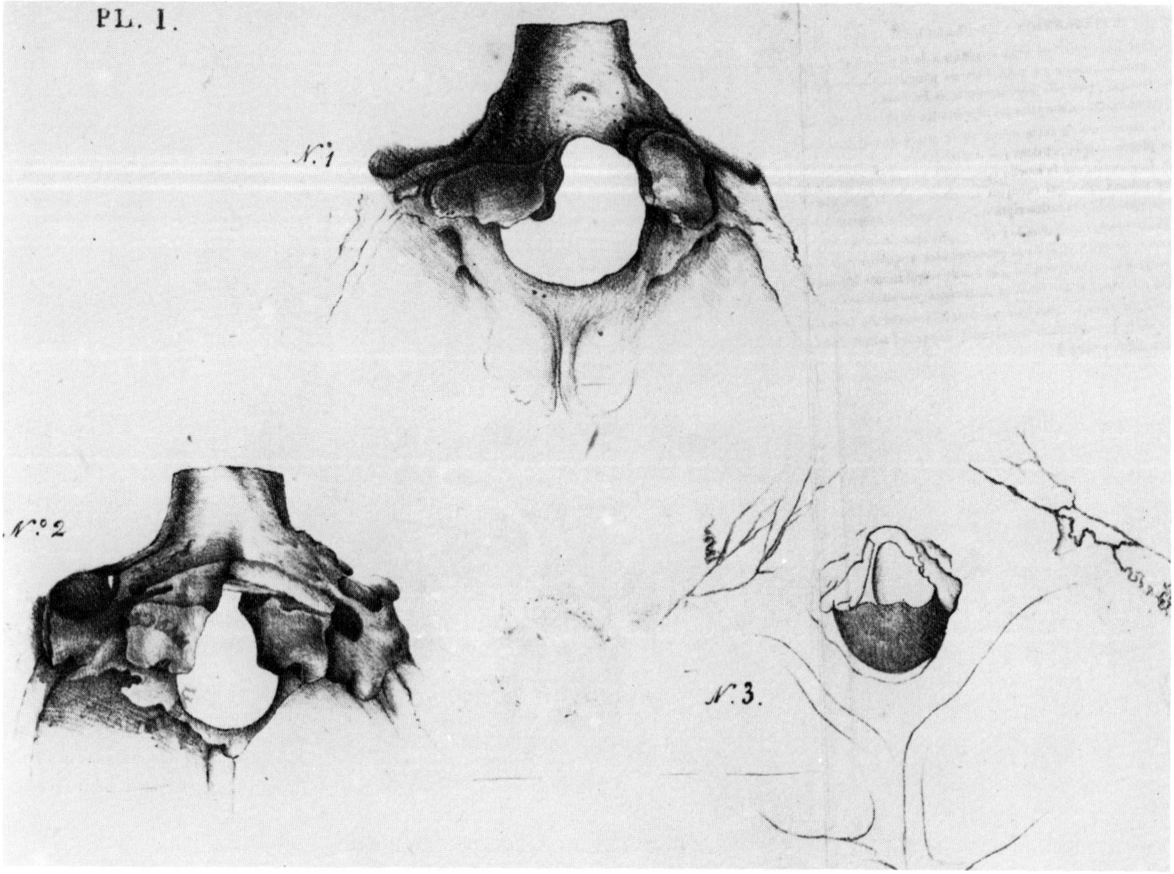

FIG. 70. Plate I of Ollivier d'Angers.[34] *No. 1* Case 23. Congenital stenosis of the foramen magnum. Anomalous development of the right occipital condyle producing a 'croissant'-shaped foramen; no disability or compression of medulla. Figs. 2 and 3. *Nos. 2, 3*. Case 22. Stenosis of foramen magnum. Onset of paraplegia two years before death, age 26 yrs. Compression of medulla with atrophy of pyramids and olives; absent posterior arch of atlas; fusion of anterior arch, odontoid and occiput; dense posterior constricting membrane. Foramen magnum reduced to fifth of its normal size. Ollivier and colleagues were undecided whether lesion was congenital or acquired; probably congenital.

internal features; anomalies of development of the cervical cord in anencephaly including bifidity, cyst formation, and absent or fused vertebrae; elongation of the fourth ventricle into the cervical cord; and absence and faults in the cord itself. In meningocele (*hydrorachis* or *hydropysie du canal*) air insufflated into the sac at autopsy reached the fourth ventricle (p. 123). Longitudinal defects and splitting of the cord may be encountered. Cavitation was not uncommon, especially in spina bifida. 'Cependant il est bien certain qu'on y a observé plusieurs fois une cavité plus ou moins large et profonde' (p. 118).

The fluid accumulating in the spine in *hydrorachis* did not always derive from the cerebral ventricles; and was not always accompanied by hydrocephalus; indeed it could be associated with anencephaly. Nowhere in this section, in the first edition, does he use the word *syringomyelia*, with which his name is associated.

He was unable to discover mention of atrophy of the spinal cord, local or diffuse, in published works. Cruveilhier had not encountered a case by 1816, but Ollivier had observed it twice (p. 140). In a 20-year-old mental defective with a paraplegia, the lumbar cord was half its normal size; the brain was normal. In an old man, five feet two inches in height (*sic*!), there was diffuse atrophy of the cord. Local atrophy could result from compression of the cord, as in spinal curvature, and from constriction of the spinal canal 'dans certains cas de rétrécissement du canal rachidienne' (p. 140). He illustrated (Fig. 70) two cases of stenosis of the foramen magnum, one congenital, the other, in which there was a paraplegia from compression of the medulla, probably acquired. Atrophy could have a mechanical or a nutritional origin ('une atonie nutritive').

The varying motor and sphincter effects of injury to different levels of the cord are well described; cervical, dorsal, and lumbar. Speech and swallowing were only affected by upper cervical lesions; the arms were largely spared when the lesion was at the first dorsal; penile erection in cervical injuries, as described by Dupuytren, Ollivier attributed to injury to the cerebellum. Convulsive movements of the limbs sometimes occurred when the trauma was penetrating (a bone splinter in the cord, or from a sharp weapon).

Compression of the cord could be acute or chronic. In trauma and in spinal caries, retraction of the paralysed limbs eventually develops (p. 220). There was some suggestion that when involuntary movements accompanied urinary and rectal retention, the cord lesion was incomplete. When there were no voluntary or involuntary movements and there was total incontinence, then the cord lesion was complete. He described the case of a young man with a traumatic paraplegia in which a dorsal laminectomy (D. 9 and 10) was carried out in an attempt to relieve the compression of the cord; his tenth dorsal vertebra had been crushed some hours previously. There was some return of sensation and sphincter function, after a few days, but his legs remained paralysed and he died twelve days later. Ollivier did not have the opportunity of examining the cord (p. 222). Trepanning the spine was obviously more difficult than the head, but it should be investigated.

Ollivier also pointed out that compression of the cord could also arise from an intervertebral disc lesion.

> Une autre cause de la compression lente de la moelle rachidienne réside dans le gonflement des cartilages intervertébraux, qui est quelquefois considerable; il parait dépendre d'une affection scrofuleuse; on le remarque assez fréquemment chez les sujets morts à la suite du *mal vertébral de Pott*. On voit dans la cavité rachidienne un bourrele transversal, saillant, qui a repoussé le ligament vertébral commun posterieur, lequel est lui-même ramolli dans le point correspondant. (p. 213)

Tumours ('tissus morbides' and 'corps étrangers') in the spinal canal, or in the meninges or spinal cord, were solid or cystic; cancer rarely affected the cord and he had not seen a case of 'fongus de la dure-mère rachidienne' compressing the cord. But he thought it would present as a gradual form of paraplegia (p. 213). Neither had he seen aneurysmal compression of the cord, although it had been reported.

Syringomyelia. This term, which Ollivier coined, does not appear in the first edition of his work. He used it in the third edition (1837) on page 202, in the chapter on congenital malformations of the cord in reference to spinal cavitation ('creusé en forme de tuyau'). Nevertheless, in the first edition

(p. 275) he describes a case of the disease, with autopsy, but omitted it from the third edition, and he referred to no further example. The case he described was not his own; he summarized one which a Dr Rullier had published in 1823.[55] He does not say whether he saw the patient, but Magendie allowed him to examine the preserved spinal cord specimen. (Magendie had commented on Rullier's original report, at the end of the article.) Ollivier did not apply the term *syringomyelia* to the disease process, but merely to the presence of congenital cavitation.

The patient, a male, aged forty-four years when he died, at the age of three years had developed a slight dorsal curvature of the spine with elevation of the right shoulder. He was quite well until aged thirty-four years when he begun to be troubled with pain, numbness, and clumsiness in his right arm. Following a fall he became worse and he gradually developed more or less complete flaccid paralysis of both arms. His head sank between his shoulders, and his arms hung uselessly by his side as he walked. His legs were little affected; he urinated normally; and his mental faculties were not affected. The hands and forearms wasted; there was pronation of the forearms and flexion contracture of the fingers, so that the nails eroded the palms. Despite this, sensation in his hands was preserved.

> Les parties contractées, conservaient toute leur sensibilité tactile; les mains ne cessaient de servir au toucher que parce qu'elles manquaient de mouvement; mais elles etaient, ainsi que le reste du membre, sensibles a toutes les différences de température extérieure et au plus léger contact. (p. 278)

So, although it probably existed, the characteristic dissociated type of sensory loss was not observed. At autopsy there was a fluid-filled cavity in the spinal cord extending from C. 5 to D. 6. The fourth ventricle contained 'une quantité notable' of fluid, in communication with that in the spinal canal; 'la valvule de Vieussens n'existait pas non plus' (p. 279). To Ollivier the case was important in demonstrating that the organization within the spinal cord was such that you could have motor involvement without sensory, and paralysis of the arms with sparing of the legs. There must be 'l'indépendance d'action des diverses portions de cet organe' (p. 284).

Multiple sclerosis. Ollivier's name is not usually associated with the early history of multiple sclerosis but he does describe a case at considerable length, without autopsy, which deserves mention. It was an example of a type of case of chronic 'myelitis' (a term he said which had only been suggested in 1820) which he had had occasion to observe.

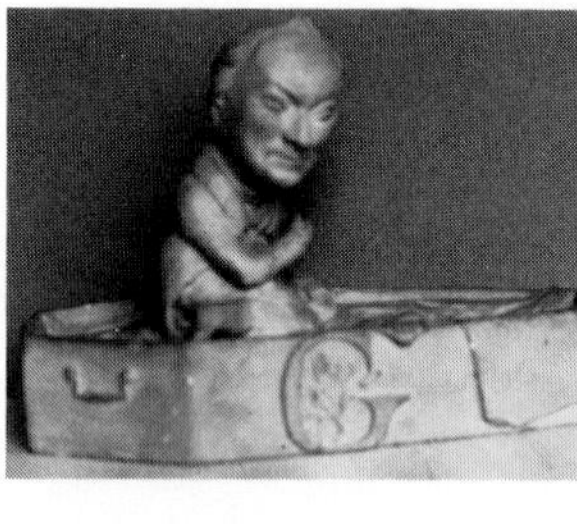

FIG. 71. A caricature statuette of Ollivier d'Angers by Jean-Pierre Dantan, the nineteenth-century French sculptor. His famous statuettes are preserved in the Musée Carnavalet, Paris. The most celebrated is that of Paganini. Ollivier took up legal medicine, hence the coffin motif. (Courtesy of the Musée Carnavalet.) Photograph by the author. (See Ollivier d'Angers in *Arch. Méd. d'Angers*, 1904, p. 7 by L. Jagot.)

His patient, a male, enjoyed good health until the age of seventeen years when, for a time, he was tired and languid. At twenty there was some weakness of the right foot; it passed. At twenty-five, for several months there was weakness and numbness of both lower limbs; it improved. At twenty-nine there was considerable paraplegia, but, again, this was followed by improvement and he was able to walk with a cane. At thirty the patient found that hot spa waters aggravated his disability and there was an acute loss of feeling in the right leg, with numbness and clumsiness of both hands. There was urinary retention; evacuation was aided by pressure on the abdomen. Writing became difficult. Sensation was not impaired in the lower limbs, but, 'une aberration très remarquable', cold water felt very hot, and when his paretic right hand touched his thigh he felt galvanic-like shocks. His condition deteriorated, his left arm became involved, speech became laboured, but his intellect and cheerfulness of personality did not suffer throughout the long illness which, had, at the time of writing, lasted twenty-six years.

This is the best documented early account of what was probably multiple sclerosis that I have encountered. One wonders whether Cruveilhier saw an autopsy; I have not been able to recognize the case history in his *Atlas*.

Ascending paralysis. Although Ollivier did not actually use this term he did briefly describe two cases of 'generalised paralysis', to which Landry referred in his classic paper of 1859, averring that Ollivier was well acquainted with 'acute ascending paralysis' (see pp. 343 *et seq.*). One of Olliviers's patients died in two days with 'generalised paralysis', a woman of thirty-one who had given birth to a child a month previously. The brain and cord were examined, but not the nerves. Nothing of note was recorded.

His second patient, a man of forty-one, took over a year to recover from acute paralysis of his four limbs. He was completely helpless within twenty-four hours and for a time there was paresis of his abdominal and thoracic musculature.

Ollivier believed that the lesion in both cases was in the spinal cord, probably some form of 'congestion'.

*

At twenty-eight years of age Ollivier appeared to be more of a pathologist than a clinician, but what he had modestly termed 'an outline' is, in fact, a book of historical importance. He drew attention to a neglected area of neurological study and undoubtedly stimulated interest and enquiry into the problems of recognizing diseases of the spinal cord. In his day, when methodical clinical examination of the nervous system scarcely existed, when so little was known of the structure of the cord, and when different modalities of sensation were not properly recognized, he could scarcely have done a better job.

Jean Cruveilhier (1791–1874). After graduating in Paris in 1816, and spending a few years in a chair of surgery at Montpellier and in clinical practice in his birthplace, Limoges, Cruveilhier was appointed to the Chair of Anatomy in Paris in 1825. This was followed in 1836 by that of Pathological Anatomy, a position he held until 1866. He was also a hospital physician and engaged in private practice.[56]

The first volume of his atlas was completed in 1835 and the second in 1842. One can only regret that it has never been translated into English. The name of Marshall Hall (1790–1857) appears on the subscribers list and in the text. He had studied in Paris and was a friend of Louis and other Paris physicians. He possibly knew Cruveilhier but it is doubtful, preoccupied as he was with his 'diastaltic nervous system', whether he would have been interested in providing an English translation. Yet it would have earned our gratitude and perhaps we might have been spared one or two of his own tiresome broadsides. One also wonders whether the gentlemen of the New Sydenham Society ever contemplated the venture. But what a task it would have presented.

Ollivier may have been dissatisfied with the way he had organized and presented his material, but compared with Cruveilhier, his efforts in this direction were admirable. Cruveilhier, of course, was dealing with the whole human body, but that, in itself, should have called for some systematic arrangement. Over the years, thirteen in all, he prepared his folios of case histories, bedside observations, 'reflexions', and illustrations, numbering them in 'livraisons' (parts), and subsequently issuing them in two volumes with the minimum of organization. Observations on the nervous system are not collected in one section but are distributed haphazardly throughout both volumes. 'Reflexions' are not necessarily restricted to questions arising from a particular case presentation; they are frequently discursive and sometimes positively erratic. Illustrations are not necessarily anywhere near the relevant text. For example, on page one of volume one, he deals with pyloric stenosis, referring to an illustrative plate that is located two-thirds of the way through the entire volume. I cannot refer to a page number because the pages are not numbered consecutively throughout each volume but thoughout each section, so that each new topic begins with page 1.

There is an index and also a table of contents in six parts, dealing with locomotion, digestion, respiration, circulation, the nervous system, and genito-urinary tract. Each part lists the subsections with references to the appropriate Livraisons and plates. I have no doubt that an owner, unlike a library reader, would be able to turn to a given topic, because over the years he would have already navigated the coast-line and explored the tributaries that would lead him to the interior and its prizes.

Volume one contains Livraisons 1–20, volume two, Livraisons 21 – 40. Cruveilhier said he divided his text into two parts; the first was descriptive 'pure and simple', the second, discussion. The coloured lithographs by Chazal, an anatomical illustrator of renown whose skill Cruveilhier acknowledges, have been universally praised. They are a delight, and some are of historical significance. But here again the reader has to bestir himself if he wishes to study them. A plate may contain a number of figures depicting a variety of lesions and he will have to seek out, in the text, the relevant legends and case-histories. It is a bit of a hunt, but amply rewarding. As Charcot once said, the *Atlas* should be '... consulted by all who desire to avoid the disappointment of making second-hand discoveries in morbid anatomy'.[57]

Lasègue[58] said of Cruveilhier's macroscopic studies that 'what he saw, he saw well, and what he said, he knew'; admitting that books so constructed do not readily become classical treatises. But, if it is a jumbled masterpiece it remains a treasure chest of neurology. In a recent evaluation, Flamm[59] concluded that although it is famous for its fine illustrations of morbid lesions of the nervous system, including original ones such as those of multiple sclerosis, auditory neurinoma, intracranial epidermoid, intracranial and spinal meningiomas, Cruveilhier's clinical observations have not been sufficiently appreciated. Flamm aptly remarked that the fame achieved at the Salpêtrière later in the century was soundly based on Cruveilhier's work. Though primarily an atlas it excels in the detailed presentation of its basic material, in the enlivening discussions, and in the appreciation of the factors involved in the task of correlating symptoms, signs, and lesions. Cruveilhier wrote that

> ... the more I study visceral lesions, the more I am convinced that, other things being equal, a particular lesion always has the same effect, manifested by the same symptoms, differences being determined by factors which have escaped observation (Liv. 32, Pl. 1 and 2).

In dealing with the nervous system he repeatedly stressed that there were consequences which resulted from two types of morbid process; destruction of nervous tissue and compression of nervous tissue, in the spinal cord as well as in the brain.

One neuropathologist[60] has said that Cruveilhier did not have 'quite the same feeling for careful clinico-pathological correlation as had the Italian masters'. To the present writer, however, he was, in the field of neurology, the prince of these physician-pathologists. He was clearly a very experienced clinician with remarkable insight. This would have been more apparent if his atlas had been better organized. An American doctor[61] who worked for him in his private dissecting room at l'École Pratique, described how impressed he was when Cruveilhier's assistants would call, 'bringing what they deemed very rare specimens of pathology'. Cruveilhier could give them 'a full account of the case and almost the symptoms the patient must have presented'.

Soury[62] has described how at the Salpêtrière, in the eighteen-twenties, it was generally taught that the grey cortex was the seat of the intellect and that the white matter was concerned with voluntary motion. In mental disorders the softening was in the cortex; when there was paralysis, it was in the central white matter. When only one arm was paralysed the lesion was to be found in or near the thalamus; when only a leg, in the corpus striatum.

Cruveilhier's training and the development of his concepts concerning the nature of tissue changes, inflammation, phlebitis, and cancer were, understandably, erroneous and afforded him no assistance in the field of neuropathology. But, theories aside, his interpretative endeavours were vigorous and perceptive, although he failed to appreciate the importance of some of the clues that were appearing concerning the function of the nervous system. On the one hand, he rejected the concept of cerebral localization, as suggested by recent studies on the frontal lobes and the cerebellum, but he accepted that of distinctive functions for the motor and sensory roots of the spinal nerves. Acceptance of the principle of the localization of cerebral function implied to Cruveilhier and others that they were endorsing the notions of Gall's cranioscopy. The existence of a speech centre he could not support from his own findings.

MALADIES DU CERVEAU (Tumeurs Cancéreuses des Méninges)

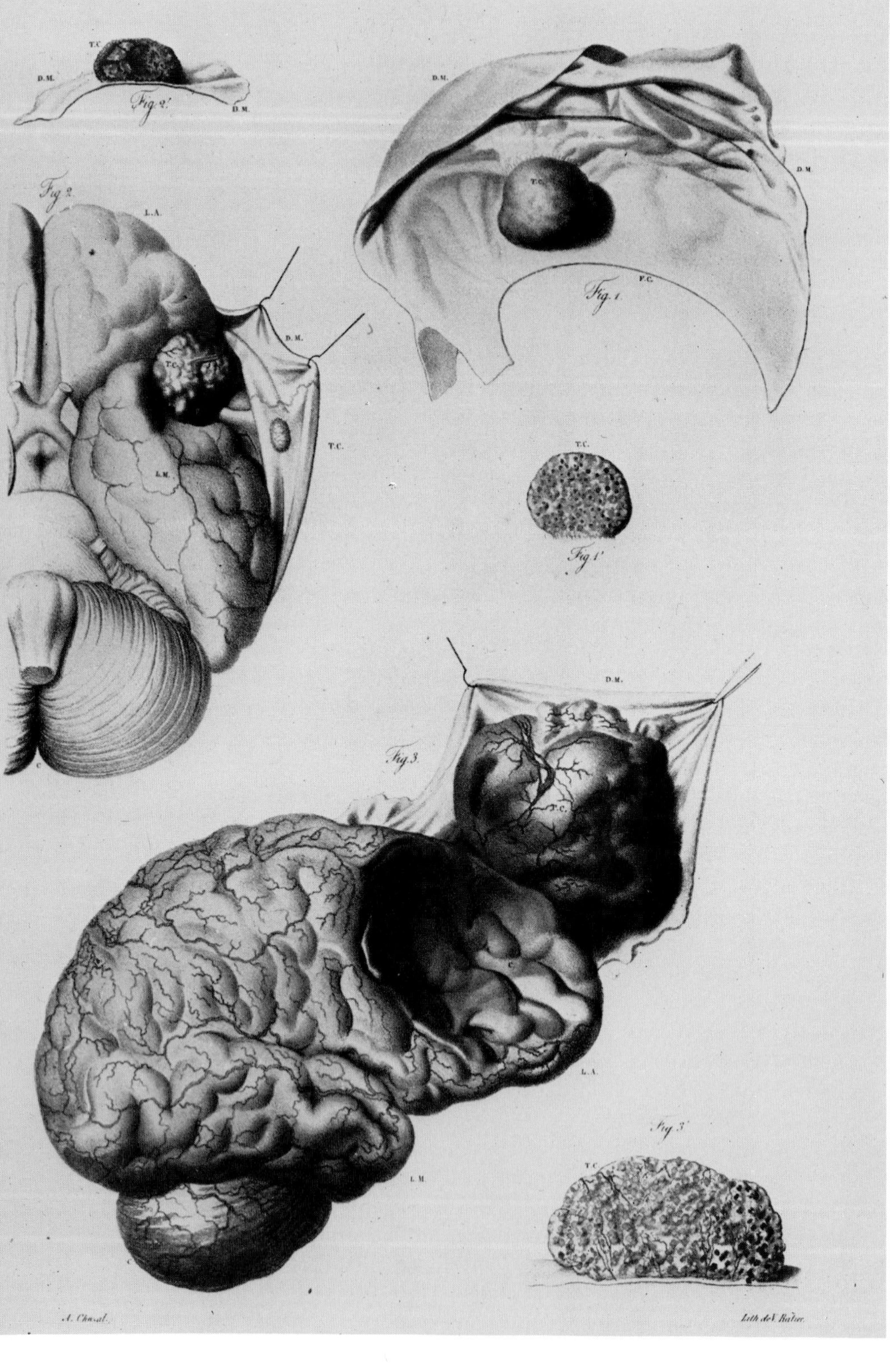

A. Chazal. Lith de V. Ratier.

In accepting Magendie, but not Flourens, there were probably many influences at work. Spinal roots were lowly items in the hierarchy of nervous doctrine. The thought of localization of function in a spinal nerve may have found easier acceptance because it did not upset the hallowed concept of the brain as a common sensorium. It was the threat to the seat of the soul, as much as anything else, which provoked such a reaction to Gall's doctrine of faculties within the brain.

With regard to the cerebellum, Cruveilhier was similarly unimpressed by Gall's theory that it was concerned with sexual function. But, as Flamm has pointed out, neither did he see any evidence to associate it with the function of coordination of voluntary motion, as Flourens had proposed in 1823. This is curious as there are several cases in his atlas in which cerebellar ataxia must have been present. His historical case of the auditory neurinoma (Fig. 74) was under his care for the last three months of her life, but ataxia goes unmentioned. Neither is it mentioned in other cases in which it was probably present, as in the cerebellar tuberculomas and basal meningiomas.

In a case of congenital absence of the cerebellum in a child of eleven years there were only defective speech and subnormal intelligence (Liv. 15, Pl. 5). Possibly this may have influenced his opinion that cerebellar lesions were not characterized by any particular features (Liv. 8, Pl. 1, 2, 3).

Intracranial tumours. Of particular interest are Cruveilhier's clinical and pathological accounts of cases of intracranial tumour – especially the meningiomas, which he called 'Tumeurs fongueuses' or 'Tumeurs cancereuses des meninges'. There is a case history with autopsy of a frontal meningioma (Fig. 72) and of a basal epidermoid tumour (Fig. 73). Cushing[63, 64] noted how Cruveilhier observed the common sites of meningiomas, and that occupied by an auditory neurinoma. In Plate 3 of Livraison 8 there are illustrations of a parasagittal meningioma and an olfactory groove meningioma. In Plate 2 (Fig. 72) there is a small convexity meningioma, a large frontal meningioma, and another in a Sylvian fissure. The right frontal meningioma was that of a schoolmistress, aged 45, with headache and failing intellect, mental apathy, weakness of left lower limb, and occasional urinary incontinence. 'She asked nothing ... refused nothing ... replying slowly to all questions ... smiling with an air of satisfaction.' There was drooping of the left corner of the mouth. Cruveilhier diagnosed a tumour on the right side of the base. He thought that the apathy resulted from the compression of the frontal convolutions disclosed at autopsy.

In considering the problem of diagnosis of tumours of the brain (Liv. 8, pp. 1–11) Cruveilhier was aware how slow compression of a hemisphere could be relatively symptomless for a long time and cited the case of a girl of eighteen who died two hours after admission to hospital (see Fig. 73). The brain 'accustomed itself' and there was a 'gradual march' of symptoms, so much in contrast to that which occurred in apoplexy. Moreover, similar lesions could have different effects, and smaller tumours might be more paralysing than larger ones. A tumour of two inches diameter might give rise to a hemiplegia, whereas one twice that size might have less effect. He also appreciated that the effects of compression were transmitted, across and

FIG. 72. *Fig. 1* (top right): Small convexity meningioma found in a man on whom Dupuytren had operated for bladder stone. *Fig. 2* (top left): Sylvian fissure meningioma; no clinical data. *Fig. 3* (bottom): Right frontal meningioma. (After Cruveilhier,[31] Liv. 8, Pl. 2.)

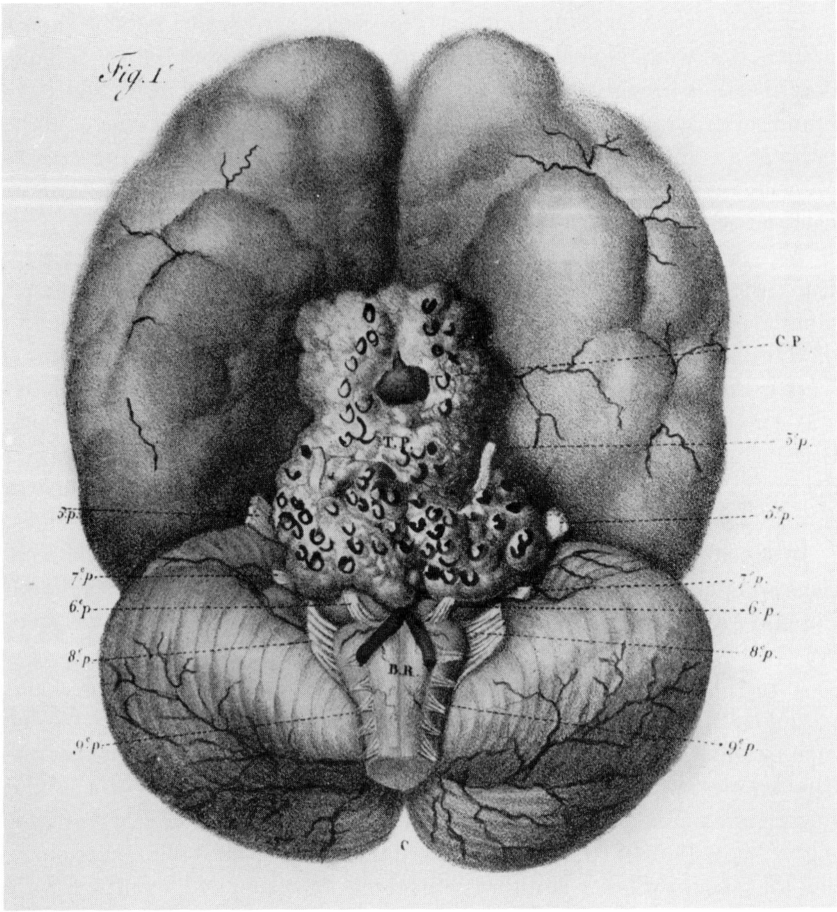

FIG. 73. Intracranial epidermoid tumour in a girl of eighteen who died two hours after admission to hospital. (After Cruveilhier,[31] Liv. 2, Pl. 6, Fig. 1.)

obliquely, to the opposite hemisphere.

There is an illustration (Liv. 25, Pl. 3, Figs. 3 and 3[1]) of gross hypertrophy of the pons, 'an extraordinary deformation'. There are no clinical data. In illustrating an aneurysm of a vertebral artery (Liv. 28, Pl. 3, Fig. 2) Cruveilhier wondered whether it would be possible to diagnose such a lesion; it would compress the medulla or pons.

Auditory neurinoma (Liv. 26, Pl. 2). A twenty-six-year-old female came under his care for the last three months of her life. She was well until nineteen, when she began to suffer from headaches and lost her hearing in the left ear; at twenty there was impairment of vision in the right eye; at twenty-one, involuntary twitching of the left cheek. Vision deteriorated so that she could not walk normally and eventually she became blind. For two years her condition was unchanged; although blind she was able to take long walks with her parents. In her last year the convulsive movements of the left side of her face grew stronger and more frequent; they spread beyond her face and were often accompanied by spasms of rigidity of the upper limbs. There was also a tingling sensation in the left cheek and increasing headache. When she came to Cruveilhier her mental faculties were well

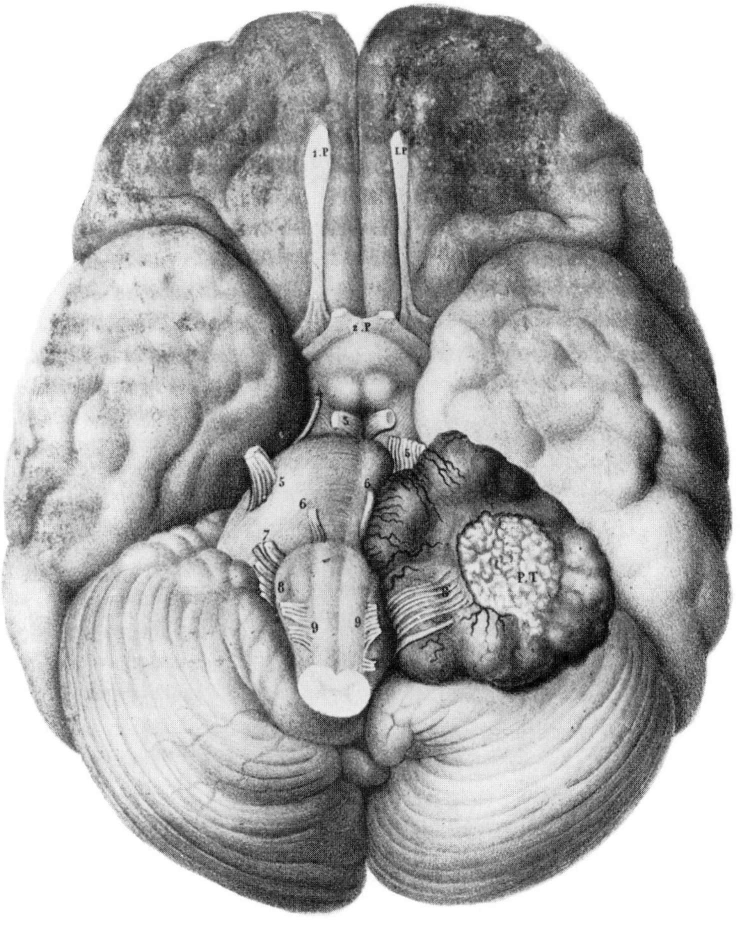

FIG. 74. Left auditory neurinoma in a twenty-six-year-old female under Cruveilhier's care for the last three months of her life. Onset with deafness on left side at nineteen. (After Cruveilhier,[31] Liv. 26, Pl. 2.)

preserved, there was no paralysis and in hospital 'she got up every day' except during her last month. She started to vomit fifteen days before her death. Cruveilhier thought she had a meningeal tumour which was compressing her brain, or one growing within its substance. He thought it was situated at the base.

At autopsy (Fig. 74) he found a large tumour in the left posterior fossa, compressing the brain stem and cerebellum, with bilateral optic atrophy and involvement of the fifth, sixth, seventh, eighth, ninth, tenth, and eleventh cranial nerves on that side. The fibrous tumour was adherent to the posterior surface of the left petrous bone and had eroded the internal auditory meatus.

Flamm has remarked on the lack of any account of ataxia in this case.[59] Although blind it is said she could walk, and in her last months in hospital she left her bed daily. Was this a genuine failure of observation, masked perhaps by the disability of blindness, or was it in any way related to his opinion that the cerebellum had no particular function? We shall never know.

Apoplexy and softening. Cruveilhier lived long enough to witness the general acceptance of Virchow's concepts of embolism and inflammation. His own views on the nature of inflammation, with its seat in the capillary bed, itself a part of the venous system, formed a poor basis for the study of softening, haemorrhage, and their relationship; not to mention their postulated link with the inflammatory process. He frequently mentions 'capillary apoplexy', in the brain and spinal cord, but recognized there were differences between red and white areas of softening. He tended to associate softening with mental change, and haemorrhage with paralysis, but he appreciated that the location and speed of development of a lesion influenced the outcome.

When discussing the case of a man of fifty-two who had been struck down unconscious and hemiplegic by a haemorrhage which had burst into a lateral ventricle he wrote, emphasizing in italics, '*Il y a une différence énorme entre une apoplexie avec perte de connaissance au moment de l'attaque et une apoplexie sans perte de connaissance*' (Liv. 5, p. 2). In pontine apoplexy paralysis tended to be complete but it was not always fatal for he had noted scars of old lesions there (Liv. 21, Pl. 5). He wondered whether the pons contained the seat of articulation as speech was so consistently affected, but it was unlikely as it was affected by many lesions – in the corpus striatum, the thalamus, and even the posterior portion of a cerebral hemisphere (Liv. 21, Pl. 5; Liv. 33, Pl. 2, pp. 1 and 2). He appreciated that a small lesion, in a crucial location, could be more devastating than some larger ones. Consciousness, power, and sensation could be separately affected in apoplexy and indeed 'Une apoplexie dix fois moindre soit dans le corps strie, soit dans la couche optique aurait entraine une paralysie complete du mouvement et peut-être du sentiment' (Liv. 5, p. 4).

Disorders of the spinal cord. When he came to discuss paraplegia (Liv. 32) Cruveilhier paid tribute to Ollivier for his excellent work but he did not think that progress in this field need be retarded by such factors as the time required or the difficulties to be faced in removing the spinal cord; 'nothing will resist the zeal of the hospital doctors and their pupils'. Paraplegia resulted from four types of lesion (Liv. 35, pp. 3 and 5): (1) alteration within the cord itself; (2) by compression; (3) by inflammation of the spinal arachnoid; (4) by immobility and joint stiffness, which produced a pseudoparaplegia.

When a paraplegia was painful it was likely to be due to compression; disease of the cord itself was usually painless (Liv. 35, p. 5). But one type tended to merge into the other. In contrast to hemiplegia, both motor and sensory loss were usually found. Clinical differentiation of the type of paraplegia was of obvious importance because of the possibility of relief of compressing lesions, as suggested by Ollivier.

The variable degree of loss of motor and sensory function was appreciated and, like Ollivier, attributed to the respective involvement of the anterior and posterior halves of the cord. No precise distributions of sensory loss are described; reference is usually made to a limb or limbs, upper and lower, and to the trunk. It was understood that there might be sensory loss in one leg and motor loss in the other. But whereas Ollivier left no actual account of sensory testing, Cruveilhier clearly realized that it was important. It is true that Ollivier occasionally mentioned feelings of heat and cold in a paralysed limb, and in the case of syringomyelia he specifically mentioned that temperature appreciation was retained as well as that of light touch. But Cruveilhier describes the tests of pinching ('pincement'), pricking with a pin ('piqûre avec une epingle'), tickling ('chatouillement'), and responses to cold and warmth. In one case he actually mentioned that he had omitted to test for temperature appreciation (Liv. 37, Pl. 5). He noted that pin-prick or tickling might provoke no involuntary retraction of a limb; even tickling the sole of the feet might elicit no motor response, unless it was roughly stroked. In the upper limbs of a paraplegic patient he mentioned that although sensory impairment was incomplete the patient could not handle a large object such as a bottle correctly, unless aided by vision; yet strong pinching was painless.

In general, formication was the commonest form of sensory disturbance, tending to precede other manifestations but subsiding when tactile sensibility was abolished. Girdle sensations are mentioned ('corset qui la gêne') and also ice-cold feelings in the feet ('entoures de glace').

He noted that sensory loss in a limb was not always distributed uniformly; it could be retained below the knee, and lost over the thigh. Tactile appreciation could be delayed for 15, 20, or 30 seconds (Liv. 38, p. 9). Or pin-prick could go unfelt, unless repeated three or four times. Sensory loss was affected in different ways. A patient might feel a strong pinch, but not the touch of a feather. Sensibility of the sole of the foot was often the last to be affected. In cord compression, appreciation of temperature was usually retained for some time. Using a 'pewter infusion pot' one often finds a sharper response to cold than to warmth (Liv. 38, p. 9).

He mentioned (Liv. 35, p. 4) the case of a paraplegic 'English lady, accused of malingering', who had lost sensation in both legs and in her right arm. 'I submitted her to tests which, even had she possessed the steadfastness of Porsena himself', she could not have sustained her stand. He was able to certify that she was a 'genuine paraplegic'.

Multiple sclerosis (Vol. 2; Liv. 32, Pl. 2, pp. 19–24; Liv. 38, Pl. 5, pp. 1–4). Cruveilhier was intrigued by strange cases of paraplegia in which at autopsy he found islands of 'grey degeneration or transformation' scattered throughout the spinal cord, brain stem, cerebellum, and sometimes the cerebrum. He was puzzled as to the nature of the indurations – 'traces of lost substance, spontaneous softening, a particular type of scarring . . . or a form of disseminated cancerous degeneration?'. In some of his cases the degeneration was more or less confined to the posterior columns; in others the pyramidal pathways were also affected. He was mainly interested in correlating the degree of involvement of sensation and movement with lesions of the posterior and anterior columns of the cord.

A fifty-four-year-old embroiderer had spent ten years in the Salpêtrière, unable to leave her bed. 'She had been seen by all the doctors of the Salpêtrière' during this time. Her illness began at 37 with numbness, first of the left, and then of the right, foot and leg. She frequently fell in the street,

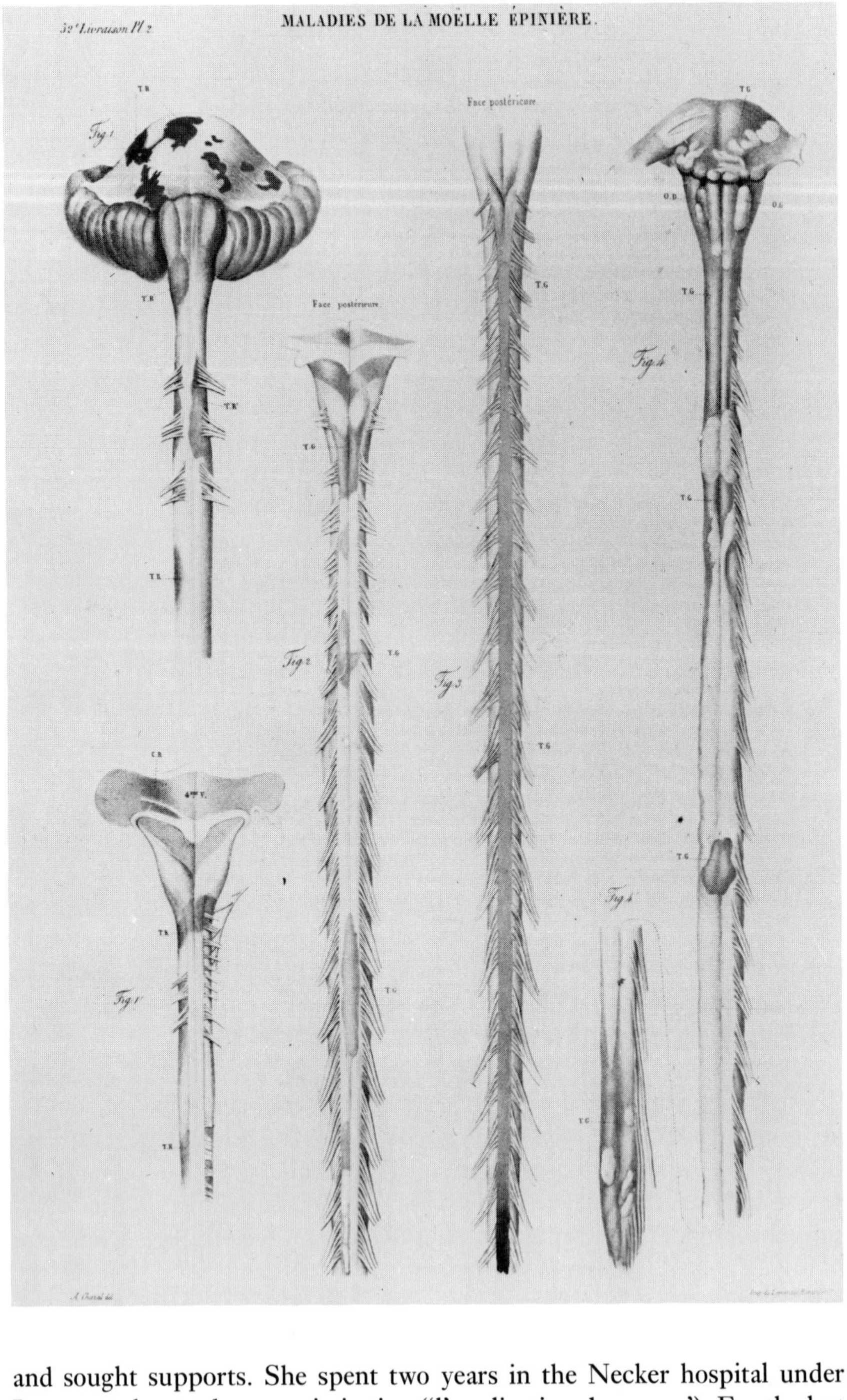

FIG. 75. 'Grey degeneration of brain stem and spinal cord.' *Fig. 1* (left): Islands of 'reddish-grey' hue in pons, cerebellar peduncles and cord. *Fig. 2* (left centre): 'Disseminated' grey lesions in another case. *Fig. 3* (right centre): Degeneration of the posterior columns; disordered gait, facial grimacing, sensory loss in hands which caused clumsiness. *Fig. 4* (right): Multiple lesions in a patient (37 years old) who died of phthisis. Paraplegia for 6 years. (After Cruveilhier,[31] Liv. 32, Pl. 2.)

and sought supports. She spent two years in the Necker hospital under Laennec who used counterirritation ('l'application de moxas'). For the last three years of her life her condition remained stationary. Her special senses were not affected but speech was weak, interrupted and accompanied by facial grimacing. Voluntary movements of her limbs were disordered and resembled those of chorea, 'as if there was a struggle between voluntary and

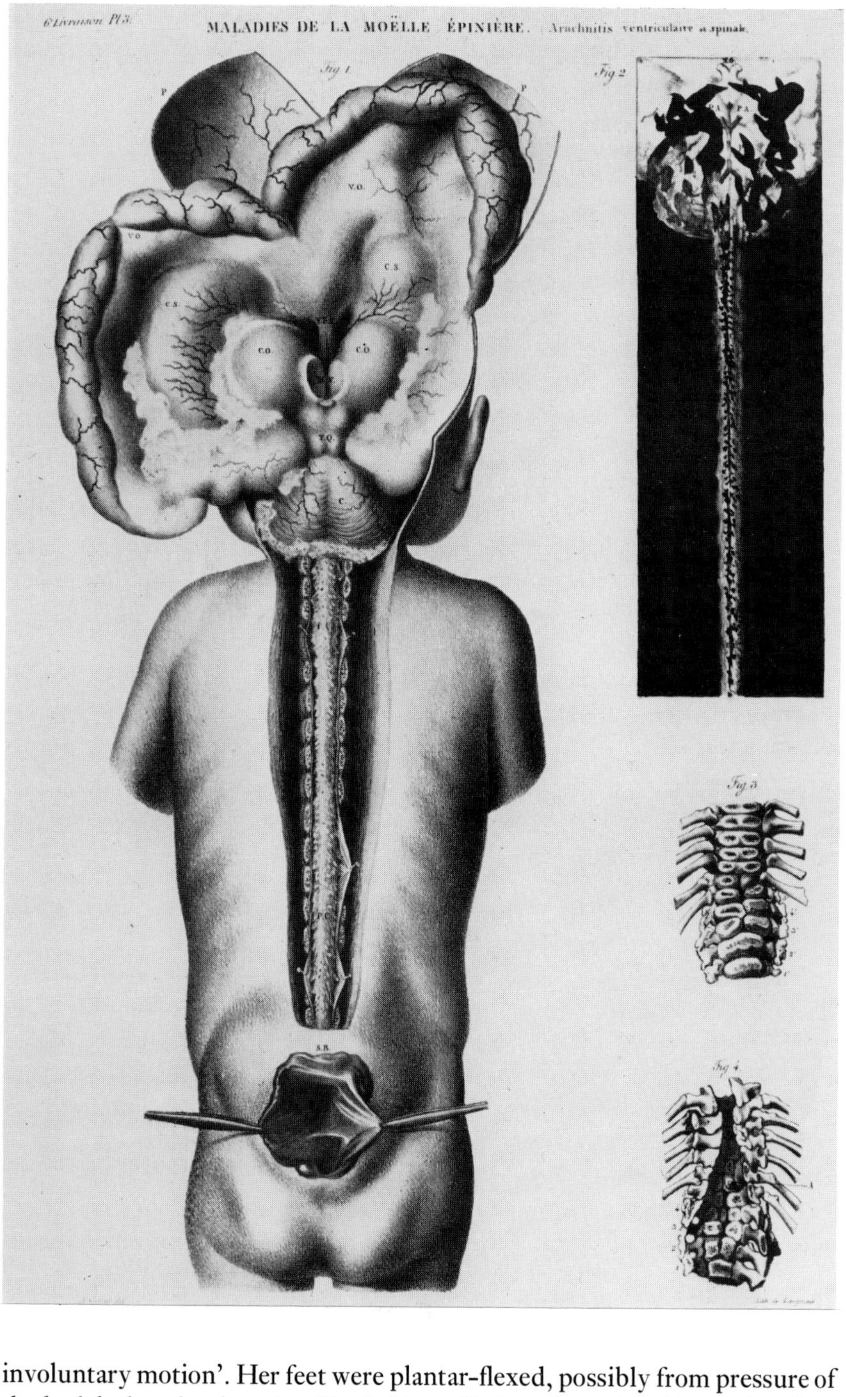

FIG. 76. Spina bifida. *Figs. 1, 2*: Spinal and ventricular meningitis in a two-week-old infant with a meningomyelocele and hydrocephalus; posterior and anterior views. V.O., lateral ventricles; C.S., corpus striatum; C.O., optic thalamus; P.A., cerebral peduncles; P, pons.) *Figs. 3, 4*: Another case of meningomyelocele in which there was diastematomyelia and the Arnold–Chiari malformation. Anterior view of dorso-lumbar spine *Fig. 3*; posterior view *Fig. 4*, showing cone-shaped bony projection from twelfth dorsal veretebra (A). (After Cruveilhier,[31] Liv. 6, Pl. 3.)

involuntary motion'. Her feet were plantar-flexed, possibly from pressure of the bedclothes, he thought. She fed herself clumsily and, with much effort, managed to take her snuff. Small things fell from her hands unknowingly. Involuntary movements of her lower limbs occurred when she was moved. At autopsy (Fig. 75), apart from some softening of the left occipital convolutions, the hemispheres, the cerebellum, and the medulla were normal. The spinal cord was atrophic and there was extensive degeneration of the posterior columns up to the level of the cerebellum. The anterior and lateral columns were not affected.

In another case in which there was blindness with paraplegia, Cruveilhier found atrophy in the optic nerves, chiasm, tracts, and the lateral geniculate bodies. Another proved to have well demarcated 'plaques' in all the columns of the cord, medulla, pons, cerebellar peduncles, optic thalami, and corpus callosum. In this case, he had noted impairment of vision, emotional lability (smiling, blushing, laughing, crying), grimacing, and irregular movements; the latter frightened her when she sat on her commode.

Although, in some of his cases, there were periods in which disability was said to be stationary, there are none in which acute episodes were followed by clear remissions and relapses as in Ollivier's case (p. 204).

Spina bifida (Liv. 6, Pl. 3) There are many examples of spina bifida and hydrocephalus, usually with evidence of infection of the sac and meningitis. In a case of meningomyelocele (Fig. 76) he noted the spread of the infection from the spinal subarachnoid space to the fourth, the third, and the extremely dilated lateral ventricles. The fourth ventricle 'communicated by a large opening, so well described by M. Magendie, with the subarachnoid tissue of the spinal cord'.

In a second case of meningomyelocele (Fig. 76), as pointed out by Flamm,[59] there is a description of the Arnold-Chiari malformation and of diastematomyelia.

At the level of the tumour, the spinal cord is divided into two perfectly distinct lateral cords; each cord giving off nerves with their double roots. A bony projection (A) in the form of a cone-shaped spine, arises from the posterior surface of the body of the twelfth dorsal vertebra, establishing the line of demarcation. Above the tumour the two cords are reunited; but they are remarkable for the complete absence of grey matter . . . (p. 2)

. . . the upper part of the considerably dilated cervical region, contained both the medulla oblongata and the corresponding part of the cerebellum which was elongated and covered the fourth ventricle, itself enlarged and elongated. (p. 2)

Cruveilhier also referred to two other cases of hydrocephalus in which a M. Sestier had observed this type of malformation of the hind-brain. All this more than fifty years before Chiari and Arnold described their cases in the eighteen-nineties.

Lastly, in disorders of the spinal cord, Cruveilhier describes and illustrates a case of spinal apoplexy (Fig. 77), one of spinal meningioma (Fig. 78), and an example of spontaneous atlanto-axial subluxation (Fig. 79).

Cruveilhier's description of degeneration of the anterior spinal nerve roots in progressive muscular atrophy is not to be found in his atlas. It came later, in 1852.[65] His patient, a thirty-two-year-old juggler, first noticed clumsiness of his right hand; he had difficulty playing his cornet and taking his handkerchief out of his pocket. The weakness spread to both upper limbs and affected speech, and swallowing. Cruveilhier noted that sensation was normal, the atrophied muscles fibrillated, and that intellect was unimpaired. In two patients he had found nothing wrong in the nervous system – Aran

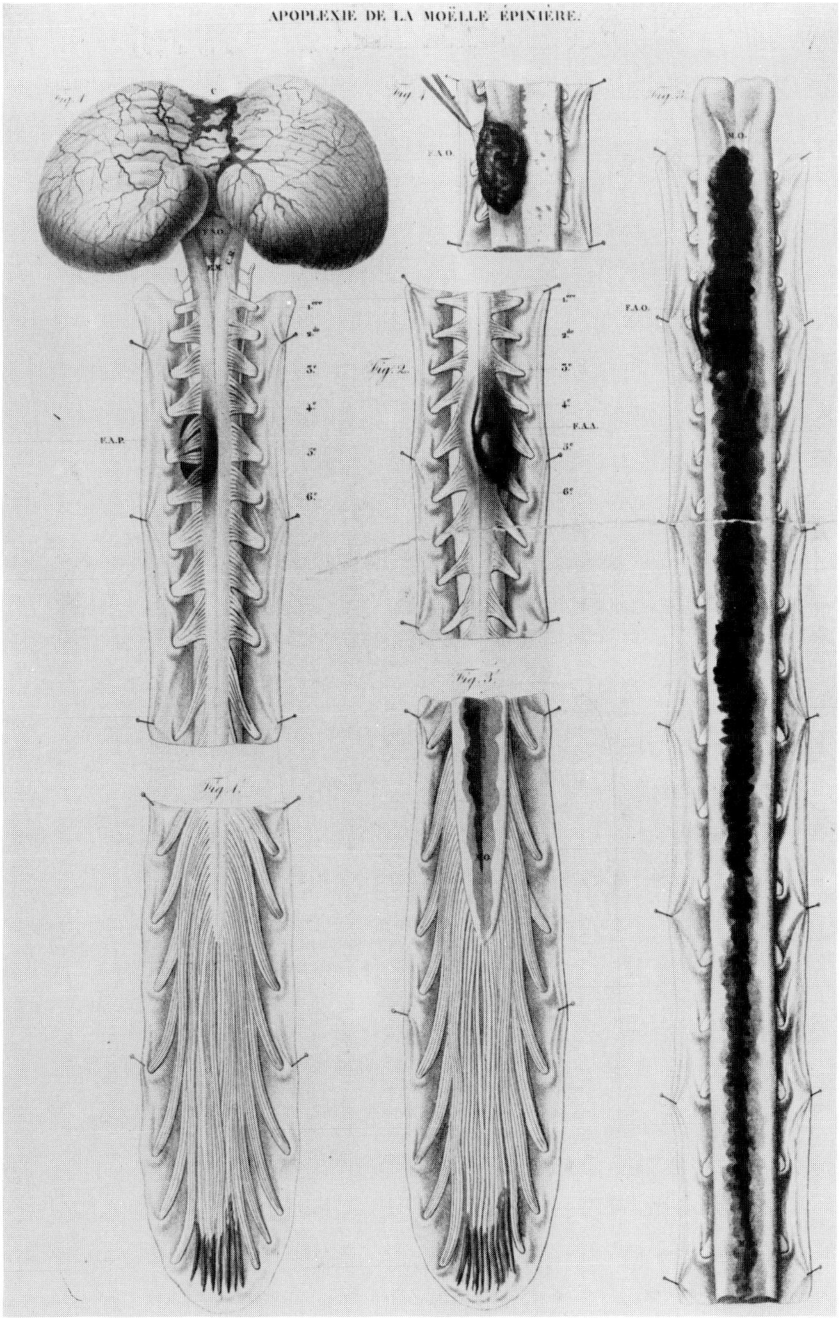

FIG. 77. Spinal apoplexy. Female student of surgery, 36 years old. Five years previously suffered an attack of severe pain in neck and left arm. A second attack began five weeks before her death. Neck rigid and tilted; left arm paralysed. Autopsy; purplish, almond-sized tumour at C. 4, 5, 6 on left side, compressing roots. *Fig. 1* (left): anterior view. *Fig. 2* (centre): posterior view. (After Cruveilhier,[31] Liv. 3, Pl. 6.)

and Duchenne, whom he mentioned, had thought the disease was primarily of muscles. But in his third patient Cruveilhier recorded that the anterior spinal nerve roots, especially in the cervical segments, were less than one-quarter to one-fifth the size of the posterior roots. It was a new species of paralysis but he did not attribute the root atrophy to degeneration of the grey matter. It was 'independent of any appreciable lesion in the spinal cord

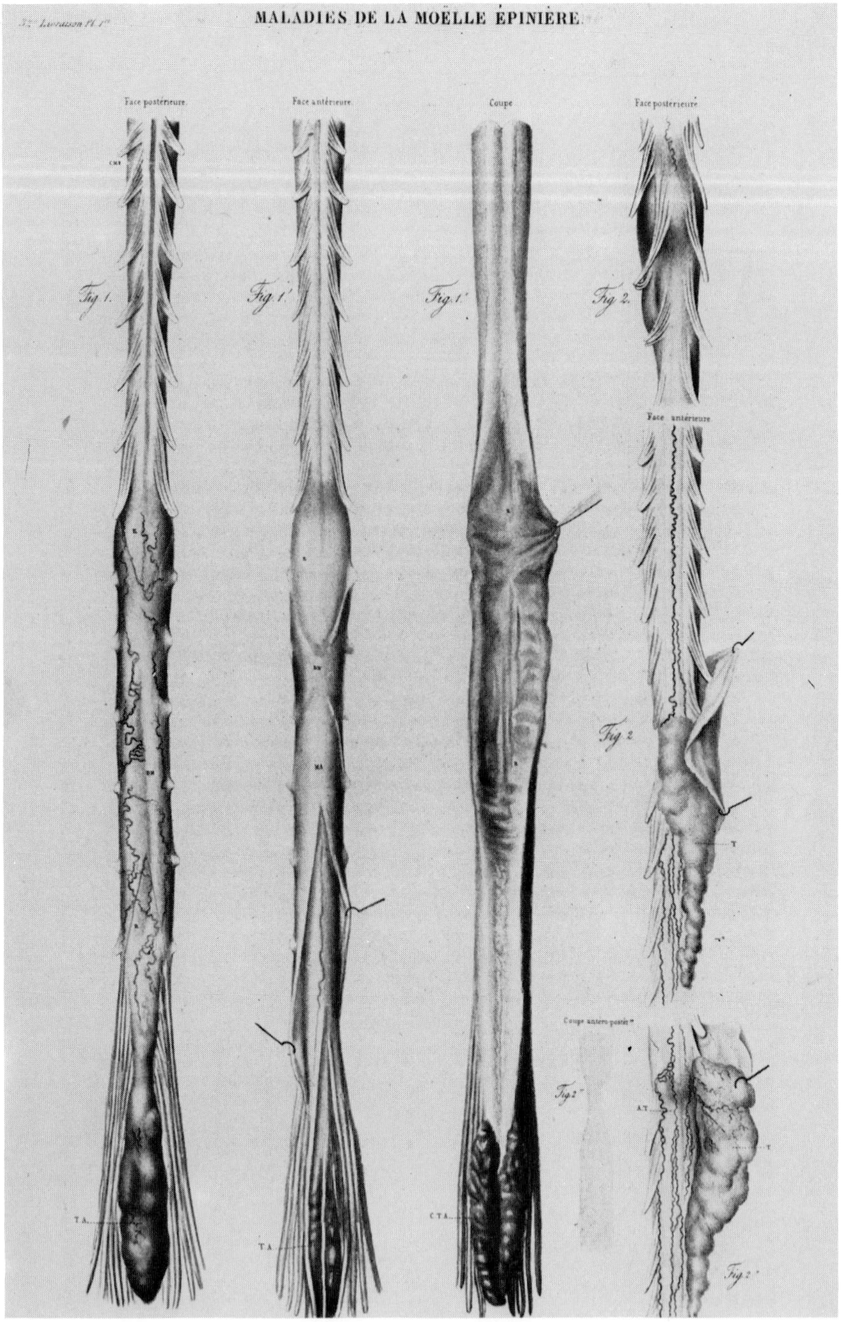

FIG. 78. *Figs. 1, 1′, 1″*: Cauda equina tumour. *Fig. 2*: Spinal cord meningioma. A sixty-year-old female knocked down by a carriage six years previously. Two years later gradual onset of paraplegia. Sensory and sphincter functions said to have been normal. Tumour compressed anterior surface of cord opposite third dorsal vertebra. Cruveilhier thought this confirmed views of Bell and Magendie that the motor pathways were located anteriorly. (After Cruveilhier,[31] Liv. 32, Pl. 1.)

. . .'. The primary lesion in the anterior horns was identified by Luys in 1860,[66] one of his histological achievements.

Cruveilhier's biographer, Delhoume, wrote eloquently about his appearance and character. He was a handsome, well-proportioned man with a smiling face and an equable temperament. 'He combined within himself

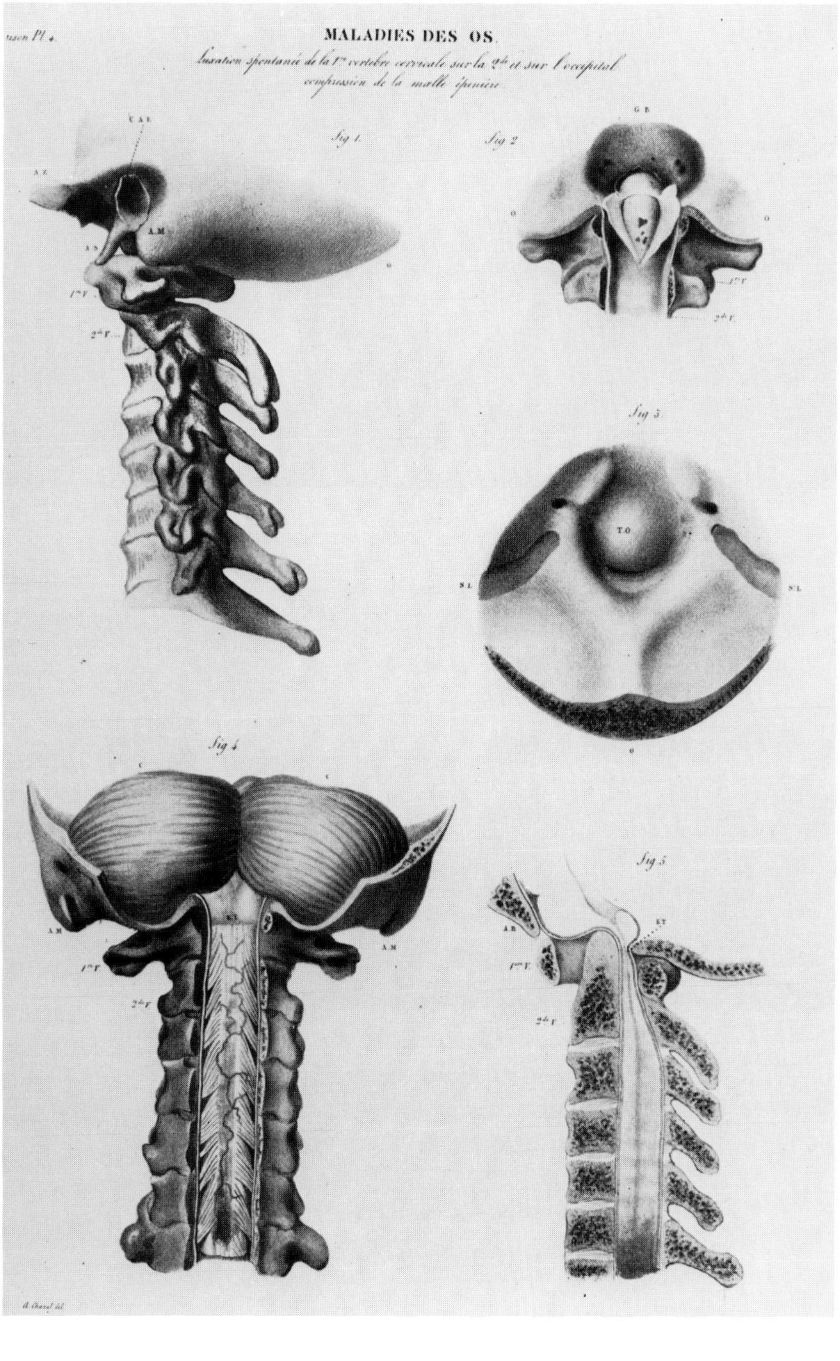

FIG. 79. 'Spontaneous luxation of first cervical vertebra.' A sixty-eight-year-old female costermonger who suddenly became hemiplegic six months previously. *Fig. 1* (top left): Atlanto-axial dislocation. *Fig. 2* (top right): Posterior surface of odontoid laid bare by sectioning of diseased annular ligament. *Fig. 3* (centre right): Constriction of foramen magnum, now semi-lunar shaped. *Fig. 4* (bottom left): Posterior view. *Fig. 5* (bottom right): Lateral view to show the degree of thinning of the spinal cord. (After Cruveilhier,[31] Liv. 25, Pl. 4.)

three qualities essential in a good doctor; knowledge, good sense, and kindness; he was an excellent clinician, with a successful practice in a distinguished society. His meticulous notes, written each day, reveal a high-principled professional conscience.'[56]

Looking back, Cruveilhier can be judged a fortunate man. Gifted

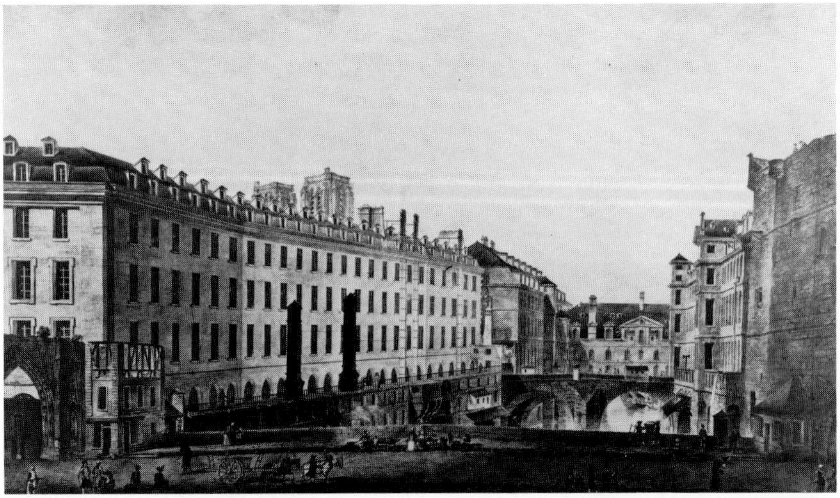

FIG. 80. The old Hôtel Dieu with the two square towers of Notre Dame above it (before the erection of the steeple). The hospital was burned down in 1772, rebuilt, and then demolished in 1877. The new Hôtel Dieu still faces the Place Notre Dame. (Courtesy of the Musée de l'Histoire de la Médecine, l'École de Médecine, Paris.)

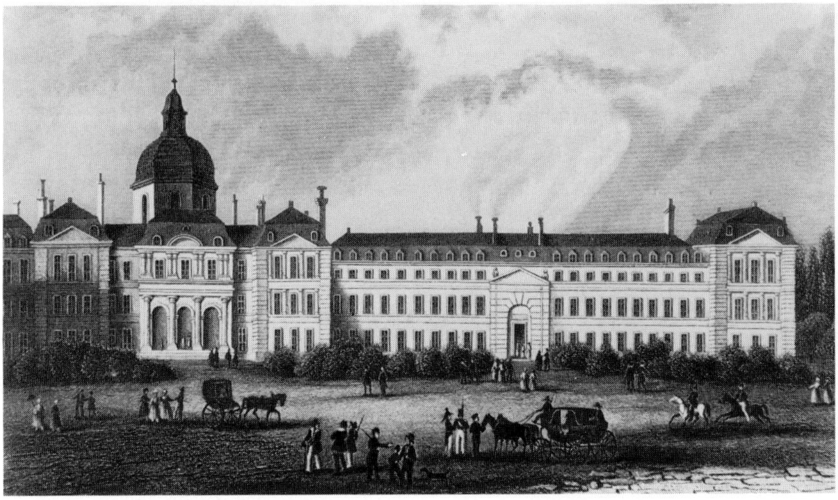

FIG. 81. The Salpêtrière in the eighteenth century. It was originally opened in 1656 as 'Hôpital General', but only for female paupers and incurables. (Courtesy of the Musée de l'Histoire de la Médicine, l'École de Médecine, Paris.)

physically and mentally, popular and successful, a university professor for thirty years in a centre unexcelled in its day, he enjoyed a long and happy life unmarred by dispute. His bequest to neurology was a rich one.

THE PHYSICIAN-PHYSIOLOGISTS 1800–1850

'My object is not to publish this, but to lecture it – to lecture to my friends – to lecture to Sir Jos. Banks' coterie, to make the town ring with it . . .'.[67] So wrote Charles Bell (1774–1842) in December 1807, in a letter to a brother, about 'My new Anatomy of the Brain ... the only new thing that has appeared in anatomy since the days of Hunter; and, if I make it out, as interesting as the circulation . . .'. Then thirty-three years of age, an Edinburgh graduate, Bell had been in London for three years, teaching anatomy. He was a good teacher, and knew it, saying that he could put his notes for a lecture on a thumb nail. Dr James Rush, son of Dr Benjamin Rush of Philadelphia, said of Bell,

Of this gentleman I thought more highly than any of the medical profession whose lectures I attended in Britain. He lectured unconnected with any Institution and his class was about eighteen!! – whilst many asses in place at the several hospitals had benches to overflowing. it pleas'd me to leave the mob and go to him.[68]

Bell's grandiose phrases about his project, with his allusion to Harvey (with whom he was later compared), were no passing fancies. In a later letter[69] he implied that he might be a 'genius', and in March 1810 he wrote that his anatomy of the brain was going to be based 'on facts the most important that have been discovered in the history of science . . . if I can but

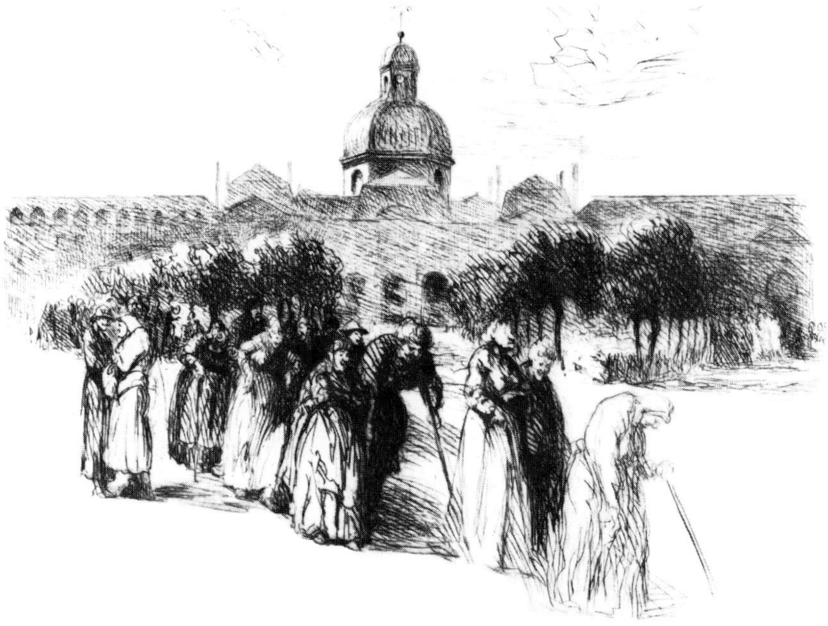

FIG. 82. Female inmates of the Salpêtrière. (Courtesy of the Assistance Publique, Paris.')

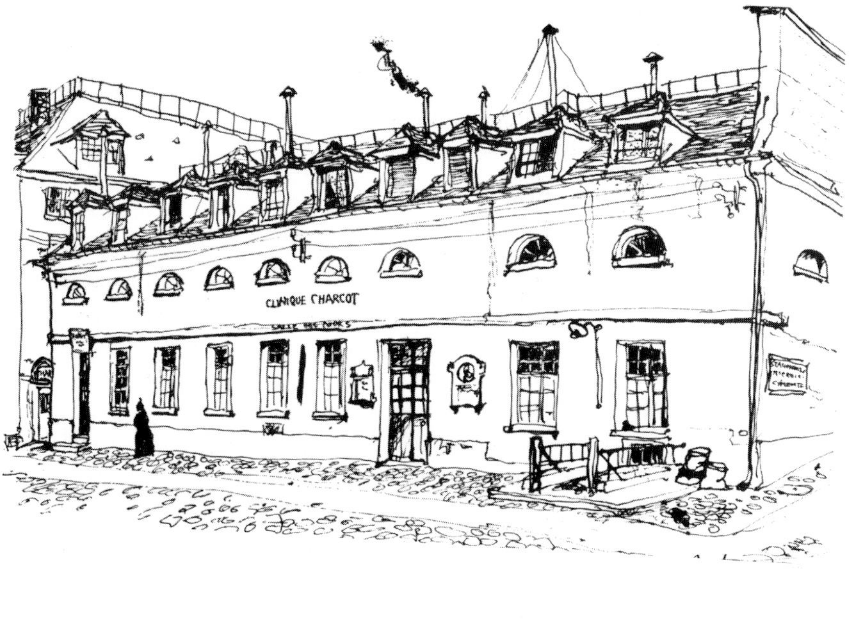

FIG. 83. The Clinique Charcot, by Zurkinden, in the Salpêtrière. Demolished in the 1950s (Courtesy of the Assistance Publique, Paris.)

sustain them by repeated experiments, I am made, and a real gratification ensured for a large portion of my existence'.[70]

Do we not scent here something more than fervent enthusiasm, perhaps an omen of things to come – a perilous degree of covert ambition and conceit? His *Idea of a new anatomy of the brain*[71] was privately printed, undated, in 1811, and circulated to a hundred of his friends, for their observations. None replied in writing.[72] Why, if he thought his *Idea* so momentous, did he not publish it? But he *never* did. Even that strange eccentric Edinburgh graduate, Alexander Walker (1779–1842), with his taste for anonymity, chose to publish his *New anatomy and physiology of the brain* (1809) in a scientific journal.[73] He was the first to suggest that one spinal nerve root was sensory and the other motor, but assigned the functions incorrectly. Bell, however, published nothing in a scientific journal until 1821. Following Magendie's articles in 1822 and 1823, as is now well known, Bell's reactions, over the years, became increasingly strange. He abused Magendie, accusing him of stealing his wares, and denounced vivisection, fraudulently altering portions of his original pamphlet and incorporating selected excerpts in new publications to sustain his argument. He was moderately successful.

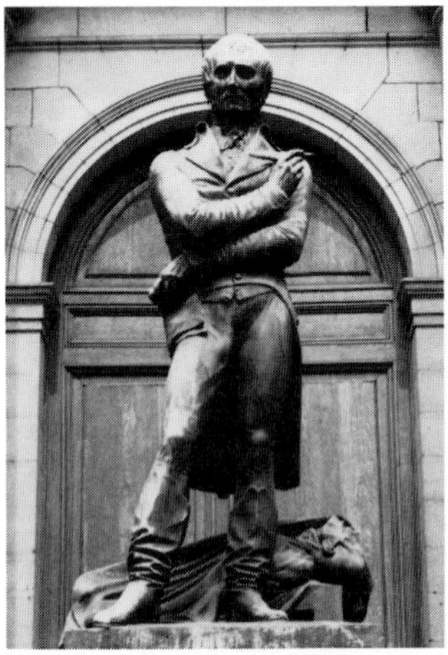

FIG. 84. The statue of Bichat (1771–1802) which stands in the entrance of l'École de Médecine, Paris. (Photograph by the author.)

When Sherrington came to write on the nervous system in Schafer's textbook of physiology in 1900, he entitled the sections on the spinal nerve roots, with sparkling brevity, 'The Way In' and 'The Way Out'.[74] Recently, Cranefield[75] has used these titles for his book on the Bell–Magendie controversy. With the reproduction of the facsimiles of the major original articles by the adversaries, excerpts from many sources, and a most detailed and comprehensive analysis of all the evidence, Cranefield's book must be the most scholarly account ever published of an historical medical controversy. On the known data, the priority question can be adjudicated without difficulty. Bell proved only that stimulation of the anterior spinal roots provoked movements and that section of the posterior roots did not. But it is equally obvious that his foremost concern was not the spinal roots but the brain. His *Idea* was about its structure and function. And over the horizon there appeared indications of the two developments which dominated neurological thought for many decades. These were the localizations of function in the brain and in the spinal cord.

'The Way in' and 'The Way Out'

Bell's pamphlet comprised two dozen pages, without illustrations, which would 'have given this Essay an imposing splendour', and without reference to any other person. He spoke as an anatomist. 'They would have it that I am in search of the seat of the soul; but I wish only to investigate the structure of the brain. ...' He intended to question the view 'that the whole brain is a common sensorium'.

He first considered the operation of the organs of sense 'as a natural introduction to the anatomy of the brain'. He stressed that 'while each organ of sense is provided with a capacity of receiving certain changes to be played upon it, as it were, yet each is utterly incapable of receiving the impression

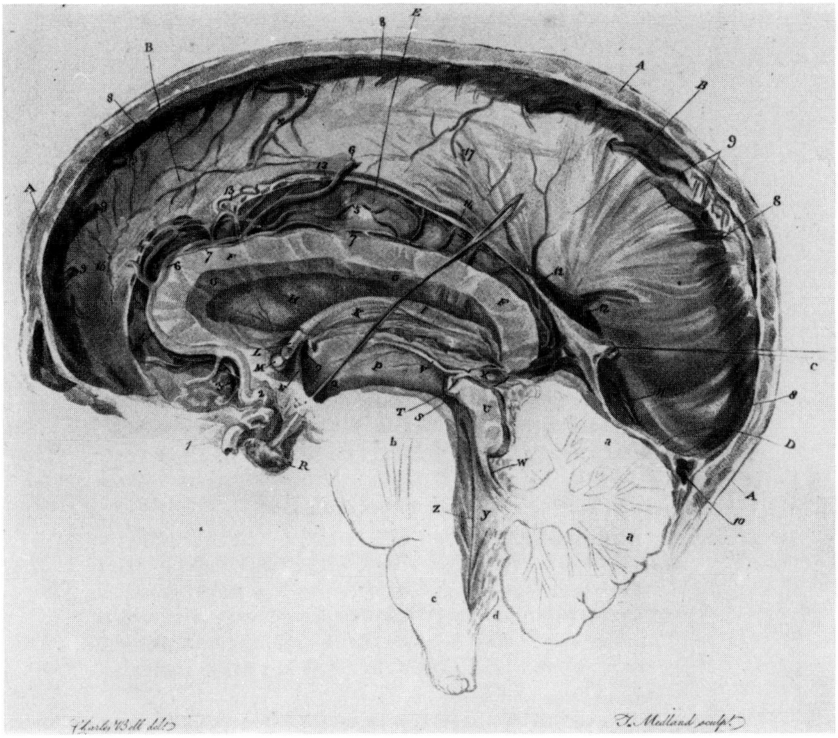

FIG. 85. Sagittal section of brain. The quill passes from the base of the third ventricle into the infundibulum; arteries, veins, and venous sinuses. (After Bell,[71] Pl. X.)

FIG. 86 (*below left*). Dissection of brain stem. To illustrate 'the great anterior column (A, B, C) which gives off the nerves of motion'. Right half of pons has been removed to disclose B. The pyramidal decussation C. (After Bell,[100] Pl. X.)

FIG. 87 (*below right*). Dissection to show sensory pathway in the brain stem A, pons; B, Fanning sensory tracts; C, union and decussation of sensory tracts; E, trigemenal sensory fibres. (After Bell,[100] Pl. 11.)

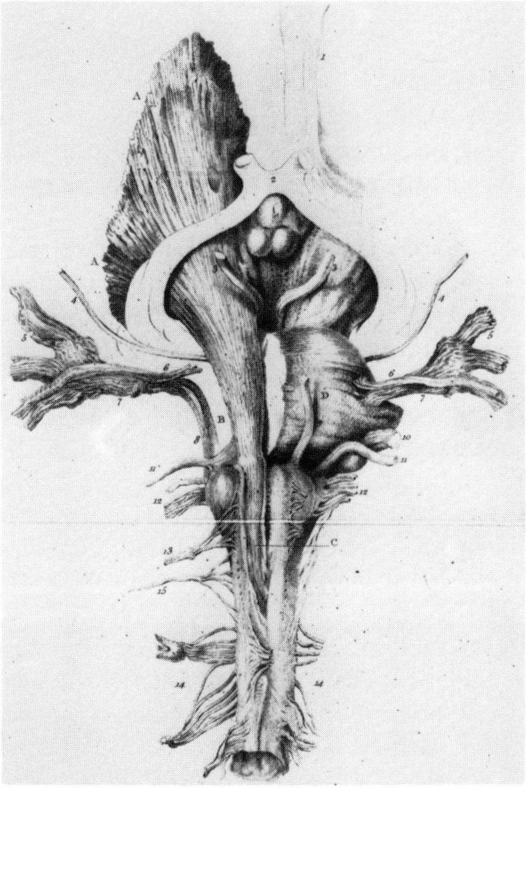

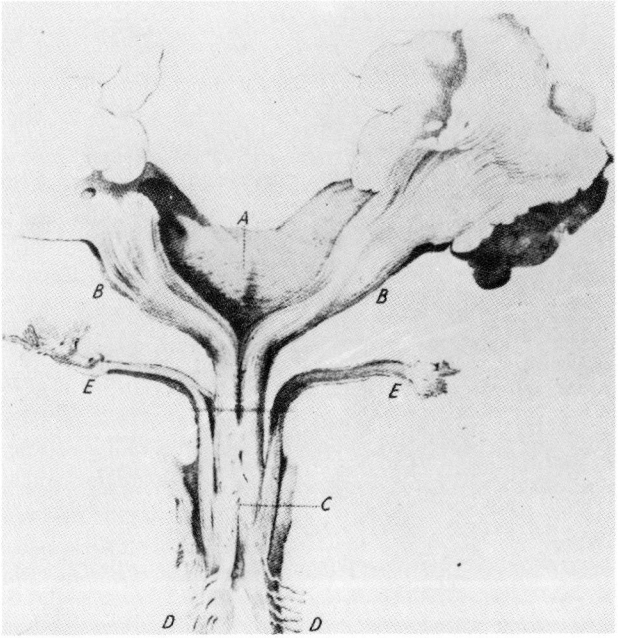

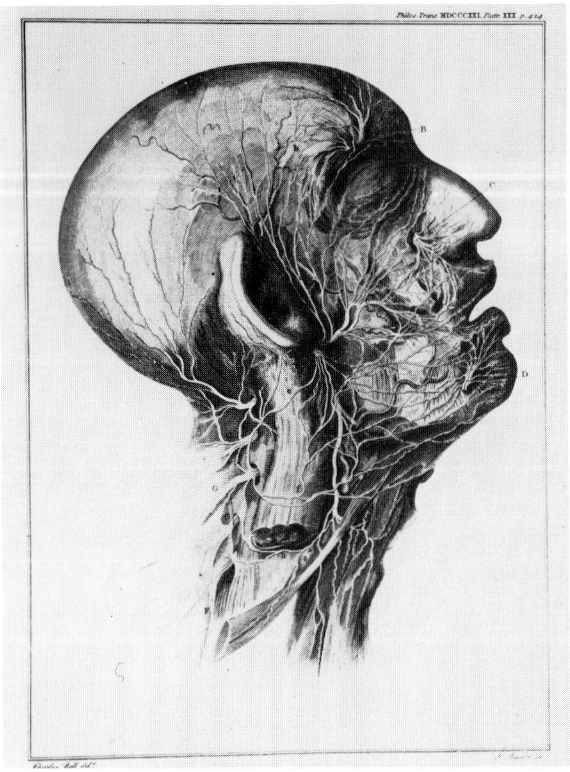

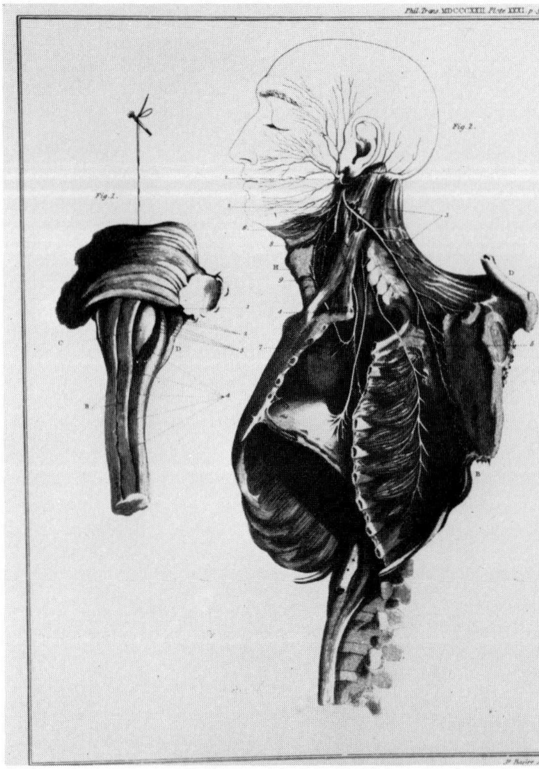

FIG. 88 (*left*). Nerves of the face. A, the seventh nerve, he named 'the respiratory nerve of the face'; F, the phrenic nerve was 'the internal respiratory nerve'; the long thoracic was the 'external respiratory nerve'; B, C, D are branches of the trigeminal nerve. (After Bell.[84])

FIG. 89 (*right*). *Fig. 1* (left): Medulla spinalis. A, pons; B, pyramidal columns; C, olive; D, restiform body; 1, 2, 3, and 4, origins of seventh, ninth, tenth, and eleventh cranial nerves. *Fig. 2* (right): Respiratory nerves. (After Bell.[85])

destined for another organ'. When one papilla of the tongue is pricked, there is a sensation of touch; pricking another may give a sensation of taste. In operations on the eye, piercing the outer coats causes more pain than touching the retina. Vision did not depend on the retina merely being much more sensitive than surface structures. 'Life could not bear so great a pain'. If light, pressure, galvanism, or electricity produce vision 'we must conclude that the idea in the mind is the result of an action excited in the eye or in the brain . . .'. The pain which is felt when the nerve of an amputated stump is touched, 'is as if in the amputated extremity'. If one wanted further proof that a peculiar sense may persist in the absence of an external organ he cited (modestly veiling it in Latin) the 'exquisite gratification of the senses' which was still possible when a chancre had destroyed the glans penis.

There were, he concluded, 'parts of the brain to which the nerves of sense tend, strictly form the seat of the sensation, being the internal organs of sense'. Other parts of the brain presided over motion and vital properties. The cerebrum contained the seats of motion and sensation, while the cerebellum was concerned with 'secret' and 'vital' forms of activity.

The brain 'had grand divisions and subdivisions'; in reality there were 'four brains', two anterior divisions (cerebral) and two posterior divisions (cerebellar). There was perfect symmetry of form and substance between right and left, with full communications to ensure 'their acting with perfect sympathy'. But between the anterior and posterior divisions 'there is no resemblance' so they must have 'distinct offices'. But 'how to put the matter to proof'?

Experiment on the brain itself was 'difficult, if not impossible'. But he remembered that, like the brain, there were four divisions to the spinal cord, for there was a deep central division, 'and also a distinction into anterior and posterior fasciculi, corresponding with the anterior and posterior portions of the brain'. He considered that he had already traced the fibres of the cerebrum and cerebellum through their crura into the anterior and posterior columns, respectively, of the spinal cord. So he thought that by irritating these columns he had an 'opportunity of touching ... as it were' the cerebrum and cerebellum.

I found that injury done to the anterior portion of the spinal marrow, convulsed the animal more certainly than injury done to the posterior portion; but I found it difficult to make the experiment without injuring both portions.

He turned to the spinal nerves, with their double roots,

On laying bare the roots of the spinal nerves, I found that I could cut across the posterior fasciculus of nerves, which took its origin from the posterior portion of the spinal marrow without convulsing the muscles of the back; but that on touching the anterior fasciculus with the point of the knife, the muscles of the back were immediately convulsed.

These two paragraphs in his essay contain the only references to experiment or new knowledge. And what did he conclude from them? Certainly not what everyone was later led to believe about the motor and sensory roots. He said

Such were my reasons for concluding that the cerebrum and cerebellum were parts

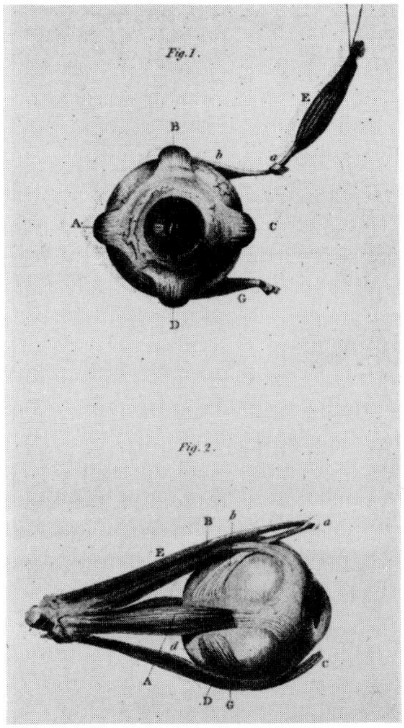

FIG. 90. The muscles of the eye. Bell describes the upward and outward rolling of the eyeball when the eye closes. *Fig. 1* (top): Anterior view A, B, C, D, the recti; E, superior oblique; G, inferior oblique *Fig. 2* (bottom): In profile A, B, D, three of the recti; E, superior oblique; G, inferior oblique. a, trochlea; b, reflected tendon of S.O.; c, d, origin and insertion of I.O. 'When the eyelids are shut, the recti or voluntary muscles resign their office, and the inferior oblique muscle gains power, and the eyeball traverses so as to raise the pupil ... This is the condition of the organ during perfect repose.' (After Bell.[89])

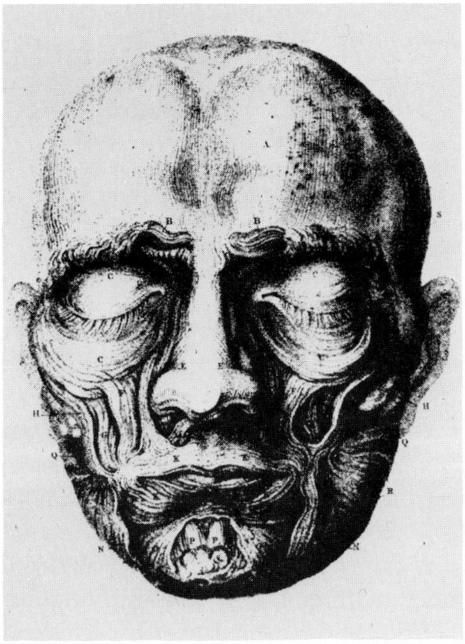

FIG. 91. The muscles of the face. Bell thought that the corrugator muscle, B, was peculiar to man, an error pointed out by Darwin. Bell wrote, 'In all the exhilarating emotions the eyebrows, eyelids, the nostrils, and the angles of the mouth are raised. In the depressing passions it is the reverse.' *Essays on the anatomy and philosophy of expression* (2nd Ed) Murray (1824).

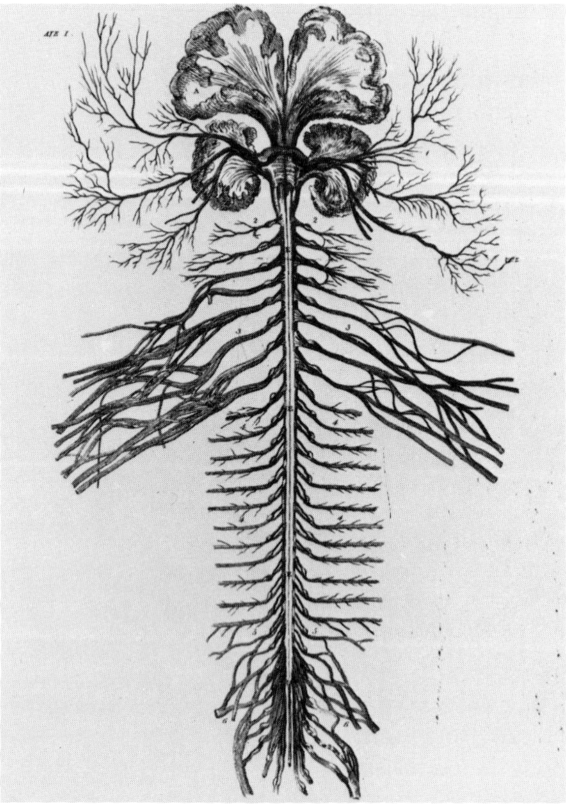

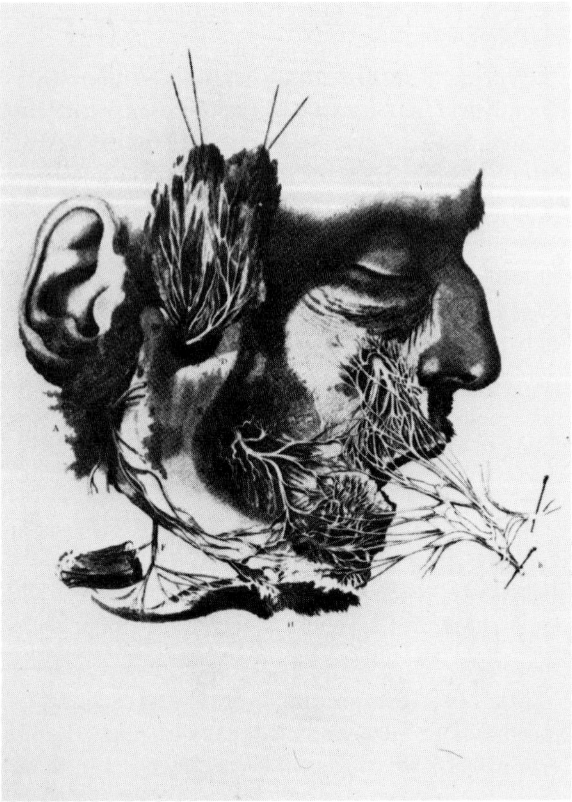

FIG. 92 (*left*). The nerves. Bell classified nerves into two systems. I; 'The original and symmetrical system, necessary to life and motion; the spinal nerves and trigeminal nerves' as here illustrated. All had double roots, with a ganglion on one of them. II; the second system was the 'respiratory nerves'. From *An exposition of the natural system of the nerves of the human body*, Spottiswoode, London (1824).

FIG. 93 (*right*). The nerves of the face. The masseter is reflected upward. B, the seventh nerve, is cut and reflected to the right 'to show its connections with the branches of the fifth on the cheek and lips. (After Bell.[86]) Three of Bell's drawings from *A system of operative surgery founded on anatomy*, (2nd, edn.) Longman, London (1814).

distinct in function and that every nerve possessing a double function obtained that by having a double root.

So, back to the brain and its grand divisions. The cerebrum united the mind to the body. 'Into it all the nerves from the external organs of the senses enter; and from it all the nerves which are agents of the will pass out.' And they passed, be it remembered, via the anterior columns of the cord and the anterior roots.

But with these nerves of motion which are passing outwards there are nerves going inwards; nerves from the surfaces of the body; nerves of touch; and nerves of peculiar sensibility, having their seat in the body or viscera.

The cerebellum, by contrast, 'governs the operation of the viscera necessary to the continuance of life'. Their nerves 'go everywhere' via the posterior columns, for 'the secret operations of the bodily frame . . .'.

Thus, what Bell was saying, was that in the anterior roots and columns there were motor and sensory fibres; and that in the posterior roots and columns there were fibres carrying 'secret' and 'vital' messages – in other words, visceral efferent fibres. But how obscured it all became with the passage of time.

With regard to his chief concern, that there was a regional organization of function in the brain, he contributed little. He noted, as others had done, that disease of the cortex caused intellectual loss, that 'the surface of the

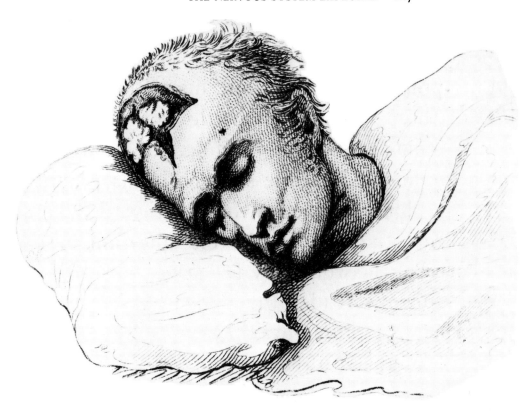

brain is totally insensible' and that 'the deep and medullary part being wounded, the animal is convulsed and pained'. As for his secret and vital process of the cerebellum, Willis (p. 70) had said as much long before. Bell clearly appreciated the principle of specific nerve energies, but here too this had been foreshadowed by Whytt.

Without agreeing that Bell's *Idea* of 1811 was the actual *Magna carta of neurology*,[76] It did, by fair means and foul, become the banner which men followed in the exploration of the pathways of the nervous system. The first, in 1822, was Magendie (1783–1855), perhaps recruited after his meeting with John Shaw, Bell's colleague, in Paris in September 1821. But between 1811 and 1822, as Cranefield has stressed, one heard no more of spinal nerve roots from Bell or any assistant, and there were ten opportunities in their published words.[77] It will be recalled that Cooke (p. 173) enquired of Bell in 1821 how he explained that paralysis could be exclusively motor *or* sensory, and in his reply Bell did not mention spinal nerve roots.

FIG. 94. 'Fungus Cerebri from gun-shot fractures.' (After Bell.)

FIG. 95. Gun-shot wound of arm. 'He was a very stout and intrepid looking fellow. He was charging with the bayonet. Musket ball struck his arm . . .' (After Bell.)

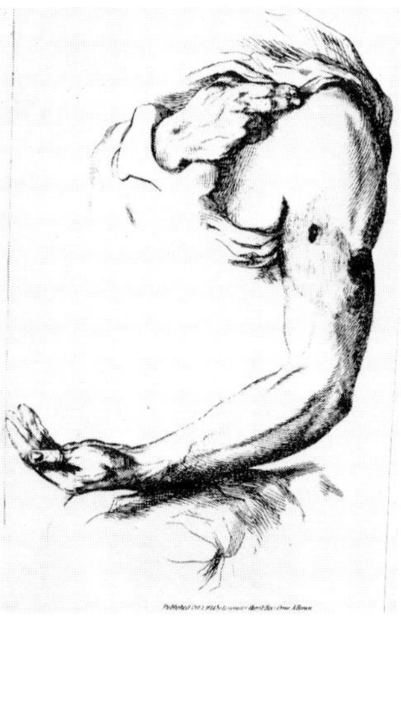

Magendie's experiments. His first publication on the spinal roots, in August 1822, comprised only three paragraphs.[78] He used six-week-old puppies so that he could expose the spinal canal without difficulty; he opened the dura mater. I quote from Walker's 1849 translation.[79]

I then had a complete view of the posterior roots of the lumbar and sacral pairs, and in lifting them up successively with the points of a small pair of scissors, I was able

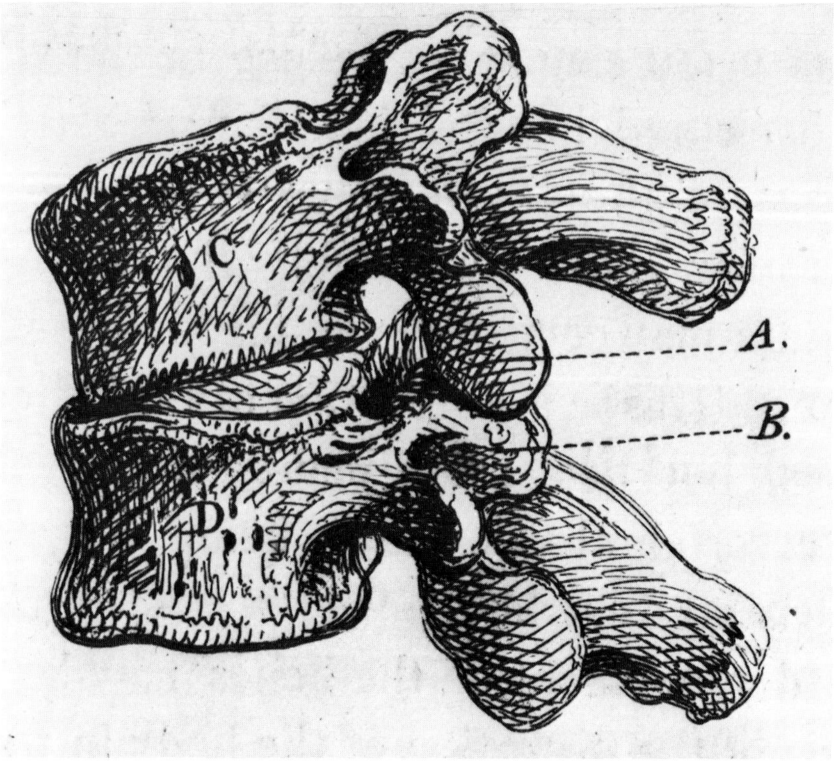

FIG. 96. 'Dislocated Vertebrae.' In the lumbar region there is 'a species of subluxation – a dislocating of the articular processes, but not of the bodies of the vertebrae, the intervertebral substance being only a little irregularly stretched'. The articulating processes, A and B, 'should lie flat on each other, instead of which their points stand opposed ... the person is bent down and unable to elevate himself. (After Bell.)

FIGS. 94–6 show three of Bell's drawings from *A system of operative surgery founded on anatomy*, (2nd. edn.) Longman, London (1814).

to cut them on one side, the spinal marrow remaining untouched.

I at first thought the member corresponding to the cut nerves, was entirely paralysed; it was insensible to the strongest prickings and pressures, it seemed to me also incapable of moving; but soon to my surprise, I saw it move in a manner very apparent, although sensibility was entirely extinct.

He repeated this experiment twice with 'exactly the same result'. Two days later he succeeded in cutting the anterior roots.

I made the section on one side only, in order to have a point of comparison. It may be conceived with what curiosity I observed the effects of this section; they were not doubtful, the member was completely immovable and flaccid, at the same time preserving an unequivocal sensibility.

Finally, that nothing might be neglected, I cut the anterior and posterior roots at the same time; there ensued absolute loss both of sensibility and of motion.

He then said he repeated and varied these experiments upon several species of animals and concluded that the roots possessed different functions, 'the posterior appear more particularly destined to sensibility, whilst the anterior seem more especially allied to motion'.

Magendie's second paper came in October 1822.[80] He presented this group of experiments in ten paragraphs. First, he employed nux vomica in view of its known effects of producing 'tetanic convulsions'. He himself had demonstrated its effect on the spinal cord in 1809,[81] and in 1822 had published his book on pharmacology. He had found that convulsions still occurred after the cord had been severed, but not when it had been destroyed.

Again, quoting from Walker's translation[82] Magendie wrote that

> ... in an animal in which the posterior roots were cut, the tetanus was complete ... in an animal in which I had cut the nerves of motion of one of the posterior members, the members remained supple and immovable at the time when, under the influence of the poison, all the other muscles of the body suffered the most violent tetanic convulsions.

Second, he employed mechanical stimulation of the roots 'in pinching, pulling, pricking these [posterior] roots, the animal gives signs of pain' [and there were weak muscular contractions].

> I have repeated the same experiments upon the anterior bundles, and I have obtained analogous results, but in an inverse sense; ... the contractions ... are extremely strong and even convulsive, whilst the signs of sensibility are scarcely visible.

He thought these findings 'seem to establish that sensation does not belong exclusively to the posterior roots, any more than motion to the anterior'.

Third, he stimulated the peripheral ends of severed anterior and posterior roots. With two exceptions, there were no effects.

Fourth, he employed galvanic stimulation of intact and severed roots, obtaining muscular contractions in each, but they were much stronger with the anterior roots.

Magendie ended by describing how, after the publication of his first paper, he had received a copy of Bell's *Idea* of 1811 and on reading it he said it appeared that 'Mr. Bell was very near discovering the functions of the spinal roots.'

Nine years later, Muller (1801–58)[83] described the results of stimulating, mechanically and electrically, the peripheral ends of the severed posterior and anterior spinal roots in the frog. He concluded that only the latter contained motor fibres, and inferred that the posterior fibres were sensory. I have depicted, in schematic form (Figs. 97–100), the experiments of Bell, Magendie, and Muller, using their own words in the legends.

In the meantime Bell, in pursuit of his ideas on the organization of the peripheral nervous system, turned to the fifth and seventh cranial nerves, but again he erred, thinking that both innervated the muscles of the face.[84–86] When his former pupil, Mayo (1796–1852), correctly ascribed the functions of these nerves,[87] Bell became involved in a second long unpleasant controversy, insisting that he had already done so and once more resorting to the alterations of his words. Bell's biographers[88] have concluded that 'beyond all possible doubt' it was Mayo who showed for the first time the true functions of the nerves of the face. 'On the Motions of the Eye' came in 1823.[89]

It is sad that the memory of these controversies still casts a shadow over the reputation of one who contributed so much to the study of the nervous system, for despite his errors and false claims, his influence must have been

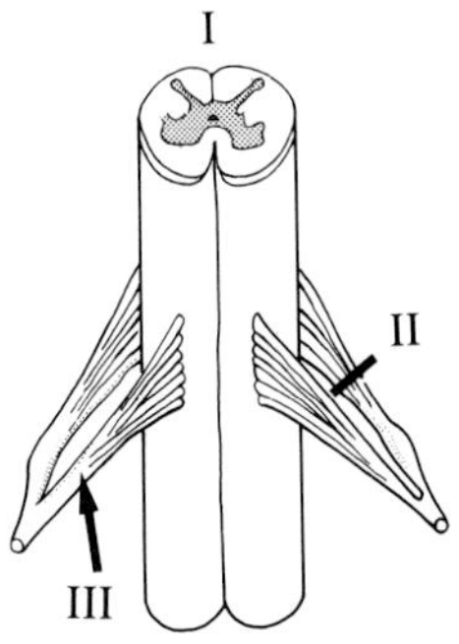

FIG. 97. Bell's experiments on the spinal nerve roots (1811). I. 'Injury done to the anterior portion of the spinal marrow convulsed the animal more certainly than injury done to the posterior portion.' II. 'I could cut across the posterior fasciculus of nerves ... without convulsing the muscles ...' III. 'On touching the anterior fasciculus with the point of the knife, the muscles of the back were immediately convulsed.'

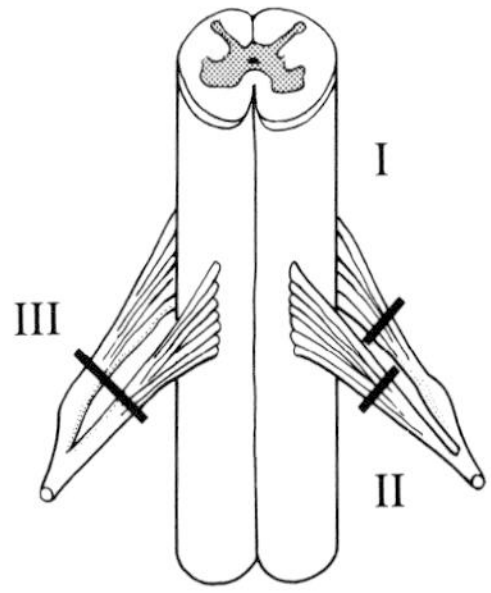

FIG. 98. Magendie's experiments on the spinal nerve roots (August 1822). I. Posterior roots; 'I was able to cut them on one side ... the member corresponding was insensible ... but I saw it move ...' II. Anterior roots; '... the member was completely immovable and flaccid, at the same time preserving an unequivocal sensibility.' III. Both roots; 'There ensued absolute loss both of sensibility and motion.'

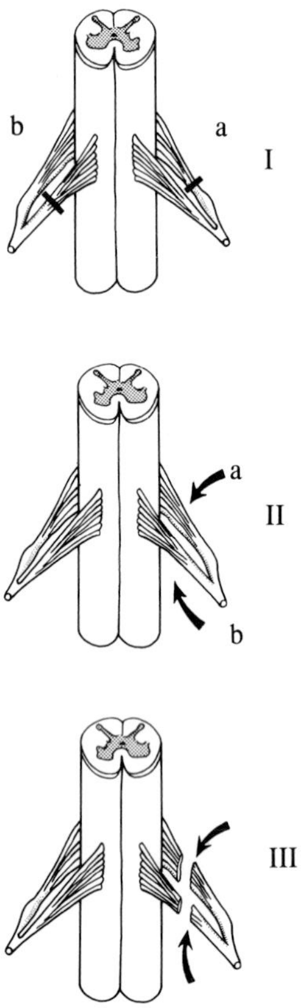

FIG. 99. Magendie's experiments on the spinal nerve roots (October 1822). I Strychninized animal. a. '... in which the posterior roots were cut, the tetanus was complete ...'. b. '... in which I had cut the nerves of motion of one of the posterior members ... the member remained supple and immovable at a time when ... all the other muscles of the body suffered the most violent tetanic convulsions'. II. Stimulation of intact roots. a. Posterior; '... the animal gives signs of pain ... contractions are slightly marked ...'. b. Anterior; '... contractions are extremely strong and even convulsive, whilst the signs of sensibility are scarcely visible'. III. Stimulation of cut roots. a. Mechanical; '... I did not observe any sensible effect from the irritation of the anterior or posterior roots thus separated from the spinal marrow'. b. Galvanic; '... I obtained contractions from each sort of roots; but those which followed the excitation of the anterior roots were in general much stronger and more complete ...'.

enormous. His book *The nervous system of the human body* (1830), in its several editions,[90] was widely read; there was an American edition in 1833,[91] while Romberg translated it into German in 1836,[92] and a French history of his life and work was published in 1859.[93]

Bell experimented, but his deductions were influenced by certain notions he held. On the other hand he was an accomplished artist, 'a Captain of anatomists' (his own phrase), and a surgeon possessed of remarkable prescience. Charles Darwin[94] wrote that Bell, in his 'Essays on the anatomy and philosophy of expression,' (1823) 'laid the foundations of the subject as a branch of science'. We have referred to his insight into the doctrine of specific nerve energy. In his essay 'On the Nervous Circle which Connects the Voluntary Muscles with the Brain' (1826)[95] he clearly anticipated the existence of 'muscle sense', and proprioceptive information, in the control of normal motion. 'Between the brain and the muscles there is a circle of nerves; one nerve conveys the influence from the brain to the muscle, another gives the sense of the condition of the muscle to the brain'. In his Bridgewater treatise *On the Hand* (1833),[96] in the chapter on muscular sense, he wrote,

When a blind man or man with his eyes shut, stands upright ... by what means is it that he maintains the erect position? ... he touches nothing, he sees nothing ... it can only be by the adjustment of muscles ... it must be a property internal to the frame by which we thus know the position of the members of our body (p. 197).

He called this 'consciousness of muscular exertion a sixth sense', but did not apparently test it in patients. Romberg may well have noted Bell's words and applied the method in his patients with tabes dorsalis.

Bell's views on the pathways in the spinal cord for motion and sensation were not based on experimentation, and over the years, as we shall see, they changed more than once (p. 268). But with remarkable skill in dissection he was able to demonstrate a sensory decussation in the brain stem (Fig. 87).

Bell's clinical papers in *The London Medical Gazette* in 1827, 1834, and 1835 reflect his wide experience, and his accounts of innervation of the eyelids,[97] facial palsy,[98] and facial neuralgias[99] are still interesting to read.

There are also many clinical summaries in the appendix to his *Nervous system of the human body*.[100] Case CLXXX (p. 431) entitled 'Partial Paralysis of the Lower Extremities' was one of muscular dystrophy. For eight years a young man of eighteen years had progressive weakness and wasting of the lower limbs, beginning in the thighs. It 'disabled him from rising; and it is now curious to observe how he will twist and jerk his body to throw himself upward from his seat'. Mounting stairs was also difficult. There was a lumbar curvature. The upper limbs were unaffected, there was no sensory loss, and sphincter functions were normal. Bell did not mention any enlargement of muscles.

Another case (CLXXXI, p. 432) was probably one of progressive muscular atrophy in a man of forty years with a three-year history of wasting of the muscles of both upper limbs. He did not mention sensation or fasciculation.

Capt. G. (Case CCXLII, p. 338) had a six-year history of numbness of the lower limbs with ataxia. His arms were normal but his urinary bladder was weak. Although 'he feels the touch of a lady's petticoat on the calf of his legs . . . he could not tell the position of his feet without looking at them'. We can suspect it was an example of tabes dorsalis.

By 1842, when Bell died, 'the prevailing doctrine of the anatomical schools' which he had set out to oppose in his *Idea* of 1811, was certainly deposed. He was correct in then asserting that the nerves of sense and motion were 'distinct thrnugh their whole course' and that there were 'divisions and many distinct parts of the brain'. And there were contemporaries who used clinical and experimental methods to probe the way in which functions were organized in the brain and spinal cord.

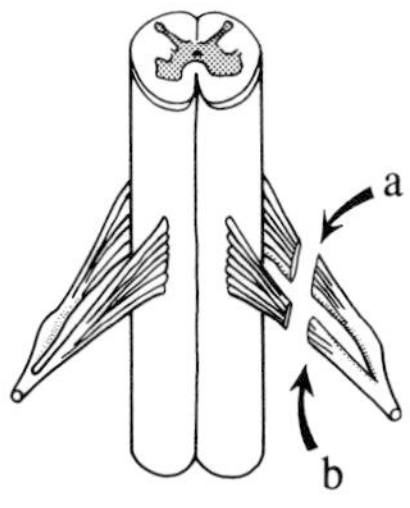

FIG. 100. Muller's Experiments on the spinal nerve roots (1831). *Mechanical*: a. Posterior: 'The end of one of the posterior roots is now seized with a forceps, and the root itself irritated repeatedly with the point of a needle; but not the slightest contraction of the muscles of the posterior extremity ever ensues.' b. Anterior: '. . . the extremity of one is seized with a forceps, and the needle is used to irritate it as in the case of the posterior root; and each time the point of the needle is applied, most distinct twitchings of the muscles take place.' *Galvanic*: 'The application of galvanism to the anterior roots of the spinal nerves after their connection with the cord is divided excites violent muscular twitchings; the same stimulus applied to the posterior roots is attended with no such effect.'

The organs of the brain

Whereas Bell submitted his essay on a new anatomy of the brain, privately, 'for the observation of his friends', Gall (1758–1828) and Spurzheim (1776–1832), in Paris, presented their memoir on brain research (1808)[101] to the Institute de France. An English translation of the committee's report on it was published in the *Edinburgh Medical and Surgical Journal* in the following year.[102]

It is an interesting document, as in its thirty-six pages it confines itself to a consideration of Gall's views of the structure of the central nervous system,

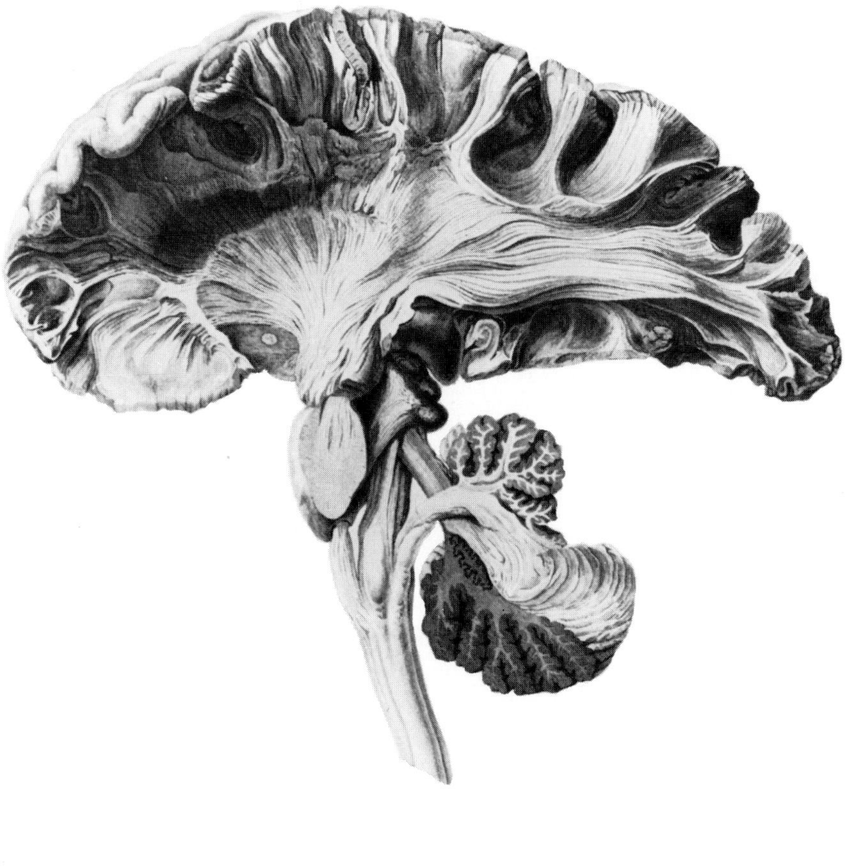

FIG. 101. Brain dissection from Mayo's *A series of engravings intended to illustrate the structure of the brain and spinal cord in man* Burgess Hill, London (1827). The main course of the white fibre tract of the brain 'disposed in three series': '(1) uniting convolutions of same hemisphere; (2) uniting convolutions of different hemispheres; (3) extending from medulla to cerebrum or cerebellum, from cerebellum to cerebrum, and from tubercular parts on the medulla to the cerebrum.'

avoiding all discussion of the popular claims for his cranioscopy, 'which are certainly not within the sphere of any academy of sciences'. Gall and Spurzheim demonstrated their techniques of dissection and observations to the committee, and as with their previous studies, observations were not restricted to the normal human brain; examinations on diseased (e.g. hydrocephalic) and animal brains were also made. The comparative approach had been an important aspect of their work. The committee reviewed the ways in which examination of the brain had been made in the past – Vesalius's technique of serial horizontal slices; Willis's procedure of elevating the posterior lobes, sectioning the fornix, and detaching the lateral parts of the hemispheres; and Varolius's introduction of first studying the base of the brain. By this last method one was able to see how 'the stem of a mushroom is fixed into its *pileus*'. It was by developing this method, they said, that Gall had succeeded so well in tracing the major white fibre tracts. They did not mention that Stensen had advocated this technique (p.98).

They next summarized 'the opinion most generally received with regard to the minute organisation of the brain' which was that the cortical substance of the hemispheres 'is a sort of secreting organ', and that 'the medullary substance' was 'fibrous' and acted as 'a collection of excreting vessels' or as 'conducting filaments'. All nerves emanated from the white matter, and the medulla and spinal cord were but large bundles of these nerves. But this concept was being increasingly questioned; why were there scattered masses of grey matter within the brain, medulla, and cord and why did the latter enlarge in the cervical and lumbar zones instead of gradually shrinking as its nerves left it? Gall and Spurzheim had certain ideas 'concerning the links and knots of which this [neural] network is composed'.

Gall and Spurzheim first explained that the grey matter was 'the matrix of the medullary filaments; wherever it exists, these filaments are produced; it exists wherever they are produced'. A white bundle which crosses an area of grey matter is always enlarged by a contribution from the latter. The spinal cord was not a bundle of nerves; the spinal nerves originated in the central grey matter. The cranial nerves did not arise in the hemispheres but in grey collections in the brain stem. The bundles of the pyramidal eminences decussated in the medulla and as they were traced upward they received fibres from structures such as the pons, the thalami, and the corpora striata. The cerebellar bundles were uncrossed and simpler. Both cerebral and cerebellar bundles terminated in 'two large expansions', the cortex of the respective hemispheres. From these 'expansions', other filaments are produced, which converged toward the midline, communicating by 'commissures', of which the largest were the corpus callosum and the fornix. Similarly, commissures had been observed between the cerebral nerves of the two sides. There were layers of grey and white matter in the cortex and 'each convolution is a kind of small purse or canal' with its inwardly directed converging filaments. The ganglia of nerves was composed of the same grey matter found in the cortex and centres of the hemispheres, in the brain stem, and in the spinal cord. It was probable that each cranial nerve had its ganglion of origin.

From all this, Gall and Spurzheim deducted that each pair of nerves formed a particular system, intercommunicating and reunited 'in the great cord of the medulla oblongata and spinal marrow'. The brain 'was reserved for certain functions, but receiving an influence from all parts of the cord, and exercising one upon them by means of their communications'.

The report went on that Gall and Spurzheim did not claim that they had discovered many new facts, 'but that the chief merit which they claim consists in the connection which they have been the first to establish between the known facts, and in the general conclusions which they have deduced from them'. The committee thought that there was nothing very new in the view that white filaments originated in the grey matter. They reserved judgement about the origin of the spinal nerves in the central grey matter. They complimented the authors on their demonstration of the origin of cranial nerves in the brain stem, facilitated by their use of 'herbiferous animals, in which the pons varolii does not cover them, since it is not so large as in man'. And they were particularly impressed by the manner in which the optic nerves were traced, not to the 'optic' thalamus but to the 'testes and nates' (corpora quadrigemina). Gall had observed that in unilateral optic nerve atrophy the corresponding 'tubercle' was also smaller, and that animal species with large optic nerves have large 'nates'. The roots of the olfactory nerve were not traced to the brain stem, but to the vicinity of the 'testes' and the internal geniculate body. There was confirmation of the general pattern of two white fibre systems, one diverging from the peduncles and the other converging toward the commissures. The decussation of the pyramidal fibres, which they recalled had been seen by Mistichelli and Pourfour Du Petit, was considered to have been finally established, but they were puzzled why so many anatomists had confused it with the transverse commissural fibres which could be seen in the depths of the longitudinal fissure of the medulla oblongata. The actual relationship between the diverging and converging white fibre tracts and the grey matter of the cortex, the committee found difficult to define, but there was no question about the commissural fibres. They also agreed that the 'ganglion' analogy between the grey matter of the cortex and that in central parts was reasonable, but that with the cranial nerve origins and the ganglia of nerves themselves presented difficulties.

In their conclusions they felt that Gall and Spurzheim had over-generalized about the probable association between structure and function of the various masses of grey matter in the nervous system and they were not convinced of 'the solution of continuity' of white matter within each convolution that would permit its unfolding, like the grey cortex itself. Finally, they deferred judgement on the view that 'there is no circumscribed place in the brain to which all sensations go, and from which all the voluntary motions issue . . .'. The anatomical questions which they had reviewed, they said, had nothing to do with Gall's physiological doctrines.

The latter, as is well known, were not truly physiological and they certainly did not emerge from anatomical studies. The theory was there before dissection began, Spurzheim himself averring that 'Gall had not yet begun to examine the brain by 1800'.[103] Neither were they deduced from animal experiment, which Gall disliked and thought ill-suited to the task of discovering the functions of the brain, although he undertook some experiments on the cerebellum after Flourens' reports in 1824.

Gall's doctrine was that the brain, being the instrument of the mind, possessed a number of organs or centres concerned with specific innate 'faculties'. Just as the senses of vision, hearing, taste, and smell had organs, so had his faculties. Why should Nature make an exception of the brain? And with the years his faculties multiplied, as he came to identify them on the surface of the brain, paired and symmetrical, by locating overlying protuberances in the skull. Despite the absurd developments of this 'organology' or 'phrenology', Gall's work nevertheless ushered in the era of the cerebral localization of function.

In the preface to the four-volume *Anatomy and physiology of the nervous system* (1810–19)[104] he wrote that 'For every discovery and especially for every new doctrine, it is customary to ask how the author came to have his initial idea.' And again and again he referred to the occasion in his childhood when he noted that prominent eyes went with a good verbal memory.

> In my ninth year my parents sent me to an uncle who was a priest in the Black Forest. To give me some competition, this uncle found another boy of my age to study with me. I was often reproached for not learning my lesson as well as my co-student. From my uncle's house my co-student and I went to Bade near Rastadt. Out of thirty class-mates there, when it came to reciting by heart, I had always to fear those who in composition achieved only the seventh or even the tenth place. Two of my new class-mates surpassed even my original fellow student in their ability to learn by heart. As they all had prominent eyes, we nicknamed them 'Cow's Eyes'. After three years we went to Bruchsal; there again, class-mates with 'Cow's Eyes' saddened me by their ability to learn by heart. Two years later I went to Strasbourg, and I continued to notice that those who continued to learn most easily by heart had prominent eyes and that some of them were quite mediocre students in other subjects.
>
> Although I had no preliminary knowledge, I was seized with the idea that eyes thus formed were the mark of an excellent memory. It was only later on ... that I said to myself; if memory shows itself by a physical characteristic, why not other faculties? and this gave me the first incentive for all my researches, and was the occasion for all my discoveries.[105]

So, on graduating in Vienna in 1795 he seems to have set about his task and soon became known for his strange beliefs. He literally looked at the human face and head. He looked at his patients, at society generally, and at portraits and busts of historical persons. He examined preserved skulls and had hundreds of head casts made. In hospitals, schools, institutions, prisons, and asylums he closely examined and recorded the configuration of the skull. He examined with great interest anyone who possessed exceptional talent, especially if it was restricted to one field. The genius and the idiot, the saintly and the depraved, the scholar, the artist, and the musician – all were material for his collection. An unusual or mishapen skull attracted him like a magnet. When he looked at a skull he was convinced he was also looking at a brain. It was farcical from the start in its uncritical abandon. It was an obsessional hunt with controls not admitted, conflicting data ignored or explained away, and only one thing being sought – confirmation of the idea. One could well imagine how a mind such as Gall's would have scrutinized the human race as depicted on our television screens. Young[106] has rightly noted the analogy between the naturalist activities of Gall and those of the evolutionists. Both relied essentially on the collection of data, but in the case of the doctrine of natural selection, experimental confirmation was forthcoming.

Out of this welter of activity he proposed the doctrine of multiple functions of the brain. He asked himself

> Is this plurality a chimera which some, deceived by the fact that no physiologist has found these organs, and seduced by metaphysical dreams, will support?. Or, would all the scholars have followed a false route?[107]

Well, some did, and others did not. The major battles were fought in Paris with such men as Lallemand, Rostan, and Andral in support. In particular there were important developments concerning two of Gall's cerebral organs – the organ of language and the organ of sex – the frontal lobes and the cerebellum.

The organ of articulate language. Intellectual ability was not determined, Gall taught, by the volume of the brain, but he focused attention on the convolutions of the hemispheres which were clearly more developed in man than other animals, and especially in the frontal regions. The convolutional pattern was not 'accidental' and in the human brain it was symmetrical and basically uniform. Each convolution was composed of grey and white matter and was distinctly demarcated. But his centres were not strictly defined; he referred only to areas of the brain surface. Not all of this was mapped and in his illustrations (Figs. 102–104) there were numerals denoting centres on the convolutions as well as on his skulls. It is strange that he did not see the possibility that the convolutions themselves might be 'centres' and it illustrates how anatomic-physiological correlation was not at the heart of his scheme.

Clinico-pathological correlation played some part, but a small one. As we have seen, bulging eyes signified a good memory. We do not know whether there was any associated goitre in his cases. The eyes bulged, he thought, because the orbits were reduced in size by the development of the inferior convolutions of the frontal lobes. He would not accept that the size of the frontal sinuses influenced the local topography and indeed came to deny their existence when defining his 'bump' of locality. Eyes that protruded were sometimes also depressed. The effects on the orbits were determined by the actual site of the adjacent convolutional development. The more anterior it was, the more likely depression of the eye would accompany its protrusion. Moreover, Gall had recognized that in the former case, in addition to possessing an excellent verbal memory, the individual was also well endowed with the faculty of language.

There were also examples of loss of speech as the result of penetrating

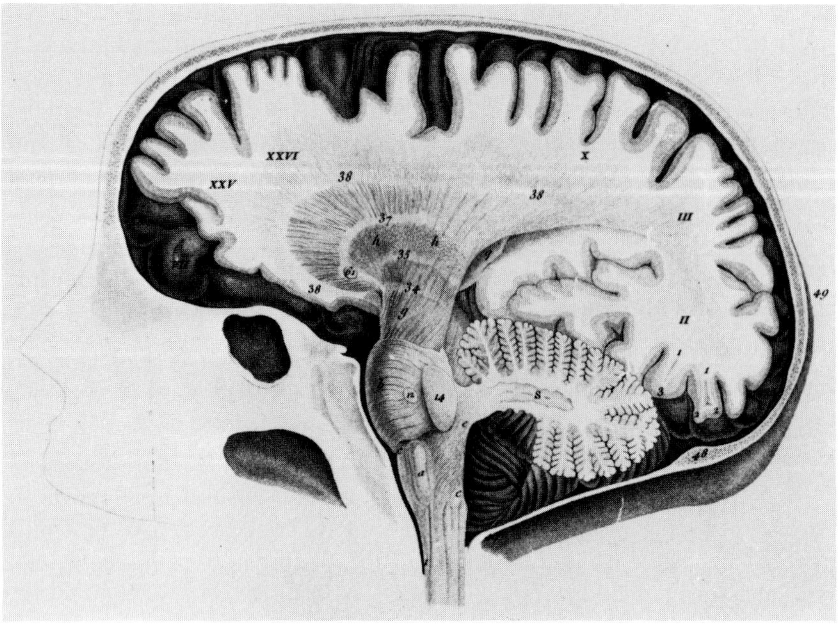

FIGS. 102–104. Illustrations from Gall and Spurzheim's Atlas which accompanied their four-volume work. With meticulous methods of macroscopic dissection, they illustrated the origins of the cranial nerves, the decussation of the pyramidal tracts and the course of the main fibre tracts in the brain. (Reil and Flourens were full of admiration for what was thus achieved.) (After Gall and Spurzheim.[104])

wounds of the forehead, usually from sword thrusts. One officer was wounded above one eye (side not mentioned) and his only disability was that he could not remember the names of his best friends. Another patient with a similar wound could not even recall his father's name. In a third there was temporary loss of sight in the left eye, anosmia, and a right hemiplegia accompanying total loss of memory for names.[108]

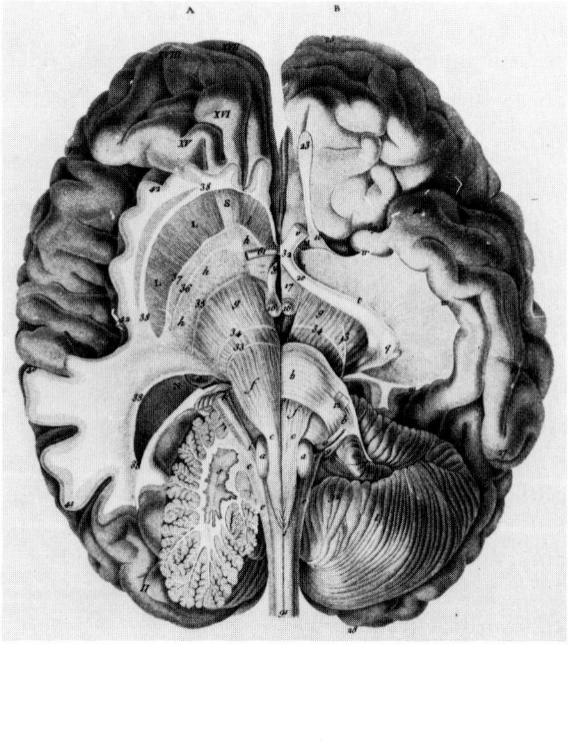

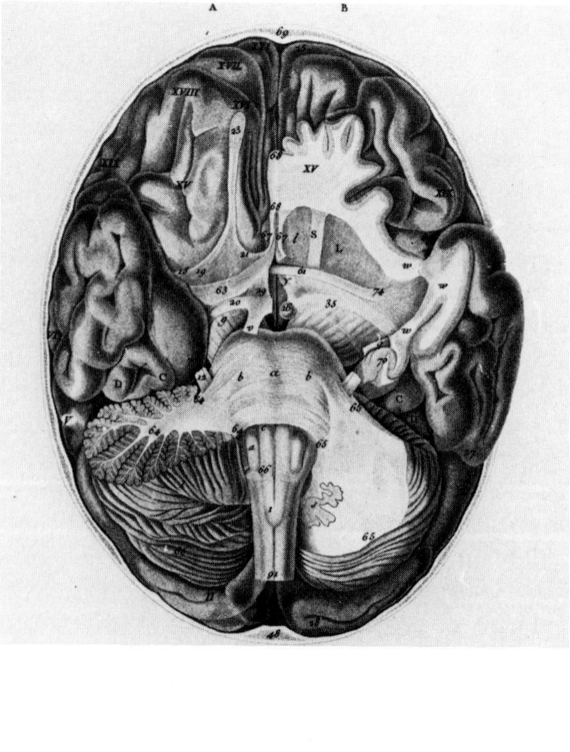

In discussing loss of speech Gall noted, as others had done, that the patient might be able to understand the spoken or written word, and the meaning of gestures. He also realized that the tongue was not necessarily paralysed.

There was no nonsense in Bouillaud's (1796–1881) evidence that speech was a function of the anterior lobes. He graduated in Paris in 1823 a few years after the last volume of Gall and Spurzheim's volumes were published. He was an ardent admirer of Gall, and a clinician imbued with the contemporary zeal for physical examination and for clinico-pathological correlation. In cardiology, as well as neurology, he made notable observations.[109]

Within two years of graduation, at the age of twenty-nine, he published a monograph on encephalitis[41] and an article on 'loss of speech'.[42] In 1822 and 1823, Flourens (1794–1867) had published two reports of experiments he had conducted on the nervous systems of animals.[110, 111] From the effects of the separate removal of the cerebral hemispheres, the cerebellar hemispheres, the corpora quadrigemina, the medulla, the spinal cord, and the nerves, he concluded, in his second report, that

> Sensation, muscular contraction, and the coordinated voluntary movements employed in jumping, flying, walking, standing still or grasping something, were all independent phenomena; deriving from the activity of distinct, separate and localised centres.

> The nervous system is by no means a homogeneous system; the cerebral hemispheres do not behave in the same way as the cerebellar, nor the cerebellum like the spinal cord, nor the cord exactly like the nerves.

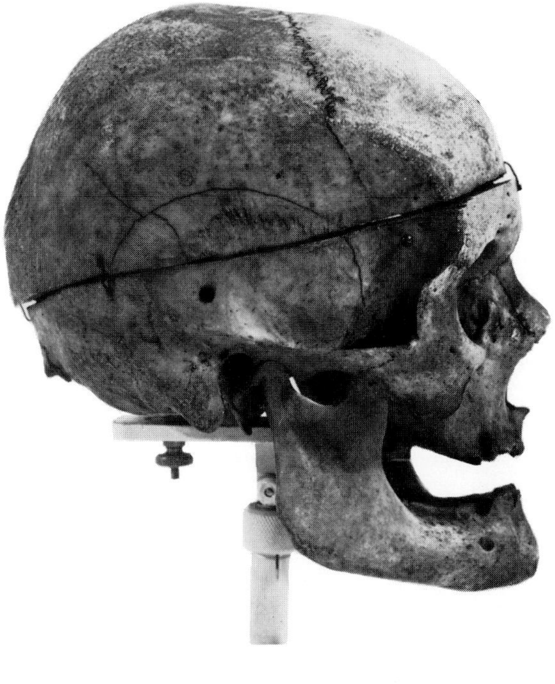

FIG. 105. The skull of Dr F. G. Gall (1758–1828). It shows nothing unusual. (Courtesy of the Musée de l'Homme, Paris.)

But it is a unique system all parts concurring, consenting and acting together; what distinguishes them is their appropriate and definite mode of action; what unites them is reciprocal action of their common energy (p. 368).[111]

In the following year, 1824, Flourens published a monograph[112] on his experimental work, concluding that, in the last analysis, the nervous system was 'a unitary system'. Unity was its cardinal principle.

Bouillaud saw that both clinico-pathological correlation and animal experiment were going to be necessary procedures for the study of brain functions. He used the former for seeking the speech 'centre'. In both of his publications of 1825 he presented a series of cases of cerebral disorders, in which he examined the location of the lesions.

In his monograph, *Traité clinique et physiologique de l'encéphalite*,[41] based on a variety of cerebral disorders that were obviously not all inflammatory, he stressed the importance of the effects of the site of a lesion on volition, sensation, intellect, and speech. In a section entitled, 'Modification of Symptoms According to the Part of the Brain Affected' (p. 273) he recalled Willis's views on the 'anterior' and 'cerebellar' functions of the brain and discussed the significance of cases in which only one arm or one leg was paralysed. There was some evidence that lesions of the middle lobe or corpus striatum affected the leg, whereas lesions of the thalamus or posterior lobes affected the arms (p. 277). He could find no clue as to what part of the brain affected the eye muscles (p. 278). In general, he considered that

The plurality of the centres devoted to motion is proved by the existence of partial paralyses, with an associated local lesion of the brain; it is obvious that if the brain were not composed of many centres, motor or conductors of muscular movement, it would not be possible to conceive how a lesion of one part could cause paralysis of one part of the body, without in any way affecting motion in other parts (p. 279).

He added that such a deduction 'appears to contradict the results of animal experiment', which were those of Flourens (p. 279).

Intellect, he thought, could remain intact if only one hemisphere was affected (p. 283); gross lesions were unsuitable for analysis. If speech was affected, testing intellect was impossible. The 'organ of articulate language' intrigued him. It may be recalled that by this time almost all the clinical forms of aphasia had been described – motor aphasia, jargon aphasia, agraphia, and alexia.[113] Bouillaud wrote,

The organs of speech must have a special centre in the brain, because speech can be completely lost in individuals without any paralysis, whilst on the contrary other patients have free use of speech although limbs are paralysed. (p. 158)

He went on to say that from his own observations and from a study of the literature,

I believe I am justified in advancing the view that the principal law giver of speech is to be found in the anterior lobes of the brain (p. 158).

Unlike Gall, he naturally felt that he should be able to show not only that anterior lobe lesions were to be found when there was loss of speech, but that 'this should be true for the inverse condition also' and that 'moreover, speech should remain, when the lesion occupied other parts of the brain' (p. 158). He appreciated that the tongue was not necessarily paralysed when there was loss of speech and he thought that 'the speech organ itself is composed of several distinct parts, each of which can be separately affected' (p. 289).

His article on 'loss of speech'[42] was undertaken to 'confirm the view of M. Gall on the seat of the organ of articulate language'. The equipotential doctrine of cerebral function proposed by Flourens, and his conclusion that the brain did not have direct and immediate control of motion, was surprising. Bouillaud felt that these views could be refuted (p. 25). It seemed simple and natural to conclude that the movements responsible for speech should have a centre (p. 27).

Bouillaud then cited three cases in which there was loss of speech, temporary in two, without paralysis; comprehension was not altered. Then, there were four fatal cases in which the lesions (abscess, softening, tumour, haemorrhage) were in the left anterior lobes in three of them, and in the right, in the fourth. In two further cases there was haemorrhagic effusion over the anterior lobes.

What he presented as 'negative arguments' comprised four fatal cases of apoplexy in which speech was preserved. In three the hemiplegia was on the left side and the lesions were in the thalamus in two, and in the middle lobe and corpus striatum in the third. In the fourth case paralysis of the right arm was attributed to a lesion in the left middle and posterior lobes. He finally quoted two cases, reported by Rostan and Lallemand, who had a left hemiparesis, normal speech, and lesions posteriorly situated.

He was thus able to conclude that there were centres in the human brain that were concerned with specific muscular movements, and that those concerned with speech resided in the anterior lobes. Sometimes loss of speech was due to loss of memory for words, at other times it was due to loss of those particular movements necessary for speech. The lesion in the anterior lobe could be in the grey or the white matter.

Andral and Cruveilhier disagreed. Andral[114] found that in thirty-seven cases showing anterior lesions, speech was lost only in twenty-one, and retained in sixteen. In fourteen other cases in which speech was lost, the lesions were in the middle lobes in seven and the posterior lobes in seven. Cruveilhier also thought loss of speech occurred with lesions in various parts of the hemispheres.

The question, whether it mattered in which hemisphere the lesion was found, was never asked. Bouillaud did not know that the normal speech in his three examples of left hemiplegia could be explained on laterality. The idea of a dominant hemisphere only emerged later in the century, mainly through the work of Hughlings Jackson, but Marc Dax, we now know, from his son's publications in 1865 and 1878, had observed the special importance of the left hemisphere in 1836.[115, 116]

Bouillaud periodically defended his concept during subsequent debates in Paris during the next four decades. He became a professor of clinical medicine in 1831 and was Dean of the Faculty of Medicine when Broca read his memorable papers 'On Loss of Speech' and 'On the Seat of the Faculty of Articulate Language' in 1861.[117, 118] In the latter Broca said that the concept 'would doubtless have disappeared with the rest of the [phrenological] system, if M. Bouillaud had not saved it from shipwreck' by his work.

The organ of amativeness. The curious location and appearance of the cerebellum had long fascinated anatomists. In their fanciful analogies Willis, Swedenborg, and others had indulged their sense of mystery about it. They were sure it was concerned with 'vital instincts', and like Marshall's spinal cord, it never slept. 'At night, while the will lies asleep, the cerebellum takes up its sceptre.'[119] For Bell, in his *Idea*, the cerebellum conducted 'the secret operations of the bodily frame'.

Once again, according to Gall, it was a boyish observation which led him to the notion that the cerebellum was the seat of the sexual instinct. This time, it was not cow eyes but bull necks that were the clues, and soon the distance between the occipital protuberances became the index of amativeness. Support of a kind was not hard to find. A man, a stallion, or a bull, had a larger cerebellum than a eunuch, a gelding, or an ox. There were plenty of examples of injury to the cerebellum, which caused testicular atrophy, as Larrey had described, sometimes even on the same side in unilateral injuries; priapism in hanging and in lesions of the posterior fossa; and eroticism, nymphomania, and perversion in various types of cerebellar lesions were gleefully noted. G. Combe, one of the two indefatigable brother phrenologists of Edinburgh, even managed to provide the information that in twenty-nine mothers guilty of infanticide, the cerebellum was very small.[120] What is more, the idea persisted for decades. Hammond,[121] in 1869, devoted half his paper on the cerebellum to this question, observing that 'there is a good deal of evidence in its favour', but deciding that it had 'no special and exclusive control over the sexual appetite'. A few years later, Ferrier[122] also felt it necessary to consider Gall's view and although he thought that a few clinico-pathological observations offered some support, he found no evidence from his own experiments and concluded that there was no foundation for the theory. Neither Hughlings Jackson nor Gowers considered sexual function merited consideration in their writings on the cerebellum, and when Holmes[123] came to describe familial degeneration of the cerebellum in 1907, he inferred that the small size of the penis and testicles in the males were associated developmental anomalies. This might be compared to the testicular atrophy we see in myotonia atrophica.

The organ of locomotion. The 'exciting developments in France' in the study of brain functions were followed with great interest in Britain. The studies of the cerebellum by Flourens and Magendie caused an anonymous writer in the *Edinburgh Medical and Surgical Journal* in 1824[124] to comment that in Britain if a man finds 'a new path of enquiry . . . he was allowed to pursue his course without disturbance or encroachment . . . [but] it was not so in France . . . where his brethren on all hands conceive themselves entitled to enter it also and to partake in the harvest along with him'. It was 'unfair . . .

but must benefit science.' Gall, it was said, was 'incensed that his organs of love were snatched from his hands to make up one poor paltry machine for regulating the baser motions . . .'. In 1823 the *London Medical and Physical Journal*[125] published lengthy extracts from the experimental studies of Rolando, Flourens, and Magendie. Certainly, the latter's 'new manifesto' for physiology – by way of experiment – was being proclaimed.

A recent Italian re-examination of Rolando's work on the cerebellum, that by Fadiga,[126] is instructive. It was first published in 1809[127] in Sassario, Sardinia, where Rolando (1773–1831) held a chair of medicine. It was a booklet of ninety pages of which thirty were devoted to the cerebellum. He used ablation and galvanic stimulation to examine the function of the cerebrum and cerebellum in a wide variety of animals. He associated both with voluntary forms of motion. Like Gall, he had a theory about the cerebellum and he proceeded to verify it. 'I believed it was destined for locomotion, and, to confirm this opinion, I undertook the following experiments.'[128] Many of his animals died, but in a kid, he was able to observe that after cutting into the cerebellum with a stilet the animal was no longer able to stand and seemed paralysed. From all his experiments he concluded that cerebellar injury impaired 'locomotive power'. Fadiga points out that in the second (Turin, 1828) edition of his work Rolando included further experimental protocols and more detailed accounts of the effects of his cerebellar ablations. He observed that an animal might 'shake', 'kneel', or tend to 'fall, sometimes on the one side, sometimes on the other'. Movements could be 'uncertain', 'hesitating', 'strange', or 'quaking'. His interpretation, however, was that he was observing paralysis, not incoordination or loss of balance. But Rolando, at least, showed that the effects were motor, ipsilateral, and that movements were unsteady, and this at a time when clinico-pathological correlation at the Salpêtrière had claimed that the cerebellum was 'le foyer central de la sensibilité.'[129]

The organ of coordination and equilibration. Rolando's book remained largely unknown from 1809 until 1822, when developments in Paris served to bring it to light. These were the systematic investigations undertaken by Flourens, and published in book form in 1824.[112] He first sectioned and stimulated nerves, then the spinal cord, and subsequently the brain stem and the cerebral and cerebellar hemispheres. The approach was Hallerian and he decided that stimulation of the distal end of a cut nerve demonstrated 'contractility'; while stimulation of the proximal end demonstrated 'sensibility'. He stimulated the exposed spinal cord by pricking and laceration and found he could produce movements of the limbs, but that as he ascended the brain stem responses began to diminish. He obtained movements from the medulla, pons, and corpora quadrigemina, but not from the substance or the surfaces of the hemispheres, cerebral or cerebellar.

Experiments on the cerebral and cerebellar hemispheres led him to conclude that removal of both cerebral hemispheres abolished volition and sensation. Removal of one cerebral hemisphere caused loss of vision in the opposite eye, and weakness of the opposite side. Removal of the cerebellum prevented an animal from jumping, flying, standing, or walking. As a result of these observations he thought that one should be able clinically to deduce the site of a lesion of the nervous system. Thus, difficulty in standing and walking pointed to a cerebellar lesion; convulsive movements pointed to a spinal cord lesion; where there was merely stupor or loss of sensibility, the lesion was in the cerebral hemispheres. In apoplexy it was understandable why there could be paralysis of movement without loss of sensation, and vice versa.[111]

Most of Flourens' experiments were conducted on birds. He mentions pigeons, hens, turkeys, swallows, owls, ducks, and the humble sparrow. Of mammals, there were dogs, cats, mice, and moles. His famous accounts of the behaviour of animals following cerebellar ablations are best remembered with respect to the pigeon and the dog. In the chapter of the second edition of his book (1842)[112] entitled 'The Role of the Nervous System in the Movements of Locomotion' (p. 37) he describes the pigeon from which he removed successive slices of the cerebellum. At first it showed only a little weakness and lack of harmony in its movements; with half of the hemispheres removed, there was agitation, and movements were brisk but ill-regulated; with total removal, the animal could no longer fly, jump, walk, or stand. Placed on its back it struggled but was not able to rise. It could still see, hear, respond to threatening gestures, and there were no convulsions.

In a dog (p. 139) there was a similar progressive loss of muscular coordination, with a zigzag gait, difficulty in turning, repeated falling, and tendency to collide with objects although he could see and hear normally. There were no convulsions, intellect was not disturbed. The disability was in lack of control and regulation of its movements.

In a pig, superficial slicing of the cerebellar hemispheres 'slightly altered the equilibrium of stance and gait'; further slicing caused the animal to 'stagger in a drunken fashion; its feet moved crudely and clumsily, normal motion was impaired and when it fell over its efforts to rise were very awkward'; when the last layers were removed 'the animal was completely unable to stand erect or to walk; it lay on its belly or on its side, often moving its feet as if running or walking, making many fruitless attempts to rise but only tumbling over again when it managed to succeed'.[111]

The disability, in all his animals, whether they typically walked, swam, or flew reminded him of the drunken gait of the human inebriate, and a sparrow made to swallow drops of alcohol behaved similarly (p. 400).

Dow and Moruzzi[130] considered that Flourens' assignment of a contralateral function to the cerebellum was not actually an error but an incomplete description of the manifestations of cerebellar deficiency in birds. He did not detect the release phenomena – extensor hypertonia – following cerebellar ablation, but that soon followed from the hands of Fodera (1793–1848) in Magendie's laboratory in 1823.

At the end of his book Flourens said that 'the art of disentangling simple facts was the whole art of experiment'. His success was not only in the technical achievement of his operations and his skill in keeping animals alive long enough to make observations, but also in making some correct interpretations. He distinguished between volition, muscular contraction, and coordination, but nevertheless, presumably because stimulation of the cerebral hemispheres failed to invoke movements, he concluded that they played no direct role in willed motion. On the other hand, he recognized that what Rolando had called 'paralysis' was, in fact, incoordination. As with Bell and Magendie, there was the customary feud between Rolando and Flourens, with Magendie defending his countryman from the charge of plagiarism. This provoked a London comment that 'The French have a most unfortunate propensity to claim every discovery and improvement as their own. . . . M. Magendie seems to have a fellow-feeling for M. Flourens, having himself been fain to give up the merit of priority to Mr. Charles Bell.'[131]

Subsequently, Flourens went on to perform experiments on the semicircular canals. By irritation and ablation he demonstrated, for the first time, their role in the organization of equilibrium.

Flourens saw that nervous function was integrated, and perhaps if he had not been so determined to expose phrenology, he would have seen that some of his own experimental results suggested cerebral localization. When Fritsch and Hitzig[133] came to report 'On the Electrical Excitability of the Cerebrum', they found Flourens' conclusions 'difficult to harmonise', and concluded their paper by saying that

> It further appears that from the sum of all our experiments that the soul is not, as Flourens and others after him had thought, a function of the whole of the hemispheres . . . but that on the contrary, certainly some psychological functions and perhaps all of them . . . need certain circumscript centres of the cortex.[133]

When Magendie turned his attention from the spinal nerve roots and the cord to the brain he soon found that anatomists were still not agreed about some important facts that would have a bearing on his experimental approach. He said 'anatomical disposition indicates that sensation is more particularly directed towards the cerebellum, and motion towards the cerebrum; but anatomy is not sufficient, unless physiological and pathological facts assist in confirming this supposition; at present, neither the one or the other have established what anatomy appears to demonstrate so evidently'.[134] When he irritated the posterior surface of the spinal cord, there was obvious pain; when he irritated the anterior surface it was 'scarcely perceptible'. Bell, it will be recalled, also initially taught that the anterior tracts of the cord went to the cerebrum, and the posterior to the cerebellum.

Turning to the latter, Magendie found that cerebellar ablation caused no loss of sensation or power. He admitted that haemorrhage was often a problem and that no doubt it tended to compress the medulla and spinal cord, but he generally confirmed Flourens' interpretations to the extent that 'the cerebellum appears to be absolutely necessary to the integrity of straight-forward motion'. One of his ducks 'swam backwards and made no other kind of progression for about eight days'.

A year later, in 1824, in a paper dealing with 'the functions of some parts of the nervous system'[135] he mentioned that he accidentally cut a cerebellar peduncle during an operation. 'I was trying to cut the fifth nerve in a rabbit before its passage in that portion of the temporal bone which anatomists call the petrous.' The animal quickly turned over and continued to do so incessantly for some two hours. The next day, while the rolling persisted, he noticed skew deviation of the eyes. 'The eyes of the animal had lost their position and their normal movement.' The eye on the operated side was directed downward, that on the other side, upward. Repeating this experiment several times he observed that the animal revolved on its own axis toward the side of the peduncular section. They did so in such a fashion that they tended to envelop themselves in the straw of the cage 'like a bottle one wishes to wrap up'. No such rotary movements followed bilateral section. This piece of serendipity served to direct attention to the phenomenon of equilibrium and the role of the cerebellum in its maintenance. Magendie asked himself 'from which side came the impulsion?' and whether he had interrupted an influence entering or leaving the cerebellum. He referred to a patient of sixty-eight, 'un grand bouveur' seized with vertigo after dining. It persisted with a continuous turning sensation 'even in bed' until he died some days later, when an extensive lesion was found in one of the cerebellar peduncles.

In 1827 Bouillaud combined the methods of animal experiment and clinico-pathological correlation in an examination of cerebellar function.[136] For the former he employed dogs, rabbits, and birds. Cauterization of the median convolutions in a dog made it 'unsteady', with 'a bizarre expression in its eyes', but without interfering with consciousness or sensibility. It had 'difficulty in eating' and 'could not coordinate the movements of its head . . . it could not turn right or left . . . and the actions of stance and locomotion were disordered'. To Bouillaud it was a peculiar sight, the dog resembling 'a live puppet'. His clinical cases – his own, those of Gall, Lallemand, and others – he recorded in two groups, as he was questioning the claim that the cerebellum was concerned with sexual function. There were patients with proved cerebellar lesions in whom penile erection had been observed, and others who had been impotent. The former were mostly cases of 'cerebellar apoplexy' one of whom had been indulging in 'plaisirs veneriens' and another who had collapsed on the quay-side in Paris 'avec des filles publiques . . . dans l'acte du coit'. He found nothing to support the notion of Gall but thought that insufficient attention had been paid to disturbance of locomotion. Vertigo and falling had been recorded in several cases, and in one young girl, who proved to have an abscess of the cerebellum, he noted 'continual oscillation of the eyes' which were turned upward.

Bouillaud concluded that the cerebellum was not just concerned with locomotion 'but with all those forces concerned with the numerous and diverse acts of posture, stance and progression'. It coordinated not just movements in general 'but those concerned with equilibrium, rest, and various modes of locomotion'. If it does actually 'furnish the elements of equilibrium to the animal machine' we might regard it not so much 'as the organ of music, like Willis' but one which 'regulates', 'steadies', and 'measures' movements, as in dancing and gymnastics. A dancer undoubtedly possesses a well-organized cerebellum. Just as intellectual activities have to be learned and remembered, so also have those concerned with the body's equilibrium. The cerebellum could well fit this role. It was clearly concerned with those spontaneous and instinctive aspects of animal life and was normally under the direction of the cerebrum.

Finally, Bouillaud wondered whether, in view of the remarkable motor behaviour of the animal deprived of his cerebellum, it might be the location of lesions in patients with bizarre disorders of locomotion. He referred to those cases in which bursts of recoiling, running, jumping, somersaulting, and so on, presented such extraordinary clinical spectacles.

*

Riese and Hoff[137] wrote that 'each division of the central nervous system – spinal cord, cortex, basal ganglia, cerebellum – has had its heroic age' and that the doctrine of cerebral localization is really 'a legitimate child of the doctrine of the seat of the soul'.

Marshall Hall and the true spinal marrow

'I beg, Gentlemen, that you will do me the favour to appoint a commission to witness my experiments, to examine my plain deductions from them, and to look over my paper with care . . .'.[138] The 'Gentlemen' were the Council of the Royal Society, the writer was Marshall Hall (1790–1857), and the 'experiments' were those he had described in a paper entitled 'On the True Spinal Marrow and the Excito-Motor System' (1837). He had read it to the Society but it was not accepted for publication, unlike his previous paper 'On the Reflex Function of the Medulla Oblongata and Medulla Spinalis' (1833).[139] As in the cases of Bell and Gall it seems that in the world of medicine, in those days, any advance led inevitably to bitter controversy.

Hall† had graduated in Edinburgh in 1812 where he had established for himself a reputation for tireless industry which characterized his whole professional life.[140, 141] He spent a year or so in Paris, Göttingen, and Berlin and then settled in practice in his home town of Nottingham where he remained for nine years. He moved to London in 1826 and developed an extensive practice, but although he lectured at various hospitals and institutions, he was never appointed to the staff of a hospital. He was made a Fellow of the Royal Society in 1832 and of the Royal College of Physicians of London in 1841. He travelled widely in Europe and America.

One product of his industry was his publications. Green[142] found that there is no complete bibliography of Hall's writings but lists two hundred items. Jefferson[143] estimated there were nineteen books and over one hundred and fifty papers. Hall had many a quarrel, some of them arising from exaggerated claims, others from lack of acknowledgement of the work of others, and actual plagiarism. He must have been a paranoid personality. Bell's fiddling of the record and controversial tactics were 'gentlemanly' in comparison with Hall's endless vituperative tirades. Both Bell and Hall seemed to have nursed the hope that history would regard them as the Harvey of the nineteenth century. Bell's work scarcely figures in Hall's conceptions, and Bell did not discuss Hall.

† Sir Edward Marshall Hall (1858–1927), the eminent barrister, was *not* the son of Dr Marshall Hall. The latter was attended in his last illness by a Dr Alfred Hall, of Brighton, who asked permission to name a son after the famous neurologist. The son became the barrister. (See *The life of Sir Edward Marshall Hall* by E. Marjoribanks Gollancz, (1929), p. 16.)

The physiologist. It is interesting that his studies on reflex action should have arisen out of the same line of enquiry – the capillary circulation – which Stephen Hales had been pursuing when he noted the effect of pithing a decapitated frog. Hall's laboratory was in his own home and he employed frogs, snakes, lizards, eels, and turtles. He subsequently wrote,

> Whilst engaged, many years ago, in my researches into the Circulation of the Blood, I incidentally observed a remarkable phenomenon; the separated tail of the eft *moved* on being irritated by the point of the scalpel. ...
>
> I soon found that similar observations had been recorded by various physiological writers, – Redi, Whytt, Prochaska, Mayo &c. &c. But I observed that, in their hands, they had remained useless and sterile, – having led to no conclusion, – having neither been traced backwards to any *physiological principle of action*, nor forwards to any *function in the animal economy*. I conceived it impossible that any such phenomenon should exist in nature without such connection, and I resolved to pursue the subject.[144]

He pursued it for twenty-five years, writing, in 1850, that he had devoted twenty-five thousand leisure hours to it, 'disentangling the maze ... [and providing] the first real step in the philosophy of involuntary motions.'[145] In doing so he devised a new nomenclature for the 'system' he had uncovered within the nervous system. This he called the *diastaltic (through) nervous system*, with its *Esodic* (afferent) and *Exodic* (efferent) nerves, and its special series of centres within the spinal cord, comprising the 'True Spinal Marrow'. But, in so doing, he succeeded in describing the functions of 'reflex action', and he described spinal 'shock'; he coined the terms 'nervous arc' and 'arcs of reflex function', and through his zeal and powers of advocacy he left physiologists and clinicians in no doubt about the significance of his discoveries. His predecessors may have contributed 'on the floor of the house', as it were, but it was Hall who put the 'Reflex' on the statute book.

His chief contributions are contained in the two papers to the Royal Society in 1833 and 1837, which he published in his *Memoirs on the nervous system* in 1837.[146] In the first paper 'On the Reflex Function' he referred to the experiments with decapitated animals made by LeGallois (1770–1814) and Flourens, saying that they had missed the evidence for reflex activity. But the inertia and want of initiative of the brainless animal had been noted and attention was drawn to the spinal cord as an organ in itself, and not just a bundle of nerves. What Hall saw in the decapitated or spinal animal was not just the persistence of motion and sensation, which could be abolished by destruction of the spinal cord, but evidence of reflex action. In a decapitated animal,

> I touched the eye or eyelid with a probe. It was immediately closed; the other eye closed simultaneously. I then touched the nostril with the probe. The mouth was immediately opened widely ... I passed the probe up the trachea and touched the larynx. This was immediately followed by a forcible convulsive contraction of the muscles annexed to it. Having made and repeated these observations, I gently withdrew the medulla and brain. All the phenomena ceased from that moment. (viii)

Stimulation of the body and tail of the same animal produced not only movements of the limbs, but also of the sphincters. The limbs and tail 'possessed a certain degree of firmness or tone, recoiled on being drawn from their position . . .'. When the cord was withdrawn, limbs, tail, and sphincters 'became perfectly flaccid' and movements in response to stimulation all ceased. Stimulation of one hind limb might result in movements of the opposite limb or of a forelimb. The message could pass across and upward in the cord. 'There is a still more interesting and satisfactory mode of performing the experiment; it is to divide the spinal marrow between the nerves of the superior and inferior extremities.' Thus, in a frog,

It was immediately observed that the head and the anterior extremities alone were moved spontaneously and with design, the respiration being performed as before. But the posterior extremities were not paralysed; they were drawn upwards, and remained perfectly motionless, indeed, unless stimulated; by the application of any stimulus, they were moved with energy, but once only, and in a manner perfectly peculiar. The stimulus was not felt by the animal, because the head and anterior extremities remained motionless at the time it was applied. Nothing could be more obvious, and indeed striking, than the difference between the phenomena of the functions of sensation and volition observed in the anterior part of the animal and those of the reflex function in the posterior; in the former there were spontaneous movements with obvious design; in the latter, the mere effect of stimulus (p. 14).

Again, if, in a decapitated frog, the spine was divided so that there were three distinct parts of the spinal cord 'each preserved the reflex function' (*Memoirs*, p. 14).

A further experiment demonstrated the 'reflex function' of the anal sphincter. In a turtle he removed the tail, the posterior limbs, with the rectum, and the lower end of the spinal cord. If water was then forced into the intestine with a syringe,

. . . both the cloaca and the bladder are fully distended before any part of the fluid escapes through the sphincter, which it then does on the use of much force only, and by jerks. The event is very different on withdrawing the spinal marrow; the sphincter being now relaxed, the water flows through it at once in an easy continuous stream . . . (p. 14)

In this paper of 1833 he concluded that reflex function 'constitutes the principle of equilibrium and tone, in the whole muscular system, and the principle which presides over the orifices and sphincters of the internal canals'. The cerebrum was the source of voluntary motion, the medulla oblongata was the source of respiratory motion, and the spinal cord was 'the middle arc of the reflex function' (p. 35). Further research into the system 'which constitutes the arcs of the reflex function' was obviously important. Reflex function could be augmented or diminished by certain poisons and rendered morbid in certain diseases such as tetanus, chorea, paralysis agitans, and certain forms of epilepsy and tremor. We could now understand, he said, how with limb paralysis of cerebral origin the sphincters may act normally, whereas with limb paralysis from lesions of the lower spinal cord sphincter function was lost.

In his 1837 paper, 'On the True Spinal Marrow,' he again explained why he thought previous physiologists were 'confused' in their deductions about the movements of decapitated and spinal animals, but conceded that Sir Gilbert Blane (1749–1834), physician to St. Thomas's Hospital, 'came nearest the truth' in his experiments with a kitten in 1788 and in his observations in an acephalous monster, and his noting that a decapitated bee could still sting. Blane had said that 'These facts show clearly that instinctive, or rather automatic motions, may be exerted, without the intervention of the *sensorium commune*, without sensation or consciousness.' Hall also noted, gratifyingly, that Muller had achieved 'similar independent results' to his own, but he differed from him in two respects. 'He thinks the cerebrum is among the central organs of reflex function; and, refers the phenomena in question to sensation' (p. 58).

There were further experiments to report, observations to be recorded, arguments to deploy, and, most important to Hall, 'new' nerves to be proclaimed: 'The Excito-Motory Nerves'.

A horse was pole-axed; it was temporarily convulsed, then lay motionless and began to breathe. A laceration of its hide brought no motor or sensory response, but when an eyelash was touched with a straw, 'the eye closed forcibly'. When the cornea was touched, 'the eye rotates'. When the anus was touched, 'the sphincter contracts, the tail is raised'. All these reflexes were abolished when 'the upper part of the medulla' was destroyed. It was the same with snakes and eels and frogs (p. 61).

Two rabbits were decapitated and in one the spinal cord was destroyed. Decapitation alone allowed 'the muscles [to] retain a certain degree of firmness and elasticity', but when the cord was also destroyed, the muscles were 'lax' (p. 93). Reflex action 'determines the tone of the muscular system'.

Then, there were clinical observations of significance (p. 63). In a case of traumatic paraplegia, notwithstanding the motor and sensory paralysis, 'when the legs were pinched, or more particularly when the sole of the foot was tickled, the extremities were retracted with considerable force'. One of his legs was 'constantly flexed' and, when straightened, it flexed up again. Catheterization caused not only erection, but flexion of his legs. Hall mentioned a paraplegic man who 'became a father' and a paraplegic woman who delivered a baby.

In an idiot, in whom at autopsy the cerebral lobes are found to be atrophic, 'the passions are not only unimpaired, but are unnaturally strong'. In the hemiplegic, surprise or emotions can move the limbs, 'so the seat of these emotions must be placed lower than the lesion'. This is not so in paraplegia, where the lesion is below the seat of the 'volitions and of the passions' (p. 94).

When strychnine is given to a hemiplegic, 'it is the paralytic limbs which first feel its influence' (p. 102).

All these activities operated through the medium of 'the true spinal marrow and the excito-motor system'. The former comprised a series of centres within the spinal cord and with its own excitor (afferent) and motory (efferent) nerves. The former were not sentient and transmitted no sensory

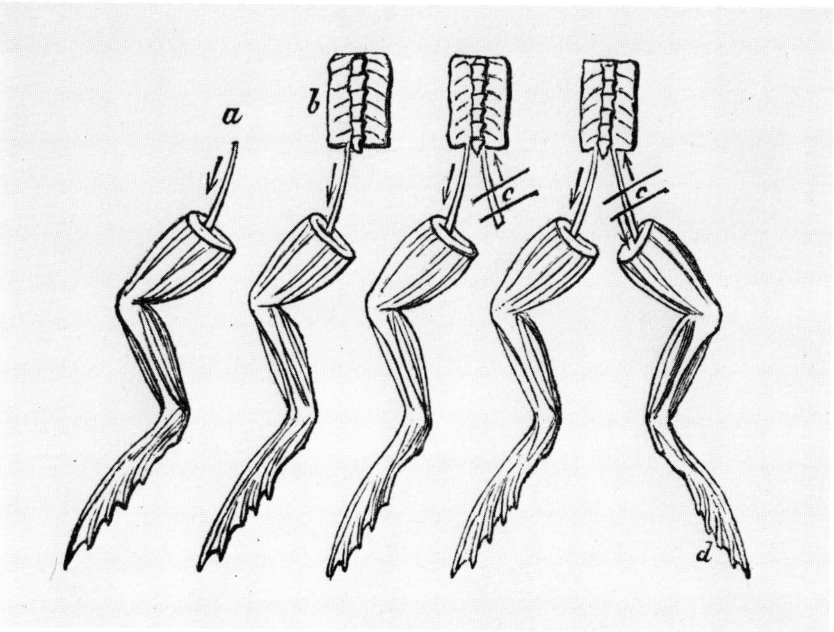

FIG. 106. Stimulation of nerve (a) or cord (b) has a 'downward' effect. Stimulation at (c) and (d) affects the same right lower limb. ('We have passed from the experiment of Haller, to that of Redi and Whytt, etc.') (After Hall.[145])

impulses; they were distinct from the sensory nerves. The latter were not voluntary and transmitted no motor impulses; they were distinct from the motor nerves. Voluntary, willed motion, and sensation, were functions of the 'cerebral' system. Reflex activity was the function of the 'spinal' system. 'The cerebral system sleeps' (p. 70); 'The true spinal system never sleeps' (p. 74). But, the latter may be influenced by the former, in fact, it was 'constantly under a certain influence of the volition' (p. 73).†

In the years following the publication of his *Memoirs* Hall continued with what he often termed his 'persevering labours'. In *A new memoir on the nervous system*' (1843)[147] we find him in his characteristic reiterative mood, 'recapitulating', 'reviewing', emphasizing the 'confusion' of others in the past (now mentioning Prochaska, but only to note how he 'confounded' everything' and drumming home the message of 'my discovery'. Had it not been for the principle of reflex actions which he had discovered 'there would have been an insurmountable obstacle to the proof of the Lex Belliana ...' (p. 91).

In 1850 came his *Synopsis of the diastaltic nervous system*,[145] a monograph 'printed at my own expense ... [in] ... the age of medical degradation'. He was proud of his term *Diastaltic*, 'as congeric with *peristaltic* ... the happy suggestion of my friend, Mr. Hoblyn'. Reflex action was '*through* the spinal marrow at its essential centre' (p. 5).

> The anatomy of the diastaltic system consists of an esodic nerve, the spinal centre, and an exodic nerve, essentially linked together, and constituting a diastaltic nervous arc (p. 36).

Reflex activity can be abolished by a lesion in any portion of the arc, but the spinal cord was 'the key-stone' (p. 31). No part of the system 'can be

† In a letter to Max Born in 1944, Einstein wrote: 'We neither of us realised that the spinal cord plays a far more important role than the brain itself, and how much stronger its hold is'. He was recalling their failure to influence revolutionary German students twenty-five years earlier (Max Born (1978), *Recollections of a Nobel Laureate*, p. 186. Taylor & Francis Ltd, London.)

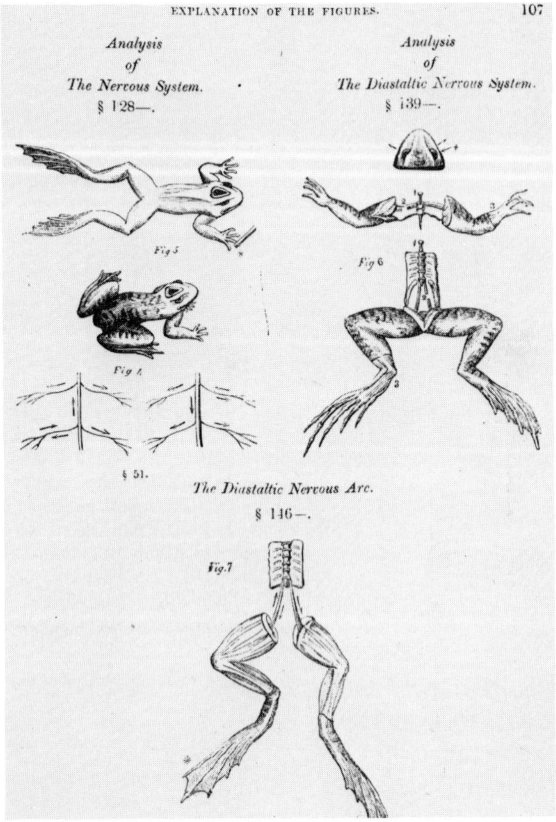

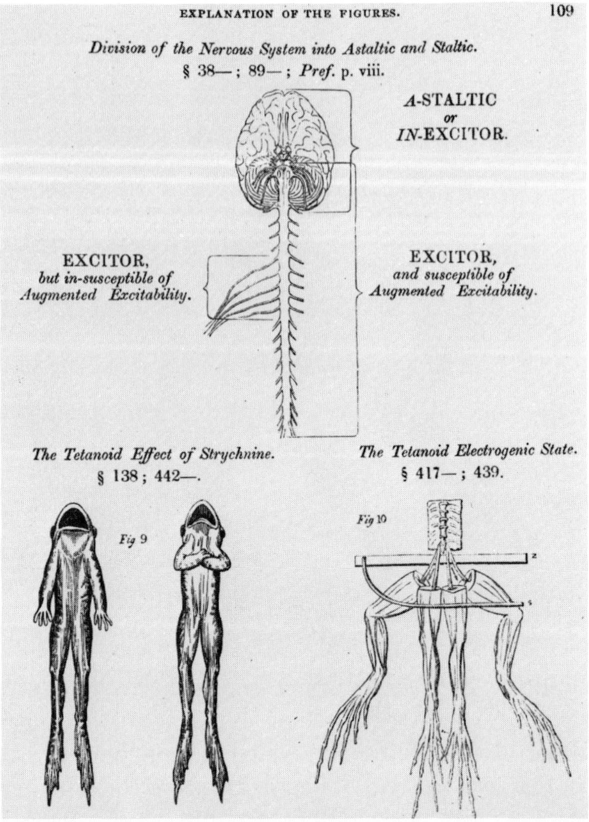

FIG. 107. Top left: A decerebrate frog moves only when touched; the limbs flex. Impulses pass in, across, along, and out from the spinal cord. Top right: A frog divided into three parts. Reflex activity is abolished by any one of: (1) remove cord; (2) divide nerves; (3) denude area of skin. Bottom centre: The diastaltic (through) nervous arc. Irritate one foot and both legs move. (After Hall.[145])

FIG. 108. Top centre: Two divisions of the nervous system – the 'cerebral' and the 'true spinal'. The former received sensations and initiated volition. The latter possessed its own nerves – excitor (afferent) and motory (efferent). They transmitted reflex activity. The divisions were separate, distinct, but were 'generally blended anatomically'. Bottom left: The reflex function is augmented with strychnine. Bottom right: The tetanoid electrogenic state, produced by the *direct* current. Contraction takes place on 'making' the circuit.

excited without telling upon *every* other ... but of what takes place *within* the structure of the spinal marrow, on which well might be inscribed the word – *mystery* – we are still entirely ignorant' (p. 13). Similarly, reflex activity could be seen to be influenced by the 'cerebral' system. There was 'the grasp reflex' of the sleeping infant (p. 15) and in the hemiplegic,[148] and the 'state of diminished excitability' or 'shock'. The diagnosis between cerebral and spinal paralysis was facilitated by reason of an understanding of these influences. In cerebral paralysis, the limbs are 'more irritable'; in spinal paralysis they are 'less irritable' (pp. 20–21).

Hall referred to a partially paraplegic patient 'who has no power of balancing himself without the aid of the eye' (p. 28). 'If a patient has lost the power of sensation in the feet, he cannot walk in the dark; the eye is essential to the due action of the muscles of the lower extremities.' He referred to Bell's 'Nervous Circle' between the brain and the muscle (p. 27) but he thought Bell's view was in error.

I believe we have no consciousness of the condition of individual muscles, or set of muscles ... the muscular sense is not in the muscle ... but in the nerve of touch, or of vision; and volition is not directed to any muscle, or set of muscles, but to the aim, object and purpose of their contraction (p. 27).

Like Bell, he also observed that patients with sensory loss in the hands were inclined to let objects fall if vision was directed elsewhere. He was impressed by the efficient manner in which control of the sphincters was normally exercised.

A sailor lies with his abdomen across the yard-arm. The pressure of the whole weight of his body is therefore on the sphincters . . . yet these sphincters do not fail in their office (p. 46).

Hall did not undertake any serious experiments with electricity. He thought Matteucci's were more 'pathological' than 'physiological'; he used 'too high a force'. But the electricity of frogs 'occupied the evenings of a winter' (p. 80).

In 1851 and again in 1852 two further monographs were published by Hall. These were *Synopsis of cerebral and spinal seizures*[149] and *Synopsis of apoplexy and epilepsy*.[150] They cannot be said to reflect any sensible application of his doctrines to the practice of medicine. Seizures resulted when some emotional or irritative influence caused a spasm of the muscles of the neck, which in turn impeded the return of blood from the brain and medulla. Tracheostomy was advised for certain cases but a hospital for epileptics should be provided, where one could 'ascertain the truth' and examine 'a series of statistics'. Psychosomatists of today will read that particularly troublesome agents were 'the Stock Exchange, speculations in commerce . . . railway property . . . the Comitia of Rome, and the mingled hopes and fears of the Senate House at Cambridge . . .'.[151]

Hall relinquished his practice in 1852 and in the following year sailed off with his wife to America, where they travelled extensively for fifteen months. He lectured, as we would have guessed, on his 'discoveries' and even managed to publish a paper on 'Experiments on the Spinal System in the Alligator (*Alligator Mississippienis*)'.[142]

By the time he died in 1857, although the vital anatomy of the reflex arc was not known, there was general acceptance of Hall's basic ideas, but no one, not even Hall, claimed ever to have seen his special nerve fibres. And his terminology died with him.

Assessing the importance of the work of a man who wrote so much, argued so much, repeated himself so much, ignored so much, and exaggerated so much – is apt to be trying. Many have commented on these lines. His paper of 1833 was immediately translated into German and appeared the following year in Müller's *Archives*. Flourens praised it and Alexander Walker in his *Documents and dates of modern discoveries of the nervous system* (1839)[73] included three of Hall's papers. In modern times, Fulton[152] wrote that Hall had 'introduced the concept that the spinal cord is a chain of segments whose functional units are separate reflex arcs'. Fearing[153] regarded Hall as 'the founder of the mechanical theory of reflex action' in his insistence on a vital connection with the cord. Riese[154] considered him 'the father of modern neurology' because 'for the first time in the history of neurology the concept of the reflex arc was adopted as a basic mechanism of nervous diseases'. Hoff and Kellaway[155] found that Hall had 'extended significantly the category of reflex actions', 'demonstrated that "tonic" actions were of reflex origin', and had 'extended the field of reflexes to include the autonomic system'. Jefferson[156] disagreed with Fearing's view that Hall's interpretations were purely mechanistic. To Jefferson, 'Hall saw what no one before him had seen, that it is impossible to put a stimulus ("an impression" he would have called it) into the spinal cord that did not have effects far beyond the anatomical segment to which the irritated nerves belonged'. Here was a foreshadowing of integration of the spinal cord. Canguilhem[157] said that it took 163 years for the idea of the reflex to become a fact – from 1670, when Willis's *De motu musculari* appeared, to 1833, on the publication of Hall's first memoir. Liddell[158] is content to give a dispassionate account of Hall's views and I could find no statement of summary to quote. Clarke and O'Malley[159] concluded that 'despite the controversies that centred about Hall's work, it is clear that he established the reflex as an essential and fundamental feature of nervous function', an opinion, I think, no modern neurologist or physiologist would care to challenge.

The following lines from Sherrington's *The integrative action of the nervous system* may justifiably be chosen to mark the significance of Hall's work.

> The edifice of the whole central nervous system is reared upon two neurones – the afferent root-cell and the efferent root-cell. These form the pillars of a fundamental reflex arch. And on the junction between these two are superposed and functionally set, mediately or immediately, all the other neural arcs, even those of the cortex of the cerebrum itself.[160]

The clinician. When Hall turned to physiological studies in London in 1830 he had already published articles on chemical and clinical topics,[142] and two books, *The diagnosis of disease* in 1817 and *An Essay on the symptoms and history of diseases*[161] in 1822. The latter was dedicated to Matthew Baillie and contains one of his many essays on the effects of loss of blood and the dangers of bloodletting. He became interested in diseases of the nervous system and in this book he included a chapter on the 'morbid states of the functions of the brain'. There is nothing in it to indicate in which direction his researches on the nervous system would follow. What he found 'extraordinary' was that the effects on the brain of 'fulness' and 'depletion', that is, congestion or anaemia, were 'very similar' although they were 'opposite states'. He also noted 'Mr. Parkinson's interesting pamphlet' on the Shaking Palsy in a discussion of tremor. On diagnosis in general he warned of the importance of distinguishing symptoms from diseases, and of describing the former 'fully and accurately'. Particular symptoms were rarely pathognomonic but 'the *kind* and *character* of the symptoms are frequently so' (p. 9). Dyspnoea, for example, was a symptom of chest disease, but how different it actually was in asthma, pneumonia, and hydrothorax.

As we know, Hall did not have the entry to hospital wards in London that Duchenne (1806–75), similarly placed without appointment, was enjoying in Paris. But then he would have been a difficult colleague, and though he applied for the Chair of Medicine at University College he was advised to withdraw. In some of his books and papers he refers to seeing patients at St. Marylebone and St. Pancras Infirmaries. He often said that there were cases that only a doctor in private practice saw, and that were not encountered in hospital wards. Privacy at the bedside encouraged closer observation. He referred to the great physicians of the day – Abercrombie, Bell, Bright, and others – but often slipping in a sly hint that their observations had been originally made by others.

In 1841 he published a book of some 380 pages, entitled *On the diseases and derangements of the nervous system*,[144] which he dedicated to Louis in Paris, 'who has accomplished for Medicine what Bacon projected for the Natural Sciences in general'. Not surprisingly, the book is a mixture of sense and nonsense. There is the inevitable recapitulation and reassertion followed by an endeavour to prove that, in comparison with Bell's work, his 'is of *still greater value* in its relation to pathology and therapeutics' (p. xi). Only personal possession of a copy of this work originally prompted me to read it; to do so in a library would be an arduous task.

The first three of the eight chapters are devoted to an account of the anatomy and physiology of the 'cerebral', the 'spinal', and the 'ganglionic' (autonomic) systems. Some idea of 'the practical applications of the physiological principles' covered in these chapters may be gathered by listing some of the symptoms and modes of therapy which Hall discusses: deglutition, choking and the stomach tube; defecation, rectal pain, tenesmus, and the rectum-bougie; sneezing, crowing respiration, and asthma; vomiting; conception and ejaculation and so on. There is a table of 'The Guards of the Orifices' (p. 58), the trifacial, the pneumogastric, and the spinal, with an account of the spasms and other forms of malfunction of *ingestion* and *egestion* they exhibit. The treatment recommended for choking (p. 79) recalls the recently recommended Heimlich manoeuvre (*J.A.M.A.* **234**, (1975), 398).

> Pressure being made on the abdomen, to prevent the descent of the diaphragm, a forcible blow should be made by the flat of the hand on the thorax. The effect of this is to induce an effort *similar* to that of expiration; the larynx being closed, oesophageal vomiting takes place, and the morsel is dislodged.

The paroxysmal rectal pain, 'generally during the first sleep, and of which I have not seen any description in medical writings' was probably *proctalgia fugax* (p. 86). In the 'ganglionic' pages, he says,

> If the sensation of the face be lost by paralysis, arising from disease of the *brain*, the eye is safe; but if the same event occur from compression or destruction of the *trifacial within* the cranium, by disease, or in an experiment, the eye ceases to be nourished, and becomes destroyed! In the former case, the nerve of sensation merely has suffered; in the latter, the nerve of nutrition, as well as sensation, has been involved in the disease or injury (p. 125).

In Chapters IV and V nervous disorders of infants and children are discussed. The foetus *in utero* is in a 'sort of ganglionic life'; the infant is under the influence of the true spinal marrow; then comes the development of the cerebral system. Congenital disorders of the brain such as apoplexy, asphyxia, idiocy, and spina bifida impede this natural progress. He quotes Cruveilhier (p. 139) stating that one-third of still-born children have apoplexy. For neonatal asphyxia Hall advocated mouth-to-mouth artificial respiration (p. 141). (His postural method of artificial respiration was introduced in 1856 and was standard practice for years.) In mentioning disorders, such as convulsions, which leave '*no* trace of pathological anatomy behind them', he stressed the value of Andral's ideas of 'a living pathology ... a subject fraught with deep interest' (p. 146). The principal *cerebral* disorders in children were encephalitis, tuberculosis, and hydrocephaloid disease, which he writes about without any reference to pathology. Then there were the croup-like convulsions, stammering, chorea, spasms, and paralysis. Chorea, needless to say, was an affection of the true spinal system, in which there was 'the want of harmony between the cerebral and the true spinal acts' (p. 195). He wondered why the limbs in infantile hemiplegia did not grow normally. 'Is it an affection of the spinal marrow, or of its nerves ...?' (p. 197).

In dealing with adult ailments, in Chapters VI and VII, he treats us to three more memoirs, before he gets down to clinical disorders. But they are quite interesting. The first is on 'Muscular Irritability in Paralytic Limbs'; the second on the 'Morbid Reflex and Retrograde Actions of the Spinal Marrow'; and the third on the 'Influence of Volition, of Emotion, and of the Vis Nervosa'.

In the first memoir (p. 207), he explains why attention to the degree of irritability of paralysed muscles is of diagnostic value. He describes the difference (without actually referring to tendon jerks, and so on) between what we would now call upper and lower motor neurone lesions. He distinguishes between 'cerebral' and 'spinal' lesions by noting the degree of 'tone', the presence of what we now term 'associated' movements, and the effects of emotion, stimulation, touching the sole of the foot, the palm of the hand, and the response to strychnine and galvanism. The 'severed influence of the cerebrum' was different from the 'severed influence of the spinal marrow'. Irritability was augmented in the former.

These differences could be discerned in paralysis of the face from cerebral and nerve lesions; in paralysis of a limb from cerebral and nerve lesions; and in paralysis from cord and cauda equina lesions.

A hemiplegic was 'able to close his hand upon a cane, although he was unable to do so without that excitant' (p. 202). Surprise, yawning, sneezing, cough, etc. cause movement in a hemiplegic limb.

In the second memoir (p. 224) he reminds us that reflex nervous arcs pass, not only across the spinal cord, but along it. Tickling the sole of the foot in a hemiplegic may induce flexion of the ipsilateral arm as well as of the paralysed leg. Another hemiplegic could not close the affected hand but 'immediately grasped any object placed in the palm' (p. 232). He alludes to the reflex grasp of the sleeping child (p. 226), and to a hemiplegic in whom slightly touching the sole of the foot caused, not only retraction of the limb, but also extension of the toes (p. 232). In paraplegia, priapism and retraction of the legs on touching the soles were now commonly observed. He discusses 'The Influence of Shock' (p. 247), explaining that both in experiment and practice it is evident 'that the reflex actions are not manifested immediately after an injury of the spinal marrow, but that they become gradually established more remotely'. And again, 'the first influence of shock is to diminish the excito-motory power' (p. 252). He did not think it a consequence of circulatory failure, but he could not explain it.

What Jefferson[162] considered 'the most beautiful description in a few words of what we mean by "spinal shock" ', comes in the final pages of this book.

In the presence of a young Parisian student I divided the spinal marrow of a frog. I pinched the toes, but there was no movement, no reflex action. My companion observed, 'Ah, c'est fini'; I replied 'Non, ce n'est pas commencé'. In a few minutes the reflex actions became obvious and in a few minutes more most energetic. We had examined the circulation previous to the division of the spinal marrow. It was most active. But immediately after that division scarcely a movement was to be seen. Like the reflex actions, however, the vigour of the circulation was gradually restored. (p. 359).

Delightedly, Jefferson remarked 'What could be better than that, "Ah, it's all over", and Marshall Hall's reply, "No, it hasn't started yet!" '

At the end of this second memoir, he refers to those cases of traumatic paraplegia in which paresis above the level of the lesion had been observed, reminding him of the reflex responses he had similarly observed above the point of cord stimulation. In the course of one quoted case history in which there was obvious lumbar displacement, the arms were contracted, and there was loss of sensation; but in the legs, the right had lost both power and feeling, whereas the left had the power of feeling but not that of motion. He found this very mysterious; if there were 'retrograde influences of the spinal marrow, we must not always conclude that the disease or injury is situated *above* the origin of the nerves affected'. Of course, the level of a vertebral injury could then only be crudely assessed, but five years later the graduating Brown-Séquard showed in his thesis how a unilateral lesion of the cord might present. Meanwhile Hall pleaded that 'in every case of cerebral or spinal disease, and disease of the nerves in their course, the condition of the reflex actions, and of the retrograde influences of the spinal marrow and nerves, will henceforth be carefully examined' (p. 251).

There is little in the third memoir on the different influences of volition and emotion that he had not already said several times previously, save that, in illustration of his ideas, he quoted the case of Lord Nelson. Normally, the emotions are under the control of the will, 'but when the latter influence is withdrawn, that of the former becomes strongly manifest'. 'Thus the agitation of Nelson's heroic mind' would never normally be revealed in his countenance, 'but the stump of his amputated arm, withdrawn from the habitual subjugation of volition, was violently agitated on many trying occasions of emotion' (p. 256). Nelson died in 1805, when Hall was fifteen years of age, so this was very unlikely to have been a personal observation.

Although he begins Chapter VII with the words 'I now proceed to treat the individual diseases of the nervous system' (p. 269) the reader soon finds that, at every turn, in the remaining pages, he reverts to a discussion, never from a fresh stance, of his own precious system of nerves. Thus, for example, he writes, 'In detailing the *symptoms* of epilepsy, I shall have to repeat all that I have said respecting the physiology of the true spinal system' (p. 323). In the sections on encephalitis, strokes, tubercles, tumours (only a dozen lines), epilepsy, tetanus, hydrophobia, and various 'spasms' there is no attempt to give a picture of the natural history of a disorder, nor to correlate symptoms, signs, and pathological anatomy. Perhaps we see here a consequence of his relative isolation from hospital life and the lessons of the post-mortem room. But we also get glimpses of the acuteness of his clinical sense, as in the case of what was probably a glomus tumour of an index finger (p. 300), how epilepsy may manifest itself 'in a momentary loss of consciousness' (p. 326), and how paralysis agitans may be 'hemiplegic' or 'general'. A young man with 'weakness and agitation of the right arm and leg ... a peculiar lateral rocking motion of the eyes ... and defective articulation', may have had spino-cerebellar degeneration.

In considering the localization of cerebral diseases (p. 283) he merely refers to earlier passages where he had quoted the findings of the Paris school, adding nothing of his own. He thought neither Flourens or Gall had shown that the cerebellum was an organ of equilibrium or generation, but compression of the medulla was probably responsible for the latter view. Convulsions were more frequent than paralysis in diseases of the cerebellum. In some instances there had been loss of balance, as in intoxication. Sensibility was sometimes affected, and if paralysis did develop in cerebellar disease, it was usually contralateral.

Organic disease of the brain could mimic insanity and lead to improper incarceration in an asylum. He mentioned (p. 296) the case of his brother who suffered from headache, and developed a right hemiplegia with aphasia, and 'erroneous ideas took possession of his mind'. He was consigned to an asylum, and autopsy subsequently disclosed a left hemisphere lesion (probably a tumour), which was not 'clot or cicatrix'. Such cases required special public facilities, where the paralysed could be cared for. He said the same about a hospital for epileptics and when the hospital at Queen Square was opened in 1860 it was for the 'Paralysed and Epileptic'.

Epilepsy could arise from any disorder within the cranium or spine (p. 319), so there was a *centric* and an *eccentric* type of epilepsy. Convulsions resulted whenever a cerebral or spinal lesion irritated the medulla oblongata.

Aetiology in nervous diseases is generally mentioned in terms of what we would now call stress, but with special emphasis always on *venus solitaria* and *venus nimia*, which were death to the true spinal system. And as for abortion and parturition, why, '*Obstetrics*, as a science, is one of the true spinal system' (p. 341).

A much larger work was promised. And also a new asylum.

Claude Bernard (1813–1878)

Whereas Magendie remained a practising physician, his assistant, Claude Bernard, spent all his time in the laboratory. 'I am not practising clinical medicine here; but I must take account of it, nevertheless, and assign it the first place in experimental medicine.'[163] He went on to say that hospitals were

> ... the first field of observation which a physician enters, but the true sanctuary of medical science is a laboratory; only there can he seek the explanations of life in the normal and pathological states by means of experimental analysis.[164]

The hospital ward was not a laboratory; the 'observational physician', to become a 'scientific physician', had to take a second step and subject his observations to analysis. This necessitated experiment. Vivisection was one type of experimentation; 'Galen may be considered its founder'.[165] 'Experimentation is only an observation carried further by artificial means – a decomposition or analysis of phenomena with counter proof etc'.[166] 'Experiment is fundamentally only induced observation.'[167]

Bernard explained that although he could understand a physician saying that he could not always rationally account for what he was doing, he nevertheless felt that if the physician 'goes on to proclaim his medical tact or his intuition as a criterion which he then means to impose on others without further proof, that is wholly antiscientific'.[168]

He considered anatomy itself 'a sterile science', its usefulness lying in the field of physiology and pathology.[169] 'What can the form of the brain or the nerves teach us about their functions?'[170] The purely anatomical point of view had been too dominating, as exemplified by Haller's view that physiology was merely 'animated anatomy'. 'To physiology, anatomy is only an auxiliary science.' As for pathological anatomy 'the changes noted in cadavers after death really show characteristics by which to recognise and classify diseases, rather than lesions capable of explaining death'.[171] Summarizing his view of medical investigation, he said,

> In a word, a physician should not hold to anatomical pathology alone, to explain the disease; he starts from observation of the patient and later explains the disease by physiology with the help of pathological anatomy and all the allied sciences used by investigators of biological phenomena.[172]

At the end of his life, he concluded,

> The experimental method is only the expression of the natural progress of the human spirit, seeking the scientific truths which are outside us. In the first place, each man has his own ideas about what he can see, and he interprets the phenomena of nature by anticipation before knowing them from experience. This tendency is spontaneous, a preconceived idea has always been and will always be, the first springboard for an investigating spirit. The experimental method strives to change this *a priori* conception, founded on an intuition or vague feeling about things, into *a posteriori* interpretation, established on the experimental study of phenomena. This is why the experimental method is also known as *méthode a posteriori* ...[173]

This 'scientific' attitude did not imply any failure to appreciate the role of the doctor in caring for his patients, for he said,

> A physician, in fact, is by no means physician to living beings in general, not even physician to the human race, but rather, physician to a human individual and still more physician to an individual in certain morbid conditions peculiar to himself and forming what is called his idiosyncracy.[174]

Neither did the 'analytic' method prevent him adopting a holistic view.

> If it is possible to dissect all the parts of the body, to isolate them in order to study them in their structure, form and connections it is not the same in life, where all parts co-operate at the same time in a common aim. An organ does not live on its own, one could often say it did not exist anatomically, as the boundary established is sometimes purely arbitrary. What lives, what exists, is the whole, and if one studies all the parts of any mechanism separately, one does not know the way they work. In the same way, anatomically, we take the organism apart, but we cannot grasp the whole. This whole can only be seen when the organs are in motion.[175]

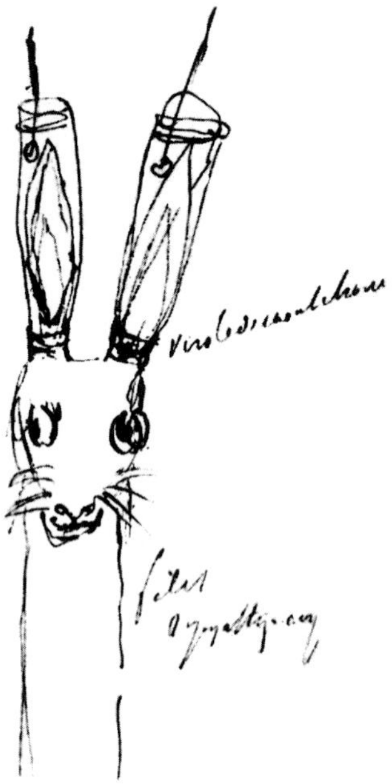

FIG. 109. Cervical sympathectomy. Claude Bernard's sketch of a rabbit with left cervical sympathetic nerve section. Ears are enclosed in glass tubes containing thermometers to register the rise in temperature in the flushing left ear. (Courtesy Musée de l'Histoire de la Médicine, L'École de Médicine, Paris.)

Experiment and criticism. The art of research is described in his famous *Introduction to the study of experimental medicine* (1865).[163] Here, with touching faith and honesty, he outlined his aims, methods, and philosophy, and from his own work he offered examples to illustrate how investigations may come about or be planned, how they may develop, and how the principles of criticism should be applied. No book of science so clearly portrays the mind of its author. It is still revered.

The starting point of an investigation may be an observation or an hypothesis or theory. An observation may be a chance one, as when he noticed that the urine of a fasting rabbit was clear. It was this that started him off on the investigations which led to the discovery of the role of the pancreas in digestion and fat metabolism – his first major achievement. A second type of observation was one that was not just happened upon, but that was induced by the investigator. Here he quoted his work on curare. He knew it could kill an animal, but no more; the mechanism was not known. Injected into a frog it paralysed the muscles of the limbs, but not of the heart, before it actually died, suggesting that the poison acted on nerve rather than muscle. Electrical stimulation confirmed this.

The starting point which led him to the discovery of the vasomotor nerves was a theory. He was interested in the influence of the nervous system on the phenomena of nutrition and temperature regulation. He knew that in peripheral paralysis, a limb could be warm or cold and that sympathetic nerve fibres 'especially followed the arteries'. Perhaps, he reasoned, it was involvement of these fibres that slowed down heat production. If so, then, if they could be cut without injuring the motor and sensory fibres, 'I should then find the part cooled by paralysis of the vascular nerves.' It was possible to do this by choosing the rabbit and the horse as experimental animals, for in them the cervical sympathetic nerves were suitably separate. What happened was the reverse of what he expected; the face and ear of the animal flushed and became warm. But, he stressed, 'without the original guiding

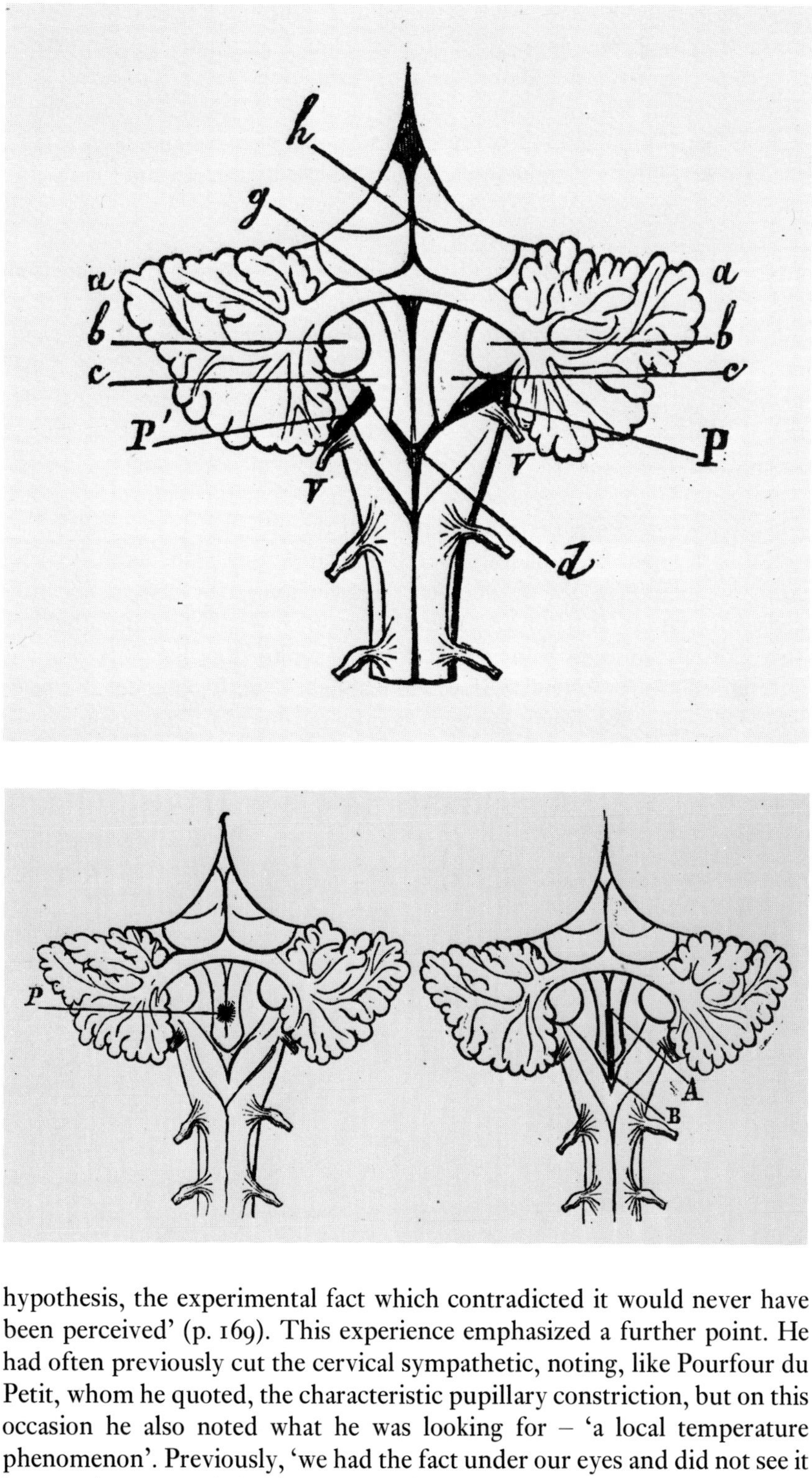

FIG. 110. Piqûre of the fourth ventricle in the rabbit. 'Rendering the animal diabetic' depended on the actual site of the puncture. Failure was frequent, but he was successful in these three examples. Top: a,a, cerebellum; b,b, auditory tubercles; c,c, olives; d, nib of calamus scriptorius; g, aqueduct; h, corpora quadrigemina; v,v, vagus nerves. Lateral lesions at P and P′ caused acute rotation, with glycosuria in one hour, persisting for six. Next day it had subsided; at autopsy the liver was free of sugar. Bottom left: Mid-line autopsy lesion which had provoked glycosuria which persisted for six hours. Bottom right: Mid-line incision (AB) which provoked glycosuria in two hours and which persisted for six hours, when the animal was sacrificed. (After Bernard,[207] Vol. 1, Figs. 51–53, pp. 405–7.)

hypothesis, the experimental fact which contradicted it would never have been perceived' (p. 169). This experience emphasized a further point. He had often previously cut the cervical sympathetic, noting, like Pourfour du Petit, whom he quoted, the characteristic pupillary constriction, but on this occasion he also noted what he was looking for – 'a local temperature phenomenon'. Previously, 'we had the fact under our eyes and did not see it because it conveyed nothing to our mind'.

When he turned from observation to interpretation, Bernard proclaimed his faith in the principles of scientific criticism. Determinism meant that in experimentation one could not accept 'contradictory' facts; 'I assert that the word exception is unscientific'. If the results of a particular experiment varied, then one must identify the conditions that were responsible. He cited the experiment in which he made a dog diabetic by puncturing the floor of the fourth ventricle (p. 173). At the time, he was trying to find out if the 'secretion' of sugar by the liver was controlled by the nervous system. Cutting or stimulating the vagi had no effect so he sought to stimulate their site of origin in the floor of the fourth ventricle. He succeeded the first time, but failed on eight or ten further attempts. He eventually found that the vital factor was the exact point of the *piqûre*. But, he said, if the reverse had happened, if the negative results had come first, he would have concluded that this theory was false. 'Yet I should have been wrong.' In the event, he found that if he cut the vagi before he performed the piqûre, he still provoked a diabetic response. We now know that the piqûre effect is a consequence of sympathetic stimulation of the adrenals.

The puzzling effects of spinal root stimulation provided Bernard with a second example of the neglect of the principles involved in scientific criticism (p. 174). It will be recalled that in 1822 Magendie concluded that sensation and motion were not *exclusively* confined to the posterior and anterior roots, respectively. It was a justifiable conclusion, but it caused confusion. In 1839, when Bernard had joined him in his laboratory, the confusion was increased because Magendie was finding that the anterior

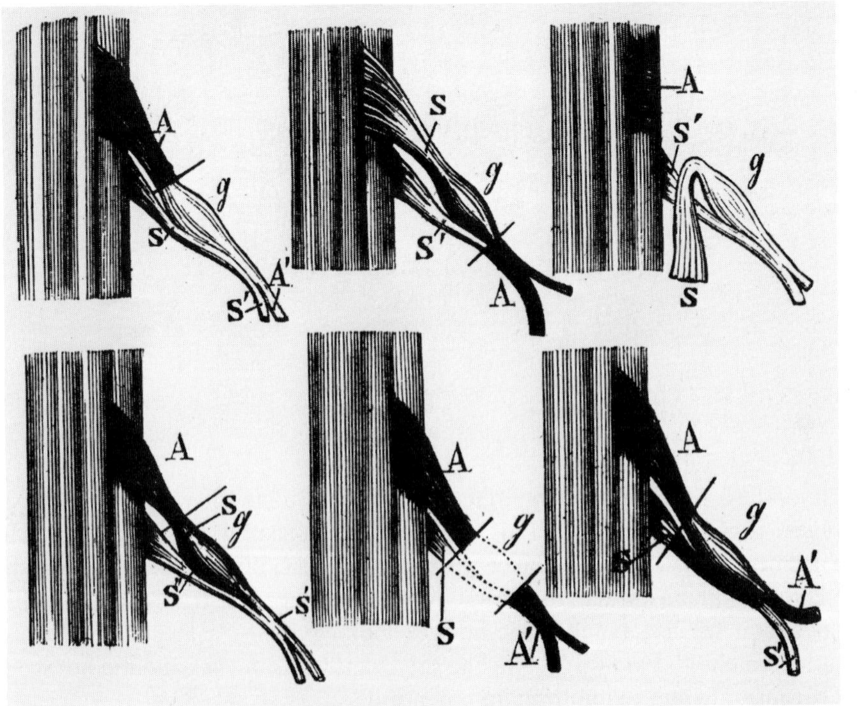

FIG. 111. The effects of sections of spinal nerve roots (at C.2). Top left: Section of the *posterior* root (A), proximal to the ganglion (g), causes degeneration only of the central (shaded) portion of that root. Top centre: Section at the *root junction*, just distal to the ganglion, causes degeneration of peripheral motor and sensory fibres (shaded). Top right: Avulsion of *posterior* rootlets at A, does not cause any degeneration in the central (reflected) portion of the posterior root. Bottom left: Section of the *anterior* root at S″ causes degeneration only of peripheral motor fibres. (In the original legend there is no reference to section of the posterior root at S; no shading of peripheral degeneration of the motor fibres.) Bottom centre: Section of *both roots* with removal of the ganglion. Peripherally, there is degeneration (A′, shaded) of motor and sensory fibres. Centrally, there is degeneration of the posterior root (A, shaded), but not of the anterior. Bottom right: Section of *both roots* just above the ganglion. Centrally, there is degeneration only of the posterior root (shaded). Peripherally, degeneration is confined to the motor fibres (A′, shaded). (After Bernard,[207] Vol.1, Fig.39, p. 237.)

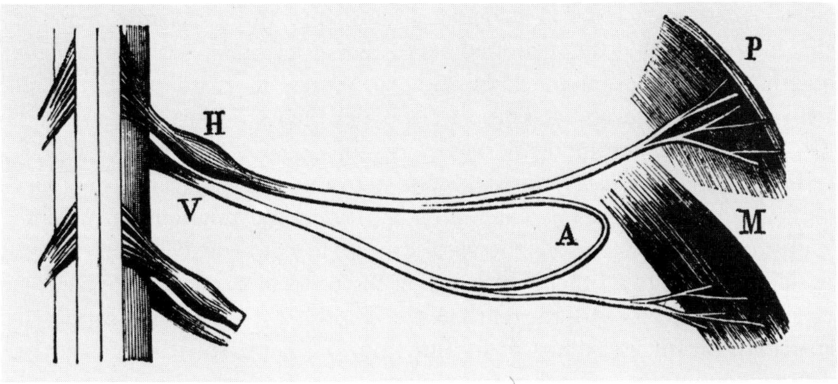

FIG. 112. 'Recurrent Sensitivity.' Its abolition by root section depends on the position in relation to a hypothetical loop (A) between the two roots. (H, posterior; V, anterior; P, skin; M, muscle.) Bernard suggested that information passed in both directions in the loop to each motor and sensory centre of the spinal cord, 'in reality an organ'. (After Bernard,[207] Vol. 2, Fig. 15, p. 462.)

roots could be 'very sensitive'. There was debate and criticism, but Bernard pointed out that much of it was ill-founded. 'We do not have to choose between the two results . . . [i.e. 1822 and 1839]; we must accept them both and merely explain and define them in their respective conditions.' Sometimes stimulation of the anterior roots was painful and at other times it was not. Bernard confirmed this and subsequently found that if time was allowed for the passing of shock, the anterior roots consistently displayed this 'recurrent sensitivity' as it came to be called. Magendie thought it might be due to the way in which some sensory fibres entered the anterior root and then looped back to enter the posterior root. But, as Cranefield[176] has pointed out, there are many possible reasons for the phenomenon of 'recurrent sensitivity' and there is no universally accepted explanation. When Magendie saw muscular contraction on stimulating a posterior root, and when he provoked pain on stimulating an anterior root, he did not make the crucial interpretation of Marshall Hall, that these were manifestations of activity in a reflex arc.

To Bernard, who returned to the problem of the spinal nerve roots on several occasions over the years, the debate made it clear that if experimental results are inconsistent one should suspend judgement; 'negative facts, no matter how numerous they may be, can never destroy a single positive fact'. Criticisim is scientific 'when it explains everything without denying anything and finds the correct causation of apparently contradictory facts' (p. 178).

The nervous system. Throughout his life Bernard stressed the importance of the role of the nervous system. 'Always pursue the idea that the physical and chemical phenomena of the organism are dominated by the nervous system.'[177] He thought the brain could be regarded as a gland; 'it receives vessels and nerves and can consequently be modified by blood and nerves'.[178] His first publication, when he was thirty years old, in 1843, was on the chorda tympani nerve.[179] Magendie had chosen him as his 'preparateur' because of his anatomical skill, and Bernard was able to demonstrate the origin of the chorda tympani in the facial nerve. When the former was cut there was unilateral loss of taste but he did not conclude that subserving taste was one of its primary functions. And it was only years later that he noticed that the sectioned nerve also reduced the secretion of saliva and that its stimulation caused dilatation of vessels in the submaxillary gland with increased secretion. These were experiments performed during the discovery of the vasomotor nerves.

In the following year came his second paper, on the spinal accessory nerve of Willis.[180] Here he was examining its functional relationship with the vagus, in the innervation of the vocal cords. He erroneously concluded that both nerves supplied them. In avulsing the roots of the accessory nerve he injured adjacent roots of the tenth nerve. To Bell, a double nerve supply to a structure meant assistance in its function. To Bernard, it suggested two different functions, probably antagonistic.

In the subsequent decade, while pursuing the investigations which led to two of his major discoveries – the role of the pancreas in digestion and fat metabolism, and that of the liver in carbohydrate metabolism – he published some twenty-seven papers dealing with the nervous system.[181] The most famous were those concerning the nature of curare paralysis (1849–52) and the discovery of the vasomotor nerves (1851–53). There were studies of the functions of the fifth, seventh, and tenth cranial nerves; he described the effects of section of the vagi on the action of the lungs, the heart, and the oesophagus. The function of the spinal nerve roots and the cerebral and cerebellar peduncles engaged his attention and he studied the effects of strychnine and atropine on the nervous system. It was a decade of unique achievement, and by the time he was forty he was famous.

The effect of vagal section on the heart was to 'not only affect the shape of the heart but alter its contractile force'.[182] The oesophagus was paralysed so that, although the animal could chew and swallow, 'food did not arrive in the stomach'. It accumulated in the oesophagus and was finally rejected, but in one or two days food was able to enter the stomach.[183] Section of a cerebral peduncle in a rabbit caused it to immediately start wheeling around; toward the side of the section when it was made below the trigeminal nerve, and away from it when the section was above the nerve.[184] Section of an inferior

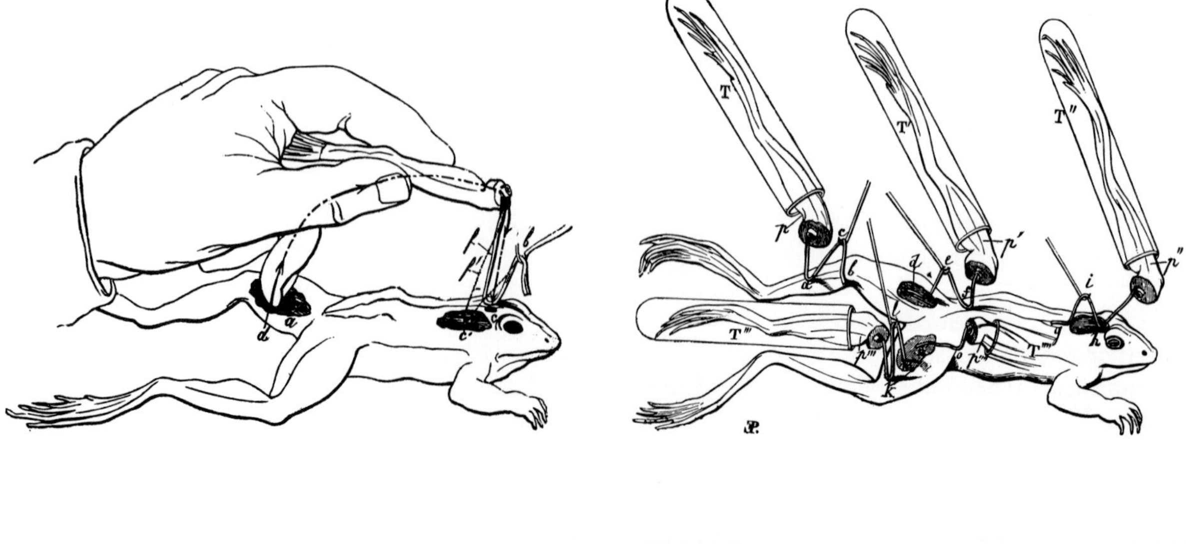

FIG. 113. 'The musculo-cutaneous electrical current in the frog.' Left: An exposed area of thigh muscle (*a*) is electrically positive (+). Skin (*c*) is electrically negative (−). A frog leg with attached nerve (*f*), a 'galvanoscopic foot', is held in one hand. The other hooks up with a glass rod, the end of the nerve (*b*). When the loop of nerve touches the skin at *c*, the frog leg twitches. The current passes through the little finger (*d*), the frog leg, and the nerve. No twitch occurs if the nerve loop touches a second area of exposed muscle (*c*′), for then, the two surfaces being positive, there is no current. (After Bernard,[207] Vol. I, Fig. 45, p. 311.) Right: With isolated 'galvanoscopic legs', muscular contraction depends on whether the contacts are made with skin or muscle. T – no contraction; T′, T″, T‴ – contraction occurs. (After Bernard,[207] Vol. I, Fig. 46, p. 312.)

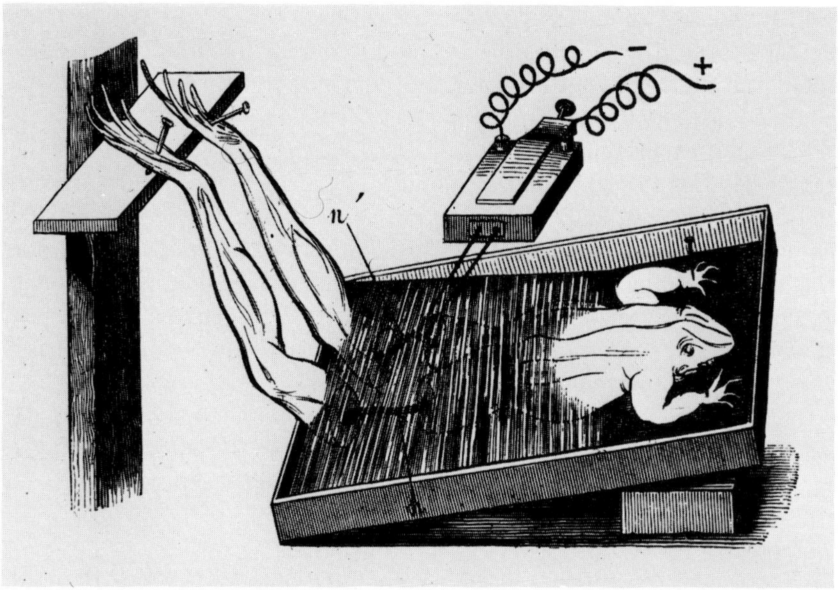

FIG. 114. In a frog preparation, when the sciatic nerves (*n* and *n*′) are the sole connection between hind limbs and trunk, dessication and inactivity can be prevented if they are immersed in a fluid such as oil, serum, or blood in an inclined tray. One limb and nerve can be placed outside the tray, for comparative tests. (After Bernard,[207] Vol. 1, Fig. 33, p. 188.)

cerebellar peduncle caused a similar rotation of a rabbit but also the appearance of albumen and sugar in its urine.[185] With regard to the motor and sensory functions he felt that, although their pathways were distinct, their functions were 'intimately linked' and that a sensory lesion affected motor function 'proportional to its extent'.[186] A deafferented frog's limb was used in an awkward fashion. Brown-Séquard (1817–94) thought that in the frog this effect was temporary.[187]

Curare. Curare proved to be a valuable weapon in Bernard's hands; it served him in his constant pursuit of physiological analysis. His first paper on it was in 1849[188] and his last in 1875.[189] By 1856[190] he had reached the conclusion that it did not act centrally, on the brain or spinal cord, nor directly on the muscles. Sensory nerves were not affected. Paralysis resulted from a selective action on the motor nerves. First, he demonstrated that it could be introduced into the stomach of a dog, without causing paralysis; it was not destroyed by the gastric juice for the stomach contents remained lethal when injected into another animal. Next, he injected curare subcutaneously into the back of a frog. When paralysis was appearing he exposed the lumbar nerves and stimulated them electrically; there was no response in the hind limbs, although direct stimulation of their muscles provoked contractions. Thus, the drug appeared to act directly on the motor nerves.

Then came his famous experiment in which he passed a ligature around the waist of a frog, isolating the hind limbs from the rest of the body, except for the sciatic nerve trunk. Curare was injected subcutaneously on the back of the frog, above the ligature. Only the hind limbs remained unparalysed. Stimuli applied to the paralysed, but still sensitive, anterior portion of the frog induced reflex movements in the posterior portion (Fig. 115a).

Bernard also showed that an arterial ligature could protect a hind limb

(a)

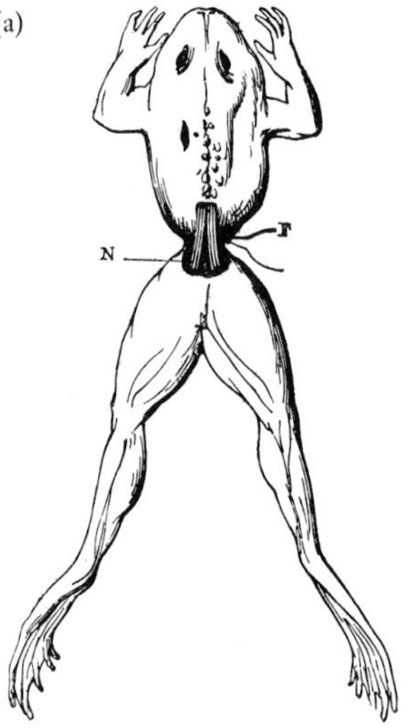

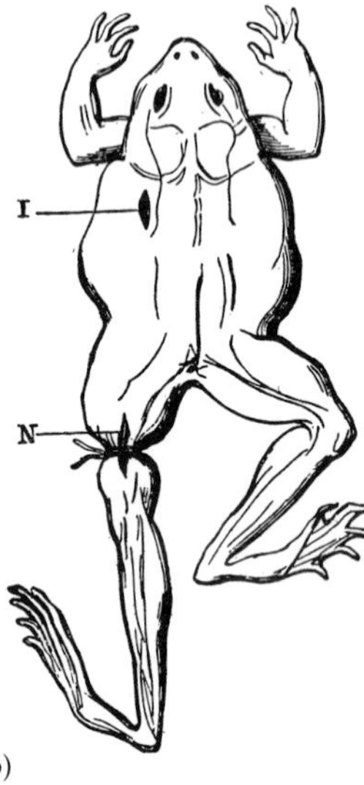

(b)

FIG. 115. The curarized frog. (a) A ligature (F) is tied around the waist of a frog, but excluding the sciatic nerve trunks (N). Curare is then injected subcutaneously on the back of the frog above the ligature. Only the hind limbs remain unparalysed. But sensation is preserved for when the forelimbs are pinched, the hind limbs twitch. (After Bernard,[207] Vol. 1, Fig. 34, p. 203.) (b) A ligature is tied around one hind limb, excluding the sciatic nerve (N). A curare injection does not paralyse this limb. But a reflex contraction could still be obtained in the other limb, by pinching it or a forelimb. (After Bernard,[207] Vol. 1, Fig. 35, p. 204.)

from the effect of a curare injection into the back of a frog. Stimulation of the lumbar nerves of the ligatured limb produced a contraction; on the other side it had no effect. But the ligatured limb responded reflexly when the paralysed hind limb was stimulated (Fig. 115b).

In these experiments the unaffected sensory nerves provided the transmission of the stimulus. Immobility, Bernard realized, could result from motor or sensory paralysis. In the case of curare, it was essentially motor. Bernard also used isolated nerve–muscle preparations to examine what happened when curare was applied directly to nerve or muscle. In 1859 he commented on the use of curare in the treatment of tetanus.[191] And just one hundred years after he first examined the poison, it was introduced as a muscle relaxant in general anaesthesia.[192]

Recently, Fessard[193] has disclosed that in one of his notebooks Bernard had written 'curare must act on the terminal plates of motor nerves' – a remarkable anticipation of the concept of junctional transmission.

The vasomotor nerves. It has often been pointed out that the part Bernard played in the discovery of glycogen and his part in the discovery of the vasomotor nerves were very different.[194, 195] In the former, his contribution was practically complete, and he immediately recognized the importance of it all. With the vasomotor nerves, however, there had already been important previous contributions; also, it was other workers, rather than he himself, who first appreciated the significance of his earlier result – the vasomotor function of the cervical sympathetic.

Although the notion of voluntary and involuntary contraction of muscle fibres was long known, it was only recently appreciated that there were two types of muscle fibre – the striated and non-striated – and that the latter could be found in the walls of arteries. Stilling (1810–79) in 1840 had actually postulated the existence of 'vaso-motor' nerves, which could involuntarily influence the circulation of the blood.[196, 197] The effects of section of the cervical sympathetic on the pupil were well known, but no one before Bernard had noted the effect on the circulation of the side of the face and head. In his first two papers[198, 199] on the subject, in 1852, it was the effects 'sur la sensibilité et sur la calorification' and 'sur la chaleur animale' to which he respectively referred in his titles. But he noted, in the first, that in addition to increase in sensation and temperature, 'the circulation was more active, and particularly apparent in the ears of rabbits'. He wondered whether this was 'the cause or the effect of the increase in animal heat'. He made a similar comment in the second paper, and suggested that the rise in temperature might not be solely the effect of increased circulation.

In the following year[200] he also commented on the observations of Budge (1811–84), the Bonn ophthalmologist, and Waller (1816–70), the English physiologist, on the innervation of the pupillo-dilator fibres of the iris.[201] They had traced degenerating sympathetic fibres, following cervical section, to a 'cilio-spinal centre' between the sixth cervical and fourth dorsal vertebrae.

Bernard also noted in this report that on the side of the section 'all the features on the corresponding side of the face appeared drawn, in consequence of the contraction of the muscles'. Galvanization of the upper cut end of the sympathetic nerve reversed the effects of section, dilating the pupil as in the Budge and Waller experiment of galvanization of the cilio-spinal centre in the intact animal.

In another paper in the same year[202] he summarized the effect of section of the cervical sympathetic nerve. In addition to narrowing of the pupil there were (1) narrowing of the palpebral fissure; (2) retraction of the globe of the eye; (3) narrowing of the nostril and mouth on the side of the section; and (4) increased temperature and circulation on the affected side of the head and face.

The true cause of the rise in temperature of the affected side of the face and head in all these experiments was, we now know, a result of vascular dilatation, a conclusion he only reached some years later. It was only when he discovered that stimulation of the chorda tympani caused not only vascular dilatation but secretion of saliva that Bernard was led to reveal that there were two kinds of nerve fibre involved; the sympathetic constrictor of blood vessels and the chorda tympani vasodilator. Thus, there were 'deux ordres de nerfs' – the vasomotor nerves.[203] But the importance of the vasodilation had been appreciated earlier by Brown-Séquard,[204] Budge,[205] and Waller.[206]

Throughout the forty-three lectures which formed the basis of his book on the nervous system[207] he stressed that the old type of ablative experiment was going to be inadequate. Function was not going to be disclosed by such crude methods. The experimenter with preconceived or fixed ideas was a danger. Disease must be produced in animals by devising experiments such as 'piqûre', in which 'rabbits were rendered diabetic' (Vol. 1, p. 397), or sectioning the vagus, which made them hungry (Vol. 2, p. 414), or the vasomotor nerves, which made them warm. The curare experiments demonstrated that the mechanisms of paralysis were probably diverse; other toxins should also be used in their study (Vol. 1, p. 196). The properties of motion, sensation, and the contractility of muscles could probably be best examined by first isolating them (Vol. 1, p. 205). Not that experimentation was the only way. Clinical and pathological studies were vital. But the best progress would be achieved by the collaboration of specialists.[208]

It was the nervous system, Bernard said, 'which inter-connects all the tissues of the organism and makes them react one upon the other'.[209] Hughlings Jackson was to refer to 'an important principle of Bernard's ... that every part of the body has some degree of autonomy, and is yet in subordination to, is directed and controlled by, the nervous system or some part of it'. He quoted Bernard's comment on the significance of the increased reflex excitability that was found below the level of a section of the spinal cord.

We find, in this phenomenon, a pathological fact which merits serious study, *all the more so because it applies to the nervous system in all its extent*. A nerve separated from its centre of origin acquires special properties, which nevertheless only differ from the normal in their excessive intensity.[210]

Hughlings Jackson was developing his concept of levels within the nervous system and of the release effects which follow injury to higher centres.

Sherrington also acknowledged a concept of Bernard's, when he wrote (on page 3 of *The integrative action of the nervous system*) that 'The nervous system is in a certain sense the highest expression of that system which French physiologists term the *milieu interne*.'

C. E. Brown-Séquard (1817–1894)

Claude Bernard's successor in the Chair of Experimental Medicine at the Collège de France, in 1878, was Brown-Séquard.[211,212] He came to Paris, in 1838, at the age of twenty-one. Accompanying him was his widowed mother, a native of Mauritius; his father, an American sailor, having been lost at sea when Brown-Séquard was an infant. Like Bernard, he also had literary intentions, but was advised to study medicine and he graduated in 1846. Few men can have written a doctoral thesis of such a celebrated nature as Brown-Séquard's. It was entitled 'Recherches et Expériences sur la Physiologie de la Moelle Épinière' and was the first of his many accounts of experimental section of the spinal cord in living animals, aimed at tracing the sensory pathways. Section of the posterior columns did not appreciably diminish sensibility and hemisection of the cord did not cause ipsilateral sensory loss.

FIG. 116 (*facing*). *Fig. 20.* A haemorrhage in one side of the spinal cord; it caused paralysis of the leg on that side and loss of sensation below the level of the lesion on the other side. (Brown-Séquard quoted this case from Ollivier.) *Fig. 22.* Decussation of lateral columns at *PD*. The anterior columns, AA, do not decussate. *Fig. 23.* Three kinds of reflex action. A sensory stimulus enters via the posterior root and ganglion (*pr* and *g*) and ascends (dotted line) to three nerves going to a gland (*g*), a muscle (*m*) and a blood vessel (*v*). *Fig. 24.* Longitudinal section of posterior aspect of the pons and medulla, to show 'the pretended decussation of the olivary columns' at CC. *Fig. 25.* Base of brain, a dissection to show cerebello-pontine fibres on left and *crus cerebelli* on right. A lesion at *h* 'causes a paralysis on the corresponding side' by a 'reflex action upon some other part of the nervous centres'. *Fig. 26.* Tumour upon the *crus cerebelli* which produced 'a peculiar kind of paralysis' on the same side. (After Brown-Séquard,[214] Pl. III.)

For the next six poverty-stricken years he struggled to gain a foothold in the field of experimental medicine, but in 1852 he gave up and went to America. By then, Claude Bernard, only four years his senior, had achieved fame with his four major discoveries. When Brown-Séquard returned to Paris in 1855 he took up clinical practice in earnest but never relinquished his activities in the experimental field. It was in the following year that he proved that adrenalectomy was invariably fatal.[213] Later,[214] he wrote that neurological research necessitated both 'experimentation upon living animals, and observation of pathological cases', and that in the case of conduction in the spinal cord 'experiments on animals could not lead to certain conclusions which I shall be able to draw from some of the pathological cases I intend relating'.[215]

Following his 1846 thesis, Brown-Séquard, in 1849,[216] made it clear that in performing hemisection of the spinal cord he was questioning the teaching of Longet (1811–71) and others, first proposed by Bell, that the posterior columns were the continuation of the posterior spinal roots, conveying sensation to the brain. Longet, a great supporter of Bell in France, considered that the posterior columns entered the cerebellum via the inferior peduncles, although admitting that cerebellar lesions did not cause sensory loss. By then Brown-Séquard had performed the experiment sixty times, usually in the dorsal cord. He found that hemisection led to 'a momentary diminution of sensitivity in the corresponding hind-limb',

Fig. 20.

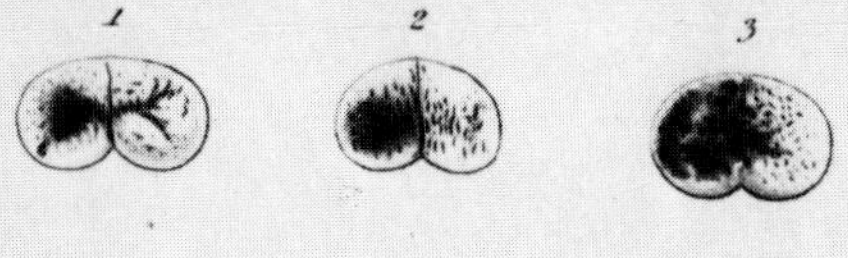

Fig. 21.

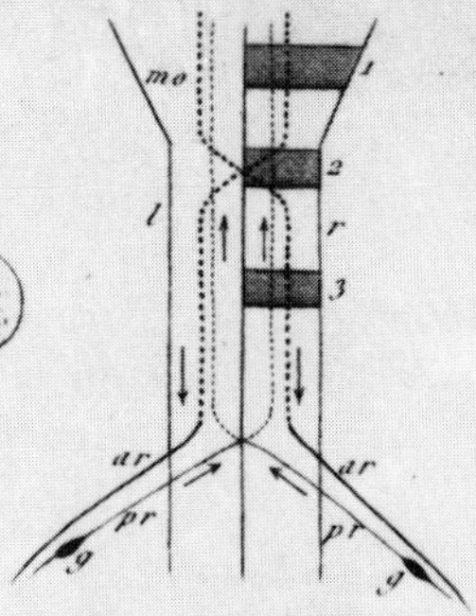

Fig. 22.

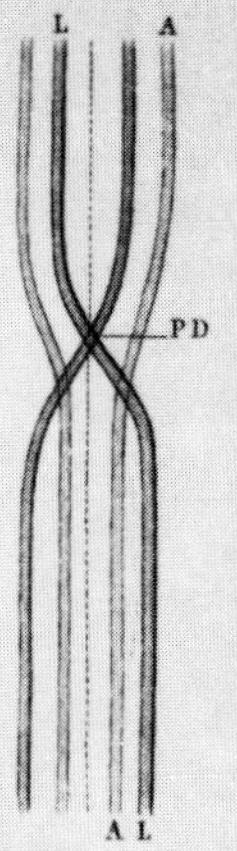

Fig. 23.

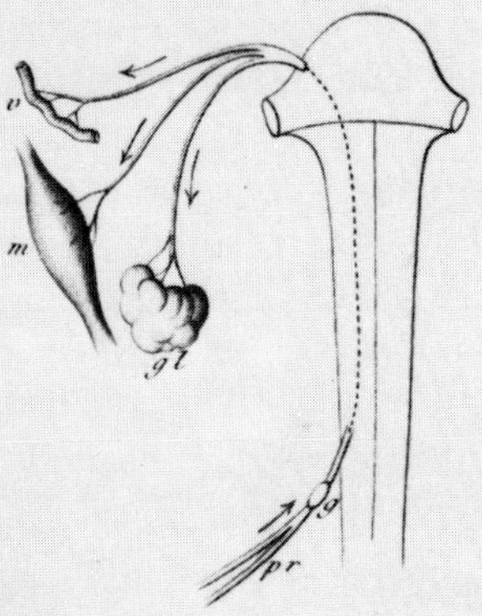

Fig. 24.

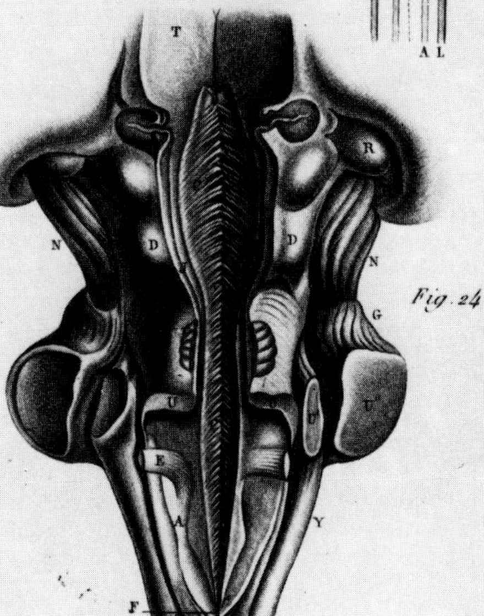

Fig. 25.

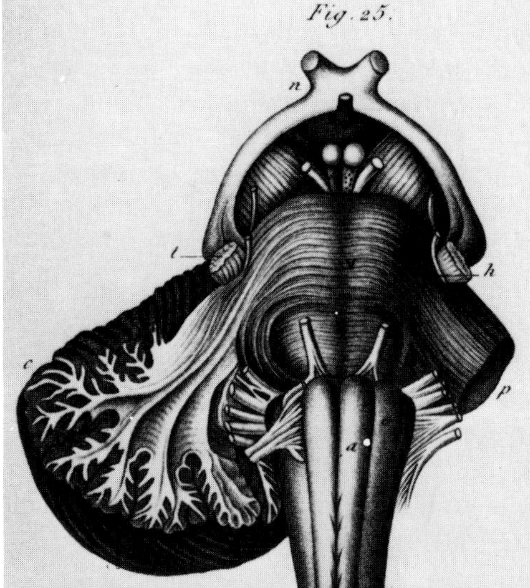

Fig. 26.

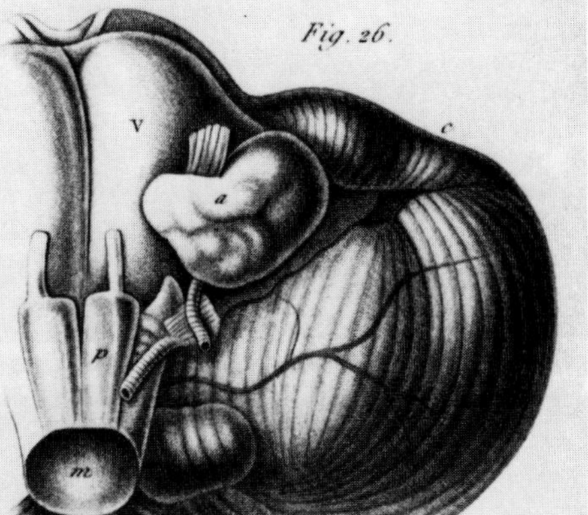

which was followed in a few minutes by 'a notable increase in sensitivity'. The contralateral limb, however, 'loses its sensitivity completely or in large part'. Although he was, of course, aware of the motor paralysis which follows hemisection and complete section of the cord, he was concerned with transmission in the posterior columns. Confirmation of the exactness of his hemisection in a guinea pig, reported in this paper, was confirmed at autopsy by Bernard. Brown-Séquard also reported that if a second hemisection is made a few centimetres below the first, on the opposite side, the sensory loss was bilateral. He concluded that 'the spinal cord thus appears to have, at least in part, a crossed function in respect to the transmission of sensory impressions'.

That he was imbued with the experimental method at this time is indicated by the fact that, immediately following this report in the Biology Society *Proceedings*, there appeared two other reports by him, one concerning the coagulability of the blood of the frog in winter, and the other on the effects of rest, motion, and galvanism on the nutrition of frog muscles.

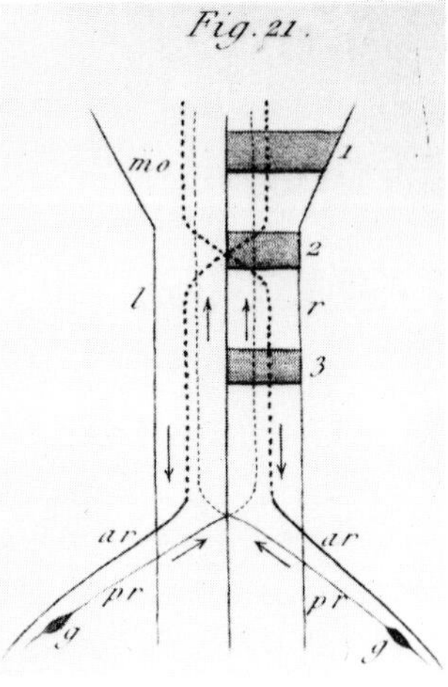

FIG. 117. Enlargement of *Fig. 21* in Fig. 116. The motor and sensory decussations in the brain stem. Lesions at 1 are above the decussation of the motor fibres. Lesions at 2 are at the level of the decussation. Lesions at 3 are below the decussation. In 1, there will be loss of motion and sensibility on the opposite side. In 2, motion is impaired on both sides; sensibility is lost on the opposite side. In 3, motion is lost on the same side; sensibility is lost on the opposite side.

The closing sentence of this 1849 report referred to the fact that Bell, by then, had withdrawn his original opinion. It will be remembered that Bell had first taught that the cerebrum was the centre for motion and sensation, with pathways in the anterior columns of the cord; the cerebellum was the centre for unconscious impressions from the body and involuntary motion, with pathways in the dorsal columns. By 1826[217] he was still teaching that 'the cerebrum has connection with the anterior columns of the spinal marrow, and the cerebellum with the posterior columns' but he now added that 'the anterior column is for motion, and the posterior for sensibility'. In 1835,[218] 'regretting that I should have expressed myself so indistinctly on the subject of the decussation of the posterior columns of the crus cerebri', Bell described that with the necessary 'delicacy of hand' the posterior column fibres could be traced from the crus, through the pons, coming together in the medulla and decussating, and 'descending continuously in their whole length, from the back of the pons to the spinal nerves'. Later, in a remarkable dissection (Fig. 87) he showed how the sensory columns decussated behind the anterior motor columns and fanned out into the cerebrum.

In his 1850[219] report Brown-Séquard demonstrated that if the hemisection was made in the cervical region there was sensory impairment in both opposite limbs. Moreover, if a second hemisection was made on the same side, then the sensory loss was nearly complete. He concluded that in rabbits, sheep, dogs, and pigs the sensory fibres decussated, not in the brain, but in the spinal cord. If any fibres did cross in the brain 'they must be very few in number'. Sensory testing was made by pinching, pricking, galvanization, and by cauterization with heat or acid.

In neither of these two reports did he mention the experiments of Galen but later, when he did, he said that 'In detailing his experiments on the spinal cord, he [Galen] does not say a single word concerning sensibility.'[220] This is correct about hemisection, but not about complete cord section (see p. 30).

In 1860, after he had joined the staff at Queen Square, he published in book form an expanded account of six lectures on the nervous system which he had delivered at the Royal College of Surgeons in England in 1858.[221] They contained, he said, 'the results of the work of almost all my life, since I began to study medicine'. They are, indeed, detailed, even tedious because of repetition, including such matters as his views on the spinal nature of epilepsy and other forgotten concepts. But his analysis of the experimental and pathological evidence concerning sensory transmission in the spinal cord is full of interest.

He first pays tribute to Bell, explaining that the importance of his work was 'not that volition and sensation have their conductors in this place or that, but that these conductors are distinct one from the other, all along from the brain to the periphery'. It was this 'principle . . . which is the great thing that science particularly owes to him' (p. 11).

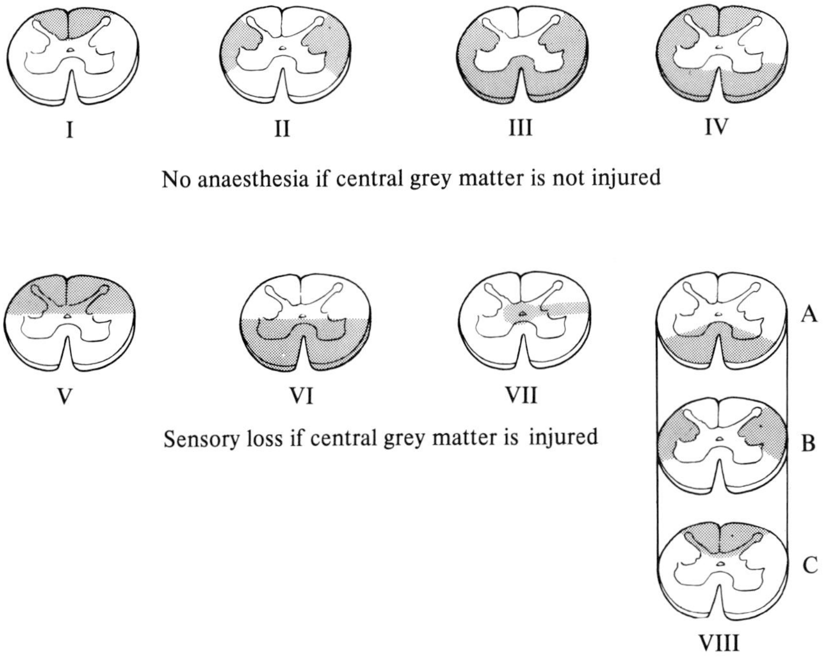

FIG. 118. A diagrammatic representation to show that loss of sensation depended on injury to the central grey matter of the spinal cord. Based on Brown-Séquard's many further experiments.

Further experiments on sensory transmission in the spinal cord. He first described experiments which showed that sensory transmission 'takes place chiefly in its central part, i.e. in the grey matter' (pp. 13–23). I have drawn illustrations of these experiments in Fig. 118. They may be summarized as follows:

I Section of the posterior columns does *not* cause distal anaesthesia.
II Section of the lateral columns does *not* cause distal anaesthesia.
III Section of the cord which leaves intact only the posterior columns does *not* cause distal anaesthesia.
IV Section of the cord which leaves intact only one lateral column does *not* cause distal anaesthesia.

But, he stressed, if during the above experiments there was any injury to the central grey matter, sensory loss occurred.

V Posterior hemisection of the cord causes sensory loss.

VI Anterior hemisection of the cord causes sensory loss.

VII Destruction of the central grey matter, with minimal injury to a lateral column, causes obvious sensory loss.

VIII If the anterior, the lateral, and the posterior columns are divided, at three different levels, so that sensory transmission can only take place via the grey matter, the hind limbs are still sensitive, though less than normally.

'These facts prove', he said, 'that the grey matter is the principal conductor of the sensitive impressions in the spinal cord.' He considered that it was in the *central* grey matter that transmission chiefly took place, and that this was achieved 'both by cells and nerve-fibres united together' (p. 23). Microscopical studies, he said, had shown that fibres of the entering spinal nerve roots were attached to cells in the grey matter and that 'these cells communicate with others in such a way that two kinds of transmission are possible, one across the cord, and another towards or from the encephalon' (p. 23).

He described further experiments which suggested that sensory root fibres could either enter the grey matter immediately, or travel a short way

FIG. 119. Experiments on the nerves, nerve roots, and spinal cord. (After Brown-Séquard,[214] Pl. I.)

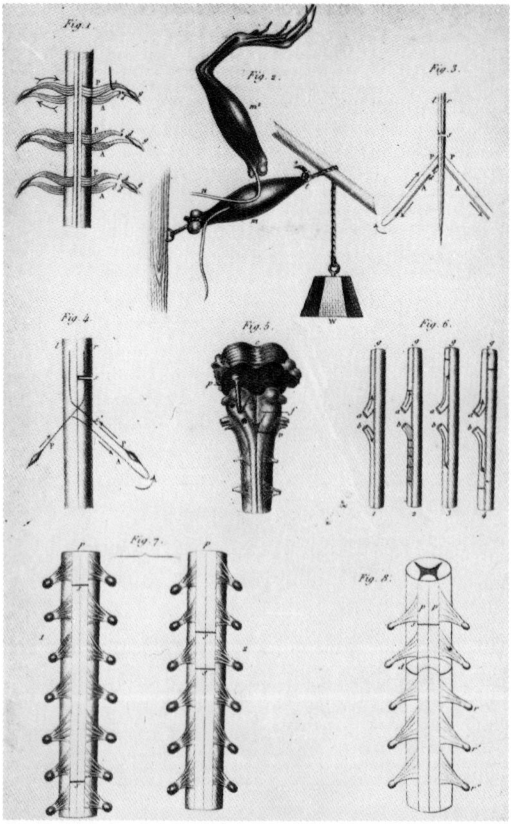

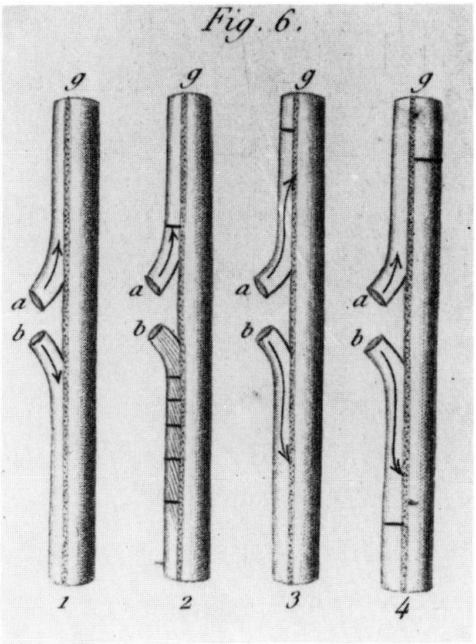

FIG. 120 (*left*). Enlargement of *Fig. 6* from Fig. 119.) 'Sections of the posterior columns of the spinal cord, and formations of upper and lower segments of these columns.' 1: Both segments remain sensitive to stimulation. 2: Section of upper segment abolishes sensitivity. 3: Section at a higher level impairs sensitivity; section at a higher level still does not impair sensitivity. 4: Section of *anterior* column does not impair sensitivity. Therefore, conductors of sensation must be leaving the posterior columns as they ascend. Similar results obtained with sections of lower segments. *g* is the central grey matter.

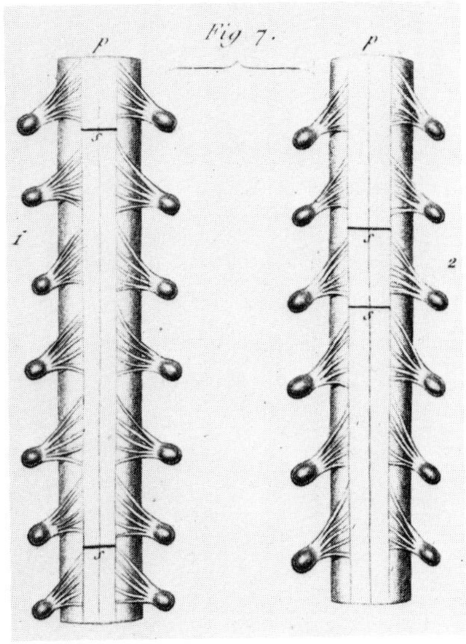

FIG. 121 (*right*). Enlargement of *Fig. 7* from Fig. 119. 'Double section of the posterior columns', at a short interval on the right, SS, and at a longer interval on the left, SS. In the former there is loss of sensibility of the posterior roots between sections; in the latter there is no loss. Therefore, incoming sensory fibres must travel short distances in the posterior columns before entering the grey matter.

in the posterior columns, the posterior horns, or the postero-lateral columns before entering it. In Fig. 119 are examples of experiments he illustrated to demonstrate these conclusions.

In more experiments (Fig. 122) he obtained evidence that sensory loss 'must depend on the section of the commissural fibres of the spinal cord . . . which cross in the median plane' (p. 33).

1. A right, lateral hemisection is made in the dorsal region; the right hind limb remains sensitive. A left, lateral hemisection is then made in the cervical region of the same cord; the right hind limb now loses much of its sensibility (Fig. 9 in Fig. 122). Conclusion: sensory fibres from the right lower limb must have already crossed from right to left below the dorsal section.

2. The two posterior columns are sectioned; sensitivity remains in the hind limbs. At the level of this section a transverse cut is made so that one lateral half of the cord is completely severed. Sensibility of the opposite hind limb now disappears completely (Fig. 10 in Fig. 122).

3. If a longitudinal section is made in the mid-line in the lumbar region, sensibility, but not motion, is abolished in the hind limbs. This was one of Galen's experiments, as Brown-Séquard recalled.

4. If a mid-line longitudinal section is made in the cervico-brachial region, sensation is lost in the forelimbs but not in the hind limbs. On now completing a right lateral hemisection at this level, sensation is lost in the left hind limb (Fig. 11 in Fig. 122).

Brown-Séquard next asked himself the question 'Is the sensory decussation complete?' The anaesthesia after a longitudinal section suggested it was. But sensory loss in lateral hemisections was incomplete. Animal experiments, he said, might reveal what relates to painful impressions, but not to those of 'touch, cold, warmth, etc.' (p. 38). He tested the responses of animals to hot and cold and he covered the head when examining touch, but

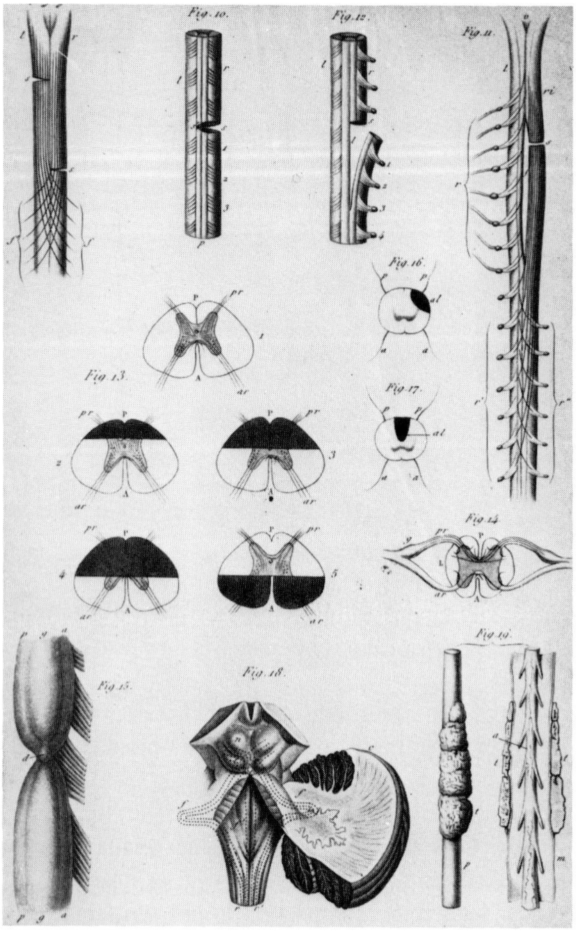

FIG. 122. The experimental section of the cord shown in *Figs. 9*, *10*, and *11* were designed to show that there was a sensory decussation in the grey matter in the median plane. (After Brown-Séquard,[214] Pl. II.)

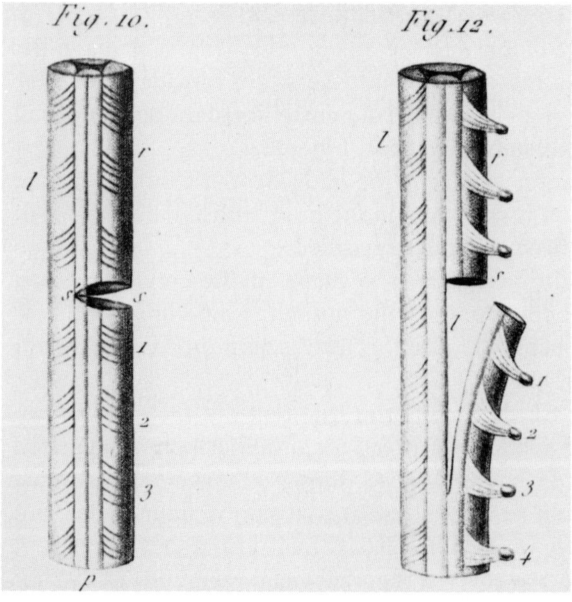

FIG. 123. Enlargement of *Figs. 10* and *12* from Fig. 122.) *Fig. 10.* Right hemisection of the spinal cord at S, after bilateral section of the posterior columns at S′. Following the latter there is hyperaesthesia below the section. When the hemisection is made there is an increase of hyperaesthesia on the right side, but sensibility disappears on the left side. *Fig. 12.* Right hemisection of the spinal cord at S, is followed by a median longitudinal section at *1*. Sensibility persists in the partly separated segments. At spinal nerve *1*, there is very slight sensibility; at nerve *2*, it is slight; at *3*, it is moderate; at *4*, sensibility is normal. The sensory decussations must take place at a short distance from the entry of the sensory root into the cord.

he came to no firm conclusions. He thought that temperature sensation was not conveyed by the posterior columns but he could not confirm Schiff's (1823–96) suggestion[222] that tactile impressions were transmitted in the posterior columns and pain via the grey matter. Clinico-pathological observations in man were going to be essential.

Schiff[223] said that his 'doctrine of the conduction of sensations' in the spinal cord was developed 'after I had conducted several hundreds of experiments', beginning in 1849, in Frankfurt. 'Right from the start', he said, 'the main achievement was the discovery of the *aesthodic* and *kinaesthodic*' modes of sensation. The former, pain and temperature sensations, crossed the mid-line in the grey matter. The latter ascended in the posterior columns of the same side.

In all these spinal cord experiments Brown-Séquard commented on ipsilateral, distal hypersensitivity in unilateral cord sections, especially those involving the posterior columns. Keele[224] has pointed out that subsequently Bechterev (1857–1927) considered that this hyperaesthesia was never taken into account. Brown-Séquard thought that it was much less when the posterior column lesion occupied several segments, as happened in injury and disease in man. This, he thought, was due to involvement of fibres which passed along these columns for some distance (p. 55).

The cervical sympathetic nerve. In his Lectures,[214] Brown-Séquard explains that in 1851 'I understood at once that the fact discovered by C. Bernard was due to the paralysis of the bloodvessels after section of the sympathetic' (p. 139). This he had been able to do because of experiments he had already carried out 'on the influence of nerves on bloodvessels'. If he was correct, he reasoned, then galvanization of the nerve would produce the reverse effects of section. This experiment he performed and reported on in America in 1852.[225] Bernard did so a few months later, not knowing of Brown-Séquard's experience, to be followed by Waller in 1853. Brown-Séquard stated (p. 142) that he was the first to demonstrate that stimulation of the sympathetic caused contraction of blood vessels, diminished flow, and reduction of temperature.

He also commented that following a lateral hemisection of the dorsal spinal cord 'we find in the lower limb on the same side most of the effects of a section of the sympathetic in the neck . . . dilatation of blood vessels, greater afflux of blood, elevation of temperature, hyperaesthesia and increase of the vital properties of muscles and of the motor nerves' (p. 144). A hemisection of the cord 'near the medulla' paralysed the ipsilateral, and contracted the contralateral limb blood vessels. But vasomotor influences could not account for all the neural effects on nutrition and secretion in normal and pathological conditions. There must be some other agency of the nervous system. Marshall Hall's '*supposed* existence of a system of *excito-secretory* and *secretory* nerves' was not based on facts.

*

In later years Brown-Séquard had much to say about the localization of cerebral functions. He conducted his own experiments on the brain and had

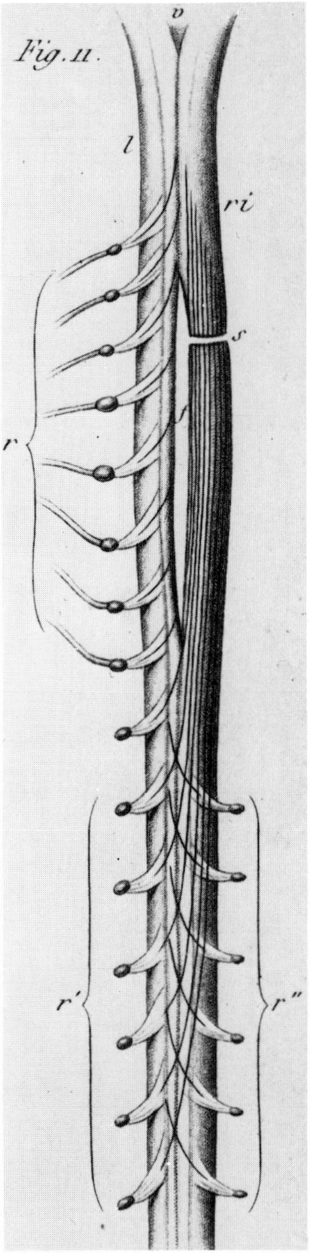

FIG. 124. Enlargement of *Fig. 11* from Fig. 122. A median longitudinal section of the cord in the cervico-brachial region, at *f*. This results in loss of sensibility in the forelimbs, but with retained sensibility in the hind limbs. A transverse section is made at s on the right side. The left hind limb then loses its sensibility: r, r′, and r″ show decussating posterior root sensory fibres.

ideas concerning ipsilateral effects, differences between the effects of cauterization and 'electricalisation', and the production of convulsions and paralysis. Many of his experimental observations were erroneous, but some of his arguments were sound.

Meanwhile, however, he was a practising, if restless, physician, and his further observations on 'Spinal Hemiplegia' will be considered later. His major experimental observations were made at mid-century at which time there were clinicians who were attempting to define and classify disorders of the nervous system and to investigate in what ways disorders of function were revealed by symptoms and signs. But little progress had been made. No Auenbrugger or Laennec had yet arrived at the bedside of the paralysed patient.

PART 4

The second half of the nineteenth century

CHAPTER 6

THE FLOWERING OF NEUROLOGY

THE NEUROLOGICAL PHYSICIANS

During the first half of the nineteenth century, despite the knowledge gained about the gross anatomy and pathology of the nervous system, the fundamental physiology of the motor and sensory systems, and the role of the spinal cord in reflex action, there were no equally significant clinical advances. Diseases of the nervous system were still largely categorized under the titles of palsy, paralysis, and epilepsy. In 1830 Bell had lamented that 'it will be long . . . before the united labours of the profession can enable the medical author to arrange the diseases of the nerves, and to describe them accurately; we are obviously in a very early stage of enquiry'.[1] Indeed, there could be little knowledge of the processes of disease within the brain, the spinal cord, the nerves, or the muscles until more was known of their component elements – their cells and fibres – and their precise distribution. But technical advances were laying the necessary foundations, mainly in the German-speaking world.

In the first decade of the century, Reil (1759–1813), in Halle, developed the technique of hardening and preserving the brain in alcohol. In the thirties came the new compound microscope with the achromatic objective, constructed by Lord Lister's father. In Prague, in 1838, Purkinje (1787–1869) published his account of the microscopic appearances of the human brain, providing the first full account of nerve cells, with their nuclei and dendrites, and the pear-shaped cells in the cerebellum. In the forties, Stilling (1810–79), in Cassel, introduced the method of cutting thin serial sections. These developments opened the way to the closer examination of nervous tissues, and, even before the arrival of staining methods in the fifties, they made it possible to identify some important features of nerve cells and fibres.

It is interesting to note that the possibility of hollow nerve fibres had still to be entertained by Schwann (1810–82) when he wrote, in 1839,

> The margin of a fibre generally presents a double outline on both sides, so that it has the appearance of a hollow tube, and the distance between the two outlines, then, denotes the thickness of the white substance . . . either this pale band is the proper nervous fibre, and the white substance only a sheath (cortex) around it (this is the view taken by Remak), or the nervous fibre is actually a hollow fibre, the wall of which is formed by the white substance. . . .[2]

Remak (1815–65) noted, in 1838, that peripheral nerve axons were in continuity with cells in the spinal cord and that some nerve fibres were not white, but grey – the unmyelinated sympathetic fibres. By 1845, Kolliker (1817–1905), was of the view that many nerve fibres were actual processes of nerve cells. There were large and small nerve cells and fibres, and he thought there was some relationship with motor and sensory functions, respectively.

The nerve cells, however, may be divided into those which are in direct connection with nerve fibres, and those which are not thus connected, but independent. ...

... in many situations [processes] undoubtedly are not prolonged into nerve fibres ... [they may] bring different regions of the central organs into mutual connection, and participate in the reflex phenomena, the sympathies, and other modes of association of the functions.[3]

By the middle of the century nerve degeneration was being used to examine the connections between nerve cells and their processes. Waller (1810–70), in the early fifties, showed that section of a nerve led to degeneration of its distal segment; this pointed to the site of origin of the anterior spinal nerve roots as being in the grey matter of the cord, and that of the posterior roots in the ganglia. Türck (1810–68), studying the secondary degeneration which followed focal lesions in the brain and spinal cord, was able to prove that the direction of tract degeneration corresponded with that of conduction – downward in motor tracts and upward in sensory.

For the clinician, however, these developments had little significance at first. The manifestations of disease of the nervous system were observed, it is true, but they could only be assessed in terms of loss of movement, sensation, or mentality. Degrees of loss were sometimes specified and unusual distributions of paralysis and numbness noted; levels of consciousness and degrees of delirium were recognized. But it was only in the last quarter of the century that 'examination' of the patient came to be a standard procedure and 'signs' were actually sought, that is, when inspection became scrutiny.

As yet there was little appreciation that lesions were not synonymous with disease, despite the tradition of Sydenham with his descriptions of the 'train of symptoms' and his concept of the natural history of disease. Although he thought the latter could be categorized like species of plants he was aware that in so doing 'we depart from nature, which is always the best guide, and indulge ourselves the liberty of conjecture'.[4] Cullen's nosology was now forgotten and Marshall Hall's divisions of the nervous system were of no immediate practical assistance. His use of an anatomico-physiological principle for classifying spinal disease, and a psychological one for cerebral disease promoted Riese to write that 'With Marshall Hall the soul entered for the first, but also for the last time, into the classification of nervous diseases.'[5]

To Magendie, medicine was 'only the physiology of the sick man' and it transpired that it was on physiological principles that the first systematic account of diseases of the nervous system was based. This was the text book by Romberg, the foremost of three mid-century treatises the examination of which will give us a picture of the neurological landscape of the day.

THREE MID-CENTURY NEUROLOGICAL TREATISES

I. *A manual of the nervous diseases of man*, by M. H. Romberg.

This was the title of the English translation[6] (to which my references apply) of the second edition (1851) of Romberg's book which had originally appeared in parts from 1840 to 1846.[7] Romberg (1795–1873)[8, 9] graduated in Berlin in 1817 with a thesis on 'Congenital Rickets',[10] a classical account of achondroplasia. Soemmerring[11] had also published an illustrated account of a still-born infant with this disease ('so-called congenital English disease (rickets?)') in 1791.

Romberg was about fifty when his book was completed and he had acquired a wide experience in the wards and autopsy rooms of the university hospital in Berlin. 'For twenty-eight years I was a physician to one of the largest unions in Berlin, in which, on average, 2000 patients presented themselves annually. ... In 1840 I was appointed director of the clinical wards of the university hospital ... from 1500 to 2000 patients apply there annually, and among them are many nervous patients.'[12] The very first sentence of the preface to the first edition was the quotation from Bell, already mentioned, about the difficulties of describing and classifying diseases of the nervous system. 'It was in the writings of English authors that I found instruction', he said. He translated Andrew Marshal's book (p. 177) on the *Morbid anatomy of the brain* in 1820, and Charles Bell's *Nervous system of the human body*, in 1832. He considered Bell to be 'the Harvey of our century'.

With respect to the task which he faced, he said physicians 'have been deterred by a fear that pathological investigations would fail to cope with the advanced state of physiological enquiry'. Yet in no other field 'has physiology exerted so great an influence ... as in the doctrine of nervous diseases'. Although he appreciated that his book could 'only serve as a stage of transition to more perfect works', he was quite certain that it was soundly based on *physiological principle.*

He proceeded to classify nervous diseases according to disorders of sensation and disorders fof motion, but, adopting Cullen's term 'Neuroses', he called them 'Neuroses of Sensibility' and 'Neuroses of Motility. These two main divisions were divided into classes according to increased or decreased sensory and motor function. Thus there were Hyperaesthesias and Anaesthesias in the sensory division, and Hyperkineses (spasms) and Akineses (paralyses) in the motor division. There were further subdivisions according to anatomical regions and levels involved. There was no attempt at pathological grouping and there were no illustrations.

Neuroses of sensibility. The manifestations of sensory disorders could only be appreciated if one kept in mind certain 'laws'. The law of 'isolated conduction' meant that adjoining fibres are not influenced by an altered state in one particular fibre. The law of 'sympathy' or irradiation referred to the way in which a stimulus is propagated to other afferent nerves. The law of 'eccentric phenomena' was one of peripheral reference of a sensation (p. 2). With regard to the speed of nerve conduction he did not think it would ever be possible to determine it 'as we do the velocity of electricity in a copper wire'. Here he was echoing his colleague Müller, whose pupil von Helmoltz actually accomplished it, in a frog, in 1850.

The hyperaesthesias (Chapters 2–17). In general the hyperaesthesias were periodic persistent disorders, which did not endanger life, but were painful and often accompanied by reflex phenomena. Compression of a nerve could be painless, but irritation was always painful. The hyperaesthesias could affect cutaneous nerves, muscle nerves, or cranial nerves. They could also involve the sympathetic tracts (the cardiac, solar, and mesenteric plexuses), the hypogastric plexus (rectal and urinary), and the spermatic plexus (testicular). The spinal cord and brain were also liable.

Cutaneous nerve lesions (Vol 1, p. 18) were responsible for the *neuralgias*, which were commoner in women, and in which pain was often accompanied by sensations of itching, formication, or heat. Points of tenderness were characteristic. Romberg referred to two reports we have mentioned – Swan's lady with the cut finger and Denmark's soldier with causalgia (see p. 191). His clinical comments are pointed. His statement (p. 30), for example, that new patients give more accurate descriptions 'than parties who have been subject to medical questioning for years past' is still one that has to be learned. There were several varieties of neuralgia affecting the face and head. In trigeminal neuralgia he had noted in one autopsy a softening of the nerve 'where it leaves the pons'; in another the gasserian ganglion was compressed by a carotid aneurysm. Migraine and migrainous neuralgia ('ciliary neuralgia') were common. In the latter photophobia was particularly troublesome, 'the eye generally weeps and becomes red ... the pain not infrequently spreads over the head and face ... these symptoms occur in paroxysms of a uniform or irregular character, and isolated or combined with facial neuralgia and hemicrania' (p. 56).

Pains in the limbs were often the result of neuralgias of the lumbosacral and brachial plexuses. In sciatica 'there must be some endemic influence' for it was 'rare' in Berlin, whereas Cotugno had said it was common in Naples. Lifting heavy weights could bring on an attack. Brodie had indicated how it should be distinguished from disease of the hip-joint. Brachial plexus neuralgia could affect one or all of the nerves of the upper limb. It should not be confused with pain referred from disease of the cervical vertebrae, which could be chronic and recurring. Herpes zoster of the upper limb was mentioned.

In a chapter (9, p. 91) entitled 'Hyperaesthesia of the Nerves of Muscular Sense' he explained that these nerves 'reconduct the sensation of action'. 'We determine the weight of objects in the hands by this sense.' Muscle pains in fevers and *Anxietas tibiarum* (mentioning Astruc and Sauvages) were examples of affections of these nerves. In *Anxietas tibiarum* there was 'a sense of painful restlessness in the lower extremities, especially in the legs and feet'. The patient 'did not know what to do with them ... though there were was relief by change of position'. This was clearly the syndrome of Ekbom or restless legs.

His nosological ideas led him to consider vertigo in this chapter, and not under hyperaesthesia of the auditory nerve; as he thought of it as a 'hyperaesthesia of a central nervous apparatus'. He defined vertigo as 'a sense of illusory movement'; it was not an actual 'hallucination'. He referred to Purkinje's studies of the effects of rotation of the head in vertical and horizontal planes. There was no mention of movement of the eyeballs.

A medley of maladies are collected together in his chapters on hyperaesthesia of the plexuses of the vagus, the sympathetic, the 'hypogastric' and the 'spermatic'. Lesions of the vagus were not characterized by 'one mode of expression like pain' but with a wide variety of peculiar sensations in the throat, chest, and stomach. There was a type of 'cardiac neuralgia' not due to 'ossification of the coronary arteries' as in the angina pectoris of Heberden (p. 126). There was also a type of 'coeliac neuralgia' which caused 'a sense of fainting and annihilation' (p. 129) reminding us of Gower's vasovagal syncope. Chronic testicular pain, in which the patient 'loses all zest for life ... and seeks castration' was a puzzling affliction. Sir Astley Cooper had apparently found the testes normal in three cases in which he had performed orchidectomy 'against his will'; he thought it was a sort of testicular tic douloureux.

Among the cranial nerves, hyperaesthesia of the optic, the auditory, the olfactory, and gustatory were quite common. In the case of the optic nerve it was difficult to know whether the lesion was peripheral or central – in the retina, the nerve itself, or in the thalamus. Sudden disturbances, 'luminous', 'chromatic', or 'scotomatous', caused much anxiety; 'only haemoptysis has such a worrying effect on a patient'. The different types of noises – susurrus, sibilus, tinnitus, or bombus – resulting from acoustic hypersensitivity, were of no differential diagnostic significance. They could arise in the brain, the auditory nerve, or the inner ear; co-existing deafness indicated a lesion of 'the nervous structures'. Noises in the head also occurred 'when there is hypertrophy of the left ventricle' of the heart.

When Romberg came to write on the sensitivity of the spinal cord and brain (Chapters 15–17) and the reason for pain in disease of these structures he confessed that 'we possess no physiological key to them'.

In disorders of the spinal cord, such as tetanus, rabies, strychnine poisoning, and hysteria, he presumed there was some hyperaesthesia in that organ. Severe 'tearing' pains in the lower limbs could arise from cord lesions, but he scoffed at the concept of 'spinal irritation' as a category of disease – 'a phantastic caricature which had been dragged into neuropathology ... by certain English physicians' and which 'had found its way across the ocean to Germany' (p. 154). Certainly, spinal cord injury, in itself, did not cause pain, although it was a feature of cord compression by tumour, or when there was inflammation, as in meningitis and myelitis. He mentioned the experiments of Longet, contested by Brown-Séquard, in which stimulation of the posterior columns caused pain.

In the brain there was some experimental evidence that 'the basal surfaces are the most sensitive' (Longet and Magendie are quoted) but 'the hemispheres were utterly insensitive'. Surgical experience confirmed this, but, as with the spinal cord, pain arose when inflammation set in. In disease of the brain, only atrophy was painless. The case reports of Abercrombie and Andral had shown that brain tumours were always painful, while those 'trustworthy observers', Rostan and Lallemand, had shown that pain was also a feature of brain softening and abscess. There was less pain in cases of haemorrhage into the brain than into other organs. Head pains were of little diagnostic value; neither the character of the pain nor its location were really helpful. They could be unilateral or bilateral, but in cerebellar disease they usually involved the whole of the head. Romberg advised his readers that just as they would always examine the thorax and abdomen in cases of pain there, so also should they remember to examine the scalp and head in patients with headache.

The anaesthesias (Chapters 18–29). Romberg made some general comments on sensibility before he embarked, in a similar manner, on a discussion of the causes and manifestations of impaired sensory functions. It was important to remember that tactile sensation diminished with age and that the two-point discrimination technique introduced by Weber in 1834 showed that there were remarkable differences according to the part of the body that was tested. With regard to temperature appreciation, he curiously thought that 'the majority of patients receive a greater impression of warmth and cold from bodies touched with the left hand than with the right' (p. 192). Tactile sensibility on the tongue may be lost, with retention of taste. Reflex responses to stimulation may be lost when there was anaesthesia, as in the loss of reflex winking when an anaesthetic cornea was touched, although voluntary winking was unaffected. In the cornea, also, the impaired nutrition of an anaesthetic part was obvious: ulceration was a danger.

With regard to the pain pathway, there is no mention, not surprisingly, of Brown-Séquard's 1851 paper, and Romberg appeared to accept that it was by way of the posterior columns, the medulla, the pons, the corpora quadrigemina to the hemispheres.

Cutaneous sensory examination required that the patient's eyes should be closed and appreciation of touch, warmth, and cold should be recorded, as well as the prick of a needle. The lesion could be peripheral as in injury to a nerve or compression by tumour. There was a condition seen in 'washer-women' (p. 207), in which there was numbness in the hands with unimpaired motility. There was tingling in the finger tips with objective sensory loss in thumb, index, and middle finger. The ailment, which was obviously the carpal tunnel syndrome, was attributed to the effect of 'ley' (i.e. lye) on the sensory nerves of the skin. In comparing the distribution of sensory and motor loss he mentioned a case of Ollivier's in which injury to the spinal cord had caused sensory loss in one leg and motor loss in the other. He also mentioned the case of Dr Vieusseux that we have described (see p. 171). Sensory loss of central distribution, without motor loss, must be rare.

In pursuing his classification he confessed that when he came to consider 'anaesthesias' of the vagus and sympathetic he had little to say. Dealing with cord lesions he referred to interference with conscious sensation and reflex activity. The latter could persist in paraplegia, despite profound sensory loss. The level of the latter was determined by the size and location of the lesion. Cruveilhier had shown that disease could be limited to the posterior columns; this occurred also in Norwegian leprosy.

The brain could be affected in terms of its function as a conductor of sensibility, like the cord, or as the organ of perception. Depression of all the senses was a feature of stupor and coma.

He was on firmer ground when dealing with the cranial nerves.

In the case of the optic nerve he used the terms amblyopia and amaurosis to mean partial and complete loss of sight. He referred to loss in the centre and periphery of the field of vision, affecting appreciation of shapes, sizes, centres, and margins of objects. Loss of colour sense could occur. In unilateral amaurosis it was essential to cover the good eye when examining pupillary activity 'as the reflex impression from the healthy eye caused a contraction of the pupil of the diseased eye' (p. 232). Loss of sight could result from a lesion in the cornea, the eye, the retina, the optic nerve or pathways, or within the brain itself, as, for example, in the thalamus, cerebrum, or cerebellum. Microscopic examination had shown that the decussation in the optic chiasm was only partial. Romberg did not mention hemianopia but referred to Flourens' opinion that a unilateral cerebral lesion caused blindness of the opposite eye.

Deafness ('acoustic anaesthesia') could result from lesions of the peripheral or central fibres of the auditory nerves. The loss could fall on the high or low tones. In determining whether the lesion was in the nerve or inner ear, he said that Müller had advised the testing of bone conduction (p. 244). Deaf people might 'look around if you stamp your feet on the ground'.

There was still some confusion regarding the nerves of smell and taste. Magendie had 'confounded sensibility of the lining of the nose' with that of olfaction; Bell had corrected him but many thought that the fifth cranial nerve served for smelling. 'We do not know what nerve performs gustatory function'; it was certainly not the twelfth. Lesions of the fifth or the ninth could affect it.

It was in Chapter 21, on 'Anaesthesia of the Muscular Nerves', that Romberg described his well-known sign. Various lesions could cause a patient to fall. In hemiplegia the tendency is to fall to the side of the paralysis. In convulsion the patient is thrown to the side opposite the lesion. Falling because of defective muscular sense was 'by gravitation'.

> I have observed that anaesthesia of the muscles alone without loss of tactile power, invariably accompanies tabes dorsalis. A simple experiment suffices to determine the fact. If the patient is told to shut his eyes while in the erect posture, he immediately begins to move from side to side, and the oscillations soon attain such a pitch that unless supported he falls to the ground. Even if the trunk is supported, if the patient be sitting and leaning against the back of the chair, the phenomenon takes place to the same extent, and he will slip off the chair. From the commencement of the tabes dorsalis as soon as the muscular power becomes diminished, this anaesthesia manifests itself; it becomes evident as the disease

progresses; and it is only towards its termination, when the muscular debility approaches to paralysis, that it can no longer be clearly distinguished. The eyes of such patients are their regulators, or feelers: consequently in the dark, and when amaurosis supervenes, as is not infrequently the case, their helplessness is extreme. Except during the last stage the skin remains sensitive; the complaints of the patient that they feel when they walk or stand as if a soft body, such as a layer of wool, intervened between the ground and the soles of their feet, must consequently be referred to the diminished muscular sense (p. 226).

The clinical features of tabes dorsalis were not described until later in his book, when he was dealing with spinal paralysis, which was a 'neurosis of motility'.

Neuroses of motility. Motor activity was voluntary or reflex and both functions were subject to disorders. Normally, also, there was a certain 'tonicity' of muscles at rest. During activity there was a central mechanism of co-ordination. Disorders of motility were classified according to the principle of exaggeration or impairment of function. Thus there were the *Spasms* ('Hypercineses') and the *Paralyses* ('Acineses').

Spasms. Romberg analysed these on the basis of the distribution of the nerves to the head, limbs, and trunk and the origin of the 'excitement' in the spinal cord or brain.

In the cranial nerve territory there was nystagmus, strabismus (spasmodic or paralytic), trismus (reflex or 'meningitic'), and facial spasms (peripheral or centrally determined), organic or 'histrionic'. Marshall Hall had noted the contracture and spasm of the facial muscles after a palsy. Spasms of the tongue were rare but they were common in the neck, in the distribution of the accessory nerve of Willis. In the upper limbs, he mentioned writer's cramp and carpopedal spasm. Brachial plexus lesions rarely caused spasms; central lesions were usually responsible. In the lower limbs the hip flexors suffered most; the lesion was usually spinal. Spasms affecting breathing (inspiratory or expiratory, laryngeal or bronchial) and vocalization were well known.

Then there were the spasms arising in the visceral plexuses – cardiac, gastrointestinal, and genito-urinary. He discussed vomiting here (Vol. 2, p. 19). He said that a cerebral origin should be suspected if there was no premonitory nausea, if it was influenced by posture (relieved by horizontal rest, aggravated in the erect position), aggravated by movement, and apparently unattended by retching or distress (as in 'a baby at the breast'). Oesophageal, anal, and vesical spasms were common. Anxiety was a well-known cause of urinary frequency, as in the case of a highwayman *en route* to the scaffold (p. 30).

A special category of spasms resulted from 'Excitement of the Spinal Cord' (p. 42). These might follow lesions in the conducting elements, the central apparatus, or in the reflex pathways. Tetanus, trismus and hydrophobia were examples of lesions of the latter kind. Hysteria was defined as 'a reflex neurosis dependent on sexual irritation' (p. 87). In the male it was transitory, but in the female 'the source is permanent'. Any disease of the spinal cord could 'exalt reflex activity' (p. 79). 'When the cerebral impulse is interrupted, and the conduction of the will arrested, the reflex phenomena not only become more evident, but they also break forth with greater force'. Romberg refers several times to Marshall Hall's experiments.

One of the spasms in tuberculous meningitis was a characteristic 'bending back of the head'. Romberg could not confirm Bright's observations relating chorea (a spasm) to rheumatic fever and heart disease (p. 54). In hydrophobia, 'the poison from the dog' chiefly attacked the medulla, causing spasms of swallowing and respiration.

Another category of spasms arose from 'Excitement of the Brain' (p. 156). He recognized four varieties; 'static', 'co-ordinated', 'psychical', and 'epileptic'. Here we have a confusing mixture of examples. Thus, static spasm occurred in disordered gait in cerebellar diseases; gesticulation, compulsive utterance, and 'locomotive' spasms were examples of co-ordinated spasm. Muscle spasms induced by some 'mental impression', as in hysteria, religious fervor, or epidemics, comprised the psychical variety. Of epileptic spasms, he wrote 'Nobody has hitherto succeeded in producing epileptic spasms in animals by lesions of the brain and spinal cord.' Marshall Hall attributed the ensuing loss of consciousness to congestion of the brain consequent on cervical spasm and jugular compression. A focal epileptic spasm might be contained by binding the limb.

Tremors (Chapter 33) are treated between discussion of spasms and paralysis. They could occur with or without disease of the nervous system. The effects of fever, alcohol, and mercury are cited and he refers to Parkinson and Todd on paralysis agitans.

Paralyses. The arrangement is similar to previous chapters. There is consideration of motor paralysis in the territory of the cranial nerves, the visceral plexuses, and spinal and cerebral paralysis.

In an introductory chapter (34) Romberg made some general observations. Diseased arteries, but not veins, of the nervous system were one cause of paralysis. A lesion might be nervous or in muscular tissue. Paralysed muscles might waste and their fasciculi might 'oscillate'. Contractures ensued from continued activity in antagonists. 'Sensory' disturbances might occur in motor paralysis. Thus a patient might complain that a paralysed limb was 'numb'. A hemiplegic patient might think there is someone or something 'lying on the paralysed side', which they try to remove or throw out of the bed (p. 252). Reflex movements in a paralysed limb may be initiated by an act such as yawning, as described by Bell and Marshall Hall.

Cranial nerve motor palsies were frequent. In the eye paralysis could affect the lid, the eyeball, or the pupil. In tabes dorsalis the latter was like 'a pin's head'. Trigeminal 'masticatory' palsy could occur with or without pain, and arise from a lesion in nerve or pons. So also could facial palsy be peripheral or central. Otorrhoea or deafness were pointers to a peripheral lesion; taste sometimes suffered. In central lesions involvement of the fifth, sixth, and eighth nerves tended to develop. In a central facial palsy only the lower part of the face was affected, and emotionally induced movements were often normal. A Bell's palsy could be misinterpreted as a stroke.

Spinal paralysis (Chapters 46–48). This had emerged as an important class of disorders 'since the despotic supremacy yielded to the brain by older authors has been overthrown'. The motor pathway lay in the anterior columns; in paraplegia there was usually some sensory loss.

When motility and cerebral insensibility are entirely lost, spinal or unconscious sensibility manifests itself... by reflex action. The sole of the foot is the part most suited to experiments of this description, we succeed best by tickling... the reflex movement usually takes place in the foot of the same side, though it may occur in both... (p. 357).

Reflex activity was much less often seen in a paralysed upper limb. In the lower limbs it tended to cease on repetition and was restored by rest. In spinal injuries it was not seen 'until some time elapses'.

An indication of the level of a cord lesion can be gained by noting the distribution of the paralysed muscles. In cervical lesions there was often dysphagia and dyspnoea; the arms were involved. The muscles of the thorax and abdomen were affected in dorsal lesions. Lumbar lesions paralysed the legs and pelvic muscles. In lesions of the cauda equina, some muscles of the legs may be spared. Lack of growth in infantile spinal palsy was a conspicuous feature. In lead palsy there was no sensory loss and the muscles wasted. There were cases, however, in which wasting was marked although there was no indication of lead poisoning.

Romberg described three such cases (p. 372): (1) A ten-year history of painless atrophy of the muscles of the right hand and forearm, and the left shoulder and upper arm; no sensory loss. (2) An attack of severe pains in the left shoulder and upper arm, with numbness of the index and middle fingers, followed, two years later, by evident weakness of the arm and wasting of the thumb. (3) Wasting, weakness, and fasciculation of the right, then the left, thumb and forearm muscles; 'widespread wasting fasciculation'; spasms and weakness of the legs; dysphagia and dysarthria. Sensation retained, 'he could feel a fly crawl over his hand'. Sphincters were normal. Romberg saw him three years later, when the patient was 41; outcome was not mentioned.

These three cases were most likely examples, respectively, of progressive muscular atrophy, neuralgic amyotrophy, and amyotrophic lateral sclerosis.

Tabres dorsalis (Vol. 2, Chapter 49, p. 395). Although there were clinical accounts of this disease, and descriptions and illustrations of degeneration of the posterior columns of the spinal cord, before Romberg's publication, his became the classical contribution. He did not, it is true, attribute the ataxia to the posterior column degeneration (which Todd had already done; see p. 301) but his declineation of the clinical evolution of the disease is nevertheless a landmark.

Early in the disease we find the sense of touch and the muscular sense diminished, while the sensibility of the skin is unaltered in reference to the temperature and painful impressions... The feet feel numbed in standing, walking or lying down... The rider no longer feels the resistance of the stirrup, and has the strap put up a hole or two. The gait begins to be insecure, and the patient attempts to improve it by making a greater effort of the will; as he does not feel the tread to be firm he puts down his heels with greater force. From the commencement of the disease the individual keeps his eyes on his feet . . . the insecurity of his gait also exhibits itself more in the dark . . .

Various pains and sensations were common – in the lower limbs, where they were 'shooting' in character, about the waist, and in the abdomen. The latter were 'gastric' or like 'colic'.

Painful sensations of different kinds almost invariably accompany the affection; the most common is a sense of constriction, which proceeds from the dorsal or lumbar vertebrae, encircles the trunk like a hoop, and not infrequently renders breathing laborious. Several of my patients have described this sensation as particularly troublesome during sleep, causing them suddenly to start up and scream out . . .

Urinary difficulties were described – a poor stream and incomplete evacuation of the bladder. Vision might fail and there was pupillary constriction.

Even when the optic nerve was not implicated I have repeatedly found a change in the pupils of one or both eyes, consisting in a contraction with loss of motion, which in one case, that of a man aged 45, attained to such a height that the pupils were reduced to the size of a pin's head.

The disease lasted from ten to fifteen years and at autopsy there was 'partial atrophy of the spinal cord', mainly in the lumbar region. The anterior columns and roots were not affected; the sensory roots and columns were shrunken; in the cauda equina there were 'empty sheaths'. As yet there were no microscopical observations. Males between the ages of 30 and 50 provided the great majority of cases. The disease had 'an evil reputation' and was associated with 'sexual excesses' and the 'campaigns of war' with their 'forced marches', 'wet bivouacs', and 'drunkenness'. One of his patients, however, was a physician who acquired the disease 'after violent emotions and severe colds, caught in the prosecution of his profession' (p. 399).

Cerebral paralysis (Chapter 50). The manifestation of disease of the brain reflected its function as the organ of the mind, and as the origin of the motor and the termination of the sensory pathways.

Softening of the grey cortex was an important cause of failing intellect, disordered speech, clumsy movements, euphoria, delusions, and dementia. In such cases the meninges were also often involved. He quoted the writings of Esquirol (1805), Calmeil (1826), and Bayle (1826) with reference to the delineation of general paresis, and he recognized that disorders of behaviour could be a result of brain disease.

In hemisphere lesions the face and limbs of the opposite side were paralysed. Lesions of the pons caused 'a peculiar combination' of ipsilateral paralysis of the face and contralateral paralysis of the limbs, the pyramidal decussation being at a lower level, in the medulla. Occasionally, brain stem lesions caused paraplegia. In infantile hemiplegia, unlike the adult variety, there was much wasting, not only of the paralysed limbs, but of the affected hemisphere. In one such case he traced the degeneration of the motor pathway from the hemisphere into the crus, pons, and pyramid of the medulla. He was not allowed to remove the spinal cord.

Sometimes, after strokes, there were multiple lesions in the hemispheres. Some were no doubt a cause of transient symptoms. Cruveilhier's autopsy of Dupuytren was mentioned. Dupuytren developed a left facial palsy during a lecture; he carried on, supporting the angle of his mouth with a finger. Previously he had had an episode of severe vertigo. Later he died of a stroke and there were several small lesions in the white matter of the right hemisphere. His intellect had not suffered because the grey cortex showed only one small lesion.

The general clinical features of disease of the brain were to some extent modified by the actual seat of the disease. If it was confined to the grey matter of the cortex, hemiplegia was uncommon. Many lesions were accompanied by swelling of the brain; Cruveilhier had recorded the lateral displacement of the median fissure. Effusions over the surface of the brain compressed it and caused paralysis. But much more knowledge was needed of the manner of radiation of the motor and sensory fibres from the corona radiata before satisfactory clinical analysis was possible.

Apart from the seat of the lesion, its 'character' influenced the type of clinical presentation. The factor of time was important; the hemiplegia of apoplexy was acute in onset, while that from cerebral compression was slow. Convulsions were more common in 'irritative' lesions, while paralysis was more common in 'softening'. Occlusion of cerebral arteries was noticeable in cases of softening and haemorrhage. Atrophy was the cardinal pathological feature in infantile hemiplegia.

The gait in infantile cerebral palsy was of the 'scissors' variety; in adult hemiplegia there was characteristic circumduction of the drooping foot.

*

A modern reader of Romberg's book will probably have mixed feelings about it. On the one hand there is the feeling that it was not, even then, necessary to push the classification he adopted to such an absurd degree, one which eventually led him to consider tabes dorsalis as a motor disability, despite his description of its essential element – a sensory ataxia. Then, too, there is little to suggest that he appreciated the importance of clinicopathological correlation, so evident in the writings of Bright and Cruveilhier. In diseases of the brain he refers to the different effects of compression and irritation, to swelling and shift of the hemisphere, to the grey matter in relation to intellectual loss, and to the importance of the 'character' as well as the 'seat' of the lesion. But these factors are only lightly touched on, or quoted. Andral and Cruveilhier and others had already discussed such matters as the significance of loss of consciousness in stroke, of the small size of lesions in crucial sites, and the problem of inferring function from a study of localized lesions. Romberg had little to say about the differences between cerebral and cerebellar lesions, for example, or between a lesion within the spinal cord and one compressing it, nor, for that matter, between disorders of the spinal cord and the peripheral nerves. The question of the localization of function within the nervous system, seen through the eyes of a clinician, was not really considered at all.

Of course, it is exceedingly difficult, and perhaps unjustified, to speculate about what the first systematic textbook of neurology might have contained in 1850. But one is left with the thought that his nosology, of which he was so proud, based as it was on physiological principle, in fact was a bit of a snare. It was a false scent which directed him away from what would have been a more rewarding trail – the correlation of symptoms, signs, and pathology.

That said, however, the modern reader will be in no doubt of Romberg's studious mind, his knowledge of the German, French, and English literature of the day, and of his careful observation and examination of his patients. We can see in him the emerging clinical neurologist.

History-taking had arrived, the course of a malady was traced, as exemplified in his account of tabes dorsalis and his stressing the importance of the time factor in hemiplegia. Careful examination enabled him to note the pupils in tabes, head retraction in meningitis, the muscular wasting in some forms of paralysis, fasciculation, anosognosia in hemiplegia, and the differences between peripheral and central facial palsies. In sensory testing he examined for touch, pain, and temperature and mentioned two-point discrimination. He did not refer to particular cases in which there was dissociated sensory loss, or refer to its possible significance, nor did he test for his 'muscle sense' by way of passive motion.

He described many forms of pains and neuralgias, indicating the features which characterized the headache of brain disease, and that of migrainous neuralgia. He referred to what we now call the carpal tunnel syndrome, restless legs, and neuralgic amyotrophy. Progressive muscular atrophy and amyotrophic lateral sclerosis may be recognized. Hemifacial atrophy he described a few years later.

Lastly, he was fully aware of the importance of the work of Marshall Hall, referring to the function of the spinal cord in reflex activity and noting that in cerebral and spinal diseases reflex activity was enhanced. He referred to the reflex movements of the arm in hemiplegia and to those of the legs in paraplegia and how the latter could be actuated by stroking the sole of the foot. We can regard him as the first clinical neurologist.

II. *Clinical lectures on paralysis, certain diseases of the brain, and other affections of the nervous system,* by Robert Bentley Todd.

What is most impressive about Robert Bentley Todd (1809–60) is that he managed to accomplish so much in the fifty short years of his life.[13] He was one of the founders of Westminster Hospital Medical School, King's College Hospital, and St. John's House training school for nurses which supplied Florence Nightingale with many of the nurses who went with her to the Crimea in 1855. At King's he promoted a collegiate system for medical students, elevating them from apprentices to university undergraduates, and introducing open medical scholarships, the first of their kind in Britain. He also instituted the office of medical dean, and was himself the first. His organizing genius transformed King's, 'reputed to be the worst in

London'[14] when he joined it in 1836, into an internationally renowned institution.

He was born in Dublin, the second son of a surgeon who had sixteen children, and was a professor of anatomy and surgery at the Royal College of Surgeons in Ireland, and subsequently its President. Todd senior died of a haematemesis, as did, in due course, his celebrated son. Todd's mother was related to Dr Oliver Goldsmith.[15] Todd was a pupil of Robert Graves and graduated in 1831 at Trinity College, Dublin, coming to London in the same year 'without a sixpence', as he later said. He obtained the post of lecturer in anatomy at one of the many small private medical schools then in existence. This was the Aldersgate Street school, near St. Bartholomew's where Marshall Hall also taught from 1834 to 1836. Todd remained there for three years, engaging also in private practice. Then followed two years at the Dean Street school, of which he was one of the founders, and which became a part of the Westminster School.

His career at King's began in 1836 when he was appointed professor of physiology and morbid anatomy at the age of twenty-seven. He held this post until 1853 but remained on the hospital staff until 1859. He died a year later in his consulting room at 26 Brook Street, Grosvenor Square. He had acquired many diplomas, degrees, fellowships, and lectureships, including FRCP in 1837, FRS in 1838, and FRCS in 1844. He gave the Goulstonian (1839), the Croonian (1843), and the Lumleian (1849) Lectures at the Royal College of Physicians.

His publications include *The cyclopaedia of anatomy and physiology*, which he planned and edited, and which appeared in four parts between 1835 and 1859.[16] His section on the physiology of the nervous system in the third volume is an admirable critical summary of contemporary knowledge.

Then there was a successful standard textbook he wrote with his colleague William Bowman in 1843, *Physiological anatomy and the physiology of man*, and a textbook for students on the *Anatomy of the brain, spinal cord and ganglions* in 1845.[17]

There were also three volumes of clinical lectures. The first, in 1854, *On paralysis, certain diseases of the brain*, etc.[18] which we shall examine; the second, in 1856, *On certain diseases of the urinary organs and on dropsies*; the third, *On certain acute diseases*, he finished shortly before he died and it was published posthumously.

Todd's book on neurology consists of twenty lectures, based on eighty-three cases, which he delivered at King's in the years 1844–54. He said that they should not be regarded as forming any sort of systematic presentation; they were based on notes made by one of his pupils, which Todd revised. My own copy, to which my references will apply, is the second edition, published in 1856; it comprises 474 pages, contains no illustrations or index, only a few references, but there is a list of the diagnoses of the cases presented.[18]

The first three lectures are on 'Paralysis'. There are seven lectures on 'Hemiplegia', three on 'Softening of the Brain', and one lecture each on the cerebral effects of 'Renal Disease', 'Syphilis', and 'Lead Poisoning'. The remaining four lectures deal with 'Facial Palsy', 'Chorea', 'Tetanus', and 'Local Hysteria and Catalepsy'.

Todd had a great reputation as a lecturer, speaking fluently and lucidly, without notes; 'his teaching was eminently demonstrative; he availed himself largely of diagrams and specimens'.[19] He showed his patients in the lecture theatre when that was possible and referred to what they had seen and discussed on ward rounds and in the autopsy room. He is said to have best enjoyed the neurological lectures. *The Lancet* obituary said that although he would be 'read of' as a physiologist, it was by his clinical lectures 'that he will live'.[13]

Each lecture begins with the customary 'Gentlemen' – and usually opens with an invitation to direct their attention to a particular subject of which there were certain examples at present in the hospital. He often gave the name of the patient, and always the age and occupation. Class distinction is noticeable; private patients were 'ladies' or 'gentlemen', often of some talent, virtue, or worth. In hospital the patient was always referred to as 'a woman' or 'a man' and many seemed to be of 'intemperate habits' or possessed of a 'syphilitic taint'. Erysipelas acquired in hospital was often fatal.

Paralysis. This was a symptom, not a disease, and usually it was motor; sensory paralysis was often temporary. Motor paralysis could arise from a disease of the nerves, which interfered with their 'conducting power', or from disease of 'the centre of volition' which reduced 'the generating power'. Poisons such as opium, lead, ether, or chloroform affected both these powers, but poisoning could also derive from diseases of the kidneys or liver, or from rheumatism or gout. Structural changes in the nervous system formed a second class – inflammation, atrophy, softening, induration. In a third class there was 'loss of continuity' by injury or haemorrhage. In the fourth class, 'compression', of 'nerve' or 'centre', was responsible; a ligature on a nerve, a depressed fracture of the skull, a clot or tumour within the cranium. The 'centre' of volition which decussated in the medulla could also be compressed in the brain stem or spinal cord.

Three cases were discussed in the first lectures; lead palsy, paresis of an arm in association with a fractured clavicle (which was attributed to bandaging), and 'hysterical hemiplegia'. The latter case may well have been one of cerebral embolism judging from the history of rheumatic fever and the sudden onset in sleep. Todd always suspected hysteria when the patient was a woman, and, in hemiplegia, if the face and tongue were unaffected, and the paralysed leg was not circumducted in walking.

Paralysis from cerebral lesions was usually hemiplegic, of acute or slow onset, and in his second and third lectures he discussed the problems of diagnosis on the basis of two cases which came to autopsy.

In the first case (Case IV, p. 25), a man of forty-nine, there was an eight-week history of left-sided headache, convulsive movements of the right limbs, followed by progressive right hemiparesis, blurred vision, and diplopia. On examination there was a right lower facial palsy, spasticity of the paretic limbs, unequal pupils, the right being the larger, with eyeballs 'constantly directed downward, with a convulsive action of the depressing muscles' (? ocular bobbing), and nystagmus in all directions of gaze ('marked convulsive twitchings' in all directions of voluntary gaze). The protruded tongue deviated to the *sound* side and this was attributed to the influence of some projecting teeth. Todd considered that the 'fixed' location of the head pain in the left parietal region and the incomplete nature of the paralysis of the right limbs, indicated a superficial lesion in the region of the left Sylvian fissure. Deep-seated lesions did not cause local pain and paralysis was usually complete. The lesion was probably 'inflammatory' because convulsive movements followed by paresis was a sequence characteristic of 'irritation' followed by 'effusion'. The early appearance of spasticity also suggested that the cerebral disease was 'irritative'; *late* appearing spasticity was a feature of destructive lesions. Todd concluded that there was an extensive meningeal, inflammatory lesion near the left Sylvian fissure.

At autopsy (p. 49) there was a mass, part soft, part indurated, with one small cyst, in the left thalamic region; the thalamus was 'double its natural size and by its great bulk compressed the crus cerebri of that side, which became flattened out by the pressure'.

These findings were all interpreted as 'cerebral inflammation', augmented by the microscopical detection of 'pus'. General autopsy findings were not recorded and no mention was made of the ears, but tumour seems more likely than abscess. In the clinical account there was no mention of speech or sensory testing. Todd admitted 'the diagnosis does not appear to have been exact'.

His second patient (Case V, p. 35), suddenly fell to the floor at breakfast. There was no loss of consciousness but she had a complete left hemiplegia. Two days later, in hospital, it was reported that the patient 'was a thin, pale ill-nourished woman, and looked at least sixty-five'. It transpired that she had been suffering from a diffuse type of headache and some drowsiness for four months. A week before admission she had felt some numbness of her left arm. There was a loud mitral systolic murmur. Todd deduced that the lesion was not meningeal, in view of the absence of signs of irritation, and the sudden and complete nature of the paralysis. It was a deep-seated lesion near the corpus striatum or thalamus. As consciousness had not been disturbed there could not have been any 'shock' to the brain, or pressure on it, so that effused blood was unlikely. The lesion was probably degenerative – 'such as white softening', and her cerebral arteries were almost certainly diseased. At autopsy (p. 52), a few weeks later, 'the disease was in the very centre of the right corpus striatum': there was cavitation and haemorrhage, and atheromatous arteries.

Todd's interpretation was that the softening was progressive and the hemiplegia a consequence of the final giving way of the fibres of the corpus striatum, with 'possibly, at the same time, the rupture of some minute vessels'. He seemed to think that it was not the rupture of an artery that caused the major event, but the rupture of nerve fibres.

Hemiplegia and softening of the brain. There were six types of hemiplegia: (1) Cerebral; (2) Spinal; (3) Epileptic; (4) Choreic; (5) Hysterical; (6) Peripheral. By far the commonest and the most important was the cerebral variety.

Todd first described the general clinical features of cerebral hemiplegia, stressing that both the clinical history and physical examination had to be adequate if a proper interpretation was going to be attempted. There were three types of case which he recognized, based on the condition of the paralysed muscles. In the first they were flaccid; in the second, rigidity was an early feature; in the third, rigidity was a later development.

Motor paralysis was most marked in the limbs. The face was usually partially affected; the patient could frown, close his eyes, smile, attempt to whistle, but the cheek sagged because of paralysis of the buccinator (which he said was also supplied by the trigeminal nerve, p. 93). Chewing and swallowing were little altered; the tongue often deviated to the paralysed side. The muscles of the trunk were rarely affected. A third nerve palsy (ptosis, dilated pupil, external squint) could occur alone, when it should be considered as an omen of a stroke, or with a hemiplegia. Sensation in the paralysed limbs was little altered but Weber's compass method should be used to compare both sides.

The cardiovascular system should be examined and a note made of the pulse rate, the state of the walls of the radial and temporal arteries, the size of the heart, and the presence of mitral or aortic murmurs. The urine should be examined for evidence of kidney disease.

The precise sequence of events leading to a stroke were difficult to comprehend but disease of the heart, the arteries, and the kidneys clearly played a significant role. Softening of the brain might be primarily degenerative, inflammatory, or nutritional (ischaemic) in origin. Occlusion of large and small cerebral arteries was of obvious importance but he was not sure about the recent concept of Virchow's and the paper by Kirkes,[20] which suggested that 'the stoppage of the arterial circulation is always caused by a plug accidentally brought from a distant part of the circulation' (p. 176). He favoured the explanation of 'a coagulum formed in the artery, promoted by an altered nutrition of its wall ...'. The word 'embolism' is not used but Todd admitted that in the case of acute hemiplegia in the young, one should always enquire about a history of rheumatic fever or chorea, and pay particular attention to the possibility of valvular disease of the heart.

Acute flaccid hemiplegia occurred with and without loss of consciousness; the latter was more likely if there was a sizeable clot in the brain. But in both, there was 'white softening, i.e. softening of the brain substance without any discolouration' (p. 196). 'The suddenness of the attack is due (as I suppose) to rupture of the softened fibres.' Coma was usually an indication of a clot of large size, or situated in some part where it can compress central and important parts of the brain' (p. 210). The prognosis was serious.

In acute spastic hemiplegia the rigidity of the paralysed muscles seemed to be present at the onset or developed 'very soon after it'. This rigidity might be slight and localized 'confined to one or two muscles' or marked and diffuse. It was more obvious in the flexor muscles than the extensors, and in the arm than in the leg. Facial muscles were rarely affected.

Concerning the muscular rigidity, he wrote,

> My idea as to its cause is, that it depends upon a state of irritation, propagated from torn brain to the point of implantation of the nerves of the affected muscles. But, you will ask, why is it that in some cases of clot the hemiplegia will be accompanied with complete relaxation of muscles while in others the rigidity of which I have spoken exists? The answer to this question is as follows; in the cases where there is no rigidity the clot lies in the midst of softened brain, and has not in any degree encroached upon sound brain; but when rigidity exists, the clot has extended beyond the bounds of the white softening, and has torn up to a greater or less extent, or irritated, sound brain. I leave this explanation to be tested by further experience and observation (p. 219).

This notion of a central 'irritating' phenomenon, and also of one of 'exhaustion' in post-epileptic hemiplegia, makes interesting reading when compared with Hughlings Jackson's interpretations, some thirty years later, of 'positive' and 'negative' effects, and the phenomena of 'inhibition' and 'release'.

Todd was particularly intrigued by those examples of acute hemiplegia in which the muscular rigidity was marked. Paralysis was usually incomplete and there was 'exaltation of the reflex actions'. Although he thought rigidity and reflex hyperactivity were due to the same cause, he stressed that the former was most obvious in the upper limb, with its flexed elbow and fingers, while the latter were better demonstrated in the lower limb. Stroking the sole of the foot elicited gross flexor response, but even tickling or stroking the palm 'will sometimes excite them' (p. 224). This type of case was most commonly seen in superficial lesions, such as depressed fractures of the skull, ruptured middle meningeal artery, and in meningeal tumours and suppuration.

> The effect is analogous to that produced by the continued action of the electro-magnetic machine . . . just as a rapid succession of electric shocks may maintain a constantly rigid condition of muscles, so may continual shocks of nervous force, due to irritative pressure, bring about a similar result (p. 227).

He conceived of lesions which could be 'irritative, as well as paralysing' (p. 231) and quoted not only from his own experience but from Abercrombie, Rostan, Lallemand, Andral, and Romberg. An irritative lesion was not necessarily an 'inflammatory' one; the latter could equally well have 'depressing an influence', like atrophy. Indeed, a lesion could pass through several stages, in this respect. Not only could hemiplegia follow a convulsion, the latter could occur in hemiplegic limbs.

In the third variety, in which rigidity was a late, progressive development, the paralysed muscles may have initially been flaccid or spastic. Here, he envisaged that whatever the nature of the initial lesion in the brain – softening, haemorrhage, or both – 'there takes place an attempt at cicatrisation . . . a gradual shrinking or contraction of the cerebral matter' (p. 245). This produces 'a slow and lingering irritation, which is propagated to the muscles' and excites them to 'contraction'. He did not wish to say that he had '*proved*' this and he suggested to his students that they should make every attempt to follow up cases of stroke 'in workhouses and other institutions where the disabled poor are received' and obtain more pathological material. It was vital 'to bring so wild and rugged a field as that of cerebral pathology into a more productive cultivation'.

When Todd came to consider the nature of the processes leading to stroke he made it clear (something others had not always done) what he meant by the term 'apoplexy'. 'By apoplexy I mean the rupture of a blood vessel, and the consequent escape of blood into the brain' (p. 95). But what could also 'rupture' were the fibres of the brain. They did so as a consequence of 'softening'. So a hemiplegia could arise from the rupture of vascular or nervous tissue in the brain. Softening of nerve fibres, of course, reduced the support they normally gave to cerebral arteries, so that, with or without disease of the arteries, haemorrhage became a danger. Hence the frequent discovery of clot *and* softening. 'White' and 'red' softening, he said, 'might be better called, *atrophic* and *inflammatory*!' The former was due to 'imperfect nourishment of the brain'. So a common sequence was 'the arteries of the brain become diseased, . . . softening takes place . . . [followed by] rupture of bloodvessels . . . or nerve fibres, and compression of neighbouring healthy brain-structure' (p. 102).

Todd's picture of what we now call arteriosclerosis is provided in the following words.

The sequence of the events may be thus described; First, the man gets into a general gouty condition, and the elimination of this morbid material gives rise to an irritation of the kidney, which at length assumes the form of gouty kidney, or, if you will, chronic nephritis; and the kidney, thus damaged and incapacitated for the perfect discharge of its function, is the great promoter of all the subsequent evils; the blood becomes still further contaminated, additional deposits to those which doubtless had already formed take place in the tissue of the heart's valves, in the large systemic arteries, and in those of the brain; the diseased arteries of the brain become insufficient channels of supply; white softening is the consequence and many of the unsupported and unhealthy capillaries at length give way; and thus all the circumstances, from first to last, fall in regular order as cause and effect (p. 114).

Todd went on to say,

The deposits in the arteries produce a twofold influence upon the circulation – by roughening the inner surface of the arterial channels they create a certain amount of direct obstacle to the flow of blood from the ventricle; and by diminishing, or nearly destroying, the elasticity of the arterial walls, they impair one of the most important forces by which the circulation is carried on in the arterial system. Thus the arteries, from being elastic yielding channels, with perfectly smooth inner surfaces, are changed into resisting inert tubes, with rough interiors. It is plain, then, . . . that the heart has to encounter great obstacles . . . hence the dilatation . . . and the hypertrophy (p. 115).

To his students, no doubt taught the traditional notions of apoplexy, that it was 'an excessive determination of blood to the brain' and 'bleeding' the inevitable therapy, these words must have sounded fresh and creative. Yet even they probably never came to use the sphygmomanometer, unless a few of them were still in practice at the end of the century. But Todd was fostering the use of another instrument – the microscope.

No more important observation has been made of late years in minute anatomy than that which showed that the minute bloodvessels are apt to become the seat of an atrophic process, in which the normal tissue (probably the muscular) of the capillary walls is replaced in great part by fat (p. 127).

He described such changes in the cerebral 'capillary vessels' of his patients who died of stroke, and in their hearts and kidneys. 'Is it, indeed', he asked, 'the primary and essential disease?' (p. 127).

Todd did not refer, in any of these lectures, to the question of localization of function in the brain. Indeed, he said, it was easier to determine the *nature* of a lesion than its actual *locality*. 'A clot in one hemisphere of the brain . . . will produce symptoms exactly the same as those of a similar clot in the substance of the corresponding cerebellar hemisphere' (p. 90). And it is intriguing, in view of the detailed nature of his accounts of hemiplegias, that he never considered the matter of loss of speech. He nearly always mentioned whether or not it was affected, signifying its degree, and if it was associated with paresis of the tongue or face. One reads – expectantly. Will he note that the lesion is usually on the left, or anteriorly? He was obviously such a gifted clinical observer that one feels that he, or even one of his students, might have stopped to ask the question – why is speech spared in one case, and not in the next? But there is no hint. There were cases of left-sided hemiplegia in which speech was 'very slightly impaired' (Case 27, p. 183), 'very imperfect' (Case 28, p. 187), in which 'we could get her to answer questions' (Case 29, p. 197), and in which 'his articulation is imperfect' (Case 22, p. 134). In cases of right-sided hemiplegia speech was nearly always seriously affected. One patient was 'speechless' (Case 32, p. 220); another 'lost entirely the power of speech' (Case 37, p. 246); and there was another who recovered complete power in her limbs 'but retaining the single peculiarity of using one word for another and of not applying appropriate names to the things she intended to signify; she never afterwards called even her own daughters by their right names' (Case 38, p. 248).

How mystifying that only Dr Dax had noticed this difference between the majority of cases of right- and left-sided hemiplegia.

Epileptic hemiplegia. Todd's paralysis, in this chapter, was described as follows:

A patient has a fit, distinctly of the epileptic kind; he comes out of it paralysed in one half of the body; generally that side is paralysed which has been more convulsed than the other, or which has been alone convulsed; but the paralysis may occur where both sides have been convulsed equally. The paralytic state remains for a longer or shorter time, varying perhaps from a few minutes or a few hours to three or four days, or even much longer. It then goes off, or improves, until the next epileptic fit, when a train of phenomena, precisely similar, recurs with like result (p. 284).

He pointed out that post-epileptic hemiplegia could occur in idiopathic epilepsy as well as in diseases of the brain – tumours, effusions, atrophy, softening, and apoplexy. It was the idiopathic variety, in which at autopsy the brain showed no significant abnormality, that led him to postulate that the paresis was a result of 'exhaustion' within the brain.

The phenomena of the epileptic fit depend upon a disturbed state of the nervous force in certain parts of the brain – a morbidly disturbed polarity ... This undue exaltation of the polar force induces, subsequently, a state of depression or exhaustion, not only in the parts primarily affected, but in parts of the brain connected with them, according to the degree of the primitive disturbance (p. 299).

Hughlings Jackson was to say in one of his papers on dissolution of the nervous system that 'On some parts I have worked for years in ignorance of what prior workers had done. I had, for example, arrived at the hypothesis of local exhaustion of nervous centres from epileptic discharges years before I knew that Todd and Robertson had stated it.'[21] A few years later in his Croonian Lectures on 'The Evolution and Dissolution of the Nervous System'[22] he wrote, in further reference to Todd's hypothesis, that the 'exhaustion' could not only involve the higher centres, 'the cells of the discharging lesion', but 'middle' and 'lowest' centres as well. 'The range of exhaustion downwards will vary according to the severity of the discharge.' Todd's words were somewhat similar in that he envisaged a local disturbance with effects in other parts of the brain. Todd had originally described post-epileptic paralysis in his Lumleian Lectures of 1849.[23]

Choreic hemiplegia. Todd also regarded post-choreic hemiparesis as a manifestation of 'exhaustion'. It resembled cerebral hemiparesis except that the face was usually unaffected, the protruded tongue did not deviate, and slight choreic movements could usually be discerned in the paretic extremities (p. 313). Distinction from cerebral tuberculosis in childhood was important. He had never seen an autopsy in a case of choreic hemiparesis but he thought that, as in epilepsy, 'exhaustion' of nerve centres was the cause.

Spinal hemiplegia. This was a rare form of paralysis; he described three cases. 'It can only occur when the paralysing lesion is seated high up in the cord just below the decussation of the anterior pyramids and where it is very exactly limited to one half of the cord' (p. 329). In the first case the cause proved to be compression from a displaced and enlarged odontoid process; in the second, the patient left hospital improved, after stiffness and swelling of his neck had subsided; in the third, Todd subsequently heard that the patient had 'caries' of the spine. Todd imagined that a tumour, clot, tubercle, or small area of softening, or any form of 'deposit' could affect one half of the spinal cord, but he had never seen any such cases.

He recalled that Bright had recorded odontoid compression in one case, and he regretted that he had not made more minute sensory examination of the paralysed limbs in view of 'Brown-Séquard's most interesting experiments' (p. 340). In the first of his three cases, which he said he correctly diagnosed, 'no difference could be observed between the two sides as regards temperature' (p. 333). In the second case 'sensibility', as measured with the compass points, was 'much more readily appreciated' in the unaffected limbs. In the third case, sensibility of the paralysed upper limb was 'decidedly diminished', but only slightly so in the ipsilateral paralysed lower limb. Spinal pain and tenderness was a feature in each case; pain was aggravated by coughing and sneezing in the third. The only reference to reflex activity was that it was 'good' in the second case. There was sphincter loss in the third.

Peripheral hemiplegia. Under this title (p. 256) Todd describes the features of what we would now attribute to diffuse cerebral arteriosclerosis. He admitted that it was not a 'correct designation' but it indicated the 'mode of access of the paralysis'. An elderly person began to complain of coldness and numbness in the extremities, followed by weakness, shuffling gait, clumsiness of the fingers, tremulous handwriting, and a tendency to stoop. With slurring of speech and 'a running gait' the picture often resembled that of 'paralysis agitans'. There was emotionality and failing mental powers. Todd had never seen an autopsy, 'as the disease generally goes on, for many years' but Cheyne had described similar cases under the name of 'Creeping Palsy' (p. 263). In one autopsy Cheyne had described diffuse bilateral cerebral softening.

Hysterical hemiplegia. When Todd came to discuss this subject (p. 264) one realizes that clinical examination was still largely a matter of observation. Any strange episode by way of disturbed consciousness, behaviour, movement, or speech immediately raised the question of hysteria. The patient was invariably a female, with ovarian tenderness, with the 'catamenia' inevitably 'irregular', and the 'physiognomy' always revealing; the 'Facies Hysterica' with its peculiar 'fullness' of the upper lip . . .[and] 'drooping condition of the upper eyelids' (p. 454).

He admitted that 'a very serious mistake would be to pronounce the paralysis from brain lesion to be hysterical' and he warned that 'a state of hysteria may co-exist with brain lesion'. But reading his case histories only serves to illustrate how incompletely such differentiations were then possible. 'The inability to excite reflex actions', for example, was one on which 'no reliance could be placed as a diagnostic sign' (p. 277). In a fatal case of a young woman of nineteen with tuberculomata in the brain, the focal and general convulsions, the hemiparesis, and the sensory loss were all interpreted as showing a mixture of the hysterical and the organic. Just as we now feel that the term 'neurosis' has become meaningless and could well be dropped, so also, reading these mid-century inherited 'received opinions' about hysteria, does one realize how superficial, still, was the scientific attitude. Women, particularly, were the patients who suffered.

Facial palsy. In paying tribute to the work of Bell he said he did not favour the designation 'Bell's Paralysis of the Face', 'for I must say that I cannot regard it as a compliment to the great names of our profession, to attach them to any of the numerous ills which flesh is heir to' (p. 66). But we can be reasonably sure he would not have protested too much about his own eponym. He did not think that Bell was correct in concluding that the eyeball turned upward in normal sleep. Only when there was forceful contraction of the orbicular muscles did this happen. He thought the buccinator muscle had two nerve supplies, one from the fifth and the second from the seventh. When taste was lost in facial palsy it 'was probably due to a coincident affection of the superficial nerves of the tongue' (p. 62). Facial palsy was 'a local palsy'; it usually recovered completely if it began to mend 'within a week'. Otitis, deafness, and parotid swelling might also be causes and there were still cases in which the nerve had been cut for the treatment of tic douloureux.

Lead palsy. The characteristic blue line on the gums in lead poisoning, which so assisted diagnosis, had recently been described by a contemporary London physician[24] and Todd repeatedly referred to the neurological features – the bilateral wrist drop, the wasting of the forearm extensor muscles, and the absence of pain and sensory loss (p. 350). He gave details of one case in which there were also episodes of convulsions and coma, following one of which the patient died. Tests for lead in brain and muscle were said to be negative. Microscopic examination of affected muscles showed degenerative changes. The nerves were not examined but Todd taught that the process of degeneration actually began in the muscles and spread into the nerves, cord, and brain. In his fatal case the brain was pale, but outwardly normal, and he had the specific gravity of various parts of it measured, but he could not draw any inference from the figures as normal ones were not fully known. Potassium iodide was useful in treatment, as it was in cerebral syphilis.

Cerebral symptoms in renal failure. Scanty or pale urine, albuminuria, the presence of cells and casts in urinary deposits – these he constantly sought in cases of cerebral disease, especially those that produced convulsions, impairment of consciousness, headache, confusion, or delirium. It was so easy, he said, 'to set the case down as one of disease of the brain'. He compared the intake and output of fluids (p. 148), and endeavoured to promote diuresis for 'when urea is retained in the blood, the brain is very likely to be affected so as to cause coma and convulsion' (p. 351). In one case the presence of urea in the blood was estimated by analysis of the serum from a blister produced on the neck; crystals of nitrite of urea were produced.

He thought that the 'constant drain of so much albumen, about 300 or 400 grains per diem' in a case of renal failure was bound to deprive the nervous system of 'its chief staminal principle' (p. 150).

A somewhat similar clinical picture – a series of convulsions followed by a fatal coma – was sometimes seen 'among puerperal women' (p. 159). 'Uterine phlebitis' was the diagnosis.

In this book Todd did not refer to his experimental researches on epilepsy, nor to his opinion on the function of the posterior columns of the spinal cord. But both deserve mention.

In his Lumleian lectures on convulsive diseases[23] he said that although stimulation of the cerebral hemispheres seemed not to 'excite motion', clinical experience suggested that 'convulsive movements may be excited by a superifical lesion of the hemispheric lobes' (p. 820). He went on to say that 'the influence of the hemispheres is most manifest for this purpose when the lesion is superficial; that is, when it affects the grey matter'. The periodicity of epilepsy reminded him of the phenomena of sleep and hibernation, in which there was a suspension of hemispheric activity. In attempting to determine what part the spinal cord, medulla, brain-stem, and mid-brain played in the production of the epileptic paroxysm, he employed galvanic stimulation. He used 'the magneto-electric rotation machine' in rabbits and found that stimulation of the spinal cord and medulla oblongata produced 'tetanic' spasms, but that stimulation of the 'corpora quadrigemina and the mesocephale' caused 'epileptic convulsions'. He said the movements consisted of 'alternate contraction and relaxation, flexion and extension affecting the muscles of all the limbs, of the trunk, and of the eyes, which rolled about just as in epilepsy'. But stimulation of the hemisphere produced nothing so dramatic.

> On inserting the awls into the hemispheric lobes, still different effects were produced by the application of the machine. I could observe nothing like true convulsions; but slight convulsive twitching of the muscles of the face took place, which were no more than what would be caused by the stimulus of galvanism acting upon the nerves of the face (p. 821).

Todd concluded that the great variation in the intensity and duration of the phenomena of epilepsy – the impairment of sensibility and consciousness, and the convulsive movements – 'depends on the nature and force of the primary disturbance in the cerebral hemisphere'. And it was not the white matter that was vital, but the grey 'vesicular matter, among the particles of the generating place of the nervous battery'.

> From all these facts, then, I infer that a disturbed state of the hemispheric lobes may undoubtedly give rise to so much of the phenomena of the epileptic paroxysm as refers to the affection of consciousness and sensibility, and that it may, *in some degree* at least, contribute to the development of the convulsions.

Todd was thus opposed to the prevailing spinal and medullary theories of epilepsy. Like Hughlings Jackson, when he began his studies on epilepsy in the eighteen-sixties, Todd believed that the seat was in the region of the corpus striatum, but he clearly also suspected that the convolutions might be involved. None of this was mentioned by Fritsch and Hitzig, or Ferrier, when they came to electrically stimulate the brain, over twenty years later. Todd's work was one of the forgotten 'prodromes' to cortical localization, so well recounted by Jefferson.[25]

Todd used to say he was an 'anatomical physician' and in his book on neuroanatomy[17] he frequently speculated on the significance of certain appearances. He noted, for example, that asymmetry of convolutions was more marked in man than in animals. There appeared to be no constancy in the differences between the right and left side, 'nor have we any clue to discover the cause of the difference between the two hemispheres, or the reason of the variation as regards predominance of size' (pp. 217–18).

He also considered the size of the columns of the spinal cord with reference to their alleged functions. 'Were the sensibility dependent on the grey matter or upon the posterior columns, as has been conjectured, it might most legitimately be expected that a proportionate development of these parts would exist in the cervical region.' Yet this was not the case; both elements were more developed in the lumbar region even though it was in the upper limbs that voluntary power and sensibility were more highly developed (p. 91).

In dealing with 'the offices of the columns of the cord' in his *Cyclopaedia*[16] he had some remarkable observations to make. He considered that anatomical and clinico-pathological evidence pointed to the fact that 'the antero-lateral columns are compound in function', serving motion and sensation. Direct experiments on the cord afforded no information on the functions of the different columns. (This was in 1847, before Brown-Séquard's first experiments.) With regard to the posterior columns all the evidence indicated that they were not concerned with ordinary sensibility. The posterior roots did not enter the posterior columns.

I have long been strongly impressed with the opinion that the office of the posterior columns of the spinal cord is very different from any yet assigned to them. They may be in part commissural between the several segments of the cord, serving to unite them and harmonise them in their various actions, and in part subservient to the function of the cerebellum in regulating and coordinating the movements necessary for perfect locomotion (p. 721q).

The attribute of locomotive power rests upon the connection of the posterior columns with the cerebellum, and the probable influence of that organ over the function of locomotion and the maintenance of the various attitudes and postures (p. 721q).

In examining a transverse section of the cord in the lumbar region, we observe a great predominance of its central grey matter; the posterior columns appear large, and the antero-lateral columns seem inadequate in proportion to the large roots of nerves which emerge from it. Now, an analysis of the locomotive actions shows, with great probability, that they are partly of a voluntary character, and partly dependent on the influence of physical impressions upon that segment of the cord from which the nerves of the lower extremities are derived. There are two objects to be attained in progression, namely, to support the centre of gravity of the body, and to propel it onward. ... The support of the centre of gravity of the body requires that the muscles of the lower extremities, the pillars of support of the trunk, should be well contracted in a degree proportioned to the weight they have to sustain. ... The stimulus is afforded by the application of the soles of the feet to the ground; it is therefore proportionate to the weight which presses them downwards. It is well known that reflex actions are more developed in the lower than in the upper extremities, and the surface of the sole of the foot is well adapted for the reception of sensitive impressions. ... All the structural arrangements necessary for this purpose are found in the antero-lateral columns. The posterior columns come into exercise in balancing the trunk and in harmonising its movements with those of the lower extremities (pp. 721q–r).

Todd, the clinician, found evidence to support this view of the function of the posterior columns of the spinal cord.

In many cases, in which the principal symptom has been a gradually increasing difficulty of walking, the posterior columns have been the seat of disease. Two kinds of paralysis of motion may be noticed in the lower extremities, the one consisting simply in the impairment or loss of the voluntary motion, the other distinguished by a diminution or total loss of the power of coordinating movements. In the latter form, while considerable voluntary power remains, the patient finds great difficulty in walking, and his gait is so tottering and uncertain that his centre of gravity is easily displaced (p. 721r).

He went on to say that in two cases, he correctly predicted that autopsy would show a degeneration of the posterior columns, and that in published reports in which there were such lesions there was always a history of unsteady locomotion, with retained superficial sensibility.

These two prescient observations of Todd – that 'superficial' lesions of the cerebral hemispheres could cause epilepsy, and that there were 'two kinds' of paraplegia – were subsequently endorsed by Hughlings Jackson and Gowers, respectively. In Todd we can catch a glimpse of the notion of 'a discharging lesion' and its 'downwards' spread, and Gowers acknowledged that the separation of the paraplegias began with him.

As Collier once wrote, 'Todd was by far the greatest neurologist Britain had produced until the time of Hughlings Jackson.'[26]

III. *The diagnosis of diseases of the brain, spinal cord, nerves, and their appendages*, by J. Russell Reynolds.

While Todd was preparing his lectures for publication, another London physician, in nearby Grosvenor Street, was also writing a book on clinical neurology, but of a very different kind. Russell Reynolds (1828–96) was not offering a text based on long experience, for he was only twenty-seven years of age when it was published a year after Todd's, and he had only been in practice a few years, and had yet to gain a teaching hospital appointment. He had graduated at University College and had the good fortune to be offered Marshall Hall's house when the latter decided to leave London in 1852. He had been a friend of Marshall Hall and was influenced by his work; he dedicated his book to him.

In his preface he explained that he was offering only a summary of what was known at the time but which constituted a 'deficiency which I felt when at college myself, and which others have often expressed to me since'. It was eventually considered to be 'the most clear and explicit account of the diseases of the nervous system that had appeared'.[27] One is reminded of another London neurologist of our own day – Russell Brain – recalling the early age (average thirty) of appointment and achievement of his predecessors at the London Hospital. He was thirty-eight when his own famous textbook was published.[28]

They both became Presidents of the Royal College of Physicians of London and Fellows of the Royal Society. Reynolds was also appointed to the Chair of Medicine at University College. He was created a Baronet in 1895.

Reynolds referred to the lack of knowledge of diseases of the nervous system and said 'We constantly hear it said that a patient has had an "apoplectic attack", a "convulsive seizure", or that he suffers from "some affection of the brain or spinal cord" and this without any further attempt at differential diagnosis.' He decided to adopt a clinical classification, and not one based on anatomical or physiological principles, because 'in the present state of medical science . . . we are far from having appreciated the nature' of the relation between symptoms and lesions. It was a matter of daily observation that similar symptoms could result from anatomically different diseases, and dissimilar symptoms from diseases identical in their anatomy.

There were three objects of diagnosis, 'locality, nature and lesion', and he proposed to arrange groups of diseases on these bases. Thus, in diseases of the brain, there were 'acute' and 'chronic' diseases. In the former they might be 'febrile' or 'non-febrile'. Non-febrile disorders were then classified according to the main feature – 'apoplexy', 'delirium', 'convulsion', and 'pain'. In 'chronic' diseases of the brain, there were three classes. Those marked by 'increased activity' (ideation, sensation, motility), 'diminished activity', or a combination of these.

Diseases of the spinal cord were 'acute' (meningitis, myelitis, tetanus, hydrophobia, haemorrhage and concussion) or 'chronic' (myelitis, meningitis, induration and hypertrophy, tumours and idiopathic paraplegia).

In the case of the nerves there were disorders that were 'structural' (neuritis, tumour) or 'functional' (neuralgia, spasm, anaesthesia, paralysis).

There was an index, some references, but no illustrations; the book was divided into four parts. In the first part, he outlined in four chapters the problems of diagnosis and classification. The second, third, and fourth parts were devoted to the brain, spinal cord, and nerves, respectively. In all, there are twenty chapters, and some 250 pages. It has a 'modern' look.

Part one. What one first appreciates is that Reynolds wrote lucidly and smoothly and with a clear aim. He wished to show in what way symptoms were related to disease.

> We can arrive at knowledge upon the diseases of the nervous system in only the same manner as upon every other subject; i.e., not by the progressive addition of element after element in a linear series, but by the simultaneous consideration and apposition of each class of truth in its relation to the others (p. 9).

Diagnosis involved examination of the relationships between locality, function, and structure. With regard to the first it was clearly essential to establish whether the disease was within or without the nervous system itself. In disease of the brain it could usually be decided which lateral half was affected and in many cases which particular portion – cortical or medullary, superior or inferior, or ventricular. There was 'much obscurity' about the functions of the cerebellum, but lesions of the centre could sometimes be distinguished from those involving the lateral lobes.

'The sensori-motor ganglia' (corpora quadrigemina, thalami, corpora striata, and pons) were commonly affected in certain diseases, such as softening, but as yet their involvement could not be accurately determined.

In disease of the spinal cord differentiation could usually be made between cervical, dorsal, and lumbar regions, but not with reference to the columns of the cord, nor between grey and white matter. Little was known about affection of the peripheral nerves, but among the cranial, there were sensory examples (e.g. the fifth), motor (the third, sixth, and seventh), and among the spinal nerves there were the different effects of sensory and motor root lesions.

Consideration of the second question – the nature of the affection – could be viewed in two ways. 'Disease' could be taken to mean 'the morbid phenomenon or process' that was present, or 'the modifications induced in the functions'. Reynolds felt that 'it is not so much the nature of these physical changes as their degree and mode of induction which determines the result' (p. 7). The difference between 'acute' and 'chronic' disorders was not just a matter of time, but also of severity.

Thirdly, there was the lesion, 'the anatomical condition'. In some diseases the tissues of the nervous system appeared to be healthy – in epilepsy, chorea, hysteria, and neuralgia, for example. In others the primary change was not in the nervous system itself but in the bloodstream. Thus, there were anaemia, hyperaemia, toxicity (extrinsic, such as poisons; intrinsic, such as 'urinaemia'), and the fevers. Lastly, there was the large group in which 'textural changes in the organs' of the nervous system were found (inflammation, softening, haemorrhage, degeneration of arteries, deposits, growths, and so on).

Summarizing his approach to the question of diagnosis he said that one sought the locality of the disturbance by way of the 'special quality of the symptoms' and their 'topographical distribution'. The nature of the disturbance required interpretation of the phenomena upon physiological and pathological grounds. The lesion was inferred not so much by the particular character or topography of the symptoms, but by evaluation of their order of development, their relation to each other, and by the identification of 'physical signs'. 'Pathological anatomy is a matter of inference only, during the lifetime of the patient'.

The elements for diagnosis. This was the term he used for the symptoms of disease, for they furnished the means by which diagnosis was made. He grouped them into two main physiological classes – mental and non-mental phenomena. The former pertained to man subjectively considered (disturbances of thought, volition, emotion, memory, and judgement), as distinct from disturbances of motility and sensibility which placed him, objectively, in relation with the external world. Volition and emotion had to be considered separately, 'as the two extremes of mental action, with ideation as their intermediating link' (p. 14).

The relation of volition to ideation was judged by observing the kind and amount of influence exerted by the will; impairment of attention, perception, recollection, and in the power of directing thought were common symptoms. 'Memory and recollection are not the same'; the former was the faculty of 'retaining', the latter that of 'finding'. They could be separately impaired.

Volition in its relation to emotion was normally one of balance, but in disease one could recognize diminished control of emotion, and diminished control of expression. The two need not co-exist.

Volition disturbed in relation to sensation caused symptoms in the perceptive sphere. It might be heightened or impaired. Loss of perception was a better term than loss of consciousness. The latter was often an assumption that later events proved incorrect; we cannot always say when the mind is inactive or devoid of self-consciousness.

The relations between volition and motility were not direct ones but when they were disturbed one could recognize such signs as the immobility of the hysteric (in contrast to genuine paralysis), excess of movement, and impaired initiation of movement.

Disturbed thought processes could only be observed indirectly in words, expressions, and actions. Ideation could be partially or wholly severed from external influences; in some forms of delirium sensation and perception persist, in others the latter are construed erroneously. The essential elements in thought processes may be separately affected. The sequence of ideas may suffer so that the patient cannot pursue a train of thought, or sequences may be too rapid to regulate. If there are none the patient is incoherent, and then one cannot judge memory.

Emotion could be considered as the source of action' and also as 'a frame of mind.' Illness may affect either. A frame of mind may be habitual or episodic. Change may be an early indication of disease.

Non-mental symptoms resolved themselves into morbid conditions of sensibility and motility and depended upon changes in one or more portions of the nervous system. Consciousness may or may not enter into sensori-motor activities.

Sensory symptoms were manifold, quantitatively and qualitatively. There were some 'new terms' to define – hyperaesthesia, hyperalgesia, dysaesthesia, hyp-aesthesia, and pseud-aesthesia (false sensations). Sensations could be misinterpreted; hot taken for cold, a single stimulus taken for two, localization misplaced.

Motor symptoms depended on the presence or absence of muscular contraction, whether voluntary, automatic, or reflex. Symptoms might be determined by 'loss of direction and combination' in voluntary movements. There may be exaggeration or impairment of 'emotion-motility', seen in the facial muscles, for example. Motility could be influenced by sensory stimuli, even in paralysis; startle can affect a paralysed limb. 'Absence of sensational guidance' (p. 35) influenced motility. A hand may be clumsy though power is adequate and cutaneous sensation is normal. So-called loss of 'muscular sense' could occur alone, in cases 'termed paraplegia'. Reflex activity and tone could both be impaired or enhanced by nervous disease, wholly or partially. Segmental reflex loss was one of the features of spinal cord lesions, as shown by Marshall Hall. Tone could alter sphincter function. It was often increased in brain disease and in paralysis agitans, and lost when there was muscular wasting.

In making some general comments on the differentiation between diseases of the brain, spinal cord, and nerves (p. 59), Reynolds referred to one difficulty of interpretation about which there was a difference of opinion. He said there were cases in which 'positive' evidence of disease of the spinal cord was sometimes associated with 'negative' evidence of disease of the brain. He cited 'hemiplegia with exalted reflex activity' as an example. One interpretation was that 'diminished cerebral power exaggerates, *per se*, the activity of the spinal cord'. Another was that the reflex activity was due to 'a morbid spinal condition ... developed either co-taneously or subsequently to the lesion of the brain'. He thought the first explanation was based on a current notion that there was 'an antagonism' between these two centres, which he did not think was true. He favoured the second interpretation and thought that in brain disease there might be some 'induced, it may be dynamic, condition of the cord'. Perhaps he was influenced by the early reports of descending tract degeneration which were then appearing, notably by Türck.

It is evident, in these introductory chapters, that Reynolds, young though he was, had given much thought to the principles involved in neurological diagnosis. His views were mature, broadly-based, and he saw that in practical terms, he had no choice but to adopt a clinical classification of disease of the nervous system.

Diseases of the brain. In presenting his diagnostic clinical classification, Reynolds defined some of his terms, and made some general statements. Although he knew that, strictly speaking, *apoplexy* meant haemorrhage he preferred to use it in a clinical sense, regardless of the actual lesion. The degree and extent of loss of function varied widely, although haemorrhage was the sole lesion. *Delirium* was of little diagnostic value in itself, and how it fundamentally differed from *coma* was not understood. Similarly one did not know what prompted the appearance of *convulsions*. All these four major symptoms of acute disorders of the brain could occur from one disease, e.g. 'softening', but 'a disease is not to be made out by either its symptoms alone, but by a conjunction of the two' (p. 67). It was just as easy to obscure progress by drawing artifical lines, as by failing to observe those laid down by nature. Names 'do not create a difference except in our own minds ...'.

In chronic diseases many different combinations of loss or exaggeration of function could occur; in the fields of motion, sensation, intellect, or emotion. The endlessly variable manner in which the resulting symptoms could be grouped was one of the major difficulties encountered by the diagnostician.

Discussion of his chapter on acute febrile diseases affecting the brain is not now profitable but one notes that he acknowledged Whytt's description of tuberculous meningitis, mentioned 'retracted head' (p. 77), and that he considered the picture in adults was different in certain respects from that in children. In the former, the onset could be by way of convulsion, stroke, or sudden loss of articulation, with little fever or 'inflammatory action'. There was sometimes 'a peculiar intellectual state' with 'mutism'; 'the patient appears to understand what is said, or asked; looks at the enquirer for a few seconds, and then turns the head away without reply' (p. 79). All rather reminiscent of akinesia with mutism. One of the most difficult problems in this acute febrile group was in distinguishing between meningitis, typhoid fever, and typhus.

Apoplexy. An apoplectic attack could result from congestion, haemorrhage, softening, tumour, uraemia, or vascular obstruction. In each case there may or may not be warning symptoms, mental or physical. They were marked in 'congestion' and usually absent in haemorrhage. To Todd 'congestion' was not real and he envisaged cardiac hypertrophy to be a secondary effect of the diseased arteries. But Reynolds did not think that hypertrophy of the left ventricle was important in relation to cerebral haemorrhage; 'the bases upon which this idea has rested are insufficient and unsatisfactory' (p. 112). 'Degeneration' in heart and cerebral vessels was 'the real link' between haemorrhage and hypertrophy. He was also sceptical about the recent concept of embolism from diseased cardiac valves (p. 114).

In ventricular haemorrhage coma was profound and paralysis often bilateral. In 'arachnoid' (i.e. superficial) haemorrhage the onset was not always abrupt and paralysis was often less marked than when the haemorrhage was in the substance of a hemisphere.

It was exceedingly difficult to distinguish between acute 'red' softening and haemorrhage but in the former there was a tendency for the onset to be less sudden, and combinations such as 'imperfect' coma with rigid limbs, deep coma without rigidity, and paralysis without loss of consciousness, would suggest the proper diagnosis (since congestion does not cause profound coma nor rigidity; and ventricular haemorrhage causes profound coma and also rigidity).

Tumour cases suffered much preceding headache, dimness of vision, and limb weakness and there may also have been a history of convulsion. Similarly, in uraemia, an apoplectic attack was usually preceded by other symptoms – general ill-health, drowsiness, depression, transient amaurosis, nocturnal restlessness, and so on.

Following recovery from an apoplectic attack the paretic muscles could atrophy from disuse but rigidity with contracture was the striking feature. Duchenne taught that the latter were a consequence of 'spinal action, increased by the fact of persistent central changes, removing cerebral control' (p. 98).

As in Todd's book there was no discussion of where the lesion might be located, apart from what has been said, and no hint of the relation of speech loss to sidedness.

Delirium. Non-febrile delirium was encountered in hyperaemia of the brain, in 'red' softening, in diseases such as uraemia, jaundice, and diabetes, and, of course, in 'delirium tremens'.

In cerebral hyperaemia, no doubt both the quality of the blood and the speed of its movement were factors at work. Delirium of this kind was usually found in the elderly, especially at night, and could affect only speech. But confusion and motor restlessness were the rule; it was rather a simple disturbance, but it might be the herald of cerebral softening.

Convulsions. He recognized that convulsions could occur throughout a lifetime without leaving a trace of abnormality in the brain. This was the idiopathic variety – the disease called *epilepsy*. Convulsions also occurred in patients with a variety of proved cerebral lesions, such as tumour, softening, or tuberculoma; they were referred to as *epileptiform* or *epileptioid*. In all types of convulsions, there were minor and major disturbances of consciousness and involuntary movement. He referred to the 'haut mal' and 'petit mal' of French authors.

In childhood, fever, the exanthemata, dentition, worms, and so on were thought to play an aetiological role, so that it was not entirely clear what the essential relation was between convulsion and a cerebral lesion. Was it a direct one, in which convulsion was 'dependent directly upon the cerebral state', or was it the result of some 'induced condition of another portion of the nervous system'? (p. 122). In childhood, for example, convulsions could be 'sympathetic in origin; i.e. that they depend upon some excess of irritation'.

Chronic diseases of the brain. Distinction from acute diseases of the brain was not as clear-cut as one would expect. A chronic disease could be symptomless until its acute fatal termination, or it could be latent, with minor symptoms of a particular nature, and suddenly manifest itself with a new variety of acute complaints. Then, too, a chronic disease could present intermittent or paroxysmal symptoms. He concluded that the division of acute from chronic was one of degree and not of kind.

So, as in acute diseases of the brain, one could classify the disturbances of function by way of exaggeration, diminution, or a combination of both. And one could consider them as they referred to mental, sensory, and motor activities.

The exact location of the cerebral lesion in epilepsy, catalepsy, hysteria, chorea, and paralysis agitans was not known, but in epilepsy and catalepsy it was 'closely related to functional derangement in the spinal cord' and in hysteria and chorea there must be 'some morbid condition of the emotional and sensori-motor centres'.

An example of a disorder in which there was '*exalted*' activity in the mental sphere was hypochondriasis; there was exaggerated ideation. In the sensory sphere, excessive activity could express itself in hemicrania, hallucinations, or illusions. Vertigo came under the latter heading and it could be objective or subjective. In the former, external objects appeared to move; in the latter, it was the patient himself who appeared to move. There may or may not be an obvious trigger. No hint of labyrinthine aetiology here.

Reynolds also used the term 'motor vertigo' to cover the disturbances of coordination observed in cerebellar disease. The involuntary movements of chorea and paralysis agitans (which was a 'bad' term because the patient was not paralysed) were also examples of excessive motor activity. In chorea there were two essential disturbances; involuntary movements and deranged voluntary movement. There was also muscular weakness. Choreic movements disappeared during sleep and they also often did so during an intercurrent fever (p. 162). There was no constant lesion found in the nervous system in chorea or in paralysis agitans but Dr Paget had recently found a lesion in the crura cerebri in a patient with a nodding head and a tendency to totter forward (p. 164). He suggested that it should be looked for in such cases.

Diseases marked by 'diminution' of function rarely existed in isolated form, and the most obvious were those in which the lesion was local and peripheral. He would discuss these when he came to the nerves. But there was one 'disease' which he thought should be considered at this juncture, and he called it 'Anaesthesia Muscularis' (p. 165). It is an account of locomotor ataxia.

This disease was liable to be 'confounded with paraplegia' and was 'most certainly a distinct morbid condition'. There was 'a diminution in the faculty of controlling movements', although power and cutaneous sensibility were intact. Neither were 'the reflective functions interfered with ... there is no exaltation of susceptibility' (which suggests that he observed that rigidity and flexor withdrawal responses were not present). The disability – a clumsiness – was most marked in the lower limbs, causing a drunken gait. It was aggravated by eye closure so it could not be attributed to a primary defect of coordination, in which 'sensational guidance' is not corrective. Reynolds concluded that in this disease there was a diminution or loss of 'the muscular sense, or the intuitional perception of muscular states' (p. 166). It could not be attributed to 'any particular organic change of a special organ ... it appears most probable (especially since this is the first change in cases which subsequently exhibit perfect paraplegia) that the *centripetal tract of fibres is affected*' (p. 167; my italics).

This account of *Anaesthesia Muscularis* is not found in the section devoted to diseases of the spinal cord, and Reynolds made no reference to similar accounts by Todd and Romberg on ataxia, although he referred to them on other topics. Romberg had described his *sign* in a chapter entitled 'Anaesthesia of the Muscular Nerves', while the disorder itself, *Tabes Dorsalis*, he placed in a section devoted to disorders of motility. He said he had first described the symptoms some ten years before the publication of his book.

The most common group of diseases of the brain, Reynolds wrote, were those in which there was a combination of increased and diminished function. It was in this section that he discussed tumours (p. 182). Symptoms which suggested the *possibility* of tumour were persistent headache, vomiting, dimness of vision, impairment of hearing, confusion, and slowly developing and often localized paresis in a patient who might periodically suffer a convulsion. There was little to guide one concerning the *nature* of a tumour, except in cases of known cancer or tuberculosis.

The *locality* of a cerebral tumour it was usually 'utterly impossible' to determine. True, one could perhaps guess which side, if the headache was localized, or the motor signs (paresis or convulsion) were unilateral. Involvement of the special senses suggested a basal rather than a superior location.

Differentiation between anterior and posterior location should also be attempted. Impairment of sight, intelligence, and articulation favoured an anterior site. But convulsions suggested a posterior site. 'Upon analysing a considerable number of cases, I find that convulsions are most frequent in tumours of the cerebellum, and that they diminish in frequency as the seat of lesion advances forwards' (p. 186).

'The differentiation of special portions of the cerebrum, or cerebellum, as the seat of tumour, is at present impossible', though there were indications that in due course this would be feasible. Some had suggested that meningeal tumours were more likely to cause pain and 'irregular convulsive movements' and that in cerebral tumours pain was less conspicuous and there was a greater incidence of motor and sensory paresis, and intellectual failure. But tumours often involved both structures and the available data did not justify this distinction.

Under the heading of 'Chronic Meningitis' he referred to the picture of general paralysis of the insane and to Calmeil's 'beautiful treatise'. In addition to progressive dementia there were such symptoms as headache, falling, limb pains, and paraesthesiae. Involvement of the muscles of the face, tongue, and eyeballs were particularly characteristic; convulsions, partial and complete, occurred, and movements of the limbs became progressively impaired. It was important in such cases to exclude uraemia and to enquire about previous head injury or syphilis.

'Chronic Softening', unassociated with apoplexy, was a grave question. Its cardinal feature was intellectual failure.

In distinguishing between tumour, chronic meningitis, and chronic softening, Reynolds suggested the following:

In *tumour*, there was intense headache, often localized; affection of the special senses; local paralyses; epileptoid convulsions; unimpaired intelligence.

In *chronic meningitis*, headache was diffuse and not marked; mental and emotional excitement were common; there were disorderly spasms and paralyses; and irregular accessions of fever.

In *chronic softening*, pain was not a feature; there was progressive failure of intelligence, motility, and sensibility.

All of which, one can only respect, coming from a young physician one hundred and twenty-five years ago.

Diseases of the spinal cord. In the twenty or more pages which he devoted to diseases of the spinal cord one gains the impression that Reynolds really had too little clinical experience for the task. He refers to Ollivier but proceeds to classify and catalogue his data in a rather tedious manner. Acute diseases of the cord were congestion, meningitis, myelitis, meningo-myelitis, tetanus, hydrophobia, and haemorrhage. Chronic diseases were myelitis, meningitis, induration and hypertrophy, tumours, and idiopathic paraplegia. In general he considered each disorder as it would affect the 'conductive' and 'centric' functions of the cord. The former resulted in defects of sensory and motor transmission, numbness, and weakness; the latter, in alteration of muscular tone, spasms, and reflex activity.

Conduction could be 'perverted' as well as impaired. In the sensory field this caused formication, sensations of heat, cold, and other dysaesthesiae, mainly in the periphery of limbs. They arose spontaneously or as a result of stimuli, such as the touch of clothes. Perversion of motility led to disordered voluntary movements.

'Centric' functions of the cord could be increased or impaired. On the motor side heightened activity caused tonic and clonic spasms. It was difficult to know whether 'centric' activity was purely and wholly reflex in character. When it was impaired there was flaccidity of muscles, general lack of tone, relaxation of sphincters, and lack of contractility to electrical stimulation. 'Diminished reflexion' was apparent; 'absence of any contraction in the limbs upon irritating their cutaneous surface' (p. 205).

Diagnosis of a spinal cord lesion actually necessitated identification of the level involved, the columns affected, and whether grey or white matter primarily suffered.

With regard to lumbar and dorsal levels the extent of motor and sensory loss was well known. In the cervical region Reynolds endeavoured to distinguish between upper, middle, and low levels. Phrenic nerve involvement in high lesions led to urgent dyspnoea; 'the unfortunate sufferer feels as if life or death depended on his exertions'. (This is one phrase which suggests personal experience.) In a lesion extending no higher than the sixth cervical vertebra, shoulder movements are spared, though forearms, hands, and fingers are paralysed. The upper limbs became involved when the lesion was 'opposite the first dorsal or the last two cervical vertebrae'. Priapism, flatus, dysphagia, defective articulation, and retention with involuntary evacuation were all common in cervical lesions.

One difficulty in trying to assess which columns (anterior, posterior, lateral) were affected was that symptoms may be referred solely to one column, yet at post-mortem others were clearly also involved. All he could say was that impaired motility suggested anterior, and impaired sensibility posterior, involvement. Clinical experience had done little to corroborate 'ingenious theories and experimental inferences'. It was much the same with reference to the grey and white matter. Clinical observation and morbid anatomy had done little 'to confirm, or refute the physiological doctrines with regard to these two structural elements' (p. 200).

Apart from his 'muscular anaesthesia', there is nothing of particular interest in the sections on chronic myelitis, induration, and idiopathic paraplegia, and in tumours he does not make it clear whether he was just dealing with involvement of the cord from vertebral lesions. He only refers to 'Tumours of the spinal column, implicating the functions or structure of the cord' (p. 220). His two groups were based on the presence or absence of general conditions, such as tuberculosis or cancer. There is no mention of tumour within the cord or compressing it.

Diseases of the nerves. These ten pages are likewise disappointing, consisting merely of an explanatory classification, with a few clinical entities, such as trigeminal neuralgia and facial palsy. Even these are poorly portrayed.

Diseases of nerves were structural (neuritis and tumours) or functional (neuralgia, spasms, anaesthesias, and paralyses). The only comment of interest is that he recognized that when Marshall Hall had used the term 'spinal paralysis' he had meant that type of paralysis which followed a lesion that had severed the muscles from their nervous connection with the spinal cord. Many had thought he had meant that type of paralysis due to a lesion of the spinal cord. A feature of Hall's 'spinal paralysis' was loss of electrical irritability, confirmed by the recent observations of Duchenne.

*

As a general introduction to the diagnosis of nervous diseases Reynolds's book must have brought some order and clarity to the students and doctors of his day. Although the classification was said to be primarily clinical, the manner which he adopted to describe symptoms and signs was very similar to that used by Romberg, but which the latter pursued too far. The best part of Reynolds's book is Part One where he defines his task and gives his reasons for his classification and his approach to diagnosis. But the text itself inevitably lacks the touch of experience and authority, so evident in Todd and Romberg. Nevertheless, its lucid and concise nature would, I suspect, have made it a popular text for an examination candidate in those days.

The pages of these mid-nineteenth-century texts illustrate what little progress had been made in the clinical examination of the nervous system since Cooke's day. Despite the discoveries of Bell, Magendie, and Marshall Hall, and the descriptions of morbid anatomists, a clinician with a patient suffering from some disorder of mentation, motion, or sensation had little to help him – certainly nothing comparable to percussion and auscultation, not to mention such refinements as 'whispering pectorioquy'. He could still do little more than assess the extent and degree of disturbance of these faculties.

Paralysed muscles could be soft and limp, or hard and rigid; some wasted, others did not. Paralysis was sometimes attended, or followed, by 'reflex excitement', 'agitation', or 'convulsion – spontaneous or induced'. Pain and numbness were variable accompaniments. Moreover, a patient might have paralysed muscles showing some of these features and others that did not, or that actually showed signs of an opposite kind. Lastly, the passage of time could influence the signs in paralysis. Wasting, in some cases, appeared to be due to disuse. In others, it transpired that the disease was actually progressive. But even when the disease was arrested there were changes in the paralysed limbs that were difficult to understand. Thus, after a stroke, the lower limb might recover much of its power and lose its rigidity, while the affected upper limb remained useless, its rigidity actually increasing, and with flexion deformity providing an additional disability. It was difficult to understand in what way such signs were the result of loss of function, especially as they could seemingly follow from lesions in brain or spinal cord. When there was no visible lesion, as in paralysis agitans or ascending paralysis, for example, the mystery was complete.

So, with only a superficial understanding of sensory paralysis, it is not difficult to see how the distinction between 'organic' and 'functional' paralysis was so hard to establish.

In *acute* disease of the brain, such as apoplexy, it was appreciated that there was a period of 'shock', with perhaps loss of consciousness, and that the hemiplegia was determined by the size and location of the lesion. But in the case of the spine Marshall Hall's conception of 'spinal shock' had yet to be fully applied to the interpretation of the physical state of the paralysed limbs. If he had turned to the examination of the 'tendon reflexes', in his studies of the reflex arc, the pace of advance might have been hastened. In *chronic* disease of the brain, as in vumour, there was little realization that there were 'general' and 'local' effects to be distinguished. Blindness, which commonly suggested the presence of tumour in a case of paralysis, could only be attributed to 'paralysis of the optic nerves'. Similarly, loss of speech was not understood.

However, in diseases of the spinal cord, as we have seen, the distinction between paralysis and ataxia was beginning to emerge, as also were the features of partial lesions. Affections confined to spinal roots were not yet recognized, and although many examples of peripheral nerve palsies were known, the concept of a multiple symmetrical peripheral neuritis lay in the future.

In general, there was some awareness that the grey and white matter of the nervous system were not equally involved in all diseased states, but the possibility of 'system' disorders had yet to be entertained.

During the third quarter of the century, the key figure in the elucidation of motor paralysis was Duchenne (1806–75). And it was largely through the continuing clinical studies of Brown-Séquard that progress was made in understanding sensory paralysis. When, to these contributions and the impetus they gave to the techniques of neurological examination, were added the introduction of the ophthalmoscope and the reflex hammer, the scene at the bedside was transformed. With the localization of the speech area by Broca in 1860 and that of the motor cortex by Fritsch and Hitzig in 1870, we approach an epoch of remarkable development in all branches of neurology.

FIG. 125. Duchenne's 'histological punch' which he used for muscle biopsy, hooking a small piece of muscle into the end of the instrument.

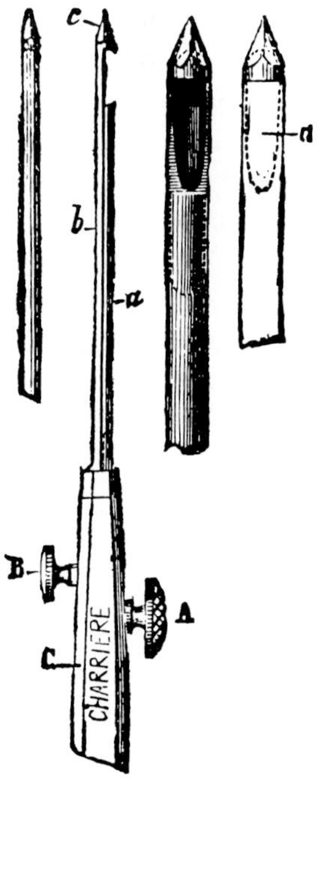

DUCHENNE ON PARALYSIS AND ATAXIA

Duchenne (1806–75), who graduated in Paris in 1831, became interested in the function of muscles when he noticed local contractions during electrotherapy for neuralgia.[29–31] He came to rely on faradic current from the induction coil invented by Faraday in 1831 and, employing moistened cloth-covered electrodes, he was able to obtain localized surface stimulation of muscles – 'sans piquer ni inciser la peau'. He became a 'néophyte électricien', studying the works of l'Abbé Nollet, Marat (familiar to us as the physician of the Revolution who was stabbed to death in his bath by Charlotte Corday in 1793), and Humboldt. He left his practice in Boulogne in 1842, at the age of thirty-six, and spent the rest of his life in Paris, pursuing his studies of neuromuscular function. He did not wish for, nor was he granted, any official hospital appointment, although he was befriended by Charcot and others. He did not want to be 'riveted' to a hospital ward as then he could not be 'a searcher'.

All he sought was access to patients and for more than twenty years he followed them from one hospital to another – and, after some criticism, also to the autopsy room. 'Sa pile et sa bobine'† was his 'principal and very modest capital', and he built up a successful private practice. He devised 'a strength gauge' or dynamometer and 'a tissue punch' for muscle biopsy (which Gowers later called a 'harpoon-trochar' or 'histological harpoon'). He learned microscopy and photography and devised splints for his palsied patients.

† voltaic cell and induction coil

He began by analysing the functions of individual muscles and muscle-groups, noting their electrical responses ('electromuscular exploration'), and what happened when there was paralysis, with or without muscular wasting. He looked for ways to assist diagnosis and prognosis. He studied the muscles of facial expression; Darwin, in his own book *The expression of the emotions in man and animals* (1872) praised him for this and reproduced some of Duchenne's photographs.

Selections of his clinical papers on the diseases he described – progressive muscular atrophy, bulbar palsy, acute poliomyelitis, pseudohypertrophic muscular dystrophy, and locomotor ataxy – are included in the third edition of his *De l'électricisation localisée*[32] which was published in English by the New Sydenham Society in 1883, and from which my references are quoted.[33]

FIG. 126 (*left*). Duchenne demonstrates the contraction of the left frontalis muscle on stimulation with the faradic current. 'Electro-muscular exploration.'

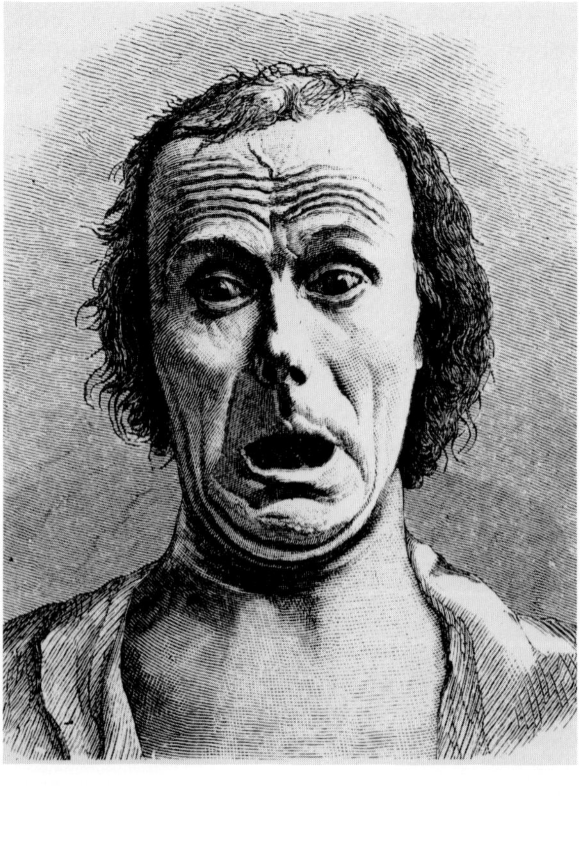

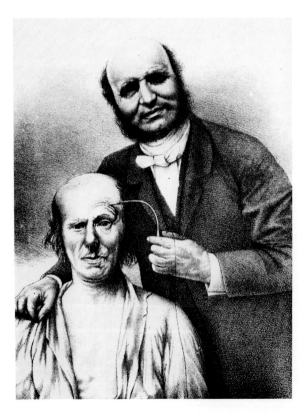

FIG. 127 (*right*). Duchenne's photograph to illustrate 'Terror'. It was used by Darwin in his *The expression of the emotions in man and animals* (1872). Bell and Duchenne thought the platysma muscle always contracted forcibly in states of fear. Duchenne called it 'the muscle of fright', but Darwin thought that was not justifiable.

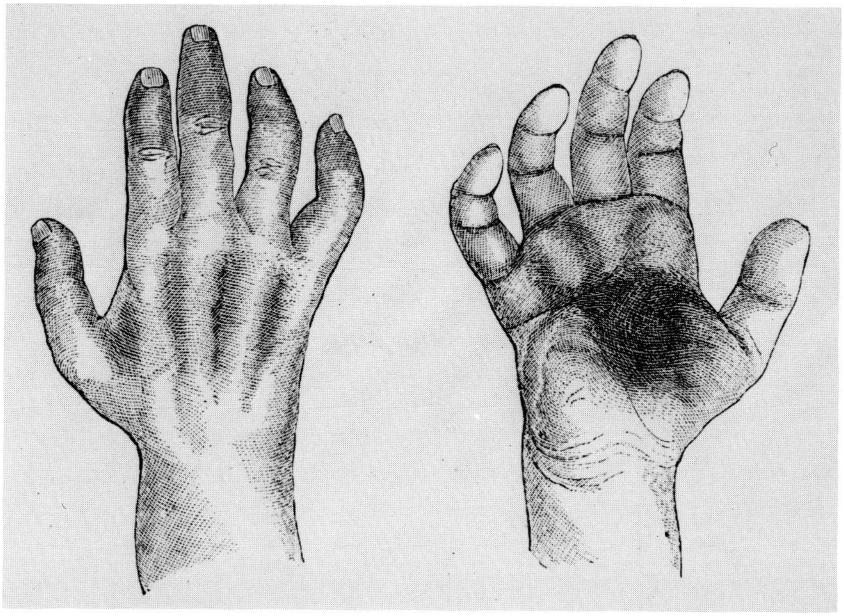

FIG. 128. A hand in progressive muscular atrophy.

Progressive muscular atrophy

What first intrigued Duchenne was that there were adult patients with paralysis of certain movements that was clearly associated 'in direct proportion' with wasting of specific muscles. It usually began in one hand and spread upward, 'the loss of power keeping pace with the diminution of muscular fibres' (p. 42). It rarely began in the lower limbs, in maybe two cases out of 159 (p. 53); and often went undetected for some time if it first affected the muscles of the trunk, as it did in twelve cases (Fig. 129). Moreover, weakness might not be noticed by the patient (who rarely mentioned that he could no longer sing, blow out a candle, or hold his breath), and wasting could be missed by the doctor. The face was usually 'well-nourished'; obesity could mask wasting. What he thought so peculiar, and what he called 'the facies' of the disease, was the way in which 'a muscle may be wasted alongside of others which are perfectly intact notwithstanding a community of nervous supply' (p. 53). Sphincters remained unaffected. Hollows were 'dissected' out where formerly there were muscle eminences, and deformities developed; 'clawed hands', 'winged scapulae', and certain types of lordosis (Figs. 130 and 131).

Affected muscles 'are often jerked by little fibrillary or partial contractions ... or little worm-like movements'. These movements were often localized and periodic, at other times they were diffuse and continuous. They were sometimes noted by the patient – 'But too much importance should not be attached to these little spasms', as they were not constant (they were absent in a fifth of his cases), they occurred in other diseases, and even in healthy persons (A 'provincial *confrère* had been much worried by them' (p. 44).

'All authors who have written on progressive muscular atrophy have said

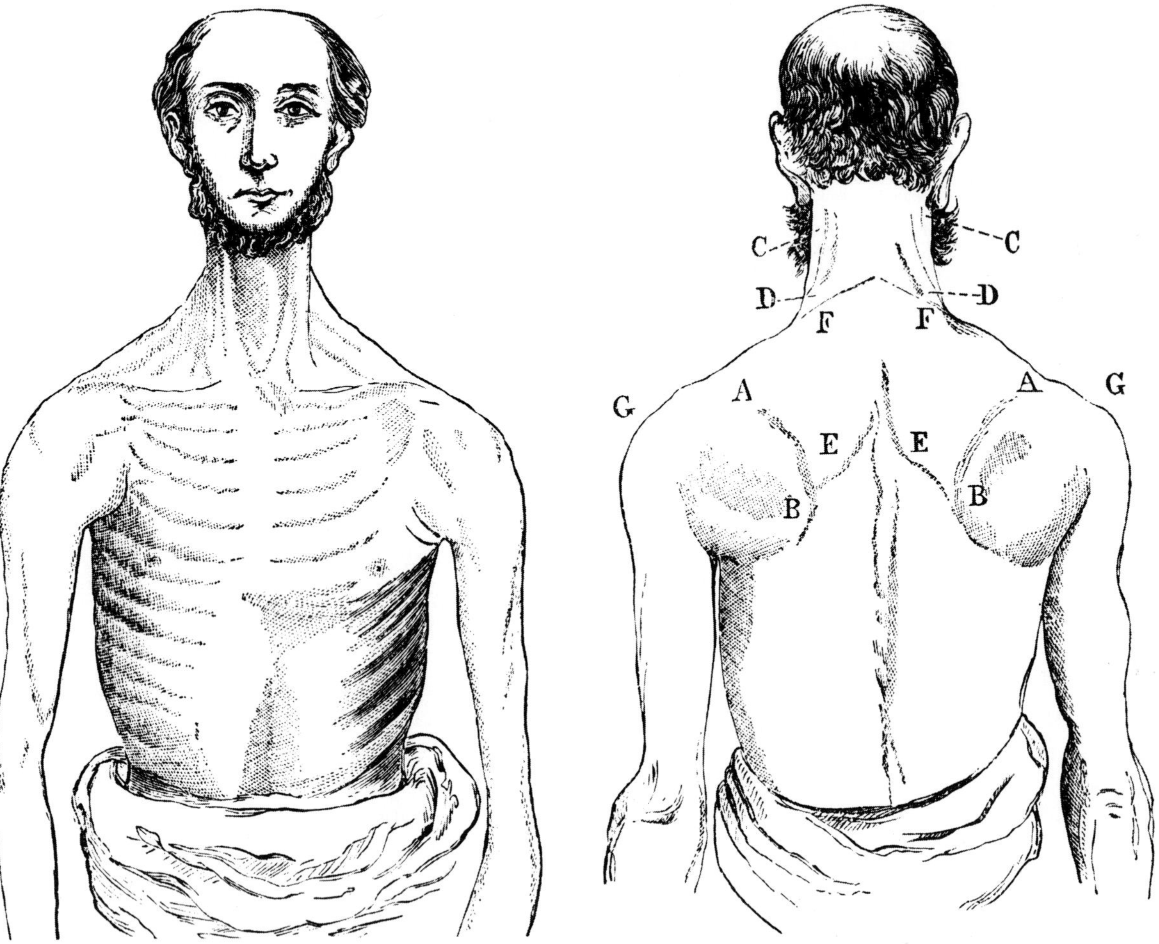

FIG. 129. Progressive muscular atrophy; to illustrate how the wasting 'attacks nearly all the superficial muscles of the trunk before reaching the upper limbs' – (*left*) anterior, (*right*) posterior.

that sensibility has always been normal in this condition' (p. 47). This was not correct, he said, for cutaneous anaesthesia occurred in patients who had rheumatic pains, which was 'a complication', or in cases in which the lesion had spread 'to the posterior horns of the cord'. Strong faradization was sometimes quite painless, and some patients 'have been badly burnt on their anaesthetic parts, without being conscious of it at the time'. Initially, of course, Duchenne had thought the disease was primarily one of muscle tissue, especially when, at the first autopsy by Cruveilhier in 1849, no spinal cord or root lesion was discovered. In 1853, however, the anterior root atrophy was noted, but Duchenne thought it was 'a secondary lesion' and he only reluctantly came to accept that the primary lesion lay in the anterior horns of grey matter in the spinal cord (p. 84). No doubt some of his cases with sensory loss were examples of syringomyelia.

It is interesting to note that with respect to aetiology he considered the possibility of over-exertion, as in workmen, the wasting 'appears first in the most fatigued muscles' – a concept that has often been discussed since his day.

Glosso-labio-laryngeal paralysis

Initially Duchenne reported these cases, an 'espèce morbide distincte', in 1868 as 'progressive paralysis of the tongue, the soft palate and the lips', but in due course he adopted the above title which had been recommended by Trousseau. By 1871 he had seen 39 cases, all in private practice, but without any autopsies. Within two months of his original memoir 'fourteen new cases were communicated to me by my professional brethren'.

It was a disease of adults which was invariably fatal in six months to three years. The intellect was not affected, sphincters functioned normally, and in only one case had he seen the disease spread to involve an upper limb (p. 154).

It usually began with difficulty in articulating 'palatal and dental sounds', and with the accumulation of saliva in the mouth so that the patient is 'continually wiping his mouth with his fingers and handkerchief'. Eventually speech became unintelligible and swallowing 'as impossible as when the tongue is depressed and the mouth kept widely open' (p. 147). Phonation eventually suffered and breathing declined. All these symptoms were due to a progressive paralysis of the tongue, palate, lips, throat, gullet, larynx, and

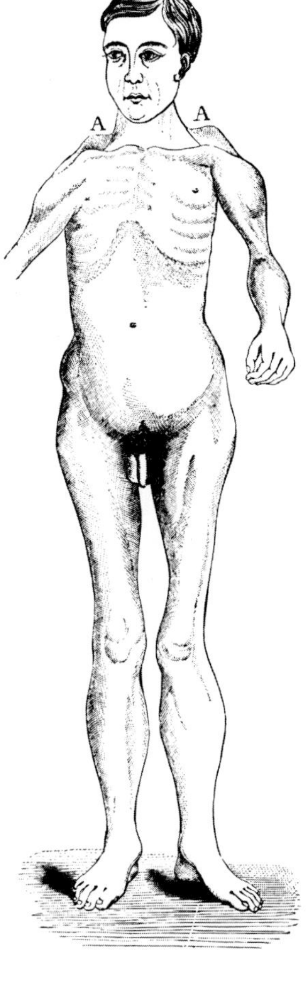

FIG. 130 (*left*). Progressive muscular atrophy; to illustrate how 'the scapulae project like wings from the thorax' when the arms are raised. The 'peculiar (fusiform) shape of the forearm' was due to selective wasting of the long supinators. It looks more like a dystrophy.

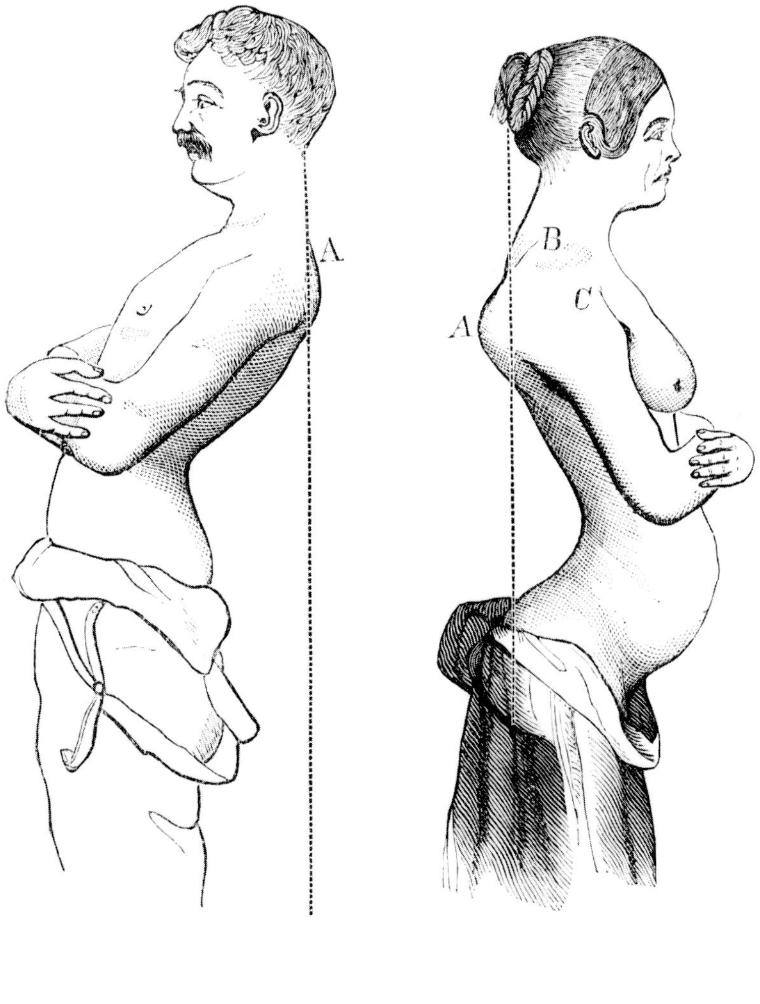

FIG. 131 (*right*). Progressive muscular atrophy; to illustrate lordosis. In the man it is due to 'a failure of the extensors of the trunk', and in the female to 'a failure of the flexors of the trunk (the abdominal muscles)'

bronchi. He did not think that the tongue wasted as it occasionally did in progressive muscular atrophy, nor did he observe fibrillation in his cases of bulbar palsy (pp. 155–6).

In the face it was the orbicularis oris muscle that was foremost affected, making the pronunciation of vowels, whistling, and kissing difficult. He had never seen involvement of orbicularis palpebrarum, zygomatic, or bucc nator muscles. Paralysis of the pterygoids made the 'grinding' of food impossible, although the patient could still 'divide it with force' (p. 149). There was no pain or sensory disturbance, and as taste and appetite were preserved, patients 'suffer the torture of Tantalus'.

Duchenne suspected a central lesion in the medulla and studied its 'intimate structure', making photographs of his sections. Lockhart Clarke (1817–80) helped him here when he visited Paris for the first international medical congress in 1867, and showed him his 'beautiful sections'. It was Charcot, Duchenne acknowledged, who showed that the lesion began in the motor neurones of the medulla, saying that 'the disease process, whatever it be, attacks the cell in the first instance' (p. 160).

Acute poliomyelitis

In the 'essential paralysis of childhood' which Duchenne described in 1855 as 'infantile atrophic paralysis', paralysis was maximum at onset. Muscular atrophy developed 'very rapidly, more rapidly than that produced by traumatic lesions of mixed nerves in the adult', and was proportional to the loss of electro-muscular contractility (p. 97). Affected limbs were cold, but not numb. He had studied 'many hundreds' of cases between 1850 and 1870 and had never seen two children affected in one family. It attacked 'rich and poor', with or without fever, and it did not 'threaten life'. In fact, he had never seen a case terminate fatally (p. 106). The paralytic stage was followed by one of recovery, often with contractures, spinal curvature, and impaired growth of a limb, including its bones. There was no sensory paralysis: bladder and bowel function remained intact.

Whereas in injuries to mixed nerves, and in lead palsies, voluntary movement tended to return before electro-muscular contractility, in poliomyelitis he had never seen this in over three hundred cases (p. 98).

In the paralytic stage, persistence of electrical activity in a muscle suggested the possibility of recovery, but in the chronic stage absence of activity could be a result of tissue changes in the muscle itself.

In the eighteen-sixties Charcot and his colleagues proved what Duchenne had suspected, that the underlying lesion was in the spinal cord, in the anterior horn cells.

Pseudo-hypertrophic muscular dystrophy

Duchenne had referred to cases in which 'hypertrophy' accompanied progressive paralysis in infancy, *hypertrophic paraplegia of infancy*, for some years prior to his classic account in 1868. 'I waited in vain for an autopsy . . . seeking an explanation of the two contradictory facts . . . of paralysis and muscular hypertrophy' (p. 171). In Germany where, he said, 'my researches

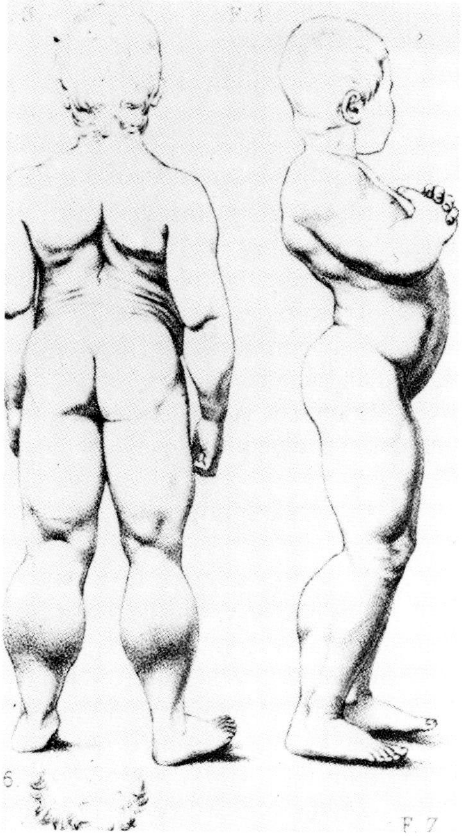

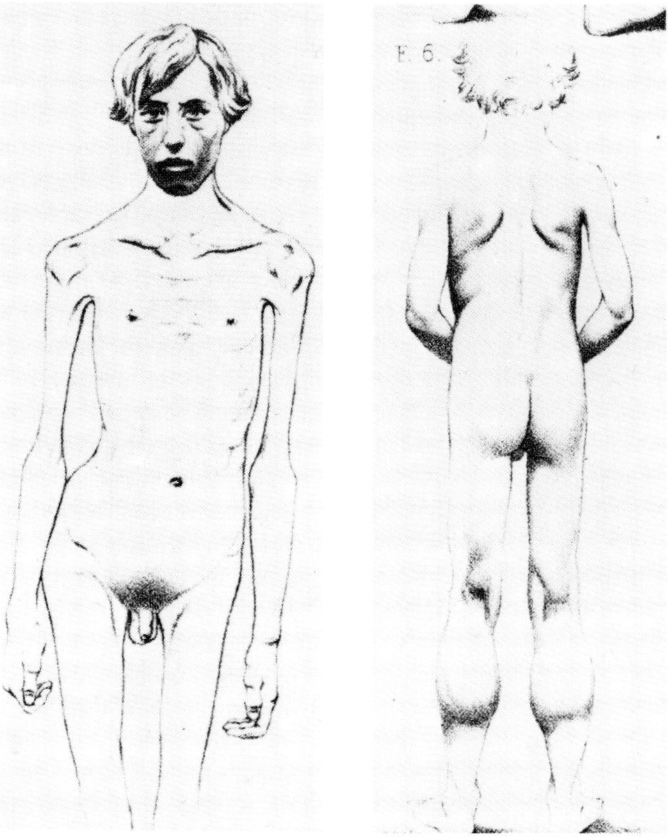

FIG. 132 (*left*). Pseudohypertrophic muscular dystrophy; to illustrate the 'exaggerated athletic build . . . and saddle-back'.

FIG. 133 (*centre and right*). Pseudohypertrophic muscular dystrophy; more advanced stages.

in muscular pathology and physiology . . . have become more popular sooner than in France' (p. 174), he learned that Billroth had found a fibro-fatty change in a piece of excised deltoid. It was this development that led him to devise his 'tissue punch', in 1865.

By 1870 he had seen some forty cases of the disease. There were three stages: (1) a period of feeble movements, (2) a period of apparent muscular hypertrophy†, and (3) paralysis. The first period lasted a few months or a year, during which there was difficulty in standing and walking, 'separation of the legs', 'waddling of the trunk', and 'lumbo-sacral curvature'. The stage of hypertrophy lasted a year or eighteen months, with enlargement usually first appearing in the gastrocnemii. Sometimes, stages 1 and 2 were 'intermingled'. A stationary period of several years commonly followed. In the paralytic stage, there was extension of weakness and wasting of muscles. The patient was usually confined to a chair or bed by 'adolescence'.

The disease was 'more prevalent in boys than girls' and 'several children of the same family' might be affected (p. 183). In the early stages the electrical reactions were normal. Muscle biopsy revealed the gradual accumulation of fibrous and then fatty tissue in the muscles, with loss of 'transverse striation' of the muscle fibres. In 1871 he obtained a number of sections of spinal cord from a case which Charcot and others studied. They

† Gowers recorded[287] that when Duchenne visited Queen Square, he thought that a child in Raphael's Transfiguration, a copy of which hung over a consulting room fireplace, looked like a case of muscular dystrophy. Gowers explained that the painting was placed there as it seemed to depict the child in an epileptic fit. In fact, there were even more 'Herculean'-looking children in other works of Raphael.

confirmed that there was no neural lesion, which German pathologists had also reported.

Progressive locomotor ataxy

Duchenne had collected data on twenty cases of the disease when he gave it this name in 1858. Later, he admitted that Romberg's *Tabes Dorsalis* of 1851 'very nearly approaches locomotor ataxy' (p. 32). But he thought, correctly enough, that Romberg had not distinguished between weakness and ataxia, despite his description of the numbness of the feet and the incoordination aggravated by eye closure. Degeneration of the posterior columns had been observed by pathologists before Romberg and Duchenne defined the clinical picture, and we have described the contributions of Todd and Reynolds in 1847 and 1855, respectively. It was Charcot and his school who firmly established the pathological lesions and added neuropathic joints to the clinical manifestations.

Friedreich's report on the clinical and pathological features of hereditary ataxia appeared in 1863.

Pupillary constriction, but not the reflex signs, was noted by Romberg and Duchenne, but the latter admitted that he had not originally recognized it regularly. One of his patients, blind with optic atrophy, used to have 'fits of pain' in the head during which Duchenne often saw the pupils dilate. He suspected that the pupillary constriction was due to a lesion of the cervical sympathetic (p. 15). He explained that when he begun regularly to use the ophthalmoscope in 1861, he found that 'dimness of sight' was proportional to 'whiteness of the papilla'. It will be remembered that Argyll Robertson described the pupillary abnormalities in 1869.

In describing the importance of excluding motor paralysis in cases of 'apparent paraplegia' Duchenne indicated that he did not just rely on observation of the capacity of voluntary movement of the reclining patient. He also tested the power to resist passive movements in each limb.

In sensory testing he found that touch, pain, and temperature were usually lost in that order: the latter was often normal. Delay in appreciation of a sensation was common; 'I have counted two or three seconds between the excitation and the perception'. In one case the delay lasted 'nine or ten seconds' (p. 11). He differentiated between Bell's 'muscular sense' and what he called 'muscular consciousness' (p. 378). Muscles and joints both possessed sensibility. In examining ataxic patients he tested ability to appreciate the weight of an object placed in the hand, to judge position and posture of a limb, and to feel passive movements of the digits and limbs. He examined these functions with the eyes opened and closed.

He thought that 'muscular' sense was really 'articular' and very disabling when it was lost.

When Duchenne died in 1875 he was recognized throughout Europe as an original medical scientist and he was honoured by many universities and societies. But in France he belonged to no university or academy. In this sense his career was unique. One can see in his work that he not only identified several important neurological diseases, but that he advanced the

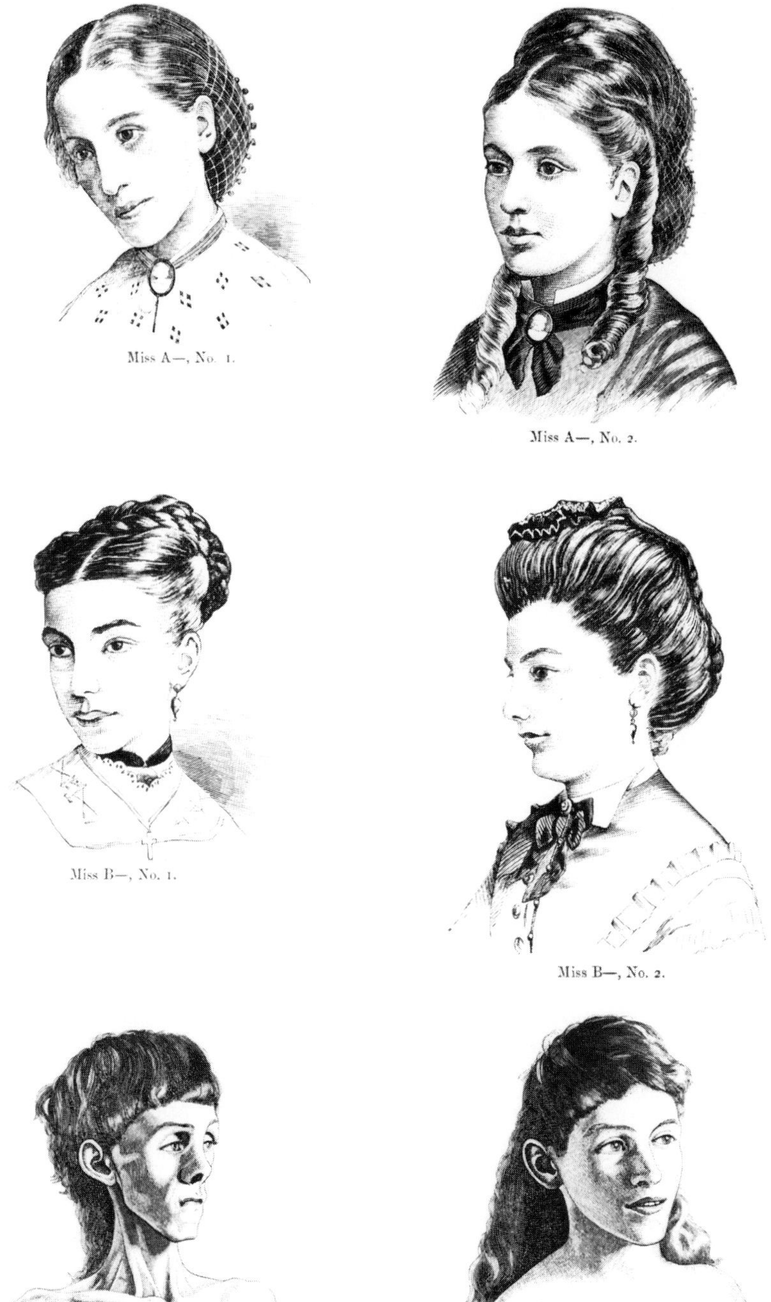

FIG. 134. Anorexia nervosa, 1874. 'A peculiar form of disease occurring mostly in young women, and characterized by extreme emaciation ...' Three patients showing the improvement with 'regular nourishment ... moral control ... relations and friends being generally the worst attendants' (after Gull[36]).

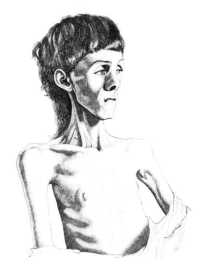

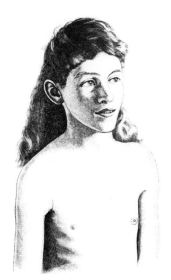

techniques of examination of the nervous system, at the bedside and in the laboratory, and played an important role in the formulation of the concept of system disorders. Anyone tempted to criticize his tardy recognition in Paris might pause to think of what would happen today in our medical establishments if there turned up, unsponsored, a brusque little man with 'un accent de terroir' and a strange box of tools. He would have to be as tough and courageous as our 'loup de mer' from Boulogne.

THE UNMASKING OF PARAPLEGIA

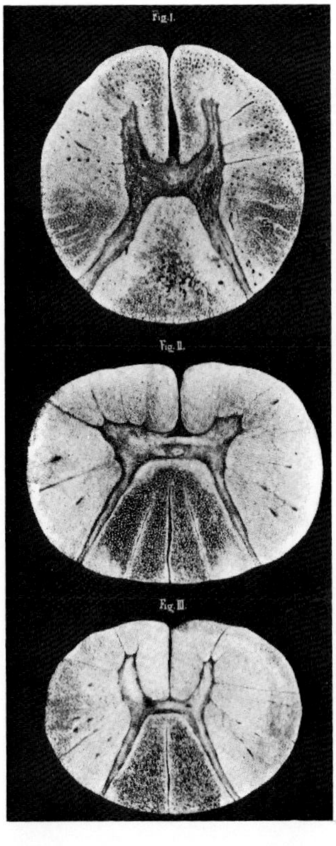

FIG. 135. Cases of paraplegia, 1858, Plates I and II (Plate II in Vol. 1 of *Collected works*, 1894). *Fig. I.* Paraplegia of five months duration. 'Remarkable atrophy of the gray substance' and 'Inflammatory degeneration of the columns'. *Figs. II* and *III*. Paraplegia of 15 months duration 'with want of control over the contraction of the muscles' of the legs. Flaccid paresis with numbness of all limbs. Posterior column degeneration in cervical (II) and dorsal (III) regions of the cord. Chronic bowel obstruction, persistent vomiting. Possibly a case of polyneuritis.

A few years after Reynolds had displayed how little was really known of diseases of the spinal cord there were two publications which showed that some progress, in fact, was being made. These were the lectures by Gull at Guy's, and by Brown-Séquard at the Royal College of Surgeons.

Sir William Gull (1816–1890) on paraplegia

Gull's 'Cases of Paraplegia' were published in 1856 and 1858.[34, 35] There were thirty-two cases, with autopsies in the twenty-nine fatal ones. These reports are important historically as they furnish us with a picture of what a first-rate clinician of the day understood of these disorders. He is famous also, of course, for his original descriptions of *Anorexia nervosa*[36], a 'Cretinoid State in Adult Women'[37] (Myxoedema) and for his 'Cases of Aneurism of the Cerebral Vessels'.[38, 39]

Gull's Gulstonian Lectures of 1848[40] had been on the nervous system and on diseases of the spinal cord, and his cases of paraplegia, ten years later, reflect his further experience. In his 1848 lectures he was impressed by the evidence for the 'segmental symmetry' of the spinal cord and he considered that there were three forms of paraplegia, with distinctive symptoms – *spinal*, *peripheral*, and *encephalic* paraplegias. In the first, motor loss always exceeded sensory loss, regardless of whether the lesion was situated anteriorly or posteriorly in the spinal cord. In the second variety, loss of sensation predominated, and the lesion was probably in the peripheral nerves. In the third type, there were also mild and often transient cerebral symptoms, which suggested the lesion was in the brain.

We can recognize the idea of polyneuritis in his second class; in the third there was probably a mixed collection of disorders, some no doubt due to 'gouty' arteries or holding venereal secrets.

Gull also used the term *Cervical Paraplegia* for cases of selective paralysis of the upper limbs, in which were probably included examples of cord, plexus, nerve, and muscle pathology.

Concerning his thirty-two cases of spinal paraplegia he said that nothing was more difficult 'than the determination at the bedside, of the causes which have given rise to the disease'. There were cases in which autopsy revealed little, even on the most careful examination with the microscope. 'Softening' and 'inflammation', diffuse or localized, were often all that could be concluded. In the future, he said, one might have to search for 'atomical', as distinguished from 'anatomical' changes in the spinal cord. He wondered why 'softening' was so commonly located in the dorsal region. But he did not believe, as some had reported, that 'acute softening' mostly affected the grey matter; the lesions were often quite superficial. A lesion could be 'partial' in two senses. You could have one confined to a segment of the cord, or to one of its columns. 'There was evidently a tendency in lesions to spread longitudinally in the cord rather than transversely through it'.

Particularly striking was the way in which a lesion could be seemingly limited to the posterior columns. He noted Brown-Séquard's suggestion that sensory loss depended on whether a considerable 'length' of these columns was diseased. There was little to favour Marshall Hall's view that they were concerned particularly with reflex functions. But Todd's suggestions were most pertinent. Gull had observed how an inability to 'regulate' motor power in the lower limbs was associated with degeneration of the posterior columns.

Direct injury to the cord could occur without any apparent vertebral damage; a fracture-dislocation was sometimes only disclosed on removing the posterior common ligament at autopsy. Haemorrhage, within the cord, or the spinal canal, was the obvious lesion in other cases. Injury was responsible for five of his cases.

There was one case (Case 13) of particular interest in which injury to the cord resulted from thoracic intervertebral disc protrusions. The patient, a young wife of thirty-three, was suddenly seized one morning with severe pain in her back, which subsided in half an hour. Next day 'almost suddenly she became paraplegic'. She was numb to the waist and incontinent. When admitted to hospital five weeks later there had been some return of power and sensibility but her buttocks were sloughing and she died three weeks later. At autopsy there was softening of the dorsal segments of the cord with protrusion of disc substance at the fifth, sixth, and seventh dorsal vertebrae and injury to the posterior common ligament. Section of the bodies of the vertebrae disclosed 'the escape of the debris of the degenerated intervertebral substance into the canal ... and so to injure the cord'.

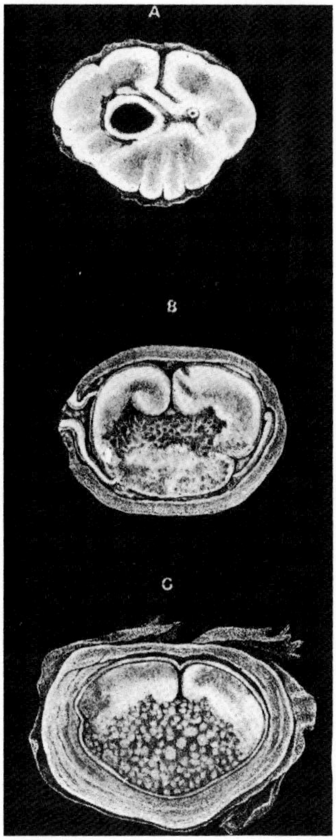

FIG. 136. Cases of paraplegia, 1858, Plate IV. Cervical cord sections from Case 29, the Guy's nurse with a syringomyelic syndrome of five years duration. Probably a cystic glioma

Injury was sometimes followed by abscess formation in the spinal canal; in other cases suppuration seemed to arise of itself. Meningeal inflammation, with thickening, vascularity, and adhesions could be acute or chronic. In one case there was a cervical 'arachnitis' which caused a fatal tetraplegia; at autopsy the cervical nerve roots were 'matted together'. Acute spinal meningitis with myelitis sometimes followed 'exposure to fatigue, wet, and cold', although 'this may appear but a vague causation for so formidable a malady'. 'Phlebitis of the vesical and pelvic veins extending to the veins of the spine, and setting up inflammation of the membranes of the cord' was another source of infection, he suggested. It could follow gonorrhoea. There were cases of 'induration' of areas or segments of the spinal cord, the majority of which were probably degenerative, but in one (Case 16), it may have been a cervical glioma. Gull does not mention any instance of recurrent paraparesis suggestive of multiple sclerosis.

'Tumour' accounted for seven of his thirty-two cases. In two the cord was invaded by vertebral malignant metastases from carcinoma of the kidney and lung, respectively. In another two the mass was intramedullary, both in the cervical cord (Cases 15 and 29). The former was possibly tuberculous, as there were also pulmonary tubercles. The other (Fig. 136) was in part cystic. The patient, a nurse at Guy's, had a long history of a syringomyelic-like syndrome, with, at autopsy, what was probably a cystic glioma.

There were no instances of syringomyelia in this series but his account of a case in 1862 may be mentioned here.[41] The patient, a man of forty-four years, died in hospital of typhus while under investigation for recent weakness, wasting, coldness, and numbness of his hands. There was atrophy of the thenar, hypothenar, and interossei muscles; upper arms were strong, lower limbs normal, and his sphincters functioned well. Although he felt his hands were numb, sensory testing revealed no significant abnormality. On the left, it was 'perfect'; on the right it was 'not so acute'. Gull made no mention of what form of sensory testing was used. At autopsy (Fig. 137) there was 'enlargement of the ventricle of the cord in the cervical region', with compression of the grey matter. Gull thought that it represented a 'hydromyelus, comparable to a chronic hydrocephalus'. He was struck by the extent of the destruction of grey matter 'without affecting sensation to any corresponding extent, and without disturbing the functions of the cord'. The retention of motor conduction, it will be recalled, was what impressed Ollivier, when he saw the extent of the cavitation in the cord. Dissociation of sensation had yet to arrive. It could not be 'recognized', like anorexia nervosa or myxoedema; it could be discovered only when sensory examination came to be based on appreciation of modalities and their separate pathways.

When Gull considered the symptoms of cord compression he stressed the significance of pain. It was nearly always present and prominent. Girdle-pain, 'a band-like constriction', was often characteristic and was more marked when there was meningeal involvement. It could be a 'referred' pain or a consequence of abdominal distension or diaphragmatic disturbance. In

(a)

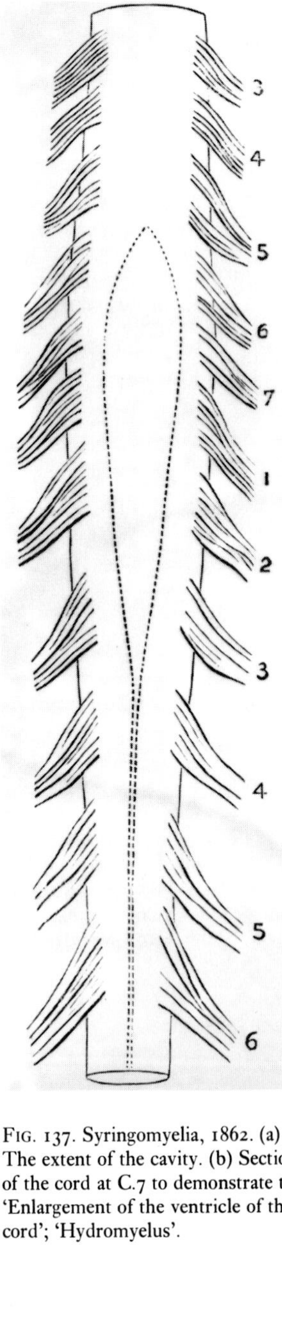

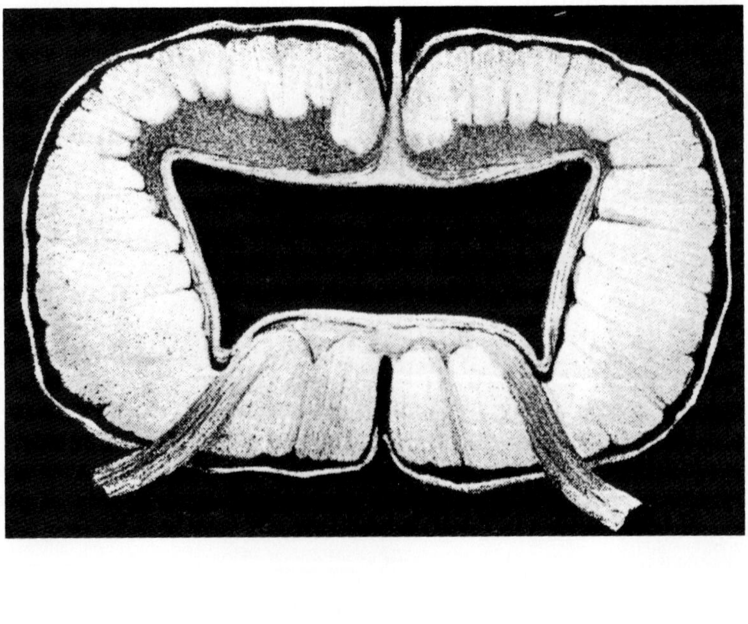

(b)

FIG. 137. Syringomyelia, 1862. (a) The extent of the cavity. (b) Section of the cord at C.7 to demonstrate the 'Enlargement of the ventricle of the cord'; 'Hydromyelus'.

the absence of pain, there were nearly always some 'varieties of impaired feeling', in the lower limbs. But what was much more striking was the developing rigidity and excito-motor activity of the weakening legs. 'Rigid extension' was followed by 'rigid flexion'. The sole of the foot was the place where a stimulus, often quite slight, most often provoked reaction. You could have an apparently hypersensitive sole, with good appreciation and localization of touch, and yet 'no amount of pinching or pricking' might give rise to pain. Gull did not actually say that in cord compression a sensory *level* was characteristic, but he did say that in a 'diffuse' lesion there was no 'distinct horizontal line limiting the paralysis'.

He described three spinal meningiomas and was sure they were not malignant, for they were discrete (one the size of a hazel nut, another like 'a boy's testicle', and the third 'large and elongated'), not destructive, and clearly only compressed the spinal cord. All arose from the inner surface of the meninges in the dorsal area, two anterior, the third posterior. Displacement of the cord was obvious (Fig. 138). Four further cases should be mentioned which were probably not spinal at all. Cases 8 and 10 read like subacute polyneuritis; Cases 17 and 20, acute polyneuritis, the latter presenting with bilateral facial paralysis. In these four cases microscopical examination of the spinal cord disclosed nothing of note and in two Gull postulated that the lesions might indeed be peripheral.

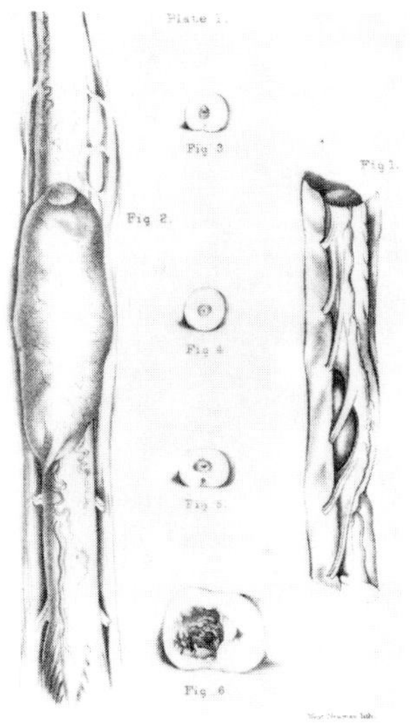

FIG. 138. Cases of paraplegia, 1856, Plate IV (Plate I in *Collected Works*). Figs. 1 and 2; 'Vascular fibroplastic tumours' compressing the cord and displacing nerve roots. Figs. 3–6; Cord sections in a case of cervico-dorsal 'nuclear growth in the gray matter'.

Lastly, Case 26 was probably one of limb-girdle muscular dystrophy (Fig. 139). He was a boy of fifteen years with painless atrophy of the shoulder-girdle muscles, lordosis, a 'vacillating' gait, and with normal sensory and sphincter functions. The wasted muscles 'showed no flickering contractions of their fibres'. He considered that because the galvanic reactions of the wasted muscles persisted, the proposed use of this test in assisting differentiation between atrophy of neural and muscular origin was erroneous. He seems to have thought that a history of a blow between the shoulders pointed to a cord lesion. Our little man from Boulogne would have been delighted to see this case, but he did not come to London until 1870, when he enjoyed identifying patients with the disorders he had described.

Brown-Séquard on spinal hemiplegia

An enlarged edition of Brown-Séquard's lectures at the college of surgeons was published in book form in 1860.[42] Having dealt with his experimental researches he looked for clinical evidence in support of his findings concerning unilateral lesions of the spinal cord.

He turned first to cases of injury or disease confined to the posterior columns of the spinal cord. He explained that in his extensive researches he 'had been hunting much more for cases that seemed to be in opposition to the theories I propose, than for those which seem to support them' (p. 90). He cited his own cases and those of others, French, English, American, and German, among whom were Ollivier, Cruveilhier, Andral, Luys, Abercrombie, Bright, Todd, and Türck. In the majority, of course, sensory examination was meagre by modern standards, and he did not always know how long before death a particular sensory report had been made. Then, too,

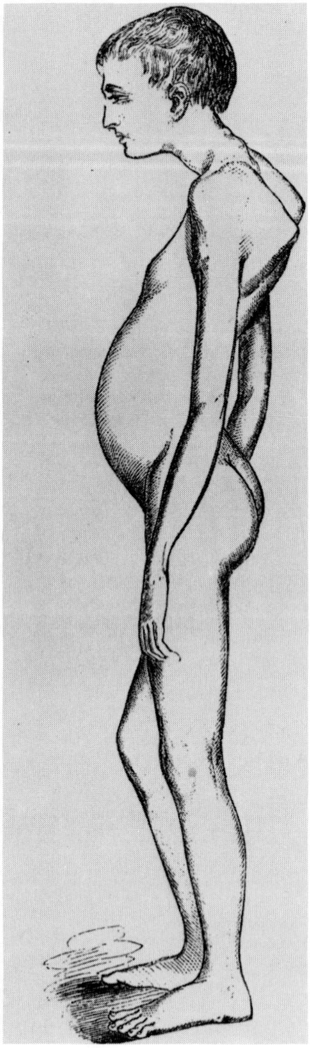

FIG. 139. Cases of paraplegia, 1858 Case 26. Reported as 'Cervical paraplegia following an injury'. Probably muscular dystrophy.

he was concerned about possible post-mortem changes in the spinal cord. In a few cases there were microscopical observations on record.

There were cases of injury (fractures and bayonet wounds), tumour, tubercles, and degenerations from which he concluded that 'if the posterior columns of the spinal cord convey sensitive impressions to the encephalon, their share in this function must be extremely slight' (p. 74). Sensory loss could not be attributed to lesions in those columns when there were accompanying lesions of the sensory roots of the spinal nerves. Sensory loss occurred when the posterior columns were spared. When the lesion in the posterior columns was longitudinally extensive there was 'a notable diminution in the power of standing and walking' (p. 55). This was a consequence of impairment of reflex movements – an activity that was channelled through the posterior columns – and of secondary effects elsewhere in the cord.

He next considered cases in which the grey matter of the spinal cord was chiefly affected or largely spared (p. 75). In the former group there were examples of haemorrhage, tubercles, tumours, and one of a syrinx ('nine English inches long'). In this case 'the upper limbs had lost their sensibility ... the lower limbs had preserved their sensibility' (p. 89). The case was obviously one of syringomyelia with progressive tetraparesis. In explanation Brown-Séquard said that sensory impressions from the lower limbs must have been conducted in the remaining elements of the grey matter, and possibly also in the anterior columns. The terms 'syrinx' and 'syringomyelia' were not used and he did not here refer to Rullier's patient quoted by Ollivier (see p. 204). He could conceive of loss of sensation with retention of power only in 'peculiar injury' affecting the grey matter, as in spina bifida or longitudinal wounds in the mid-line of the cord.

In reviewing those cases in which there were proved unilateral lesions of the spinal cord he described the syndrome we now associate with his name. He contrasted it with the features encountered in unilateral lesions of the pons and medulla. Again, it was largely instances of tumour, haemorrhage, and penetrating wounds which disclosed that 'a transversal section of a lateral half of the spinal cord causes a loss of voluntary movement in the corresponding side of the body, and a loss of sensibility in the opposite side' (p. 105). Such cases, he said, were not rare; others had mentioned them, including Cooke and Bright. In a unilateral lesion of the pons the motor and sensory loss were on the opposite side. In unilateral lesions of the medulla the results depended on the level in relation to the decussation of the motor pathway. He illustrated these diagnostic points in a diagram (Fig. 117).

In a further series of lectures in 1868,[43] by which time he said he had collected data on some twenty cases of 'hemi-paraplegia', there was accumulating evidence to confirm his main deductions. In London, Paris, and in America he had hunted them down and he paid tribute to colleagues (among whom was Hughlings Jackson) for their assistance. There were no new cases in which he had autopsy findings. Stab wounds provided some of the most clear-cut examples, and Hughlings Jackson providing drawings of one of the weapons. (One is left wondering whether, somewhere in earlier

Italian writings, some account of stiletto wounds of the spine records the striking clinical effects.)

When Brown-Séquard referred to loss of 'muscular sense' in a paralysed limb he meant 'the power of directing movements'. This was usually associated with superficial hypersensitivity and, for some time, vasodilatation. He did not appreciate the nature of the sensations transmitted by the posterior columns. He did, however, note that in the trunk, anteriorly and posteriorly, the junction between normal and altered sensation was not in the mid-line; he realized that there was overlapping innervation from each side.

In some cases he noted that recovery of motor power preceded and exceeded that of sensation, unlike what occurs in nerve injury.

In the *Anatomies of pain*[44] Keele has told the fascinating story of the discovery of the spinothalamic tract, in which Brown-Séquard played such an important initial role. It was revealed when, in addition to his pioneering experiments, histological studies demonstrated the relation between nerve cell and fibres in the posterior root ganglion, the crossing of the afferent sensory fibres in the anterior commissure, and the ascending Wallerian degeneration in the posterior and antero-lateral columns of the cord. When he came to review the contributions of experiment to the tracing of the sensory pathways in 1886, Gowers,[45] whose own clinical and pathological observations were so important, and who first described the 'antero-lateral ascending tract', said that the experiments of Schiff (1823–96) and Voroschilov (1842–99) also 'deserve the greatest weight'. Schiff's suggestion that not all sensory modalities travelled by the same pathway was a vital point. Voroschilov's spinal cord sections proved that the sensation of pain was carried in the antero-lateral ascending tracts. Gowers thought there were 'no important facts' to oppose this view but that it had yet to be finally established whether tactile sensation travelled in the posterior columns; 'muscle sense' certainly did. 'The path for sensations of temperature is still unknown' but it was presumably near that of pain.[46] It is still not accurately known.[47]

The advent of the tendon reflexes

We have seen that for a long time physicians had observed movements of a reflex nature in healthy and in sick people. They were generally interpreted as normally serving a protective function. In paraplegia and in hemiplegia they appeared to be alike, consisting essentially of brisk, spontaneous or induced movements of flexion of a limb. Muscular rigidity was a common accompaniment. Clinicians had also noted such things as sphincter troubles, loss of the pupillary light reflex, absence of a blink reflex in Bell's palsy, flexion of a hemiplegic arm on yawning, and the grasp reflex. But the most commonly reported reflex abnormality was abrupt flexion of a paretic lower limb on touching or stroking the sole of the foot. This was about the sum total of observations of reflex abnormality in diseases of the nervous system until 1875, when Erb (1840–1921) and Westphal (1833–90) turned from these 'superficial' or 'cutaneous' reflexes to the 'tendon reflexes'. It is interesting to recall that in Ferrier's *Functions of the brain*,[48] published in 1876, the only references to human reflex activity were in connection with the grasp reflex of the sleeping infant and the plantar reflex in health and in paraplegia.

One can be sure of course that the 'kick' of a knee had not passed unobserved by laymen or doctors before 1875. Many a hemiplegic must have noticed its exaggeration on the affected side. Indeed, in the opening sentence of his paper, 'On Some Motor Phenomena Produced on Tendons and Muscles by Mechanical Means,' Westphal[49] referred to a patient with cerebral symptoms and a spastic leg who, in 1871, drew his attention to the way the leg jerked forward when it was tapped just below the knee-cap. No doubt Westphal was not the only doctor who had been asked about the knee-kick. A hypochondriac would want to know if it meant anything sinister; the hemiplegic, if it was a sign of recovery. Just as one wonders whether Marshall Hall ever looked for it, so also one can speculate why, when the plantar reflex had been known for generations, no one before Babinski (1857–1932), in 1896, realized the diagnostic significance of *extension* of the toes.

Erb's paper was entitled 'On the Tendon Reflexes in Health and in Diseases of the Spinal Cord'.[50] He, too, it transpired, had been in the habit of testing and recording the 'patellar-tendon-reflexes' for several years and had come to the conclusion that they were more reliable for the clinician than the cutaneous reflexes. He submitted his paper to the editor of the German *Archives of Psychiatry and Nervous Diseases*, only to learn that the editor himself – Westphal – was preparing a similar publication, and they agreed on simultaneous publication. Westphal explained this in a footnote on the first page of his paper. But he did not use the term 'tendon-reflex'; indeed, he did not think the 'knee-phenomenon' was a reflex. In that, he was in error, although Erb's term also proved to be inaccurate.

Erb's opening remarks do not suggest that he actually anticipated the great interest he would arouse in the neurological world. 'I do not think', he said, 'that I shall be saying much that is new to my professional colleagues.' But although he felt that most of them would have known about these reflexes, he had found the literature was 'fairly silent about the matter' so that he decided to publish his experiences. At the end of the paper, he seemed equally cautious about the role these reflexes would play in diagnosis, although he clearly cited the possibilities.

He described the familiar technique of crossing the legs when the patient was sitting and how, using the fingers or a percussion hammer (a rubber-tipped hammer used for examination of the chest), a tap on the patellar tendon would provoke an 'immediate, lightning-like, clear and obviously reflex contraction of the quadriceps' muscle. 'It was uncommonly difficult to suppress this reflex voluntarily.' Erb found that there was no response to tapping the patella itself, nor when the adjacent skin was tapped or pinched, nor when a raised skin-fold was tapped. Tapping the quadriceps itself, if heavily done, sometimes provoked a response, but this was clearly a local, mechanically induced contraction. He also observed that electrical stimulation of the patella tendon did not produce the reflex. Lastly, he observed, the tap on the tendon had to be sharp; slow pressure, for example, was of no use, although patellar clonus could be induced by a sudden downward thrust of the knee-cap when the patient lay relaxed on a bed.

Erb also mentioned reflexly induced contractions of the sartorius, gracilis, adductors, and biceps femoris muscles, noting that the reflexogenic areas were larger than in the case of the quadriceps. But the 'foot-clonus' seemed more interesting. Here there was a 'rhythmical clonic movement of the foot which persisted as long as pressure was maintained' on the sole of the sharply dorsiflexed foot. 'Even slight stroking of the toes or their getting caught up in the bedsheets is sufficient to cause the most exquisite cramp.' It could even be apparently spontaneous. Slow passive dorsiflexion of the foot did not provoke it. Passive plantar flexion could arrest it. Sometimes the entire leg would shake with the response, and it could spread to the opposite leg. Erb came to the conclusion that the clonus was due to a stimulation applied to the achilles tendon. If the patient lay on his bed to one side, and his knee was bent and his foot held slightly dorsiflexed, then a light tap on the achilles tendon would produce a visible contraction of the calf muscles. As with the patellar reflex, neither stimulation of adjacent skin nor slow pressure on the tendon was effective. The tap had to be sharp; repeated taps set up clonus. A single stimulus produced a reflex contraction of the calf muscles, which in turn set in motion further reflex activity.

In the upper limbs Erb noted the responses on tapping the tendons of the triceps and supinator longus but he did not mention any biceps reflex.

He knew that Charcot was well acquainted with the ankle clonus but he could find no reference to it, nor to the tendon reflexes in the writings of the eminent Leyden (1832–1910). He wondered what relationship these phenomena might have with the spinal epilepsy of Brown-Séquard.

Erb concluded that the physiological explanation of these tendon reflexes would obviously necessitate animal experimentation. What was their relationship to spastic phenomena? Why were they enhanced in patients with diseases of the spinal cord? What were the effects of involvement of the white and the grey matter? They should assist us in determining the level of a spinal cord lesion because 'reflex arcs' were obviously implicated. Erb had already noted that they should be helpful in cases of spinal cord compression. He mentioned three such cases with kyphosis; two dorsal, one lumbar. In the former the patellar, adductor, and biceps femoris reflexes were exaggerated. In the latter, the patellar and adductor reflexes were absent. In locomotor ataxy Westphal had noted that the knee and ankle phenomena were absent.

As Schiller[51] has written, 'Erb and Westphal had hit upon the unique spot in the body where scientific purity and simplicity reign because only two neurons are involved in the [knee] reflex ... While neither reflexes nor hammers in themselves were much newer than pitchforks, they helped in the construction of a new edifice; the functioning nervous system as an assembly of interdependent and hence variably active reflexes, each one inhibited or enhanced by others'.

In England, a few years later, Gowers[52] was reporting on the frequency, form, strength, and speed of response of the 'tendon-reflex phenoma', which, in the case of the patellar tendon, he later named 'the knee jerk'. He observed, like others, that in locomotor ataxy, where there was damage to the posterior nerve roots, in progressive muscular atrophy, where the lesion lay in the anterior grey matter, and in cases of 'old meningitis', where there was damage to the anterior roots, and in the disease of muscle itself, namely, dystrophy, the knee jerks were diminished or lost. He also confirmed that they were excessive in 'lateral sclerosis' of the spinal cord.

Gowers also quoted the results of the animal experiments and clinical observations of Tschirjew, made in Berlin, in 1878. He proved that the knee jerk was a true spinal reflex, abolished by cutting the femoral nerve, or the spinal cord where it emerges.† Cord section above this level led to an exaggeration of the reflex. Gowers also examined the 'ankle clonus', in forty cases, employing a graphic method. He compared his tracings with those of the knee jerks and decided that in ankle clonus, stimulation of the calf muscles was direct and not itself a reflex; it could be a normal phenomenon, 'excessive in disease'.

The debate whether these tendon phenomena were true reflexes went on for some twenty years. Waller[53] in 1890 and Foster[54] in 1897 still did not consider them as such. Two of the main difficulties lay in the belief that there were no nerve fibres in tendons, and that the speed of response made conduction to and from the spinal cord an unlikely event. However, nerves were found in tendons, and spindles in muscles, and it was learned that a tendon reflex was really a muscle-stretch reflex. The tendon transmitted the stretch stimulus to the muscle but it was not, in itself, essential. A muscle without a tendon – such as the masseter – proved to have a reflex. These physiological disputes did not seriously worry the clinician in his use of this new tool, despite the period of 'inflation' which characterized their early application.[55]

The manner in which the discovery and introduction of the tendon reflexes accelerated the study of diseases of the spinal cord may be seen, for example, by looking at the appropriate section in the book on diseases of the nervous system by Samuel Wilks (1824–1911).[56] It was a standard work, published in 1878, but largely a reprinting of lectures which had been delivered ten years previously at Guy's Hospital. Thus, the description of paraplegia was written just a few years before the advent of the tendon reflexes. Although he mentions that he had included 'additional material' in the ten-year interval, such as the discovery of the motor cortex in 1870, there is no mention of tendon reflexes. Diagnosis of the various forms of paraplegia is considered much as it had been by his senior colleague William Gull, twenty years previously. Wilks, in 1878, was fifty-one, an experienced, eminent physician with an interest in neurology. He had written on the 'pathology of nervous diseases',[57] on 'alcoholic paraplegia',[58] on 'cerebritis, hysteria, and bulbar palsy,'[59] and other neurological topics.

He did not identify that the paralysis from alcohol resulted from peripheral neuritis; he thought it was a disease of the spinal cord. One of his

† The knee jerks were abolished by an injection of cocaine on the occasion of the first lumbar puncture. But the actual target was the genital reflexes (Corning, J. L. (1885) *N.Y. Med. J.* **42**, 483).

four cases of bulbar palsy[59] has been considered to be the first recorded example of myasthenia gravis,[60] but Critchley[61] has suggested that it was more probably one of post-diphtheritic neuritis. There is insufficient data in Wilks's account to be dogmatic about the diagnosis but a record of the tendon reflexes would have been helpful. The patient was a girl with 'general weakness' and 'lethargy', rather than 'actual paralysis', who was observed in hospital for a month. She was able to walk about, but every movement of her limbs and speech was performed so slowly and deliberately that 'hysteria' was suspected. There was a sudden deterioration and she died of bulbar palsy but microscopic examination of the medulla revealed no abnormality. There was no mention of a previous sore throat, nor of numbness of her extremities, and her limbs were not paralysed when the bulbar palsy developed, so that myasthenia is more likely.

In his 1878 book Wilks devoted 120 pages to diseases of the spinal cord and he stressed that paraplegia was not a single affection but 'a useful term for including many cases which no doubt will one day submit to a further analysis' (p. 198). The inner structure of the cord then being gradually revealed indicated that various types of paraplegia could emerge. The mode by which the nerves were connected in the cord was only partly known, but the differences between paralysis and ataxia were being detected, and sensory loss could be 'dissociated' (p. 185). (He said this had been known to Erasmus Darwin, a hundred years previously, in connection with an Edinburgh patient who could appreciate warmth in a leg, but not pain.) There was no connection between brain and skin 'except through the grey matter of the cord'. Disease of the grey matter was likely to cause sensory paralysis of some kind, while disease of the white matter resulted in a motor paralysis. Thus, injury, and disease spreading from the vertebral column, were more likely to cause a motor paralysis. On the other hand an effusion of blood within the cord primarily affected sensation. He did not think that one man's spinal cord functioned exactly like that of another. Like the brain, spinal cord centres 'become educated' (p. 17) and are 'regulated, excited or arrested by cerebral influence'. The reflex-like actions of the ticket-clerk at Charing Cross Station daily reminded him of the 'automaton action of the spinal system'. In motor paralysis, Wilks saw its 'seat' in the cord, not the brain. 'We look to the spinal marrow as the seat of all paralysis . . . it has not been clearly proved that a lesion of a convolution will produce paralysis of any part of the body while the ganglion below is healthy' (p. 20). In disease of the 'brain proper' there was loss of 'perception and voluntary effort', 'delirium', and 'dementia'. 'True paralysis is associated with disease of the spinal cord' (p. 30).

With regard to the excito-motor hyperactivity of the spinal cord in paraplegia, it was most obvious, he said, when the lesion in the cord was inflammatory. Pain, spasms, and rigidity sometimes combined to produce a picture like a 'tetanised frog'. 'In the human subject if the foot be touched, there is not the same reflex action as in a case of paraplegia (p. 8).' The only other reference to reflex activity in his book is when he writes on the 'doctrine of reflex paralysis' (p. 230). It was a term employed to explain cases of spinal paralysis in which no lesion could be found. It was postulated that in such cases the cord was 'paralysed' by some external irritation possibly arising in bladder, bowel, or womb. But in those cases of paralysis without cord lesion there were clear examples of polyneuritis, a syndrome not then recognized, and one in which loss of tendon reflexes proved to become a valuable diagnostic indicator.

Among the listed diseases of the spinal cord we find those in which muscular wasting was a cardinal feature, such as poliomyelitis (infantile paralysis) and progressive muscular atrophy, in both of which destruction of anterior horn cells was the essential lesion. Bulbar palsy was also recognized as an occasional accompaniment of the latter. Myelitis, acute and chronic, was described and 'insular sclerosis' (i.e. multiple sclerosis) had been separated from that other ailment characterized by tremor – paralysis agitans. In multiple sclerosis the tremors were not continuous 'and do not come into play unless volition is acting upon the muscles'. There was no sensory loss or impairment of sphincter function, and although Wilks made no mention of the tendon reflexes he did say that 'if the foot is struck, or firmly bent, a tremor will sometimes take place passing through the whole limb'. Paralysis agitans was considered, without explanation, as a spinal cord disease, although the pathology was not known, and in one of his cases was found to be normal.

The clinical and pathological features of these diseases of the spinal cord had largely been described in the late 1860s, mainly in Charcot's school. Tendon reflexes do not feature in their original accounts. In amyotrophic lateral sclerosis Charcot emphasized the contrast between the flaccid, atrophied and fibrillating musculature of an upper limb with that of the rigid, paralysed, but unwasted lower limb. In his early cases he noted that tapping the forearm muscles provoked movement responses, but there is no mention of tendon reflexes. A few years later he observed that they were generally exaggerated in the upper and lower limbs, although in the former he referred only to the triceps and supinator reflexes – and not to the biceps.

No upper limb tendon reflexes were mentioned by Erb in 1874 when he described the clinical features of injuries to the brachial plexus.

In describing locomotor ataxia (p. 284) and how it differed from simple motor paraplegia, Wilks quoted how Duchenne used to get one of his ataxic patients to carry a student on his back across the lecture room, to illustrate the retention of muscular power in the lower limbs. The obvious lesion lay in the posterior columns and posterior spinal nerve roots, but opinions differed on how the ataxia arose. Some said the lesion impaired peripheral sensibility; others that it interfered with the connections between one portion of the grey centres and another; or that the link with the cerebellum was lacking. Wilks questioned the existence of Bell's 'muscular sense' as no one had yet shown that sensory fibres entered muscles, which were 'almost devoid of feeling'. But he admitted that 'something equivalent to it' was there, perhaps in our bones and ligaments, 'since we should otherwise be in the position of the statue, or the patient with ataxia'. (He went on to discuss whether the appreciation of rhythm is dependent on hearing or some other sense, and recounted his consultations with the principal of a deaf and dumb school in the Old Kent Road!)

But also among the disorders classified by Wilks as of spinal origin were *alcohol paraplegia* (p. 265), *diphtheritic paralysis* (p. 233), *peripheral paralysis* (p. 235), *acute ascending paralysis* (p. 225), *recoverable paraplegia* (p. 228), as well as our old friend *hysterical paraplegia* (p. 236) and that new ogre *the railway spine*. In each of these affections the new tendon reflexes subsequently enabled the physician to make much sounder diagnostic judgements.

The emergence of multiple neuritis in all its forms (polyneuritis) will be recounted later. Wilks's cases of 'recoverable' paraplegia were certainly not due to multiple sclerosis, whatever they may have been, and the Victorian epidemic of railway spine, in which not only paralysis but mental loss ensued, merits a treatise in itself, if only as a chapter in our social history. The term was still in the index of Gowers's textbook in 1886 although he never took up the old concept of 'spinal irritation' which Romberg had complained of but which, in America, was still impressing Hammond[65] at the end of the century.

As for hysterical paraplegia it could be distinguished from 'real paraplegia' as the patient did not look ill, and no bed sores or incontinence developed (p. 371). One can only think how dangerous it must have been, one hundred years ago, to be a girl with some weakness of her limbs. But then, it was such a predominantly male society, that in his lecture on bleeding, I am sure Wilks's students did not think it amiss when he recited lines from Henry V's speech at Agincourt, a verse from the 'Charge of the Light Brigade', and spoke proudly of the 'handful of men the other day who reconquered India' (p. 97). He was, after all, rebutting the doctrine that not only might diseases change, but men also. He reassured his students that at any rate, the British male members of the human race showed no sign of 'impoverishment or deterioration'.

But, to return to our tendon reflexes. In essence, they became the practical demonstration of the truth of Marshall Hall's teaching. Where the lesions in the reflex arcs were known – as in dystrophy, poliomyelitis, and progressive muscular atrophy – loss of tendon reflexes could be understood. When diseases of the spine, the meninges, or the cord involved the sensory or motor spinal roots, segmental reflex loss could be explained.

But for decades it was usually only the knee jerks that were *routinely* examined. In his textbook, Gowers,[45] for example, in 1886, did not refer to loss of the ankle jerk in sciatica (Vol. 1, p. 84), nor of the biceps or triceps reflexes in lesions of the upper limbs (Vol. 1, p. 67). In his table (Vol. 1, p. 142) depicting the segmental arrangements of the spinal cord, the only deep reflexes listed were the knee and ankle jerks. However, he drew attention to the recently described 'jaw jerk' (Vol. 1, p. 150). Beevor[66] had published an account of a case of amyotrophic lateral sclerosis 'with clonus of the lower jaw'. He induced the clonus, which he likened to the 'chattering of the teeth in the cold or in a rigor', by quickly depressing the lower jaw teeth with his fingers. In a note with the article, De Watteville suggested that 'the masseteric tendon reaction' he called 'the jaw jerk'. Gowers said that an American physician (Morris Lewis) had also described it, in 1886, as the 'chin reflex'.

Explanation of reflex abnormalities only really came when histo-pathological studies demonstrated how lesions disrupted the chain of communications within the spinal cord. In the case of loss of reflexes, of course, sometimes no lesion was found; it was in the nerves themselves. In the majority of cases of cord diseases there was exaggeration of reflex activity, and it was the pyramidal tracts that were eventually implicated, either directly or as part of a descending degeneration. Thus it was learned that the old 'excito-motor phenomena' of the lower limbs in paraplegia were identical with those in the upper limb of cerebral hemiplegia.

If loss of reflexes meant that the reflex arcs were interrupted, what of exaggerated reflexes? It obviously implied that the arcs were intact, but it was easier to understand the former than the latter. It was conceivable that in *acute* diseases of the spinal cord or brain, reflex hyperactivity was a result of 'irritation of the motor centres'. But in *chronic* disease it was more likely to be due to 'loss of control'. For a long time it was known that *superficial* reflexes could be voluntarily suppressed, so that the idea of cerebral inhibition was not new. Unilateral loss of cutaneous reflexes (the plantar, the cremasteric, and the abdominal) had been observed in cerebral lesions. On the other hand, a cerebral lesion appeared to exert the same effect on tendon reflex activity as did a spinal one. But cerebral lesions never abolished deep reflexes, as they often did cutaneous ones. Lastly, it was apparent that alteration of tendon reflex activity after a cerebral or spinal lesion was not an immediate effect, as with cutaneous reflexes, but a delayed one. The transient reflex manifestations of Marshall Hall's 'spinal shock' were now observed in man, and in more detail.

The delay in the appearance of reflex hyperactivity in a pyramidal lesion might conceivably be a result of the ensuing descending degeneration influencing the activity of the reflex centres in the grey matter of the cord. Alternatively, it was possible that little control was habitually exercised, and that hyperactivity was 'a release' phenomenon, which gradually increased. Exaggeration of a knee jerk, and ankle clonus, after unilateral convulsion was considered by Hughlings Jackson[67] to be due to released hyperactivity consequent on 'exhaustion' in higher centres. Loss of knee jerk after a convulsion Gowers considered to be due to 'exhaustion' in lumbar centres.[68]

Spastic paraplegia. This was the term that came to be applied to those cases in which paraplegia was associated with muscular rigidity, exaggerated knee jerks, and ankle clonus. It could arise, not only in an acute manner, from injury, myelitis, or compression, but in an insidious manner, and without any form of sensory loss.

When Heine (1799–1879)[69] originally described infantile paralysis in 1840, he also referred to cases of *paraplegia spastica cerebralis.* A few years later, Little (1810–94),[70] himself afflicted with an equinus deformity of his

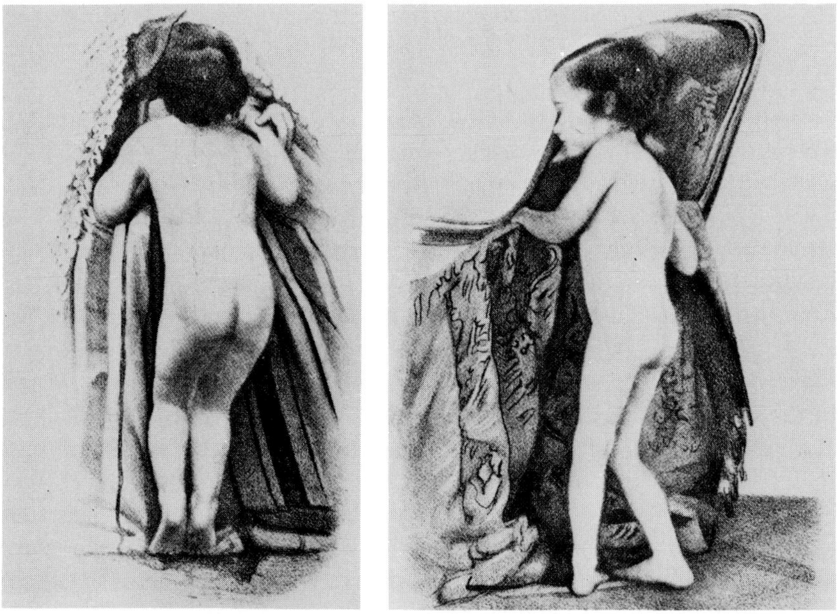

FIG. 140. Little's disease, 1861. Case XLVII (left) and Case XLIII (right). Congenital cerebral spastic diplegia.

left foot, began to publish his accounts of children with 'congenital spastic rigidity of the limbs', which he concluded were often due to injury or anoxia at birth. By 1861 he had seen two hundred cases. He had performed no autopsies on cases that had survived infancy or childhood but he imagined that the sustained spasticity must have been due to 'a certain amount of chronic myelitis'.[71] He had seen a case at the London Hospital in which a similar 'general spastic rigidity of the upper and lower extremities' had commenced 'after adult age'. Autopsy had shown 'a chronic meningitis and myelitis'. He considered that in his 'congenital' cases, both brain and spinal cord could be implicated in the birth trauma. Marie wrote that 'For a long time the researches of Little were almost unknown to neurologists'.[72]

Erb was one of the earliest to write an account of a chronic form of *spastic spinal paralysis*, and both he, Charcot, and Gowers entertained the possibility of a 'pure' primary lateral sclerosis. In 1875,[73] the year of his account of the tendon reflexes, he referred to sixteen cases. He was concerned to learn at what stage of the disease the tendon reflexes became hyperactive; they were considerably increased in five out of six cases which he saw early enough. He also noted that they were 'very much exaggerated' in the upper limbs 'in the earliest stages of paresis'. But pathological confirmation of a 'primary lateral sclerosis' was never forthcoming. Erb actually mentioned 'multiple sclerosis' in the differential diagnosis, observing that in his sixteen cases there was 'no trace' of 'ataxia' or 'voluntary trembling' which were 'so characteristic of multiple sclerosis'. Nevertheless, it is commonly agreed that multiple sclerosis, amyotrophic lateral sclerosis, and perhaps syphilis explained the majority of these cases of primary lateral sclerosis. Perhaps one day *Lathyrism* may be shown at autopsy to be a rare but genuine example.

Ataxic paraplegia. Gowers employed this term to denote those cases in which 'there was a combination of paraplegia and ataxia, and consists in combined disease of the posterior and lateral columns'.[74] Despite the obvious ataxia and positive Romberg test, the pupils were normal, there were no lightning pains or sensory loss, and the knee and ankle jerks were usually exaggerated, so that distinction from locomotor ataxia could be made. The cause was unknown but Marie suspected a vascular origin.[75] The occasional presence of sensory loss, absent knee jerks, and cerebral impairment suggest that some cases, at least, were examples of the 'subacute combined degeneration of the spinal cord' described in 1900.[76]

Compression paraplegia. Pain had long been considered a prominent feature of the paraplegia resulting from chronic compression of the spinal cord. With the understanding of the 'reflex arc', of 'secondary degeneration', and the advent of the 'tendon reflexes', the cardinal features of slow compression came to be recognized. There were two classes of phenomena – the root symptoms and the cord symptoms. At the level of the lesion, sensory symptoms comprised pain and hyperaesthesia, while on the motor side there was weakness, wasting, and spasms. Alteration of arm reflexes were not usually recorded. Below the lesion, opinion differed as to the degree and extent of the sensory loss. The majority of observers considered that motor loss could be complete with little or no sensory loss. But all were agreed that spasms and rigidity and hyperactive plantar reflexes were a conspicuous feature.

Widespread sensory loss, with an upper level usually related to 'hips', 'xiphisternum', or 'nipples', was usually recorded only when the paraplegia was more or less complete.

Though suspected during life, the actual features of spinal cord tumour compression were only seen at autopsy. Gowers (Vol. 1, p. 416) devoted sixteen pages to the subject and illustrated 'gliomas' in the cord, and subdural and extradural 'sarcomas' and 'myxomas' compressing the cord. Tumours arising within the cord were less likely to give rise to root pains, spinal pain and tenderness were less common, and the symptoms were often bilateral from the first; muscular atrophy was also more common. The symptoms and signs of a meningeal tumour depended to some extent on its position in relation to the cord. Lateral compression might produce 'crossed' sensory loss; mid-line compression had bilateral effects, usually motor, but occasionally ataxic, from interference with the posterior columns.

In cervical lesions, Gowers did not mention the tendon reflexes of the upper limbs, but in dorsal lesions he said the 'trunk-reflexes' (abdominal) might be lost, and that in tumours of the cauda equina, knee and ankle jerks disappeared. Exaggerated knee and ankle jerks were otherwise invariable. Curiously, when considering the level of a lesion, he made no reference to the importance of determining the 'sensory level' – although it is obvious enough that it was appreciated.

On the treatment of cord tumours Gowers wrote these prophetic lines.

It is highly probable that Surgery may ultimately be able to cope, in some degree, with meningeal tumours. Modern methods render the opening of the spinal canal far less formidable than it formerly was, and the removal of a tumour from the membranes of the cord would involve less immediate danger of serious consequences than the removal of a tumour from the brain (Vol. 1, p. 432).

He did not have long to wait. A year later, in 1887, he made a diagnosis of a laterally situated, non-malignant, extramedullary tumour in the mid-dorsal region and Horsley (1857–1916) successfully removed it.[77] This famous patient, Capt. G., was the first such in history. Aged forty-two, a business man who travelled extensively, he had sought relief for 'intercostal neuralgia' for some three years, in London, China, Shanghai, and Constantinople (this was the heyday of Empire) and had taken the baths in Aix-la-Chapelle and wintered in the south of France. The pain was intermittent, severe, little relieved by morphia and situated in the left scapular region. Early in 1877 he began to lose the power in his left leg, then his right. When Gowers saw him on 5 June he was paraplegic with loss of 'cutaneous sensibility of all kinds as high as the ensiform cartilage'. His legs were rigid and 'clonus could be obtained with great readiness in the muscles of the calf and front of the thigh'. The bladder was distended.

Gowers reasoned that 'The gradual onset of the paralysis, the affection of one leg before the other, and the long-preceding signs of nerve irritation at the level of the lesion, made it practically certain that the spinal cord was damaged by compression and that the cause of the compression was outside the cord itself'. Horsley saw the patient at 1 p.m. on 9 June and operated, in the presence of Gowers and Ballance (1850–1930) at 3.30 p.m. that day, at the National Hospital, Queen Square. Horsley had judged that the sensory loss had reached as high as 'the fifth dorsal nerve'. At laminectomy (Fig. 141), D.4 to 6, and incision of the dura, no abnormality was seen, so the exposure was extended to D.3 to 7. Nothing abnormal came to light, and,

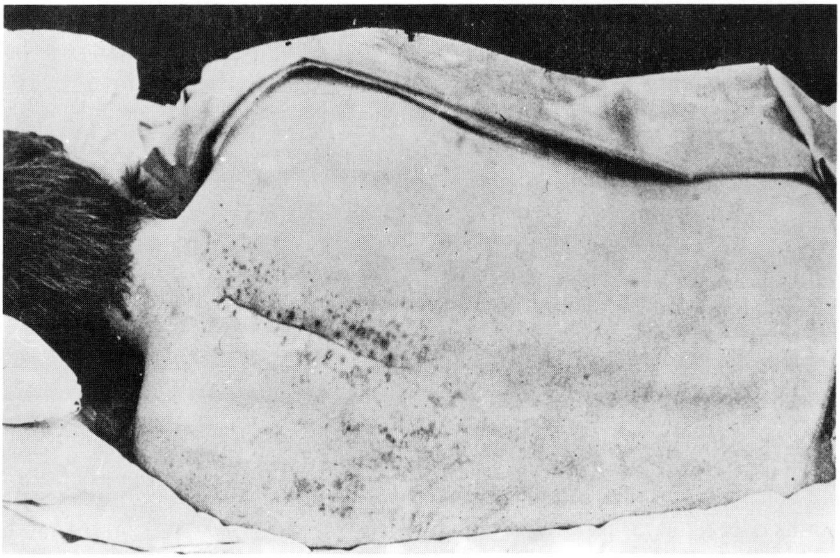

FIG. 141. The laminectomy incision in Gowers's and Horsley's patient of 1887; the first successful diagnosis and removal of a spinal cord tumour.

urged by Ballance, Horsley now removed the second dorsal laminae, and caught sight of the lower end of a tumour on the left side. On removing the first dorsal laminae it was exposed and 'detached', proving to be an encapsulated benign nodular growth, about one inch in length and a half an inch in width. It was actually sited four inches above the level of anaesthesia.

Power began to return to his legs some twelve days later and in the ensuing months progress continued and by the end of the year 'he could walk three miles with ease'. A year after the operation he was working energetically – up to sixteen hours a day!

Gowers and Horsley concluded their account of this historical event by reviewing the features of fifty-eight published cases of spinal meningeal tumours. The majority were in the dorsal region, benign, and apparently removable. The *march* of the symptoms was clearly 'Pain, Motor paralysis, Sensory paralysis'. Unfortunately the exact localization of the pain in relation to the position of the tumour was infrequently described. Precise determination of the level of the pain would materially assist diagnosis. The *uppermost* border of the anaesthesia or hyperaesthesia was a vital sign. The tumour was nearly always higher than was clinically estimated.

The discovery of the knee jerk was, after all, an item of clinical research. There is a story[78] of how Benjamin Jowett (1817–93), renowned Master of Balliol and inventor of the tutorial system, and an opponent of research ('a mere excuse for idleness'), one day asked for an example of 'research'. All that could be quickly recalled by an undergraduate was the recently discovered 'knee-kick', which was thought might be an indication of the state of health. Jowett did not believe a word of this and said 'just give my knee a tap'. 'The little leg reacted with a vigour which almost alarmed me, and must, I think, have considerably disconcerted that elderly and eminent opponent of research'.

MULTIPLE NEURITIS

The term 'multiple neuritis' was coined by Leyden[79] (1832–1910) in 1880 when he authoritatively established what had been debated for many years. Namely, that there was a disease which paralysed, not by attacking the brain, the spinal cord, or the spinal nerve roots, but the nerves themselves. Moreover, it was the peripheral extremities of the nerves that were first affected. It was really the 'end' of a rather long story.

We now know that the first account of a disease which proved to be a multiple neuritis was that provided by Bontius in 1642 in his account of beriberi.

> It is a kind of paralysis, or rather tremor; for it penetrates the motions and sensations of the hands and feet indeed sometimes of the whole body ... movement and sensation particularly of the hands and feet are depraved, and they are weak; and in them is felt very often a tickling ...[80]

The effects of alcohol in causing a painful paralysis and numbness of the limbs were noted by Lettsom (1744–1815)[81] in 1787 in London and, independently, by Jackson[82] (1777–1867) in 1822 in Boston, USA. They both commented on the peculiar, smooth, shining appearance of the skin of the hands and feet, their exquisite tenderness, the general helplessness of the patient, and the wasted lower limbs. Lettsom made no suggestion about the site of the lesion, but Jackson considered it lay in the skin and muscles. His account made little impression, for an American reviewer of Wilks's book on diseases of the nervous system, in 1878, wrote, in reference to 'Alcoholic Paraplegia', that 'it was not recognised in this country'.[83]

Roberts F. Graves (1796–1853)

The possibility of a lesion at the periphery of the nervous system in some cases of paralysis was, in fact, suggested by Graves in 1843, in the first edition of his *Clinical lectures.*

> In a word, may not the decay and withering of the nervous tree commence occasionally in its extreme branches? and may not a blighting influence affect the latter, while the main trunk remains sound and unharmed?[84]

Gull quoted these lines in 1848 when he suggested there was a class of parapelgia he called 'peripheral' (p. 322).

Graves, a gifted man with a talent for languages, graduated in Dublin in 1818. He travelled extensively in Europe and on one journey he joined up with the artist Turner in the Alps and Italy. In 1828, in Paris, he observed an epidemic of what was clearly some form of acute polyneuritis. It was described by Chomel[85] in the same year. Graves wrote,

> One of the most remarkable examples of disease of the nervous system commencing in the extremities, and having no connection with lesions of the brain or spinal marrow, was the curious *epidémie de Paris*, which occurred in the spring of 1828. Chomel has described this epidemic in the 9th number of the *Journal Hebdomadaire*, and having witnessed it myself in the months of July and August of the same year, I can bear testimony to the ability and accuracy of his description. It began (frequently in persons of good constitution) with sensations of pricking and severe pain in the integuments of the hands and feet, accompanied by so acute a degree of sensibility, that the patients could not bear these parts to be touched by the bed-clothes. After some time, a few days, or even a few hours, a diminution, or even abolition of sensation took place in the affected members, they became incapable of distinguishing the shape, texture, or temperature of bodies, the power of motion declined, and finally they were observed to become altogether paralytic. The injury was not confined to the hands and feet alone, but, advancing with progressive pace, extended over the whole of both extremities. Persons lay in bed powerless and helpless, and continued in this state for weeks and even months ...
>
> At last, at some period of the disease, motion and sensation gradually returned, and a recovery generally took place, although, in some instances, the paralysis was very capricious, vanishing and again reappearing.
>
> The French pathologists, you may be sure, searched anxiously in the nervous centres for the cause of this strange disorder, and could find none; there was no evident lesion, functional or organic, discoverable in the brain, cerebellum or spinal marrow ...[86]

Graves viewed this as an 'instance of paralysis creeping from the extremities towards the centre ... can anyone . .hesitate to believe that paralysis ... may arise from disease commencing and originating in the nervous extremities alone?'

There can be little doubt that this experience made a deep impression upon the young Graves. His recollection, 15 years later, came in a lecture entitled 'The Pathology of Nervous Diseases', one of the thirty-eight contained in his book. The theme of his lecture was that disease of 'the circumferential parts' of the nervous system, of 'the nervous cords themselves' had been neglected by pathologists and that for too long, enquiry had centred on the brain and the spinal cord. In another lecture, entitled 'Paralysis', he said he wished to draw attention to 'some of the obscurer forms of paraplegia' (p. 623). He cited cases of acute paralysis of the lower limbs after fevers, gastrointestinal disorders, and exposure to cold and damp. (Many of his patients came from those who enjoyed 'field sports'; duck-shooting, in particular; others were labourers in quarries or waterways.) He recalled the common experience of how 'the handling of snow or immersing your hands in freezing mixtures' tended to cause loss of power and sensation. In many cases, weakness of the lower limbs was not noticed until the patient got out of bed; pain and numbness had not been prominent.

'In what way', he asked, 'does paraplegia arise from inflammation of the bowels?' (p. 630). Others must have observed such cases 'although no author has as yet written upon the subject'. In lead and arsenic poisoning there was gastroenteritis followed by paralysis of limbs, but in the case of lead he felt that the latter was a direct effect of the poison and not a consequence of the gastrointestinal disorder.

In these obscure cases 'there was considerable variety in the rate of [its] progress'; there were acute, subacute, and chronic varieties. There was even a relapsing variety.

Graves cited (p. 641) one patient, a man of twenty-three, who suffered for years with sudden episodes of 'incessant vomiting', abdominal pain, and collapse. Eventually they were followed by numbness and weakness of the lower limbs. There were pains and 'severe twitches' in his limbs. Ultimately, after a particularly severe attack he developed 'a state of almost total paraplegia'. His legs wasted and were numb and remarkably cold. For some months before his death he was completely paraplegic. At no time were there disturbances of cerebral or sphincter function. A complete autopsy was carried out, 'we scrutinized every part of his system with the most anxious care'. There was no trace of abnormality in any organ; brain and spinal cord were entirely normal. 'We examined the large nervous trunks that supply the lower extremities' and found nothing to explain the illness. But Graves felt sure that it had 'implicated the nerves of the lower extremities'. Perhaps it was porphyria; in the attacks the urine was 'turbid and scanty', but there was no mention of a reddish colour.

In another case (p. 645) of acute paraplegia, which had begun overnight, and was fatal in eleven weeks, the spinal cord was again found to be quite normal. But 'Dr. Stokes observed that he thought the cauda equina appeared to be slightly softened'.

Graves thought that acute *spinal* paraplegia was more sudden in onset, with sensory loss that was more marked than in these obscure affections of the periphery of the nervous system.

Aside from these observations and ideas of a peripheral neuritis he also believed that in some way the concept of *reflex paralysis* had to be entertained. Disease of intestine, bowel, or urinary bladder, might 'be propagated towards the centre, and hence, by a reflex action, to other and distant parts' (p. 624). But some of his examples read strangely when compared with his accounts of the kind mentioned above. For example, there was the young scholar who developed cystitis after catching a fish-bone in his throat, which first set up an oesophagitis. And there was the medical student 'travelling through Wales on the outside of the mail', in a keen wind. The onset of impaired sight, a few days later, was attributed to retinal disturbance 'in consequence of an impression made on the facial branches of the fifth pair' by his recent exposure.

One's own impression of Graves's place in the history of this subject is that it is a pretty sound one. Perhaps he might have done more by way of documentation if he had held his views about the concept of peripheral neuritis for all those years. But Gowers[87] was scarcely justified in drily remarking that although Graves 'long ago suspected that many cases of paralysis were due to disease of the nerves' he had probably missed lesions of the cord which modern methods would have disclosed. And Viets,[88] in his historical review, was, I think, rather dismissive in referring to Graves's contribution as 'a rather casual note'. He quoted only Graves's recollection of the Paris epidemic. In his introduction to the French translation of Graves's book, Trousseau (1801–67) said that Graves had 'created the class of peripheric or reflex paralyses, and he has clearly established the relations existing between these paralyses and acute diseases'.[89]

But what of the Paris epidemic which had seemingly set Graves on this trail?

Auguste-Francois Chomel (1788–1856)

Chomel was a member of an old medical dynasty in Paris. His father is credited with the first description of post-diphtheritic palatal paralysis in an epidemic in 1749. Chomel junior succeeded Laennec (1781–1826) as Professor of Clinical Medicine at the Charité in 1827. He became a leading Paris physician and a year after his election to the professorship the editors of one of the many Paris medical journals, a weekly periodical, decided, in their ninth number, to begin summarizing Chomel's lectures at the Charité.[85] The idea was to record cases of interest in his wards and to discuss their significance much as the young Hughlings Jackson and Jonathan Hutchinson did in London in the 1860s in their 'Reports from Hospital Practice'.

The first hebdomadaire summary, in November 1828, was not signed and was mainly devoted to Chomel's lecture on the epidemic, 'still without a name', which had been rife in Paris since the spring of that year. It was first recognized in the Marie-Thérèse Infirmary but had spread to many parts of Paris, and was particularly common in the densely populated, poorer quarters around the Hôtel-de-Ville. 'Nearly a quarter of his [Chomel's] hospital beds' at the Charité were taken up by patients with this 'obscure malady'. It was not restricted to patients of any one class, nor to areas that were low-lying and humid. Neither was it related to the location of the 'many new constructions' in the city; indeed, 'not one case' was reported from recently completed streets.

There was no mention of the numbers of cases comprising the epidemic, nor the age or sex incidence, nor the mortality rate. But infants were spared. On the whole it appeared to be 'peu grave', and varied in its course and severity. There was no formal division into acute, subacute, chronic, or relapsing types, but the impression is gained that such was the case.

The general health of the patients was usually 'satisfactory'; appetite and digestion were good, there was no fever, but some patients suffered sore throats, vomiting, or diarrhoea.

The cardinal symptoms affected the extremities of the limbs. There were intense pains in the hands and feet, followed by numbness and weakness. Not all limbs were equally affected, although generally speaking disability was symmetrically distributed. The pains were sharp, intermittent, and paroxysmal, provoked by touch or pressure, worse at night, and often caused the sufferers to cry out and disturb their neighbours. Tenderness of the feet led to the discarding of shoes and the adoption of 'sabots' or woollen slippers. Some wore gloves to protect the hands. There were sensations as of 'crawling ants' and of 'walking on needles'.

In the hands and feet there was both hypersensitivity and numbness. On the one hand, the least contact with an object might cause sudden discomfort and force a patient to drop anything he had picked up – one patient described how he could not handle a knife or tolerate the contact of bedclothes on his feet. At the same time the numbness was such that a patient might not be able to identify an object by touch; the distinction between a key and scissors, for example, might be impossible. In some cases the sensibility of the feet was so impaired that a shoe might fall off without the patient being aware of it, nor of the coldness of the pavement. The steps of a staircase sometimes felt as if they were made of something soft and were giving way under the patient.

These sensory phenomena were followed or accompanied by weakness and clumsiness of the movements of the limbs, especially of the fingers and hands, toes and feet. Flexion and extension of the digits were impaired, and handling small objects was difficult; fastening buttons, for example. Movements of the digits were 'restricted by sensations like first degree burns'. The gait looked awkward, the feet were lifted up and put down in a flat-footed manner; the feet did not appear to grip the ground and the toes dragged. Some patients walked with their legs separated 'as if they had some affection of the genital organs'.

In severe cases there was paralysis of the limbs. 'They lie stretched out in their bed, the two arms alongside the body; a limb lifted up falls back when it is let go; the wrists droop from the forearms, and the fingers from the hands. The toes in a posture of flexion.' At times there were sudden pains in the extremities which cause them to tremble or start, but not in any convulsive manner.

In addition to these obviously neuritic manifestations there was a second group of signs. These were cutaneous. They were not constant, however, and bore no direct relation to the severity of the sensory or motor loss. 'The most remarkable is the inflammatory redness, the erythema extruding from the feet and hands'. These areas of distal erythema were often sharply delimited in the hands and feet, spreading, sometimes in a linear-fashion, to the fingers and toes. Sweating, blister formation, and desquamation were observed. Sometimes the tissues of the pulps of the digits were swollen and thickened, at other times they were remarkably smooth and soft, 'finer and glossier than was natural'. In general the body surface was not affected by any discoloration or eruption but in one lady 'the skin of the nipples became detached in the form of a little cap which remained in place by adhering at points on its circumference'.

There was one further strange form of change in the skin. This took the form of 'a black colouring of the skin, partial or general'. It was seen in only a few subjects but at the time of the report there was no actual case in Chomel's wards. Patients who remained paralysed in bed for long periods suffered an obstinate oedema of their limbs.

It was stressed that although the pains appeared to arise 'in the tissues of the skin', in many the latter was quite normal. In one severely paralysed patient death came suddenly from respiratory failure a few hours after she had eaten heartily. An autopsy was performed by Dr Louis. 'The spine was opened, the nerves were dissected and followed to the tips of the fingers and toes. Not only was nothing found to explain the death, but neither was there any explanation for the paralysis'. In a second autopsy, Dr Andral found no abnormality. 'All types of lesion eluded us'.

When Graves recalled this epidemic he did not mention that the nerves had been examined; he referred only to the negative examination of the brain and spinal cord. Yet it is clear that Chomel strongly suspected that the lesion might lie in the nerves.

As to causation, Chomel saw nothing to suggest that 'poor quality wine', plumbism, or ergotism were responsible. 'One conjectures in vain', he said. That it was an epidemic of acute polyneuritis is obvious enough, but whether it was toxic or infective it is not possible to say. Poisoning by arsenic, silver, or mercury may be reasonably excluded on clinical grounds, and as for infective polyneuritis, there seems to have been a greater incidence of cutaneous manifestations than we now meet. We can but join Chomel in his perplexity, hoping also that like 'Pink Disease' and the 'Royal Free Disease', admittedly more nebulous than Chomel's, it will not return to torment us.

Octave Landry (1826–1865)

It is rather curious that Landry,[90] at the age of thirty-three, was able to say, in his famous paper on 'Acute Ascending Paralysis' in 1859 that, in addition to the details he gave on the case which came to autopsy, 'I have observed four cases which were similar to the case described.' Nobody would be surprised to learn that he had also uncovered five more in the literature, of course, because ascending paralysis is a rather rare but dramatic illness, and likely to be reported. But there, in Paris, Duchenne had already been toiling for seventeen years delineating various forms of muscular paralysis. If he saw a case of ascending paralysis he certainly left no recognizable description of it. We can recall that he thought some cases of progressive muscular atrophy recovered, and that sensory loss was an occasional finding. Syringomyelia, as already mentioned, may have explained some such cases. Perhaps others were neuritic.

Landry's patient was a man of forty-three, a paver by occupation, who was periodically ill for more than a year before his final illness. There were fevers, chills, malaise, loss of appetite, and, on one occasion, pains in his limbs. In the spring of 1859 he had 'pulmonary congestion' and was at home for two months. He was purged, bled, and blistered; his doctor advised 'une diète sévère', and for eighteen days he took no food. He improved, returned to work for a week, and, finding himself generally weak, and with 'formications in the tips of his fingers and toes', he took himself off to hospital. 'On June 1st, he walked from Boulogne-sur-Seine to the Hospital Beaujon without difficulty', a distance I judge to be about five miles. He died there three weeks later, after an illness lasting some five to six weeks.

Landry's account of the illness still makes excellent reading. It is much more detailed than the majority of neurological case reports of those days and he brings out the distinctive features of paralysis arising in the periphery, and the absence of those signs which were associated with spinal and cerebral disease. The limbs remained 'supple', there were no cramps or pains, no involuntary spasms, no rigidity, muscle wasting or contractures. The sphincters functioned normally and there was no spinal pain. To the end, he remained alert, his responses even 'more clear and lucid', but although 'his expression was calm' he appeared apprehensive about his prospects.

Meanwhile, however, the paralysis was ascending. He had difficulty in moving about, and on one ward round, when he tried to stand by his bed, he had to be supported by two persons. In bed he could raise his legs. Indeed, the contrast between his helplessness and the lack of signs of illness was puzzling. Dr Gubler, into whose service the patient had been admitted, was, from the start, suspicious about the genuineness of the paralysis, and remained so for some two weeks.

But in the third week of the illness when his lower limbs were virtually paralysed, there were sinister developments. There was fever, cough, and difficulty in breathing, speaking, chewing, and swallowing. He had trouble in moving his trunk and shoulder muscles. His fingers were clumsy and weak.

Landry recorded the ascent of the formications and sensory loss, 'like a band around the affected parts'. At first there was only slight loss on the soles of the feet, and even on the day he died, when his motor paralysis was now 'generalised', sensory loss was slight. Touch was lost in the feet but little impaired in the upper two-thirds of the lower limbs; it was absent in the finger tips and impaired in only the lower third of the upper limbs. 'Pain and temperature sensation were not altered anywhere'. Appreciation of passive movement was lost only in the toes and feet. There were areas over the trunk where his ability to identify the difference between 'simple touching and rubbing of the skin' and between 'light' and 'heavy' touch was impaired or lost.

He was fortunately spared any of the usual depletory treatments in hospital; his limbs were massaged and given electrical stimulation, and he was provided with 'substantial nourishment' by way of 'côtelettes & vin de Bordeaux'.

Autopsy, as in the previous cases, revealed no abnormality in the nervous system. It included microscopic (not just macroscopic[91]) examination of sections of the spinal cord at different levels and also of a soleus muscle. Thus, the vital examination of the nerves was omitted. This is a little surprising in view of the way he so carefully recorded the ascent of the motor and sensory paralysis, and how he indicated the difference from spinal paralysis. Perhaps the fact that the nerves retained their excitability to electrical stimulation influenced him. The statement that 'reflexes could not be elicited' referred, of course, not to tendon jerks, but to responses obtained on superficial stimulation, usually, as we have seen, of the soles of the feet. The cord sections were inspected by 'Messrs. Bourguignon, Gubler, Ch. Robin and myself'. Might not the young Landry have hesitated to suggest examination of the peripheral nerves? Possibly, but unlikely, in view of his statement that 'the muscles were deep red', so that the opportunity of taking a specimen of nerve was surely there.

In the second part of his paper, in which he discussed the general picture he had formed in his mind, based on the five personal and five recorded cases, he first stressed how innocently such a dangerous illness could begin. There were three deaths (not two as often stated[88]); two at the height of the paralysis and another after several months of fluctuating illness. The rapidity of the ascent varied greatly, from hours to one or two weeks; there could be fluctuations during the course of the illness; return of power, usually in a manner inverse to the way it ascended, could be halting. Peril seemed ever present. Death was usually sudden.

In two cases the onset followed exposure to cold and in another two, during convalescence from fevers, which must, he thought, 'play some role in the pathogenesis of the paralysis'.

At the end of Landry's paper, Dr Gubler added a note, a column in length, which is usually omitted in translations and abstracts of Landry's account. Gubler complimented Landry on his observations and pointed out how Landry had warned him that the patient was going to die. Gubler admitted that he was not at first convinced of the 'paralysis' and believed that, although he had found no clinical evidence of active tuberculosis of the lungs, he felt that there was a 'tuberculous diathesis' with some defective innervation of the limbs. He was reminded of other cases of paralysis he had seen after fevers like typhoid, in women after childbirth, and in long severe illnesses. He thought there might be some link between cases of this kind and diphtheritic paralysis, and also with cases of 'septic illness' and 'croup', in which profound weakness was a common sequel. He concluded

> Thus post-diphtheritic paralysis could be a secondary effect in a large number of diverse illnesses which had in common that of exhausting the nervous system, weakening the constitution and reducing the level of the vital forces, all of which could lead to permanent defects of innervation.

At that time, of course, the pathology of diphtheritic paralysis was not known, but in coming so near to the truth, we can still wonder why those peripheral nerves went unexamined.

As we now know, in the ensuing years, 'Landry's paralysis' became something of a 'bogy-syndrome'. There was much debate and confusion, even long after it was established that ascending paralysis could be due to multiple neuritis. There were further case reports but the concept was resisted, although Duménil (1823–90),[92, 93] in Rouen, had provided the first histological proof of its existence. There were various explanations why a spinal cord could remain 'normal' in acute ascending paralysis, even on microscopic examination. Wilks,[56] for example, suggested that 'There may be a state in which the so-called reflex paralysis has occurred, in which the cord is in no way structurally altered, and therefore may at any time recover its function.' Alternatively, it may be because 'the effects of the inflammation have not had time to display themselves'. Wilks referred to nine cases of 'acute ascending paralysis' which he had seen. All died within four to thirty days, seven within twelve days. The spinal cord was examined in six. In no case was there any macroscopic change. Microscopic study was made in four; in one there was no abnormality; in a second 'it was thought that slight degenerative changes could be perceived'; in the third and fourth cases there was 'degeneration throughout all the tracts'.

Wilks described acute ascending paralysis in the section of his book dealing with diseases of the spinal cord. He referred to the fact that no one 'both in this country and on the continent' had discovered 'any abnormal changes'. He did not mention Landry's or Dumenil's names, but the book, it will be recalled, was in the nature of a collection of lectures. In the section on 'Nerves' there is no mention of multiple neuritis.

'Peripheral Paralysis', 'Alcoholic Paraplegia', and 'Diphtheritic Paralysis' are all considered in the section on the spinal cord, but in the first he refers to 'the doctrine . . . where the nerves are not injured at their source, but in the course of their distribution'. 'Reflex paralysis' and 'exhaustion' of the spinal cord centres are hypotheses he entertained in such cases. In alcoholic paraplegia the possibility of a peripheral neuritis was not considered; he supposed there was some form of 'chronic meningomyelitis'. (The literature of the era emphasized, rightly or wrongly, that it was in the female sex that most cases of alcoholic neuritis were seen. The language employed in describing the 'vices' of the 'unfortunates' was much like that used in descriptions of hysteria. The 'inferiority' of the female was unquestioned.) In diphtheritic paralysis, also, the possibility of a neuritic lesion was not mentioned; 'exhaustion of the cerebrospinal centres' and our old friend 'reflex paralysis' are the only explanations suggested. He mentioned one fatal case of diphtheritic paralysis in which an autopsy was obtained but 'no morbid changes were found in any organ'.

Wilks admitted that the concept of 'reflex paralysis' was purely hypothetical. It was used, he said, to explain various types of paralyses especially those in which no lesion was discovered at autopsy. 'A paraplegia induced by an external irritant' was also 'styled *reflex paralysis*'. Those cases in which there was complete recovery could also be included. But, although Wilks clearly expressed 'the greatest difficulty' in adopting the reflex hypothesis, and was perfectly aware of the features of ascending paralysis, he did not really see that what was missing was information about the nerves themselves.

A decade later, Thomas Buzzard (1831–1919),[94] then fifty-four, and on the staff at Queen Square, said of Landry's acute ascending paralysis that it was one 'of which I know little, save what I have read'. Yet he described cases of 'acute and subacute multiple neuritis', noting bilateral facial paralysis in two, and how the knee jerks disappeared in one case and reappeared with recovery of the paralysis.

Like Wilks, Gowers[95] also placed acute ascending paralysis in a section on the spinal cord. He observed, however, that 'the most careful and skilled examination has failed to discover any morbid change in the spinal cord'. He also knew that the tendon reflexes tended to disappear, and commented, like Gubler, that 'the malady to which acute ascending paralysis bears the closest analogy is diphtheritic paralysis'. By then, of course, the neuritic nature of the latter had been demonstrated, in the palatal nerves, the anterior spinal nerve roots, and in the peripheral nerves, by the Paris school in the eighteen-sixties and seventies. Neuritis had also been demonstrated as the lesion responsible for the paralysis of lead and arsenic poisoning, and in leprosy and beriberi.

In 1893, in their comprehensive treatise *On peripheral neuritis*, Ross and Bury[96] dealt in great detail with the contributions subsequently discussed by Viets. They analysed the literature on acute ascending paralysis and found that, at that time, there were 90 reported cases with 52 deaths. There were 42 autopsies. The medulla and spinal cord were examined microscopically in 26 and were found to be 'completely normal' in 14. Spinal nerve roots and peripheral nerves had been examined microscopically in only nine, but there was evidence of neuritis in six. Ross and Bury concluded that Landry's paralysis was 'an acute form of multiple neuritis' (p. 3).

They pointed out that the first mention of loss of the knee jerk in this condition was made by Westphal in 1876 (p. 69). By 1893 the state of the knee jerk had been reported in sixteen cases and in all it was completely lost. The cutaneous reflexes were recorded in only 24 of the 90 collected cases; they were lost in 14. The 'reflex of the sole' was usually one of these. They had an interesting observation to make concerning the position of the great toe in paralysis of the feet in subacute multiple neuritis (p. 102). The great toe did not always drop. Sometimes it assumed a position of hyperextension.

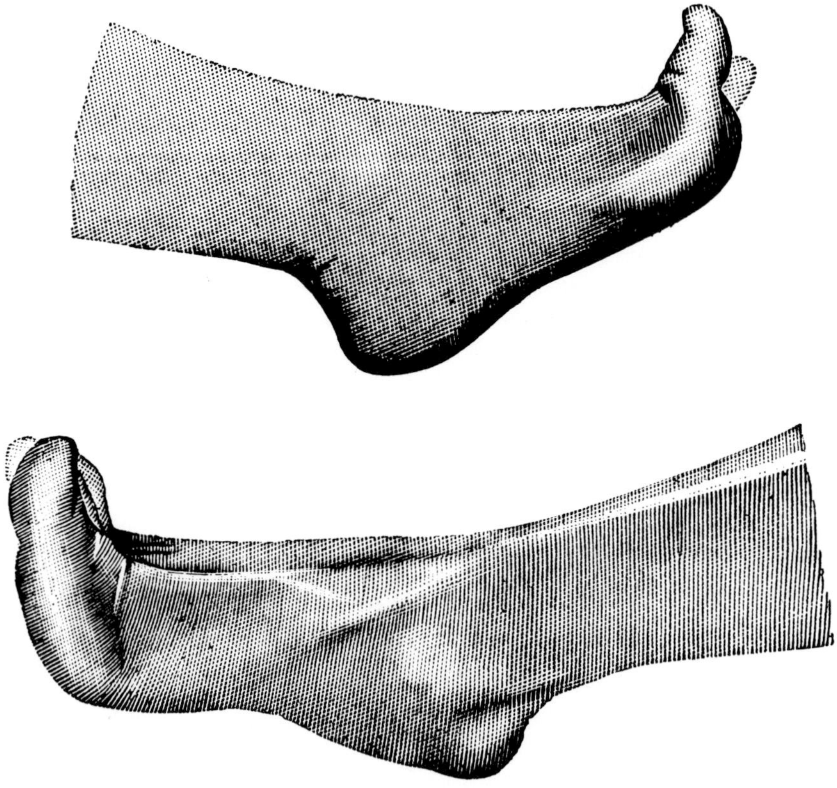

FIG. 142. (*upper*) The extended position of the great toe in multiple neuritis, described by Ross and Bury in 1893. 'The same attitude is met with in spastic paralysis'. (*lower*) Hyperextension of great toe in transverse myelitis, 'due to active spasm of its extensor'.

This they attributed to the imbalance that arose between the flexors and extensors of the toes consequent on the stretching of the paralysed extensors. This extension of the great toe might suggest that the lesion was in the lateral columns of the cord, as 'the same attitude is met with in spastic paralysis' (Fig. 142). Babinski's sign was still eluding 'capture'.

So confusion persisted. Even in 1940 Kinnier Wilson,[97] who seems to have thought that Landry had merely published a single case report, was writing of 'Landry's spinal syndrome' and 'the polyneuritic type of Landry's syndrome', adding that 'The conception of a self-contained Landry's paralysis has been reduced almost to vanishing point.'

The merit of Landry's paper was that it drew attention to a clinical syndrome of acute ascending paralysis for which there was no spinal explanation. To Landry it was an illness 'without apparent lesion of the nervous system'. If ever a gate had been opened in neurological exploration, here was one. Despite his young age, he was not to see how things would develop for he died of cholera six years later in the Paris epidemic of 1865. His illness lasted only forty-eight hours and he was attended by Charcot.[98]

Louis Duménil (1823–1890)

Landry and Gubler would no doubt have seen the article entitled 'Motor and Sensory Peripheral Paralysis Affecting the Four Limbs' which appeared in 1864 in the same journal that had carried their own communication. It was by L. Duménil[92] of l'Hotel-Dieu, Rouen, and if they read it they may have realized that it contained the clue to their own speculations, for it provided the first evidence that diffuse paralysis could result from disease of the peripheral nerves.

Duménil's patient was an old man of seventy-one, a former stone-cutter, with no history of alcoholism, who was admitted complaining that for some weeks he had been troubled with tingling sensations in his toes, and then in his left foot and right arm. His condition deteriorated and he developed flaccid paresis of his limbs, more marked distally, with wasting of the musculature and impairment of superficial sensation. The paralysis did not ascend in such a striking and symmetrical fashion as in the Paris patient and the sensory loss was not of that pattern which later came to be called 'glove and stocking'. At first it picked out the left ulnar nerve, the right median nerve, and the outer aspect of both legs, later spreading upward. There was more atrophy than in Landry's case, the thenar and hypothenar muscles on the right side practically disappearing. The deltoids were notably involved.

'Electrical exploration with the apparatus of Duchenne' revealed loss of faradic response in many distal muscles of the limbs. When the patient died of pneumonia five months later, he was not as completely paralysed as Landry's patient.

At autopsy there was no disease of the viscera apart from the consolidation of the lungs, but there was widespread wasting of the muscles of the limbs. Neither the brain, the spinal cord, nor the roots of the spinal nerves showed any abnormality to the naked eye.

Similarly, inspection of the nerves showed nothing abnormal except that 'the terminations of the collateral nerves of the toes' were 'more transparent' than usual, the significance of which was thought to be questionable. Nevertheless, Duménil asked a colleague with histological experience, a Dr Georges Pouchet, to make a microscopic examination of some nerves and muscles from the four limbs. In the latter he found obvious loss of transverse striation of the shrunken fibres. He found 'a genuine atrophy of the medullary substance of the peripheral nerve tubes', especially evident in areas where muscle atrophy and sensory loss had been most pronounced. The preserved but unstained nerve specimens, cutaneous and muscular, were examined by Pouchet without knowledge of whether they came from paralysed or unaffected parts. There was no doubt that the microscopic signs of nerve degeneration were most marked in the periphery and they correlated well with the clinical findings.

Duménil referred to Charcot's and Vulpian's recent demonstrations of degeneration of the palatal nerves in diphtheritic palsy and to Rokitansky's opinion that there was a class of case in which there was an apparently spontaneous atrophy of peripheral nerves. Duménil believed that in his case it was the primary lesion and that it began in the distal terminations of the nerves to the skin and musculature. He admitted that he had not proved how far up the trunks of the nerves the atrophy had progressed and that he had not examined the roots of the spinal nerve with the microscope. But the evidence all pointed to lesions arising in the extreme periphery of the nervous system. He did not mention Landry.

In a second, longer paper, two years later, Duménil[93] gave a detailed account of three further patients with 'peripheral paralysis' due to 'neuritis' and he summarized six published case reports. In his first case the neuritis began in a sciatic nerve, spreading to all four limbs over the course of five years, and leading to death from bulbar palsy and respiratory paralysis. Microscopical examination of the cord, spinal nerve roots, the trunks of peripheral nerves, and their terminal branches disclosed an atrophy of the neural elements with a proliferation of interstitial tissue. (Viets[88] erred when he said there was no autopsy in this case.) In the cord there was degeneration of the posterior columns and of the posterior horns of grey matter; the posterior spinal nerve roots were more affected than the anterior.

His second and third patients both recovered, after many months. Among the six cases he collected from the literature only one fits the picture of a polyneuritis. He quoted Swan's lady with the injured finger (see p. 191), a case of third nerve palsy following a facial neuralgia, a case of brachial neuritis, one of median neuritis, and one of sciatica.

He paid tribute to Graves for originating the concept of peripheral neuritis and to Todd for pointing out that the paralysis of lead poisoning was neuritic in nature. He thought the 'eternal question of Hallerian irritability' was now solved and he particularly noted how Claude Bernard had shown that the lesion in curare paralysis was in the nerve. He knew of Weir Mitchell and nerve injuries in the American Civil War and observed that the smooth, shining, tapering fingers in upper limb injuries were just what he had seen in his second patient. Lastly, he suggested that the cases which Gubler, Landry's chief, had described as paralysis of convalescence and post-febrile were probably examples of peripheral neuritis. But again there is no mention of Landry.

Duménil asked where the neuritic process actually began. 'In the periphery or the centre?' And was it 'ascending or descending?' All the evidence, he thought, clinical and pathological, pointed to the periphery, where Graves had envisaged it. It did not always ascend in a symmetrical manner and its rate of spread varied considerably. There was clearly a chronic variety – 'a chronic neuritis'. A fatal outcome was usually a consequence of involvement of 'essential' nerves such as the vagi.

He concluded his classical contribution with the following words.

> There is a class of spontaneous peripheral paralyses due to an atrophy of the nerves. In a certain number of cases, if not in all, the responsible morbid process is inflammatory.
>
> These paralyses can affect sensation and motion with equal intensity, either simultaneously or successively, and in the latter case motion appears to be affected by reflex action. They are often limited to one portion of the branches of one or several nerves, and do not necessarily correspond to the anatomical distribution of the trunks.
>
> They may be accompanied by alterations in the nutrition, not only of the muscles, but also of the skin and joints, as in paralyses from nerve injury.

The responsible morbid process may follow an ascending course and extend to the spinal cord, leaving unquestionable, substantial traces. Pathological anatomy amply confirms Graves's opinion.

According to Gowers (p. 91), Duménil's observations attracted little notice, and it was not until Grainger Stewart's publication in 1881 that multiple neuritis came to be adequately recognized in the English-speaking world. Stewart's paper was entitled 'On Paralysis of Hands and Feet from Disease of Nerves'.[99] In the works of Wilks, Hammond, Leyden, Erb, and others he said he failed to find a satisfactory clinical account of the disease, although it was obvious that these writers had encountered similar cases, and he had noted Leyden's recent paper. He quoted Duménil's papers as providing the earliest references, and Joffroy's[100] as giving a historical survey of the localized and general forms of neuritis, with the concept of 'interstitial' and 'parenchymatous' lesions.

Stewart reported three cases, one with autopsy. He thought the clinical picture was 'quite distinctive'. Sensory symptoms usually preceded motor; the tendon reflexes disappeared; the muscles wasted and the skin of the hands and feet become thin and glossy. 'The process may take weeks, or perhaps months, to arrive at its full development.' Improvement usually begins in the upper limbs. Recurrences had been reported and he had had one patient who suffered three attacks within a few years. In severe cases the disease spread to the spinal cord, as in his fatal case. Here, although to the naked eye the peripheral nerves were normal, there was a striking 'breaking up of the axis clinders'. The 'lower stretches of the nerves' were most affected; 'the cords of the brachial plexus, and the sciatic' showed but little change. The cord lesions occupied the columns of Goll and superficial parts of the lateral columns. He interpreted these as forming, not the primary lesions, but secondary ascending ones, though he was puzzled about the relative sparing of the proximal portions of the peripheral nerves.

Stewart suspected that in the past many cases of peripheral neuritis had been diagnosed as 'spinal congestion, slight myelitis, or such like'. He speculated that there might be selective involvement of motor or sensory nerves, when mixed nerves were affected, so that there might be variation in the clinical presentation. In the former there would be a picture 'closely resembling Landry's acute ascending paralysis'. He appeared to think that in this condition there was no sensory paralysis and that no lesion is found at autopsy in the nervous system, whereas in multiple neuritis, there is sensory loss and well marked pathological changes. But he thought 'the processes may, on further examination, turn out to be related to one another . . .'. These comments remind us of what confusion had followed Landry's report.

It is not inappropriate to end this account of the history of multiple neuritis by referring to the contribution made by Korsakoff (1853–1900), whose third and last paper has been translated by Victor and Yakovlev.[101] In each of his communications Korsakoff was stressing, not only the association of mental disturbance with alcoholic neuritis, but that the syndrome could arise in many ways. He had encountered it after infections and parturition, in tuberculosis, malignancy, and in different types of grave illness. The weakness and ataxia of the lower limbs, with the mental confusion and disturbed memory, might be mistaken for 'natural weakness, exhaustion of the nervous system or cerebral anaemia'. The course and outcome depended on this aetiological background. Whatever was actually poisoning the body must be affecting, not just the peripheral nerves, but also the brain. Although the nature of the causative 'toxic substances' was not known, he conjectured that they could be endogenous as well as exogenous.

Perhaps further researches will show that this disease is not only a disease of the nervous system but also a general disease, and one most probably depending on the development in the organism of some noxious substance disturbing the nutrition of the tissues, but chiefly the nervous system.

Like Wernicke's encephalopathy, Korsakoff's syndrome proved to be a nutritional disorder of the nervous system, just as did the beriberi of Jacob Bontius.

THE EYE-MIRROR

'I think it the luckiest thing in my medical life, that I began the scientific study of my profession at an ophthalmic hospital.' Those words were spoken by Hughlings Jackson (1835–1911) as he began a lecture on 'Ophthalmology in its Relation to General Medicine' in 1877.[102] He went on to say that 'the nerve of the most special of all the special senses goes to the eye, and the end of it can be seen by the ophthalmoscope'.

It had taken centuries for man to see into another's eye.† Why the pupil was black was a mystery. The ancient notion that the eyes were radiators of light was related to the observation that the eyes of some animals shone at night. Not until the nineteenth century was it realized that in complete darkness they did not shine and that to see into an illuminated eye the observer had to stand in the path of the emerging rays.[103]

Blindness was originally divided into two varieties, according to the clarity or clouded appearance of the pupil (e.g. glaucoma for glaucos, greyish-green). Night-blindness[104] and colour-blindness[105, 106] were identified in the eighteenth century, as was the true nature of cataract.[107]

During the nineteenth century the optical properties of the different portions of the eye were worked out, and the lesions of the opaque cornea and of glaucoma, and the anomalies of astigmatism and refraction, were elucidated. Although, in England, Cumming (1812–86) and Babbage (1792–1871) obtained glimpses of the interior of the eye, it was Helmholtz's[108] (1821–94) invention in 1850 of the 'Eye-Mirror', later to be named the ophthalmoscope, which revolutionized ophthalmology and also, subsequently, neurology. His instrument (Fig. 143) consisted of mirror-plates, set at an angle, combined with a concave lens. It was mounted with a holder for one lens, which had to be changed for eyes with different refractions. The basis of the modern instrument soon followed, with its silvered mirror and central hole, and with a revolving disc to carry a series of lenses.

† J. E. Robert-Houdin (1805–71), the famous Parisian prestidigitator, founder of modern conjuring, learned in several sciences, including optics, devised an ophthalmoscope with which he was able to examine his own retina.

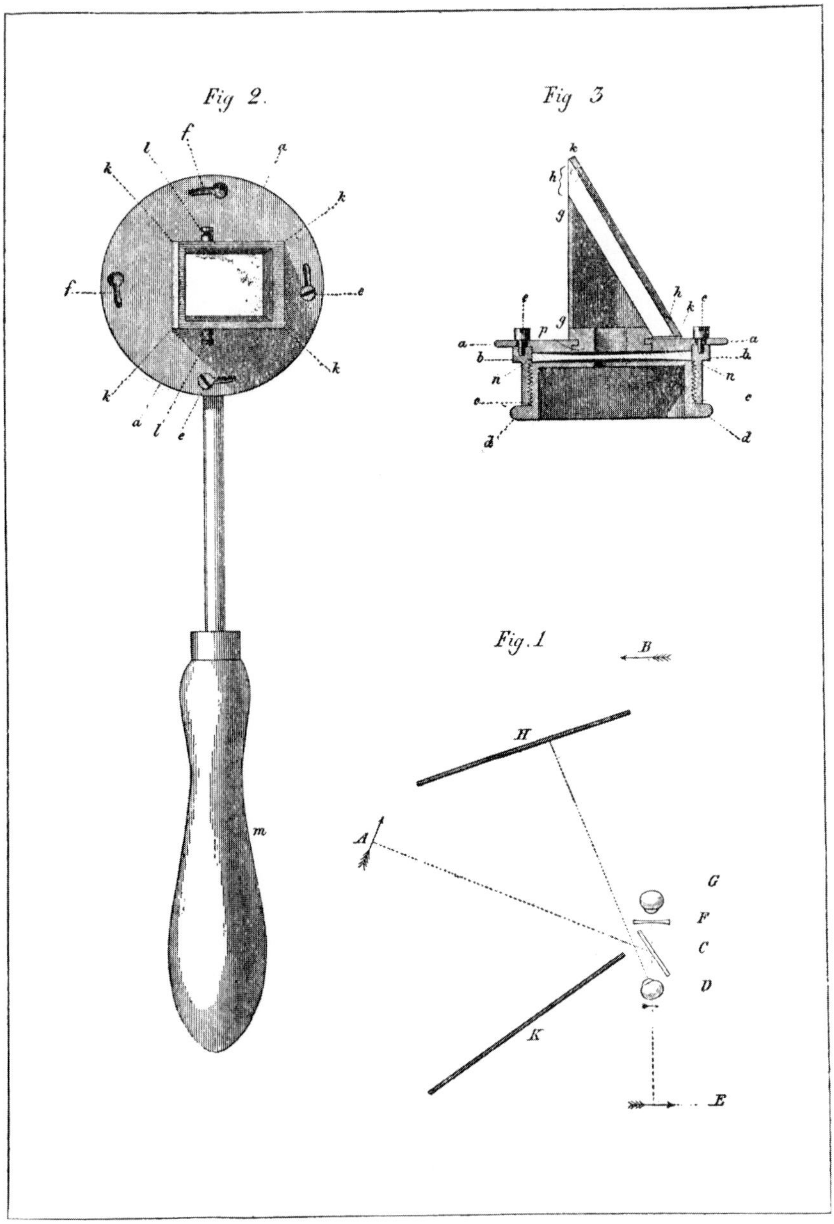

FIG. 143. Helmholtz's 'Eye-Mirror', 1851, was a triangular instrument with an acute angle at the top. Mirror-plates on the side of the triangle reflected light into the eye of the patient at an angle of fifty degrees. *Fig. 1.* A is the source of light; C, a mirror-plate; D, the observed eye; G, the observing eye. H and K are objects of gaze. *Fig. 2.* The instrument mounted on a handle. *Fig. 3.* The instrument in horizontal cross-section.

Helmholtz's hopes for his instrument are interesting to recall.

In brief, I believe that I may hold the expectation not to be exaggerated, that all the alterations of the vitreous body and of the retina which, until now, have been found in cadavers, will also permit of recognition in the living eye – a possibility which appears to promise the most remarkable advances for the hitherto undeveloped pathology of this structure.[108]

Within a few years, in Vienna, the changes in the optic discs of patients with tumours of the brain were being recorded. Türck (1810–68) described retinal haemorrhage and von Graefe (1828–79) bilateral 'optic neuritis'.

The latter also described embolism of the central artery of the retina. The first atlas of the fundus, by Liebreich (1830–1917), was published in 1863 and translated into English in 1870. In 1875 Gowers[109] translated the text of another German atlas of the fundus.

The first English book on the use of the ophthalmoscope was published in 1871 by Allbutt (1836–1925).[110] He was interested in neurology and had studied under Duchenne in Paris in 1868.† He was later to introduce the short modern clinical thermometer and the sphygmomanometer to Britain. He dedicated his book to Hughlings Jackson, saying, 'It was about the same time, I think, that you in London and I in Leeds began to use the ophthalmoscope in the investigation of cerebral diseases.' He went on to say (p. 9) that 'The number of physicians who are working with the ophthalmoscope in England may, I believe, be counted on the fingers of one hand.' One of them was Gowers, whose own book *Medical ophthalmoscopy* appeared in 1879.[111] Hughlings Jackson's interest in ophthalmology had been stimulated when, through the influence of his friend and fellow Yorkshireman, Jonathan Hutchinson (1828–1913), he became associated with the Royal London Ophthalmic Hospital at Moorfields, in 1859. They had both begun their medical studies at the York Medical School, and Hutchinson had been working at Moorfields since 1854.

Initially, direct and indirect methods of inspection of the fundus were used, the source of illumination coming from a candle, oil lamp, or gas mantle. The electric ophthalmoscope was not developed until the late eighteen-eighties.[112] Many of the early instruments were cumbersome but gradually the basis of the majority was the concave mirror with a central perforation, mounted on a handle.

Hughlings Jackson first wrote on the use of the ophthalmoscope in 1863[113] when he was twenty-nine years of age, and through his association with Moorfields he was able to pursue his studies for many years. In all he published at least forty papers on ophthalmoscopic appearances, six in 1863 alone, one of which was on the retina during sleep. He never grew tired of advocating the use of the instrument and of stressing its importance.[114]

In an 1863 paper entitled 'Observations on Defects of Sight in Brain Disease'[115] he pointed out that the cause of blindness in tumours of the brain was 'white atrophy', of the optic discs. It was possible to see at autopsy that in some cases this was due to compression of the optic nerves, chiasm, or corpora quadrigemina but in others, in cerebellar tumours, for example, the explanation was difficult. It might be produced by the effects of 'general pressure' or 'reflex irritation' which contracted the blood-vessels of the retina. Transient blindness before an epileptic fit might be due to retinal arterial spasm, such as was supposed, in the brain, to be responsible for epilepsy itself. He had seen cases of sudden, complete, but transient blindness, for which there had been no explanation; possibly it was 'an epilepsy of the retinae'. Optic atrophy was also sometimes found in paraplegia; the cause was quite obscure. But although optic atrophy was 'what is found in nearly all cases of amaurosis in cerebral disease', there were some in which the optic papillae were 'swollen, ill-defined and blood being

† 'It was a wonderful experience to watch the gradual unravelling under his [Duchenne's] discerning eye of the several kinds of palsy which he described to the world later' (From *The Right Honourable Sir Thomas Clifford Allbutt* by Sir H. D. Rolleston. Macmillan (1925). p. 16.)

diffused near them'. He had seen 'a well-marked case of this kind'. This was a humble beginning to what proved to be a major contribution to the subject.

By 1871[116] he was able to say that it was 'optic neuritis' that was 'the commonest ophthalmoscopical condition in cases of cerebral disease'. It developed in stages, it was 'almost invariably double', sight could remain normal or fail in a 'paroxysmal' way, and it was 'not a localising symptom'. Just as hemiplegia pointed to the *position* of intracranial disease, so did optic neuritis point to its *nature* – to cerebral disease which was 'gross' or 'coarse'; 'I mean a lump or something'. In 1886 he had suspected that optic neuritis was more common in left hemiplegia. He had been comparing loss of speech with loss of sight, as symptoms of cerebral disease, and like others, was noting that the former usually occurred in right hemiplegia. Optic neuritis did not occur in epilepsy of the idiopathic variety, nor in chorea, cerebral thrombosis, or embolism. If the swelling of the disc subsided 'the descent to atrophy begins'. There were, therefore, two kinds of atrophy; primary or 'progressive', because it was atrophic from the beginning, and 'consecutive', that is, to the neuritis. He then described how they could be distinguished.

But as to the cause of optic neuritis and how it was to be distinguished from 'the swollen disc (Stauungs-papille of Graefe)', there were difficulties, shared, of course, by Allbutt, Gowers, and others.

The terms 'optic neuritis' and 'swollen disc' derived from observations of von Graefe[118] (1828–70) that in some cases of cerebral tumour with swollen discs, the optic nerves themselves showed no naked eye signs of inflammation, whereas in meningitis with swollen disc, Virchow had shown that the nerves were inflamed. There was 'a descending neuritis' which affected the retina as well as the actual papilla. Von Graefe thought that swelling of the disc in tumour was an effect on the circulation of the eye due to raised intracranial pressure, and to obstruction of the venous return from the eye by compression of the cavernous sinus. This mechanical effect might be intensified by the unyielding character of the sclerotic ring. The 'stauungs papilla' (*stauung*, a damming back) was characterized by vascular distension, gross swelling of the disc, and retinal haemorrhages. Allbutt proposed the term 'choked disc' for this appearance.

In his 1871 paper Hughlings Jackson admitted that he sometimes could not tell the difference between 'optic neuritis' and a 'swollen disc', although 'that there are two different things clinically I have no doubt'. He considered three 'hypotheses' to explain how optic neuritis was produced by a cerebral tumour. Did the tumour destroy some 'centre of sight'? He rejected this because he did not believe in any such centre in the hemispheres, 'although I do believe that the optic and all other nerves are represented – perhaps I should say re-presented – in the cerebral hemisphere in very complex groupings'.

> A tumour does not 'cause' amaurosis because it has *destroyed* so much of the hemisphere, but because it has led to secondary changes . . . Loss of speech *is* caused by *destruction* of certain processes superintending speech. The amaurosis is not caused by destruction of any part superintending sight.[116]

The second possibility was that a tumour 'led to pressure transmitted to the optic nerves and venous sinuses at the base', as suggested by von Graefe. But this was unlikely because you could have a small tumour with bilateral optic neuritis, and a large one, without. 'I believe, then, that the intracranial disease does not lead to optic neuritis by causing increased pressure within the head.'

The third hypothesis was that the tumour acted as 'a foreign body' which produced a state of 'irritation' within the brain. This could possibly be transmitted to the optic nerves 'by the intermediation of the arteries and their vasomotor nerves' as proposed by Brown-Séquard. But he did not feel happy about this either. 'I confess that optic neuritis is a very great puzzle.'

But he was sure of three things. (1) Optic neuritis was often present even though the patient could read small print. (2) In tumour cases there was a wide degree of variation of optic neuritis, and in any given case it also varied with the stages of the disease. (3) When there was *severe* and *continued* headache 'you should never omit to use the ophthalmoscope'.

Allbutt[110] (p. 57) told how you could have an 'astonishing' degree of swollen disc without any disturbance of vision. For him there were three main causes of choked disc: meningitis, hydrocephalus, and tumour. 'Choking' was confined to the disc. In optic 'neuritis' the nerve itself was affected. But was it inflammation? 'Vascular extensions do not make inflammation any more than the railways of the Force in Abyssinia made the war' (p. 59). He was uncertain about 'descending neuritis'.

Brain tumours, Allbutt said, were not very common and it was difficult to keep track of patients with them. 'I can not even now count more than eight cases which I have watched from first to last in life, and have examined after death' (p. 115). He was then thirty-five. But he had made a catalogue of cases published at home and abroad and had concluded that tumour was nearly always attended by optic neuritis. He analysed the incidence of optic neuritis according to the site of the tumour. He listed them as hemispheric (convexity, base, anterior, middle and posterior lobes; corpus callosum, corpus striatum, and optic thalamus), brain stem, and cerebellum. He concluded that although the ophthalmoscope may unexpectedly reveal the presence of a tumour 'the occurrence of optic signs is so uncertain that the ophthalmoscope will give no encouragement to the practitioner who takes it in the hope of making careful thought and quick sense unnecessary' (p. 177). Nevertheless, he felt it was an invaluable clinical instrument. Allbutt used it in homes as well as hospitals. 'There are very few houses in which I find it difficult to make an ophthalmoscopic examination.' If there was no 'gas pendant', a candle or lantern could be used. He had 'a black silk curtain' on his instrument which fell around the orbital region of the patient. (The author remembers that as a student his professor of medicine used an umbrella with a black curtain hanging from its rim; the patient held the umbrella.)

Allbutt thought that the situation of an intracranial tumour had much to do with the production of retinal changes. In tumours of the anterior fossa, the more basally situated were more likely do so. In the middle fossa it was 'hard to see how the optic nerves could escape'; a normal fundus practically excluded tumour there. When tumours arose in the cerebellum ('to which no definite function had yet been appropriated') optic neuritis and optic atrophy were very common. Similarly with the pons. This was probably due to pressure on the corpora quadrigemina and the development of 'ventricular and subarachnoid dropsy'. He studied the records of 100 cases of cerebellar and 40 of pontine tumours.

He was not sure that the distinction between 'primary' and 'consecutive' optic atrophy, described by Hughlings Jackson, was wholly reliable, but just as with swollen discs he was 'amazed' to see how well a patient could read despite having discs that were dead white and glistening.

In Bright's disease, Allbutt reminded his readers (p. 213), there were two types of blindness. In the first, 'uraemic amaurosis', it was transient and the retinae were normal. In the second, it was insidious and you would find the signs of 'albuminuric retinitis'. This distinction could not be made before the introduction of the 'eye-mirror'. He described the 'spots' of degeneration' 'the streaks' of haemorrhage, the 'exudates', and the 'stellate' surround of the macula. Failing vision was no forerunner; the retinal lesions were already there. He could offer no explanation for involvement of the retina in disease of the kidney. Were they causally related or were both due to some other 'precedent'? Arterial degeneration itself was unlikely but hypertrophy of the heart might play a role. Allbutt did not mention blood pressure. Sphygmomanometry came later.

Allbutt had some mistaken views about the optic fundus in epilepsy and spinal injury, not to mention menstrual disorders. In the first he suspected that vascular changes occurred in the retina during the convulsion. He had managed to study six cases, two of whom 'were daemonising during the hours of attendance'. The anaemic or hyperaemic retinal changes were usually transient, but in long standing cases of epilepsy there was a tendency to chronic hyperaemia. 'I have often said that I thought I could pick out an epileptic by the appearance of his disks and retinas, from a row of healthy persons' (p. 80).

There was 'a curious connection' between the retina and the spinal cord. Optic atrophy was often seen in acute and chronic diseases of the spinal cord; it was found in myelitis, insular sclerosis, and progressive degenerations, as well as in the well-known locomotor ataxy. But it did not occur in spinal injury. Here, however, you could often see signs of 'hyperaemia'. He said he found vascular changes, not in those cases of injury which proved fatal within a few weeks, but in those who developed 'chronic spinal disease' as a consequence. Here, I think, we are dealing with that old familar 'railway spine'.

As a whole, Allbutt's book still reads well, his style being discoursive and forthright. But it does not compare in thoroughness or accuracy with that of Gowers eight years later. Allbutt did not think illustrations were necessary, in view of Liebreich's recent edition in English translation. There is an appendix with 123 case summaries of varying value, which includes descriptions of the fundal changes he thought he saw in mania and melancholia. He provided no index.

By 1877 Hughlings Jackson was convinced that 'without an extensive knowledge of ophthalmology, a methodical investigation of diseases of the nervous system is not merely difficult but impossible'.[102] The value of 'specialisation' was nowhere better portrayed than by the rise of the ophthalmological surgeon. The student of neurology should seek his 'direction'. General physicians seemed still unconvinced of the value of the ophthalmoscope and they were not clear about the wide range of retinal appearances that were quite normal. Even in epilepsy, where he had not found any characteristic abnormality, he still felt the subject required continuing study. He had now abandoned the term 'epilepsy of the retina' but in both epilepsy and migraine there were 'local discharges of cerebral convolutions', which affected vision and might be accompanied by visible retinal changes. He said that Virchow had predicted that the effects of embolism would be seen in the eye, four years before von Graefe actually did see them. Embolic phenomena in the retina might indicate the cause of a sudden hemiplegia. It was not uncommon for the ophthalmologist to be the first to detect the existence of renal disease. Just as retinal haemorrhage may exist without affecting sight, so also was it possible that small cerebral haemorrhages could be symptomless. At autopsies of Bright's disease 'we see in the brain just the sort of change we saw during life in a part of the nervous system easily looked at.'[102]

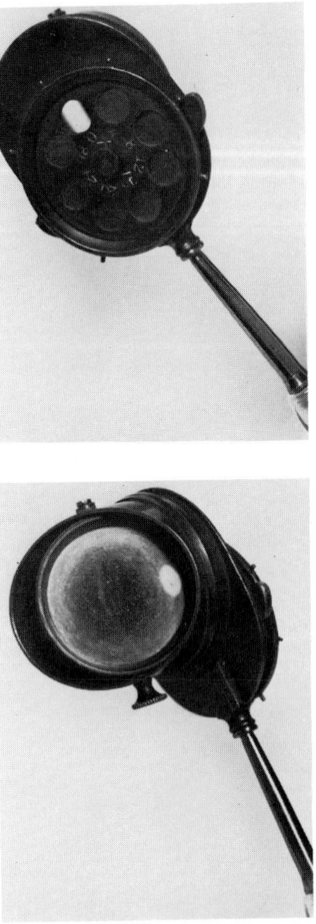

FIG. 144a. An ophthalmoscope used by Hughlings Jackson. (Courtesy of The Institute of Ophthalmology, London).

Hughlings Jackson, in the same paper, drew attention to 'the minute observations' Dr Gowers had made of the fundal changes in Bright's disease. He had found that there was typically an increased arterial tension, with retinal arteries 'distinctly smaller than normal'. Small vessels may be seen, associated with hypertrophy of the heart, before any albuminuria was present. But retinal arteriolar contraction was not always present when there was high arterial tension so that it could not be the only cause of raised tension. Gowers had also noticed the presence of miliary retinal aneurisms, like those Charcot had described in cerebral haemorrhage.

The ophthalmoscope should be used by all physicians in a routine fashion. In 1885,[119] in his last address on the topic of ophthalmology in diseases of the nervous system, he said that Argyll Robertson's (1837–1909) bequest to neurology in 1869 was repaid, as it were, by the neurologists Erb and Westphal when they demonstrated the diagnostic value of loss of the knee jerk. But on this occasion it was not ophthalmoscopic appearances that were on his mind, but the ways in which the neurologist and the ophthalmologist could integrate their studies and investigate how diseases of the nervous system caused manifestations at various 'levels'.

Gowers was a skilled instrumentalist. His very first publication was entitled *A safety hypodermic syringe*, in 1872, and, as is well known, he invented a haemoglobinometer and improved the haemocytometer. His first papers containing reference to the ophthalmoscope were in 1875. In his book on *Medical ophthalmoscopy* of 1879 he described how the ophthalmoscope he used had been made for him 'from a design of my own'. He even described how a student could make one for himself 'at the cost of a few pence', as he considered that ophthalmoscopy was a part of practical

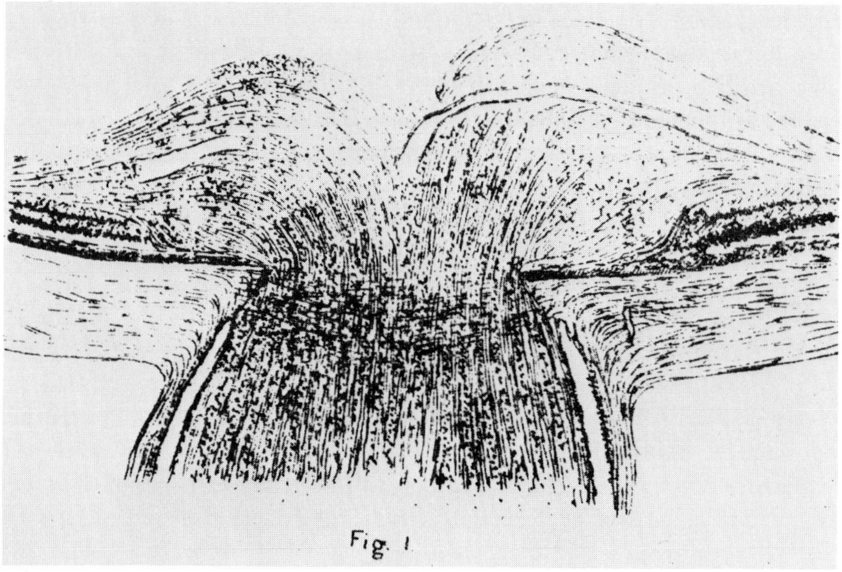

FIG. 144b. The optic disc in papilloedema. The disc swelling was asymmetrical; the margin of the retina was displaced from the edge of the choroid; the nerve sheath behind the lamina cribrosa was scarcely distended. (After Gowers,[111] Fig. 1 from Plate XIV.)

physiology which should be learned early. Usually the student 'only succeeds in seeing the optic disc just before he leaves the hospital'. The student's eye-mirror could be made from 'a piece of looking-glass, two inches long by one wide ... [with] paper pasted on the back of it and over one-half of the front'. A small hole was then made in the paper at the back, opposite the middle of the uncovered part of the mirror, and the silvering scraped away at the spot. With this, and a three-inch lens, 'the fundus, disc and vessels can be clearly seen'.

Gowers was also an excellent artist and he illustrated his book with his own drawings; there were 16 plates, two of them coloured. In four he showed the histological appearances of sections of abnormal discs and fundi. There is an appendix of 85 pages containing case notes of sixty patients and an adequate index.†

In Part 1 he described the 'changes in the retinal vessels and optic nerve, etc. of general medical significance'. In Part 2 he dealt with the 'changes in special diseases'.

He pointed out that 'in no other structure of the body are the termination of an artery and the commencement of a vein presented to view' (p. 7). He reminded his readers that 'the red lines spoken of as retinal arteries and veins are not the vessels themselves, but the columns of blood within them'. The vessel walls only became clearly visible when the direct method of examination was used, and when there were structural changes in the walls. He had never been able to see actual atheroma of retinal arteries, but thickened walls and minute aneurisms could be detected and increased tortuosity noted. He had seen no spasm of vessels during an epileptic convulsion and the normal variations made detection of 'anaemic' fundi very questionable. Venous congestion was seen in local disturbances such as retinal vein thrombosis, intracranial thrombosis, and in diseases of the heart

† Page references are to the second edition, 1882.

and lungs. Similarly, haemorrhages could arise from local or general disease; as a consequence of raised pressure, arterial or intracranial, and in Bright's disease, diabetes, and diseases of the blood. The central retinal artery was said to be 'terminal', without anastomoses, but Gowers thought he had seen signs of anastomosis after embolism. The latter was most often the result of mitral disease but it was also seen in atheroma of the aorta, in fevers, in pregnancy, and in Bright's disease.

The two major changes in the optic discs were characterized by increased vascularity or signs of inflammation, and diminished vascularity and signs of wasting. In the first there was congestion, swelling, 'neuritis', or 'papillitis'. In the second, atrophy; this could be primary, or follow congestion, neuritis, or choroiditis and retinitis.

He disliked Allbutt's term of 'choked disc' because he did not think that mechanical impediment to the return of blood from the eye was the explanation. The 'strangulation' occurred in the papilla itself and was not mechanically induced by raised intracranial pressure, distension of the optic sheath, or pressure by the sclerotic ring (p. 77). Neither was there any evidence that optic neuritis was a consequence of some reflex vasomotor influence, as had been suggested. Gowers favoured the 'descending neuritis' concept, obvious in meningitis, and found more commonly than many appreciated in tumour. When he came to deal with brain tumours he said 'encephalic tumours do not cause neuritis by the direct effect of their mass on the intra-cranial pressure' (p. 136). He was impressed by the absence of optic neuritis in hydrocephalus, which, he thought, could not be explained by the slowness with which the pressure was raised, for the growth of many tumours which caused optic neuritis was equally slow. He said 'The facts of medical ophthalmoscopy certainly make it difficult to connect papillitis with increase of intra-cranial pressure' (p. 70).

Optic neuritis was *the* ocular lesion in intracranial tumour; it was present in about four-fifths of cases (p. 135). But it did not seem to be related to the site, size, or nature of the tumour, or even to its rate of growth. Optic neuritis was not a constantly associated condition in the history of a cerebral tumour; it was a transient event. A tumour might exist and cause symptoms for years before optic neuritis was produced. It was usually bilateral. Gowers did not think there was any point in trying to classify optic neuritis into different varieties according to hypothetical modes of origin. One could only grade its stages. When it was developing, other symptoms and signs often appeared, but acuity of vision, fields of vision, and colour vision could all remain unaffected. Increase in the size of the blind spot was proportional to the size of the disc swelling.

The atrophy left by optic neuritis, the consecutive type, could not always be diagnosed with certainty. Although concealment of the lamina cribrosa was a valuable sign, evidence of previous neuritis might be very slight, with the edge of the disc quite clear-cut and the vessels only slightly narrowed. Simple optic atrophy was far less common in intracranial tumours.

Locomotor ataxy was the commonest disease of the spinal cord in which optic atrophy occurred; probably one in six developed it. The degeneration of the optic nerves usually stopped at the chiasm. The atrophy could develop well before any symptoms of spinal cord disorder made their appearance. There was progressive loss of the peripheral field of vision; acuity could be preserved for a long time. On the other hand, loss of colour vision was nearly always an early symptom. The degeneration in the cord and in the optic nerves was seemingly independent. Optic atrophy was rare in lateral sclerosis of the cord, but amblyopia, often without signs of atrophy of the disc, occasionally occurred in insular sclerosis (i.e. multiple sclerosis). Gowers did not here (p. 168) stress how 'frequent and important' was loss of sight in this disease, as in his textbook seven years later (Vol. 2, p. 512).

When dealing with injuries of the spine, he said that much of what had been written about optic disc changes was 'the result of an affection of the mind of the observer, rather than of the eye observed' (p. 169). Litigation and 'railway cases' were responsible for much of what had been claimed, but he thought Allbutt had shown that hyperaemic changes occurred, especially with high injuries.

Gowers had closely studied the fundi in chronic kidney disease (p. 181) and found that narrowing of the arteries was a characteristic feature. It seemed to be independent of any other retinal change and he thought it was due to contraction, although degenerative changes in the walls of the vessels also occurred. Irregular dilatation of the retinal capillaries, and aneurismal dilatations could be seen. The well-known features of 'albuminuric retinitis' were probably the most frequent ocular changes to come under the notice of the physician. The retinal changes corresponded in time with the development of cardiac hypertrophy, and the haemorrhages resulted from the increased arterial pressure and the degeneration of the vessel walls (p. 191). The question of differentiating albuminuric retinitis from the optic neuritis of tumour, from degenerative neuro-retinitis, diabetic retinitis, and from the fundal changes of pernicious anaemia and leukaemia are carefully considered.

In the various forms of meningitis, then so common, Gowers found that disc changes were most likely to occur when the inflammation was basal, as in tuberculosis and syphilis. In the former, tubercles of the choroid were less frequent in meningitis than in 'general' tuberculosis. But changes in the discs were present in about half of the cases of meningitis.

With regard to epilepsy Gowers said 'I have examined very carefully about a thousand epileptics' (p. 172). He found no significant abnormality, even immediately after a convulsion. Neither had he seen the chronic hyperaemia of discs described by Allbutt in longstanding severe epilepsy. In like vein he did not think that in insanity, mania, or melancholia – apart from general paralysis of the insane – there were any fundal changes, as had been alleged.

Finally, with typical thoroughness, Gowers included a page on 'The ophthalmic signs of death'. They provided 'the most unequivocal signs of death'.

As the heart's action is failing, the arteries may be observed to diminish in size (Arlidge). On the cessation of its contractions, the diminution in their size becomes more marked. A few minutes after death the capillary redness of the disc disappears, and its surface becomes of papery whiteness, in which, however, the central cup, if present, may appear of still more brilliant whiteness. ... The veins may present normal characters, or may, like the arteries, quickly become indistinct upon the disc ... Commonly the columns of blood within them soon become interrupted and broken up into segments, which give the vessels a beaded appearance. ... In the course of half an hour, sometimes in ten minutes [the arteries] are irrecognisable ... the choroid [fades] ... [there is] commencing opacity of the retina ... accompanied by a red spot at the macula lutea (Gayet) ... similar to that seen in the embolism of the retinal artery.

... generally after five or six hours, the progressive opacity of the media prevents further observations (p. 255).

As Hughlings Jackson said, 'Dr Gowers is so good an ophthalmoscopist.'

A decade later, in his textbook of neurology, Gowers was still of the opinion that in brain tumour, 'the optic neuritis is certainly not produced by the mechanism of increased intracranial pressure' (Vol. 2, p. 470). He thought that 'more than one mechanism' was involved, including 'tissue irritation' in the optic pathway, 'distension of the sheath of the optic nerve by fluid from the subarachnoid space', and 'meningitis' extending from the tumour to the optic nerves.

The swelling of the optic disc head in cerebral tumour was still referred to as 'optic neuritis', 'papillitis', or 'choked disc' until the classical paper of Paton and Holmes[120] in 1911. Their study, 'The Pathology of Papilloedema', was based on 700 cases of cerebral tumour. They examined the eyes at autopsy in sixty cases of papilloedema; fifty from brain tumour, and ten from miscellaneous conditions. Their object was to interpret the features of papilloedema in terms of the histological changes they found.

They found no evidence that papilloedema was an inflammatory process nor that it was 'a descending oedema spreading from the brain'. They found nothing to support the vasomotor theory. 'Our observations establish the fact that papilloedema is an oedema of the nerve-head due to two factors – venous engorgement and lymph stasis' (Fig. 145).

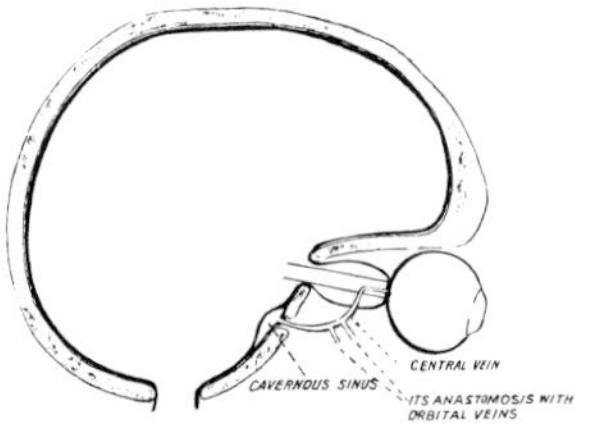

FIG. 145. The connexions of the central vein of the retina. (After Paton and Holmes,[120] Fig. 21.)

In our opinion therefore, the oedema of the papilla that constitutes tumour papilloedema is in the first place due to the venous engorgement that results from the rise of intravenous pressure that is necessary in order that circulation should be maintained in the intravaginal portion of the vein where this is subjected to an increased sheath pressure. The increased sheath pressure is also the origin of the second factor, the obstruction to the lymph drainage from the papilla.

Few serious students of modern neurology would not enjoy reading this famous paper or fail to admire the care and thoroughness with which the authors marshalled their data and debated their findings in the light of the prevailing theories of 'optic neuritis'. It is one of the 'jewels' of *Brain*.

THE BIRTH OF AMERICAN NEUROLOGY

In Europe, as we have seen, neurology was evolving, albeit slowly, in the first half of the century. Progress accelerated in the third quarter. There was no actual 'birth'. In America, however, it is possible to speak of its 'birth' with some justification.

Garrison[121] said 'The War of the Revolution was the making of medicine in this country', and it can equally be said that the Civil War was the making of American neurology. Two men played an outstanding role – Silas Weir Mitchell and William Alexander Hammond. Pearce Bailey[122] wrote that 'The team of Hammond and Mitchell virtually placed neurology on the medical map of the United States, and they were towers of strength in its early growth.' There were others, of course, during its nascent period in the eighteen-seventies and eighties who played vital roles, but they were rallying, as it were, to the banner raised by Mitchell and Hammond.

Silas Weir Mitchell (1829–1914)[123, 124, 160]

Mitchell was born in Philadelphia in 1829, the seventh physician in three generations. His father, John Kearsley Mitchell (1793–1858), was a practitioner in that city; he had been born in Virginia, educated in Scotland where he had been sent as a boy on the death of his parents, and was a graduate of Edinburgh Medical School. Weir Mitchell's paternal grandfather, Dr Alexander Mitchell, had emigrated from Ayrshire to Virginia. The great grandfather, a revenue collector, was said to have been a friend of Robert Burns and the Mitchell alluded to in a poem 'To Mitchell on asking for a loan'.[125] Mitchell's father was a professor of chemistry at the Philadelphia Medical Institute and later occupied the chair of medical practice at Jefferson Medical College.

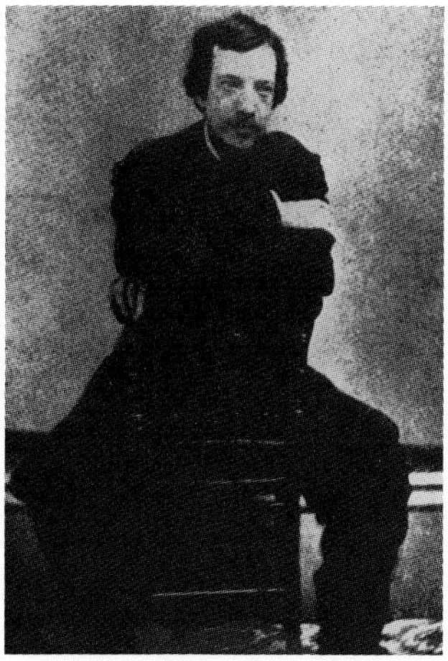

FIG. 146. Silas Weir Mitchell, age 33, 'Contract Surgeon' at Turner's Lane Hospital, Philadelphia during the American Civil War, 1861–5. (Reproduced by permission from *Silas Weir Mitchell; his life and letters* by Anna Robeson Burr, 1929, Duffield, New York.)

Silas Weir Mitchell graduated in medicine in Philadelphia after a two-year course in 1850 when he was twenty-one years of age. He spent a year in Europe and met many of the eminent medical men of the day: in London, the anatomist, Richard Quain, the physiologist, William Carpenter, Sir James Paget, and William Jenner. In Paris, where he caught smallpox, he bought a microscope (there was only one such instrument in his hospital even in July 1887, and that was Osler's) and thought the teaching there was unsatisfactory (classes of 250 or more for some lectures). He seems not to have been impressed by anyone in Paris other than Claude Bernard. He said that the latter advised him: 'Why think when you can experiment' – an aphorism generally attributed to John Hunter addressing Edward Jenner.

For the next decade, 1851–61, he assisted his father in practice. The latter wished him to take up surgery but an essential tremor of his hands, which lasted all his life and affected his writing, persuaded him to remain in medicine.

The 'contract surgeon' in the Civil War (1861–1865). Recalling the Civil War years, shortly before he died in 1914, Mitchell spoke of the horrors he had witnessed. Three million troops were involved, 200 000 died of wounds and 414 000 of disease.[126] Hospitals, ambulances, and a medical corps had virtually to be created. Mitchell described how Hammond created huge pavilion-style hospital complexes. In Philadelphia they provided 30 000 beds, in Washington 26 000. After the three-day battle of Gettysburg (1863)

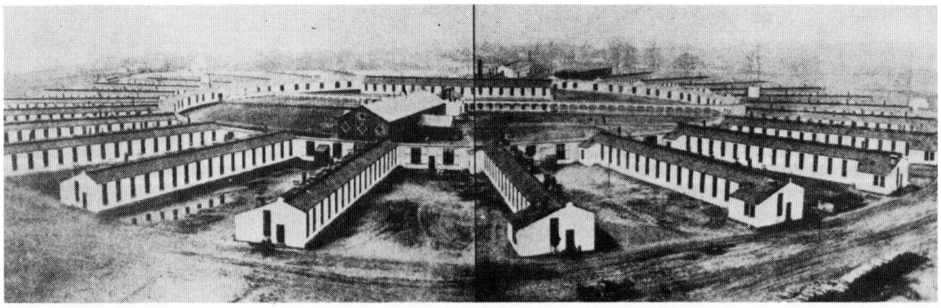

FIG. 147. Jefferson Military Hospital, Indiana. One of the many large pavilion type hospitals constructed during the American Civil War under the direction of Surgeon-General W.A. Hammond (Reproduced by permission from *Doctors in blue; the medical history of the Union Army in the Civil War* by G. W. Adams, 1952, H. Schuman, New York.) There were 24 pavilions and 2600 beds.

27 000 wounded required attention; they were dressed and under shelter twenty-four hours after fighting had ceased. Mitchell contrasted this performance with that of the ten days this took at Waterloo (1815). In Philadelphia 28 per cent of amputations and 61 per cent of trephine cases died. Scurvy, erisypelas, and hospital gangrene were major terrors.

It was against such a background, employed as 'a contract surgeon' while continuing his medical practice, that Mitchell came to be in charge of a 400-bed hospital for nervous diseases in the suburbs of Philadelphia at Turner's Lane. Here, with the collaboration of George Reed Morehouse (1829–1905) and William Williams Keen (1837–1932), came to be written a classic of medical literature entitled *Gunshot wounds and other injuries of nerves.*[127] It was only 164 pages in length and contained not a single illustration. In the preface to his larger work, *Injuries of nerves and their consequences,*[128] Mitchell wrote that the organization set up by Hammond 'enabled us to classify in distinct wards the numerous cases ... never before was there such

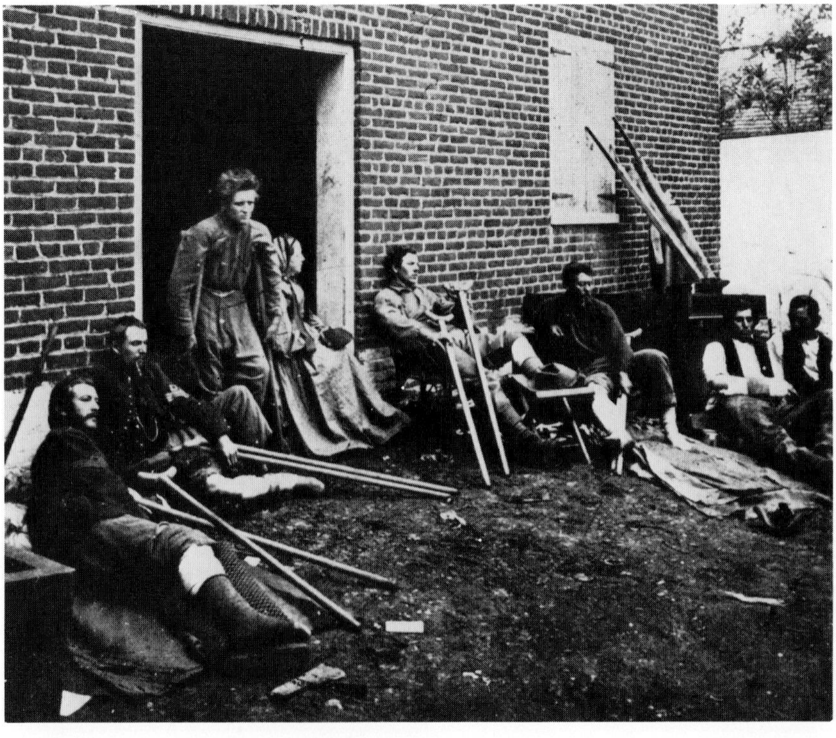

FIG. 148. Wounded Union soldiers, photographed by Mathew B. Brady, 1863. Medical photography was unfortunately not used. (Reproduced by permission from *Mr. Lincoln's camera man* by Roy Meredith, 1946, Scribner's, New York.)

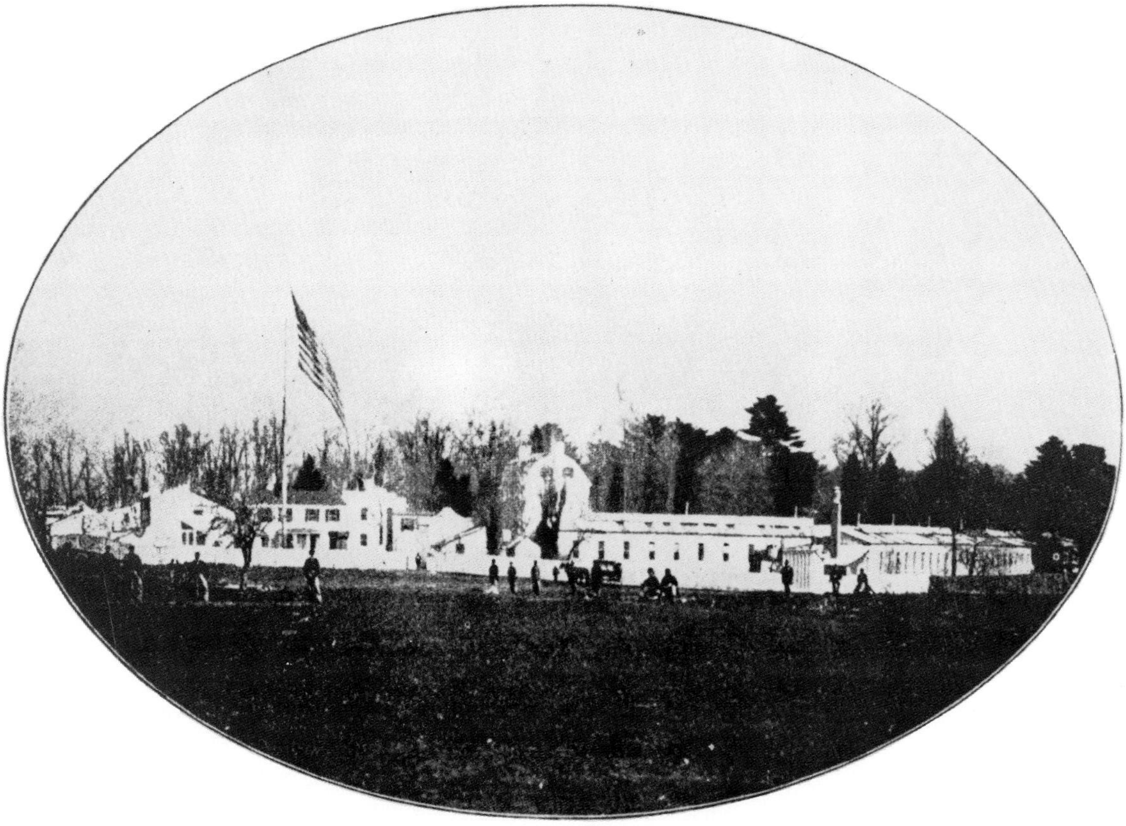

FIG. 149. Turner's Lane Hospital, Philadelphia, where the first classic study of nerve injuries was made. (Reproduced by permission from *Silas Weir Mitchell; his life and letters* by Anna Robeson Burr, 1929, Duffield, New York.)

an opportunity for the study of nerve lesions ... a multitude of cases, representing every conceivable type of obscure nervous disease was sent to us'. In 1914 he said: 'There were cases of amazing interest – epileptics, every kind of nerve wound, palsies, singular choreas and stump disorders'. Detailed notes on epilepsies and exhaustion were destroyed in a fire. 'To this day I cannot think of it without regret.' The hospital was a 'Hell of Pain'. In one year 40 000 injections of morphia were given.[129]

Turner's Lane Hospital deserves to be remembered and not only in the United States of America, for it, surely, was the birthplace of American neurology. The hospital formed the subject of Middleton's excellent Fielding Garrison Lecture.[130] Middleton was able to trace the progress of certain of the wounded soldiers through the original case notes preserved in the Library of the College of Physicians in Philadelphia. The accounts were such that often from the moment of injury the effects could be studied. The attitudes and reactions of the wounded were graphically depicted; the shock, the spasms, the sensations, the pain, paralysis, or numbness and whether the man fell or lost consciousness. Then followed the minute recording of the motor, sensory, and 'trophic' consequences. Many interesting items emerge. In a series of 91 wounded soldiers, a third experienced no pain. Mitchell never saw a bayonet wound. There were only a few notes of wounds of cranial nerves, presumably because of the high mortality rate of

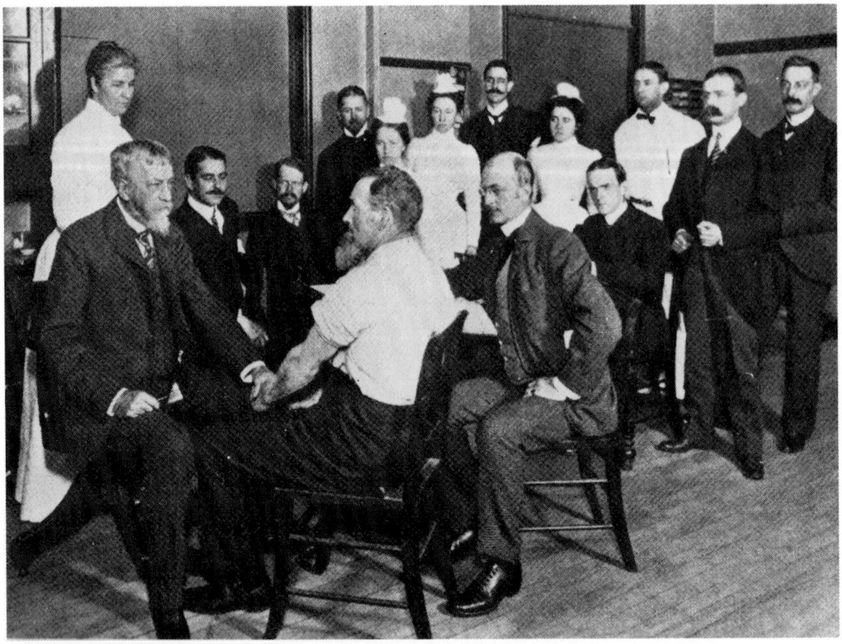

FIG. 150. Silas Weir Mitchell examining a Civil War veteran in 1902 at the Infirmary for Nervous Diseases in Philadelphia. (Reproduced by permission from *Silas Weir Mitchell; his life and letters* by Anna Robeson Burr, 1929, Duffield, New York.)

head injuries. The disagreeable odour of sweat from an injured limb was noted.

Of the trio that made this hospital famous, one, Morehouse, passes from the historical scene at the end of the war. He returned to his practice in the city of Philadelphia and Weir Mitchell said that 'what he did not go on to do is still to me a matter of wonder, interest, and friendly regret'.[130] Keen went on to study in Paris and Berlin. Claude Bernard was greatly excited to hear his account of the ptosis, miosis, and flushed cheek which followed a wound of the superior cervical sympathetic ganglion.[131] This was recorded on page 40 of the 1864 book on nerve injuries,[127] thus antedating Horner's classical publication.

> The pupil of the right eye is very small, that of the left eye unusually large. There is a slight, but very distinct ptosis of the right eye and its outer angle appears as though it were dropped a little lower than the inner angle. The ball of the right eye looks smaller than that of the left. . . . The conjunctiva of the right eye is somewhat redder than that of the left and the pupil of the right eye is somewhat deformed, oval rather than round . . . [in warm weather] his face became distinctly flushed on the right side only and pale on the left. . . .[127]
>
> We ourselves are of the opinion that this case was a case of injury of the sympathetic nerve and if so it is probably the only one on record.[127]

Mitchell referred again to this case in his 1872 book (p. 318) and regretted that although they had compared the temperature on each side of the face *during repose*, they did not do so when the face was flushed by exertion. Mitchell also observed that there was no abnormal retinal appearance on ophthalmoscopic examination by a Dr Dyer.

Keen eventually became Professor of Surgery at Jefferson Medical

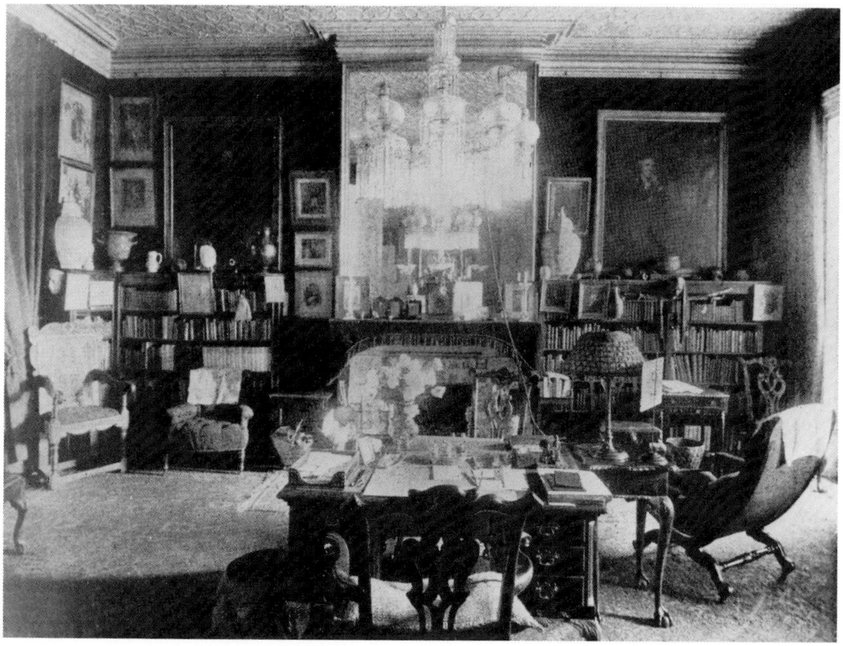

FIG. 151. Silas Weir Mitchell's consulting room in Walnut Street, Philadelphia. Harvey Cushing said it was 'a delight', dominated by two portraits – of Harvey and Hunter – and with a bust of Dante, a Keats death mask – and many first editions of famous books. 'Mitchell was vain but he had much to be vain about.' (*Harvey Cushing; a biography* by J. F. Fulton, 1946, Blackwell, Oxford, p. 226). (Reproduced by permission from *Silas Weir Mitchell; his life and letters* by Anna Robeson Burr, 1929, Duffield, New York.)

College and in 1888, at the First International Congress of American Physicians and Surgeons, which Horsley and Ferrier attended, Keen reported the successful removal of three brain tumours. With C. K. Mills (1845–1931) he used the faradic current to explore the cerebral cortex in his patients and Horsley said at the congress that his 'American colleagues had gone farther than we have in Europe' in that field. Middleton pointed out that Keen had the unusual distinction of being the only medical officer who had served in both the Civil War and the First World War. During the latter he published a book entitled *The treatment of war wounds.*[132] He lived to the age of ninety-five years.

The war saw no significant advances in surgical technique[133, 134] but it turned the attention of Mitchell and Hammond to disorders of the nervous system and made them America's first neurologists, while Keen became one of her first neurosurgeons. The segregation of soldiers with heart complaints in another pavilion at Mitchell's hospital enabled Da Costa to write his classic account 'On the Irritable Heart'. He told Mitchell, years later, that he wished he had not surrendered all his notes to the Medical Department in Washington, as instructed, at the end of the war. Mitchell and his colleagues, on receipt of that order, frantically copied as much as they could. The war gave to medicine the terms 'causalgia', 'phantom limb', and 'irritable heart' and it is not unlikely that the term 'neurasthenia' was similarly born. This was coined by George M. Beard (1837–83) in 1869 when he was lecturer in nervous diseases at New York University. He had served as an assistant surgeon in the US Navy during the war. His paper was entitled 'Neurasthenia or Nervous Exhaustion' and he wrote: 'The specific name is now, I believe, for the first time presented to the profession ... what anaemia is to the vascular system so is neurasthenia to the nervous system ... both can be cause or effects of illness.'[135]

'Nostalgia' was an officially acceptable diagnosis during the civil war.[136] The official medical history of the war recorded 'a total of 5,213 cases of nostalgia among the white troops of the North during the first year of the war'.[137] Rosen[137] says that the term was coined in 1678 by Johannes Hofer of Basel 'to signify the pain which the sick person feels because he is not in his native land ... I have called it nostalgia (from *nostos*, return to one's native land, and *algos*, pain or distress).' It was a well-known ailment among continental European armies of the eighteenth century, and sometimes referred to as 'The Swiss Disease'.

After the war the term 'nervousness' began to appear in medical and lay literature and there were subsequently many comments to the effect that 'nervousness' was a particularly American trait. In the editorial in the first issue of the *Journal of Nervous and Mental Diseases*, in 1874, the increase in nervous disorders in the United States was attributed to 'mental occupations ... the relentless demands of journalism ... large commercial enterprises ... speculation ... exciting literature ... stimulants and sedatives ... etc.'.

When Gowers' textbook was reviewed in that journal by B. Sachs he said: 'We are astounded that but one page out of 1357 should be devoted to neurasthenia. The author denies the justice of considering neurasthenia to be a clinical entity. The "Morbus Americanus" ... is as clear a conception as is hysteria.'[138]

Nerve injuries. In their 1864 monograph, Mitchell, Morehouse, and Keen state how they seized their opportunity 'since never before in medical history has there been collected for study and treatment so remarkable a series of nerve injuries ... nowhere were these cases described at length in the textbooks, and, except in a single untranslated French book, their treatment was passed over in silence. ... In the great monographs on military surgery, this defect is still complete, that wounds of nerves are there related rather as curiosities and as matters for despair' (p. 10). A close analysis of some 120 cases of nerve injuries formed the basis of this publication and 'no labour has been spared in making these clinical histories as perfect and full as possible'; the authors go on to say that: 'Those only who have devoted themselves to similar studies will be able to appreciate the amount of time and care which we have thus expended' (p. 12), a remark that will be endorsed by any doctor who had war-time experience of nerve injuries.

The burning pain suffered by some of his patients, which he later termed 'causalgia', was described so vividly and precisely that the words used (p. 101) have been quoted and requoted in many countries and have become part of the language of medical history.

> It is a form of suffering as yet undescribed, and so frequent and terrible as to demand from us the fullest description ... it was described as 'burning', 'mustard red-hot' or as 'a red-hot file rasping the skin'. ... In these parts, it is to be found

most often where the nutritive skin changes are met with, that is to say, on the palm of the hand or palmar face of the fingers and on the dorsum of the foot; scarcely ever on the side of the foot or the back of the hand. . . . The part itself is not alone subject to an intense burning sensation, but becomes exquisitely hyperaesthetic, so that a touch or a tap of the finger increases the pain. Exposure to the air is avoided by the patient with a care which seems absurd, and most of the cases keep the hand constantly wet, finding relief in the moisture rather than in the coolness of the application. Two of these sufferers carried a bottle of water and a sponge, and never permitted the part to become dry for a moment.

As the pain increases the general sympathy becomes more marked. The temper changes and grows irritable, the face becomes anxious and has a look of weariness and suffering. The sleep is restless . . . the rattling of a newspaper, a breath of air, another's step across the ward, the vibrations caused by a military band, or the shock of the feet in walking, give rise to increase of pain. At last the patient grows hysterical, if we may use the only term which covers the facts. . . .

Cold weather usually eased these pains; heat and the hanging down of the limb made them worse. . . .

The temperature of the burning part we have always found to be higher than that of the surrounding parts. . . . (p. 104).

Finally (p. 108) they write: 'We have again and again been urged by patients to amputate the suffering limb' and they admit that perhaps their readers 'may feel that we may be supposed to have exaggerated somewhat in delineating these hitherto undescribed neural disorders' or that there has been 'a desire on the part of the patient to magnify his pains'.

Mitchell proposed the term 'causalgia' for this burning pain of nerve injuries in a later publication in 1867 'in accordance with the suggestion of my friend Professor Robley Dunglison'.[139] In the first account of the syndrome, in 1864, he considered the cause of the pain 'was at first sought for among reflex phenomena. It then seemed to us probable that a traumatic irritation existed in some part of a nerve trunk and was simply referred by the mind to the extreme distribution of this nerve'. Further study suggested that 'the irritation of a nerve, at the point of wound, might give rise to changes in the circulation and nutrition of parts in its distribution, and that these alterations might be themselves of pain-producing nature'.

'Causalgia, in my experience gets well in time', he wrote (p. 282), but thirty years later his son Dr John Kearsley Mitchell (1869–1927) followed up fifteen of his father's patients and found several in whom pain had not subsided.[149]

The aggravation of pain by weather continued to interest him. In 1877 he published a paper[140] on the subject based on meticulous records in the case of an army captain who had sustained a gun-shot wound of a foot in 1864, requiring amputation below the knee three hours later. Pains began six to nine months later and the patient had plotted his 'neuralgic curve' for three years, in relation to weather, before Mitchell first saw him in 1874. Their further studies did not reveal any single factor – temperature, barometric pressure, weather (clear, cloudy or rain) – that could be related to pain. But it was clear to them both, and to many others of his patients, that 'falling pressure and rising humidity' were closely associated with the onset or aggravation of pain. 'There is no reason to doubt the popular view which relates some pain fits to storms.' This is one of the first studies of its kind.

Richards,[141] in an interesting account on the origin of the term 'causalgia', traced Mitchell's first use of it to an obscure account in a volume, edited by Austin Flint, of the United States Sanitary Commission Memoirs, in 1867. This volume is entitled *Contributions relating to the causation and prevention of disease, and to camp diseases*; Chapter 12, entitled 'On the Diseases of Nerves Resulting from Injuries', is by S. Weir Mitchell. In this chapter he explains that 'I felt that it would be well to give it some more convenient name than merely "burning pain". A colleague named Dunglison suggested "causalgia".'

Dunglison (1798–1869), a medical graduate of Edinburgh, emigrated to the United States and ultimately became the Professor of the Institutes of Medicine in the Jefferson Medical College of Philadelphia.[141, 142] He was a medical lexicographer which is presumably why Mitchell turned to him for a name for the 'burning pain'. He was given a name of Greek derivation but there was never any definition. This only came when the characteristics of causalgic pain were defined in 1920 by the Nerve Injuries Committee of the Medical Research Council.

After the war Mitchell continued to study nerve lesions of all kinds following up his old patients, experimenting on animals and on himself, and in 1872 he published his major work entitled *Injuries of nerves and their consequences*, which he dedicated to William A. Hammond 'whose liberal views created the special hospital which furnished the chief experience of this volume'. This monograph and that of Tinel (1879–1952)[143] in the First World War were the two books that were eagerly sought by doctors who had to cope with nerve injuries in 1939–45, a subject which invariably suffered neglect in peace time. It is extraordinary that Mitchell should have again neglected any form of illustration. The Civil War, as is well known, was the first to be extensively photographed. Matthew Brady[144] and others left photographs of the wounded, and their activities were such that Mitchell must surely have heard of them and seen some of the striking photographic plates. But although he apologizes for the lack of pathology in the 1864 book he does not mention the lack of illustration in either.

The 1872 book itself comprises 377 pages, in 14 chapters. Of the anatomy of the peripheral nervous system he wrote (p. 28) that 'the intricate interlacing (of plexuses) seems to be merely an arrangement for interchange of fibres, since those which enter the plexus acquire in it no physiological properties which they did not previously possess'. He recalls the observation of Hilton, in 'Rest and Pain', that 'one of the elements of protection to nerves, that in most instances the motor nerves enter their respective muscle on the underside, so that the whole thickness of the muscle is interposed between the nerve and exterior sources of injury' (p. 29). He refers to Schwann's microscopical studies of nerve, to Waller's experiments on the effects of compression, freezing, and section, to Schiff's observations on the reunion of nerve fibres, to Rokitansky's account of the pathology of neuritis, and to the clinical descriptions of Swann and Duchenne.

He deals fully with the question of the existence or otherwise of 'trophic nerves'. He wrote that: 'When the physiology of the vasomotor system was first elucidated by Claude Bernard and Brown-Séquard and Schiff and others it was supposed that it would enable us readily to explain the many obscure phenomena arising from nerve wounds'. But: 'I have made many attempts to bring about trophic changes in the face by irritating and partially wounding the sympathetic, but my efforts have uniformly failed' (p. 32). Atrophy was the only inevitable consequence of complete nerve section (p. 33) but in partial lesions trophic changes in skin, hair, nails, areolar tissue, and muscle are found (p. 38). He did not think these tissue changes were dependent upon the existence of trophic nerves. The 'justification for their existence lies in an apparent necessity for their presence . . . [Duchenne said] if we had no knowledge of such nerves, we should be forced to invent them . . . The phenomena of nerve wounds, as I have seen them, lend no conclusive report to the theory' (p. 36).

Mitchell did not 'look upon pain as a distinct sense with afferent tracts peculiar to itself' (p. 40). 'I have repeatedly chilled or froze the ulnar nerve in myself with ice, or ice and salt' (p. 59); he thought that: 'Acute neuritis [was] . . . probably of extreme rarity as an idiopathic affection' (p. 61). He found that 'rapid or slow pressure upon nerves present distinctive differences of very striking character, so that while the former is apt to occasion most severe and positive suffering, the latter may sometimes cause extensive muscular wasting without sensory loss of any kind whatsoever' (p. 108).

He endeavoured always to identify whether there was 'commotion, confusion, compression, or partial division' of a nerve. Seddon[145] has commented that Mitchell described 'neurapraxia' as, for example, in the following case: 'A man is shot in the thigh, the ball passes near the sciatic nerve, and instantaneously the nerve is paralysed; within a few minutes, or at the close of a day or a week the volitional control in part returns, but finally there may be left some single group of muscles permanently paralysed.'

In dealing with 'remote symptoms' he noted the rarity of tetanus; 'none in 200' cases of nerve injury, an unexpected observation (p. 147). Cutaneous eruptions, including herpes, he did observe (p. 153). He quotes the account of glossy skin in association with neuralgia, as previously described by Denmark. He also refers to the observations of Paget[146] and his description of glossy skin in intractable neuralgias (p. 157).

He opens the chapter on sensory lesions (p. 179) with the statement that 'the sensory functions of nerves are affected by wounds in such a manner as to be lessened, exalted or perverted' and he goes on to describe the subjective and objective findings in a way which clearly demonstrates the meticulous care with which the patients were examined. 'When, indeed, there is hyperasthesia for pain, we are apt to find it associated with lessened or lost power of tactile appreciation' (p. 179). He likened hyperaesthesia to 'sensory tetanus' and advised that 'the most delicate test of all is to touch the tips of single hairs . . . plainly enough felt during health', mapping out the results 'on previously prepared drawings' (p. 182). He writes of 'incessant questioning and repeated examination' and the preliminary use of pencil point and feather. He describes the difficulties in using the aesthesiometer of Weber and in assessing two-point discrimination. Defects in tactile localization were recorded and he comments on how necessary it is not to allow the patient to make the slightest movement of the part being tested.

Delay in the appreciation of sensation he found more characteristic of cord or brain lesions. In nerve lesions 'if a touch were felt at all, it was felt with no remarkable delay' (p. 225). He estimated time with 'a watch beating quarter seconds, or still better by a metronome'. The effects of cold and prolonged immobility on the results of sensory testing are noted. He cited cases in which motor loss was complete and sensation spared and others in which overlapping of nerve distribution was apparent. Sensory function preceded motor during recovery. In treatment: 'Of acupuncture in traumatic neuralgia I have nothing good to say; it was repeatedly used by our staff, without the slightest advantage' (p. 268).

'Trick' movements in muscle testing are not described but the difficulty in distinguishing muscular contracture from paralysis is stressed. The nature of a nerve impulse, he reported, was regarded 'as some form or manifestation of electricity', but he thought that the rates of transmission were different and that they were not identical: 'The electrical states which arise during nerve disturbance are merely manifestations related to the states of nervous activity ... dependent ... upon molecular alterations' (p. 43).

Although he considered idiopathic neuritis a rare disorder Mitchell thought it 'one of the most common consequences of nerve wounds' (p. 61). But he was only once able to produce it in a rabbit. In man he diagnosed it when there were developments such as fever, rigors, pain, redness, and tenderness along the path of a nerve and he conceived the process as sometimes spreading to adjacent nerves and plexuses. It could become chronic. When his 1872 book was translated into French in 1874, Vulpian (1826–82)[147] wrote a twenty-page preface based on a 'superficial examination of the work' which he generally praised. Vulpian had never been able to produce neuritis experimentally and doubted the conception of a spreading process from a traumatized nerve. He agreed with Mitchell that the 'trophic' lesions did not require the invention of special nerves for their explanation. It is probable that much of the neuritis seen by Mitchell was the result of wound infection. Carbolic acid was used to clean out infected wounds in those days, before Lister's antiseptic surgery and the discovery of bacteria, but it was not used to sterilize fresh wounds and the surgeon's instruments. Lister's papers began to appear in 1867 and for a time there was considerable confusion about the 'germ theory' and the practical requirements of 'antiseptic surgery'.[148]

Tinel commented on Mitchell's conception of 'ascending neuritis'. He thought it must be 'very rare' ... [its] 'exact nature completely baffles us' (p. 81). He thought it may have been due to infection.

In the chapter on the remote effects of nerve injuries Mitchell describes cases of 'curious inflammatory states of joints' of the affected limb (p. 168).

The nature of the injury did not seem to be the determining factor. He suspected that joint involvement often went undetected as it usually occurred some time after the injury. It might affect just one finger joint or involve every joint in the hand, or one articulation in the limb. The swelling lasted some weeks or months and then usually subsided, leaving some residual stiffness. He thought the recent paper by Charcot in 1868 on neurogenic arthropathies was relevant. Indeed he quoted a paper by his father, J. K. Mitchell,[150] in which were described cases of spinal lesions 'followed by inflammation of joints below the point of spine affected'. But a study of this paper does not suggest that Mitchell senior should be regarded as really antedating Charcot in the concept of neurogenic arthropathies. The title of the 1831 paper was 'On a New Practice in Acute and Chronic Rheumatism'; four patients with 'caries' or 'curvature' of the spine developed rheumatism in the limbs and failed to respond to treatment until attention was directed to the spine where leeches and cupping were applied. Mitchell senior published a further paper on the subject of spinal treatment of rheumatism in 1833[151] and both were referred to again by Weir Mitchell[152] in a paper entitled 'Spinal Arthropathies'. He quoted Charcot's reference to his father's 1831 contribution in which Charcot said Mitchell senior was the first to describe rheumatism 'in the paraplegia connected with Pott's disease'. Weir Mitchell wrote, 'To an American physician belongs the long forgotten credit of the discovery that an obvious spinal cause may produce rheumatism'. I have studied these publications and came to the conclusion that there was nothing to warrant the view that the concept of neurogenic arthropathies could be attributed to Mitchell senior, and was relieved to find subsequently that an American physician had also come to the same conclusion.[153]

Turner's Lane Hospital became known as the 'Stump Hospital' and the last chapter in Mitchell's book of 1872 is entitled 'Neural Maladies of Stumps', which were listed as 'chorea, neuralgia, neuritis and sclerosis'. These phenomena, he rightly averred, had been 'almost entirely neglected' and he proceeded to describe them in his customary graphic fashion. He referred to Ambroise Paré's observation 'that the absent limb is felt as if existing' and he said the 'hallucinations are so vivid, so strange, and so little dwelt upon by authors, as to be well worthy of study'. In 90 cases of amputation he found but four in which there was never what he came to term 'a phantom limb ... a sensory ghost of that much of himself, and sometimes a most inconvenient presence, faintly felt at times, but ready to be called up to his perception by a blow, a touch, or a change of wind'. He described the time of appearance of the phantom after amputation, its size, shape, position, and apparent movement, its singularly incomplete duplication of the original limb, and its mode of shrinkage proximally. He noted how wearing an artificial limb influences the phantom or restores one that has disappeared. One soldier said: 'If I should say I am more sure of the leg which ain't than the one which are, I guess I should be about correct'. Mitchell faradized stumps and was able to 'conjure' up a phantom and induce movements in its digits.

These observations on the phantom limb by Mitchell excited the interest of Hughlings Jackson who referred to his 'magnificent work'. He pondered their significance and referred to them many times. He thought that the dominance of the hand or the foot, and individual digits, in the phantom limb suggested 'the order in which lost parts remain most vividly represented in consciousness ... almost exactly the order in which parts physical do fail in dissolution of the nervous system'.[154] Referring to the faradization observations, Jackson wrote:

A man loses his arm by amputation just below the elbow; he knows nothing of anatomy, and yet when the end of his ulnar nerve is faradised (the stump being healed) he describes the *movements which we should see* if we faradised the ulnar nerve in a healthy man. Obviously these '*movements*' of the lost limb are the result of excitation of *motor* centres roused into activity by incoming currents from the sensory nerves contained in the ulnar nerve stump.[154]

When he gave the first Hughlings Jackson Lecture in 1897, he wrote:

Here is some indirect evidence that parts, those of the arm at least, having small muscles are more represented in the highest level than are the parts having large muscles. Now perhaps will be understood what I meant when I spoke of nervous arrangements in the highest level for manipulatory and other "voluntary" movements having psychical concomitants (so-called "ideas" of movements).[155]

Mitchell, too, endeavoured to interpret his observations. He concluded:

When we will a movement, there arises coincidentally ... impressions as to the force of the act and the position of the parts which we will to move; so that given the volition, there springs up in the mind a consciousness as to the act and its qualities ... certain nerves carry centrally, during motion, impressions which, with those nascent in the centres when the act is willed, go to complete the general knowledge as to motor activities (p. 359).[128]

It is curious that nerve suture received little consideration in treatment although Mitchell carried out animal experiments. He concluded that regeneration began in the distal segment of a cut nerve.

Reflex paralysis. In December 1940 Professor J. F. Fulton, on returning to the United States from the bombed cities of England, chose 'Neurology and War' as the title for his Weir Mitchell Oration of the College of Physicians of Philadelphia.[156] With the current problems of shock and blast injuries in mind he referred to the historic importance of the paper entitled 'Reflex Paralysis', by Mitchell, Morehouse, and Keen (1864), published as 'Circular No. 6' from the Surgeon-General's Office in Washington. Fulton had it reprinted for the occasion.[157] In this short 'pamphlet' of twenty-three pages the authors considered the pathogenesis and nature of shock, its cardiovascular and nervous aspects, and the phenomena of loss of consciousness and paralysis in soldiers whose injuries were confined to the limbs. Concussion, 'commotion', or 'shock' to a nerve or plexus were clearly conceived as probable explanations for paralysis of a limb in the absence of demonstrable nerve injury. They reported seven cases in which wounds exerted a temporary paralysis of a part of the body that was *not* injured. The term 'reflex paralysis' seemed specially to be applied to such cases:

Case 1. A wound of the muscles of the neck causing paralysis of both arms.

Case 2. A superficial wound of the right thigh causing paralysis of the right arm and left leg.

Case 3. A wound of the right thigh, with probable 'commotion' of the sciatic nerve, and reflex paralysis of the right arm.

Case 4. A wound of the right testicle and paralysis of the right anterior tibial and peroneus longus muscles.

Case 5. A superficial wound of the left thigh with sensory paralysis of the right thigh.

Case 6. A wound to the right thigh and paralysis of the right arm.

Case 7. A wound of the right deltoid causing paralysis of the right upper limb.

Such cases were rare – seven examples out of 60 cases of nerve injuries – and the authors concluded that a wound might temporarily paralyse a distant 'nerve centre' like 'a strong electric current' or 'a stroke of lightning'. They concluded that 'the condition called shock is of the nature of paralysis from exhaustion of nerve force'. Fulton considered that their views of the role of the nervous system in shock were 'nearly a hundred years ahead of their time'. But it is difficult to agree with the statement by Haymaker[158] that the term 'reflex paralysis' was 'given to the sudden motor loss resulting from wounds of the brain, especially the forebrain where motor centres, Mitchell and his collaborators reasoned, surely must control muscles of the opposite side, an observation anticipating Fritsch and Hitzig's announcement by about five years'.

Today the term reflex paralysis is rarely used. It does not appear in Sunderland's[159] or Seddon's[145] books, and Weir Mitchell's latest biographer, the neurologist R. D. Walter,[160] shares my doubts on the importance of the concept.

The civilian neurologist. When the war ended in 1865 Mitchell was thirty-six years of age. He returned to his practice in Philadelphia and was a regular contributor to the medical societies and journals of the day. The following selections from his neurological papers will give some idea of his wide clinical interests.

The cerebellum: In 1869 came his account of 'Researches on the Physiology of the Cerebellum',[161] based on a six-year experimental study of the effects of lesions produced in pigeons, rabbits, and guinea-pigs. He produced 260 'irritative' lesions by means of needles, the application of cantharides, and by freezing, or the injection of globules of mercury into the cerebellum. He also performed 87 ablative experiments. He quoted the experimental observations of Rolando, Flourens, and Magendie and the clinical opinions of Brown-Séquard ('who had no firm opinion'), Vulpian ('unable to assign any positive function'), and Luys, who considered the cerebellum to be 'an apparatus for generating nerve force'. Mitchell thought clinical experience generally discounted Flouren's view that the cerebellum was the organ of 'coordination', because the ataxia of cerebellar lesions was not necessarily permanent and because 'loco-motor ataxia is a spinal disease'. He quoted Magendie's opinion that equilibration was 'an office trivial for its size', although we now credit Magendie with this conception of its function Rolando's view that cerebellar ablation disclosed ipsilateral motor disturbance and that cerebellar function was concerned with 'the intensity rather than the regularity of muscular acts . . . resembles my own views'. Mitchell succeeded in keeping some of his pigeons alive for some weeks or months after operation and he observed that the initial drunken ataxia tended to subside but that 'the pigeon was incapable of prolonged exertion'.

In assessing the value of Mitchell's contribution that the cerebellum augments and reinforces movements and that some form of compensation takes place in chronic lesions, one should remember how obscure were the current views concerning cerebellar function in 1869. Luciani's classical monograph was not to appear for more than another twenty years in 1891. Meanwhile, Hammond[162] also experimented on the cerebellum, concluding that 'it has no special or exclusive function of any kind' but he felt impelled to mention the persistence of the notion that the organ was related to sexual function.

Hemichorea: Although his friend Hammond had introduced the term 'athetosis' in 1871, Mitchell preferred to speak of hemichorea. His paper[163] on post-choreal paralysis and preparalytic chorea contains no reference to the work of Little,[70, 71] but he clearly recognized the significance of 'intra-uterine palsies' and noted that the more complete the infantile palsy the smaller the danger of chorea, and that residual chorea was often the main disability 'after full muscular power is restored'. Osler, who also worked in Philadelphia from 1884 to 1889, acknowledged Mitchell's writings when he came to publish his own important monographs, *The cerebral palsies of children*[164] which he dedicated to Mitchell and *On chorea and other choreiform affections.*[165]

The knee jerk: Bannister (1844–1920),[166] one of the two founders and editors, in 1874, of the *Journal of Nervous and Mental Disease*, published in the journal, in 1878, a paper on the 'Diagnostic Significance of the Tendon Reflex'. In 1886 Mitchell and a colleague, M. J. Lewis, published a study of the knee jerk.[167] They found that reflex activity varied during the day and that the knee jerk could be exhausted. They also found that it could be enhanced by many small voluntary acts, such as closing the eyelids, moving the scalp or ears, or by frowning, winking, or rolling the eyes. The knee jerk could sometimes be elicited in the supine position when it was absent in the sitting posture. 'Tone', they concluded, 'was like the tuning of a muscle in preparation for an act'. McHenry[168] says that Mitchell 'was among the first to test the tendon reflexes as part of the physical examination' and that he introduced the method of recording the knee jerk using the symbols KJ + for an exaggerated knee jerk; KJ + + for an excessively exaggerated knee jerk; and KJ − for a depressed knee jerk.

Erythromelalgia: We have seen that when Mitchell coined the term 'causalgia', he described it without defining it. This is also the case with his invention of 'erythromelalgia'. He was rather keen on introducing new terms; fear of cats became 'ailurophobia', the title of a paper he wrote in 1905.[169] In causalgia and erythromelalgia he stressed the 'burning' character of the pain so that definitions become important. After decades of discussion, the general agreement reached about the essential features of causalgia has not, however, been achieved in the case of erythromelalgia. Mitchell said[170] that this was 'a rare vasomotor neurosis of the extremities'. He described sixteen cases, all males, who suffered from pain in the feet – 'burning', 'aching', or 'throbbing' in character, associated with flushing or redness. It was aggravated by warmth and in erect or dependent posture and relieved by cold and a horizontal position. He mentioned 'a brief, unnoticed paper', of 1872.[171] In his *Clinical lessons on nervous diseases*[172] he refers to measurements of the surface temperature of the affected feet and he considered that when they were in the dependent position the temperature often rose. He used terms such as 'flushing', 'throbbing' of arteries, 'heat', and a 'vascular storm' when describing 'attacks' of 'red neuralgia' and he was clearly under the impression that there was acute arterial dilatation consequent on a vasomotor lesion.

In 1933, Lewis[173] concluded that Mitchell had mistakenly interpreted the physical signs and that the concurrence of redness, swelling, throbbing, burning, and a sensation of heat were not in themselves necessarily indicative of increased peripheral blood flow. Indeed he considered that 'Erythromelalgia is a term that should be abandoned as the name of a disease.' It was no more than a peculiar condition that could arise in a number of diseases. Lewis thought that it was 'an interesting and important illustration of the difficulties which can arise out of the attempt to identify a hitherto undescribed disease upon the basis of a group of symptoms; the method is sometimes unavoidable and when successful helps progress; but when it fails it may impede progress'.

Lewis' paper probably served further to reduce the frequency with which the diagnosis was made; textbook accounts dwindled and shrank. But the dilemma continues. Smith and Allen[174] did find that skin temperatures were raised in attacks and they thought that the syndrome could be primary (idiopathic) or secondary (related to nervous, peripheral vascular, or other diseases). They reported that aspirin relieved the pain. In 1964, Catchpole[175] was able to relieve a patient by prescribing the anti-serotonin agent, methysergide, although there was no rise in the serotonin content of blood draining from the patient's feet when they were warmed. Babb *et al.*[176] state that the diagnosis was made 51 times at the Mayo Clinic in the decade 1951 to 1960. There were 30 primary and 21 secondary types. Skin temperature studies in 31 patients were positive in 26; that is, increasing the skin temperature induced the distress and reducing it brought relief. Of significance is the fact that it transpired that the syndrome antedated the appearance of myeloproliferative disorders, particularly polycythaemia vera, in 10 cases.

Abramson[177] considers that although no pathological basis for the disorder has yet been discovered it appears to be 'a definite clinical entity'.

Lewis, of course, was writing as a 'clinical scientist', and the notion of a malady that was rare, intermittent, never clearly defined, readily mimicked by other disorders, and without known pathological basis was one which he no doubt found peculiarly unsatisfactory. Ekbom's syndrome of 'restless legs' is equally strange and unprecise, but the toiler at the bedside knows the dangers of trying to tidy up reality too determinedly.

Toxicology. Mitchell's pre-war interest in toxicology and pharmacology continued after the war. McHenry[178] records that 'He published at least ten physiological and about twenty-five pharmacological papers.' The latter author quotes the noted American physiologist W. H. Howell as stating that 'before the establishment of laboratories in the seventies probably the most significant name from the standpoint of physiological investigations is that of Weir Mitchell'. When he was sixty-seven years of age Mitchell published a paper in the *British Medical Journal*[179] describing his personal experiences in experimenting with the drug 'mescaline'. He noted the euphoric and hallucinogenic properties of the drug and said, 'I predict a perilous reign of the mescal habit when the agent becomes attainable.'

Monographs. His *Lectures on the diseases of the nervous system, especially in women* (1881) was appreciated by Gowers. Gowers said that Mitchell's style served 'as a model on which to frame my own style of medical description'.[180] Mitchell dedicated his *Clinical lessons on nervous diseases* (1897) to Hughlings Jackson. Neither was reviewed in *Brain*.

The successful practitioner was meanwhile writing popular medical books such as *Wear and tear; or hints for the overworked* (1871); *Fat and blood; and how to make them* (1877). The latter went into eight editions and was translated into French, German, Italian, Spanish and Russian.[124] In 1888 came his *Doctor and patient*, another very successful popular book.

Fame in Europe came with these publications and with accounts of his 'Rest Cure' or the 'Weir Mitchell Treatment' for 'nervous debility', a term he made universally known. There were Weir Mitchell Institutes in Europe. His treatment of seclusion, bedrest, feeding, massage, and exercises was still mentioned in textbooks when I was a student. It is now generally recognized that his success was largely due to his personality, the training he gave his nurses, and the general discipline was not difficult to establish in a masculinist society.†

Doctor and patient is replete with reflections of his status and success. In his introduction he writes 'scarce anyone can have seen more of women' with nervous disorders than himself (p. 9). In this pre-Freudian era the complexities of all the factors at work in causing neurosis obviously intrigued him. 'The priest hears the crime or folly of the hour, but to the physician are oftener told the long, sad tales of a whole life, its faraway mistakes, its failures and its faults . . . the causes of breakdowns and nervous disasters and consequent emotional disturbances and their bitter fruit, are often to be sought in the remote past. He [the doctor] may dislike the quest, but he cannot avoid it' (p. 10). Writing of excessive sympathy by the doctor he mentioned the old Quaker lady who said after a consultation: 'Thee will

† A modern American female view of Mitchell's 'Rest Cure' is sardonically expressed in a recent book, entitled *For Her Own Good; 150 Years of the Experts' Advice to Women*, by B. Ehrenreich and D. English (Pluto Press, 1979).

do me a kindness not to ask me to see that man again. Thee knows that I don't like my feelings poulticed' (p. 46). The features of anxiety neurosis are vividly depicted – 'the indecisiveness . . . irritability . . . unreasonableness of temper . . . restlessness . . . giddiness and fear of walking out . . . sense of fatigue so that the grasshopper is a burden' are all there, as if from the pages of a current text. Mitchell pointed out that the apparently strong and healthy may also succumb, if the strain is sufficient, for 'we are all neatly ballasted'. Mills[181] thought that Mitchell was 'one of the greatest of our psychoanalysts'.

In 1894 he was gravely concerned at the 'isolation from the mass of the profession' of the psychiatrists of the day. In a frank address to the semicentennial meeting of the American Medico-Psychological Association[182] he complained of the lack of scientific investigation in the 120 public and 40 private asylums in the United States. He contrasted the lack of progress in psychiatry with what 'our few neurologists have done'. Of asylum life he said: 'Upon my word I think asylum life is deadly for the insane.' 'Where is', he enquired, 'the mysterious therapeutic influence to be found behind your walls and locked doors?' His outspoken address was widely reported and reveals the combination of scientific and humanistic philosophy which characterized his whole life.

But there remains another aspect to the career of this remarkable man – the world of letters. In 1880, at the age of 51, he published his first novel – the first of nineteen. I have read two of them: *In war time* (1884) and *Hugh Wynne, free Quaker* (1896). The latter, according to his biographer[124] was a best-seller and sold 500 000 copies, and has often been compared to *Henry Esmond*. 'His income from his pen was at times as large as from his practice', said Sir William Osler.[183] The copy of *Hugh Wynne* I read and enjoyed was a school edition published in 1922. The wife of a professor at Dartmouth College, New Hampshire, told me that it was prescribed reading in many schools and she herself could remember the summer she read it in her teens. It is a long flowing narritive of Philadelphia in the period of the War of Independence, peopled by famous men of the day, civil, military, and medical as well as by fictitious characters, all depicted against a background which the author vividly brings to light. Written today, its author would also be enjoying film and television rights.

One of Mitchell's three biographers[124] wrote that 'He was almost a genius. His contemporaries believed he was one, an opinion Mitchell came to share.' Sir William Osler[183] knew him for thirty years and said: 'Of no man I have known are Walter Savage Landor's words more true – "I have warmed both hands at the fire of life" – we have to go to other centuries to find a parallel to his career . . . in the combination of a life devoted to the best interests of science with literary and social distinction.'

Harvey Cushing,[184] speaking of the rise of neurology in the nineteenth century in the schools of Berlin, Paris, and London, said: 'Had the luck of academic preferment fallen to his [Mitchell's] lot, a purely American school of neurology immediately contemporaneous with that of Charcot might well have come into being'. But Mitchell's failure to achieve a chair at Jefferson Medical College in 1864, and later in the University of Pennsylvania, called forth from his old friend Professor Oliver Wendell Holmes the comforting words that 'Perhaps it is hardly desirable that an active man of science should obtain a chair too early, for I have noticed . . . that the wood of which academic fauteuils are made has a narcotic quality which occasionally renders the occupants somnolent, lethargic, or even comatose.'[124]

Seeing the tall patrician figure of Weir Mitchell passing one day before Independence Hall in Philadelphia, a friend said: 'He and it match each other pretty well.'

William Alexander Hammond (1828–1900)

Like Mitchell, Hammond also was the son of a physician. He was born in Annapolis, Maryland, and studied medicine at New York Medical School, graduating in 1848 at the age of twenty. After a year's hospital service he entered the US Army as an assistant surgeon, serving at various frontier stations in New Mexico, Kansas, and Florida.[185–188] During a visit to Europe he made an intensive study of military hospitals and asylums.

The Surgeon-General. Hammond resigned from the army in 1860 and spent a year as professor of anatomy and physiology at the University of Maryland, Baltimore, but rejoined the army on the outbreak of the Civil War in 1861. The Army Medical Department was quite unprepared for war. Its chief, Surgeon-General Lawson, was over eighty and he presided over an antiquated organization with only ninety-eight officers,[133] few hospitals, and no ambulance service or nursing corps. But the lessons of the Crimean campaign were known and the agitation of influential public citizens led to the establishment of the US Sanitary Commission, but not without resistance in Washington, where President Lincoln was afraid of 'a fifth wheel to the coach'. The Commission, acting not unlike a Red Cross service, was appointed on the understanding that it would not 'meddle with regular troops'. Hammond was eventually appointed as Surgeon-General, in April 1862, largely through the urging of the Commission. But he held this post only until November 1863. During these months this 'big, burly and genial man' initiated projects and reforms which eventually transformed the medical services of the army. A gigantic programme of hospital building was undertaken, largely of the pavilion-type, with 'ridge ventilation', and central administration. Special hospital and ambulance corps were created and at Washington he organized medical supplies, transportation, and medical and hospital reports and statistics. He wrote a book on military hygiene, a manual for military surgeons, inaugurated the *Medical and surgical history of the War of the Rebellion* and edited the *Reports of the Sanitary Commission.*

Hammond had wanted to found an Army Medical School but was removed before he could. It was created in 1893 and is now known as the Walter Reed Army Institute of Research. But he did succeed in establishing an Army Medical Museum, which grew into the Armed Forces Institute of Pathology.

But this driving force emanated, as one might suspect, from a personality likely to indulge in tactless decisions and high-handed actions. 'He had a voice so powerful that it could be heard up wind in a hurricane.' McHenry records that after a visit to a Philadelphia hospital: 'The staff made up their minds that a more arrogant and pompous man never visited the hospital.'[187] Jealousy over his initial appointment and resentment at his sweeping proposals and didactic commands built up during 1863, and culminated in a clash, mainly over the purchasing of medical supplies, with Secretary of State Stanton. He was demoted but he demanded and eventually obtained a court martial in 1864. He was charged with 'conduct to the prejudice of military discipline' and 'unbecoming an officer and a gentleman' and found guilty.[186]

'Penniless and in debt' he set up practice in New York City as a neurologist and psychiatrist and in a decade or so became Professor at the University of the City of New York and at Bellevue Hospital Medical College. By 1878 he had sought and obtained annulment of the court martial proceedings and sentence from Congress and the President of the United States. His rank of Brigadier-General was restored and his full-length portrait in uniform now hangs in the Army Medical Library in Washington, which he had helped to create. He died in 1900 and was buried in Arlington National Cemetery, Washington, DC with full military honours.

The New York neurologist. Hammond met Mitchell before the war in Philadelphia. They collaborated in an experimental investigation of the effects of a South American arrow poison in animals.[189] This paper, entitled 'Experimental Researches Relative to Corroval and Vao; Two New Varieties of Woorara, the South American Arrow Poison', is thus of historical interest, as it represented the first collaboration of the two men who founded American neurology. They concluded their report as follows: 'No statement has been made in this essay, and no conclusion deduced, of the accuracy or truth of which we at least are not fully satisfied. How far this may be the case with others we cannot say; and, at all events, whatever be the fate of these researches, we shall at least have had the pleasure of the pursuit', words that presaged the liveliness of everything they wrote in the future.

During the war, Mitchell and Hammond both became increasingly interested in diseases of the nervous system, organic and psychological, and with the establishment of a special hospital for nervous disorders in Philadelphia, American neurology was born. When the American Neurological Association was formed in 1875, Mitchell was elected first president, but he did not accept. Hammond became president in 1882. The Semi-Centennial Volume of the history of this association, published in 1924,[190] contains accounts of the early meetings, the scientific programmes and discussions that were held, together with biographies and bibliographies of its members. There is no comparable publication in Britain.

Athetosis. At that inaugural meeting in 1875 Hammond presented the patient on which (with one other he had been told about) he had based his description of 'athetosis' in 1871. This was in his textbook, *A treatise on diseases of the nervous system,*[191] in which he wrote:

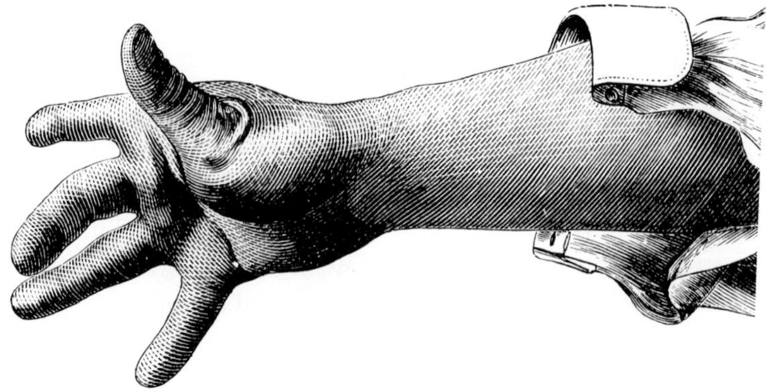

FIG. 152. Athetosis; 'without fixed position'. (After Hammond,[191] Fig. 24, p. 328.)

Under the name athetosis, I propose to describe an affection which, so far as I know, has not heretofore attracted the attention of medical writers and of which two cases have come to my knowledge. It is mainly characterised by an inability to retain the fingers and toes in any position in which they may be placed, and by their continual motion. From these phenomena, I have applied the term 'athetosis' to the disease, having as yet had no opportunity of ascertaining by postmortem examination the nature of the lesion to which the symptoms are due. (p. 654)

He coined the term 'athetosis' from the Greek, meaning 'without fixed position'. Concerning the site of the responsible lesion he wrote:

The phenomena indicate the implication of intracranial ganglia, and the upper part of the spinal cord. The analogies of the affection are with chorea and cerebrospinal sclerosis, but it is clearly neither of these diseases. One probable seat of the morbid process is the corpus striatum. (p. 661)

Ramsay Hunt[190] recorded that at the 1875 meeting Hammond said that 'The motions of the fingers continue also through the night, and to that extent modified his original description of the disorder.' But examination of Hammond's original account shows that, from the first, he thought the movements did not cease during sleep. When the patient was admitted to hospital the resident physician reported to him that 'they [the movements] occur not only when he is awake but when he is asleep'. In the account of the meeting reported in the *Journal of Nervous and Mental Diseases* (1875, **2**, 377), Hammond said 'The motions of the fingers *continue through the night*, and in this respect the description given must be modified' (his italics, not mine). Denny-Brown[192] said that 'Hammond insisted at first that athetosis should continue in sleep, which it seldom does.'

Gowers[193] reported the first autopsied case of athetosis, in which there was an old cerebrovascular lesion in the optic thalamus. A few years later,[194] in the first number of *Brain*, he said that lesions in or near the optic thalamus were the most common autopsy finding in athetosis, or 'mobile spasm', a term which he preferred. But, in six out of the ten cases he mentioned there was no impairment of sensibility. Later, in his textbook[195] he said that 'Since the optic thalamus is not in the motor path, disease limited to this must produce the symptom, indirectly by disturbing the function of the motor cortex.'

Hammond's forecast, in 1871, of a lesion in the corpus striatum in athetosis is often regarded as a historical landmark in the concept of the role of the basal ganglia in the aetiology of involuntary movements. At that time, however, the motor centres were thought to reside in the corpus striatum; the primacy of the convolutions was not established.

In 1886, Hammond's son, Graeme M. Hammond,[196] who in turn became president of the American Neurological Association in 1898, had some strange observations to record on his father's original athetoid patient. He described how he first saw him in 1882, the athetosis having begun in 1865. G. M. Hammond stretched the median nerve of the affected arm by open operation 'at the inner edge of the biceps' by placing his finger under the nerve so that 'strong traction was brought to bear on it'. Not only did the movements of the hand and foot cease, but his arm pain and convulsions subsided. The patient was an alcoholic, subject to convulsions, delirium tremens, and prolonged bouts of unconsciousness, after one of which his athetosis had appeared. There were three months' relief, so that Hammond repeated the manoeuvre in 1884 (with four months' relief) and again in 1885 (with sixteen months' freedom, up to the time of his report). He wondered why an operation on the arm should affect the foot and concluded: 'I don't know.'

In 1890, G. M. Hammond described the autopsy on this famous patient.[197] There was a scarred lesion extending from the posterior portion of the thalamus and internal capsule forward to the lenticular nucleus. He wrote that the sparing of the motor tract 'was further evidence of his theory that athetosis was caused by irritation of the thalamus, the striatum or the cortex, and not by a lesion of the motor tract'.

Not unexpectedly, the term 'athetosis', although it was an actual chapter heading in Hammond's book, was not quickly adopted. Gowers preferred the term 'mobile spasm', although he referred to Hammond's term, while Mitchell ignored it and spoke of 'hemichorea'. Charcot[198] considered that 'they are simply choreiform movements'. He thought Hammond's definition imperfect because 'The movements of the fingers are performed slowly ... moreover, the athetosis does not always remain limited to the muscles which move the fingers and toes; sometimes, in fact, the entire hand and foot are affected ... some muscles of the face and neck are stirred by choreiform movements, simultaneously with those of the hand and foot.' Charcot concluded that 'athetosis is only a variety of post-hemiplegic chorea'. When Dana,[199] of New York, came to publish his own textbook of neurology in 1892, he did not use Hammond's original woodcut of the athetoid hand, but one from Strumpell in Germany. It was not as good as Hammond's.

The textbook. Hammond's book *A treatise on diseases of the nervous system* was published in 1871. It comprised 750 pages with forty-five illustrations and was arranged in five sections – diseases of the brain, the spinal cord, cerebrospinal diseases, diseases of nerve cells and of peripheral nerves. In the first section he deals with cerebrovascular disorders, aphasia, sclerosis (diffuse and multiple), tumours, and insanity. The second section includes

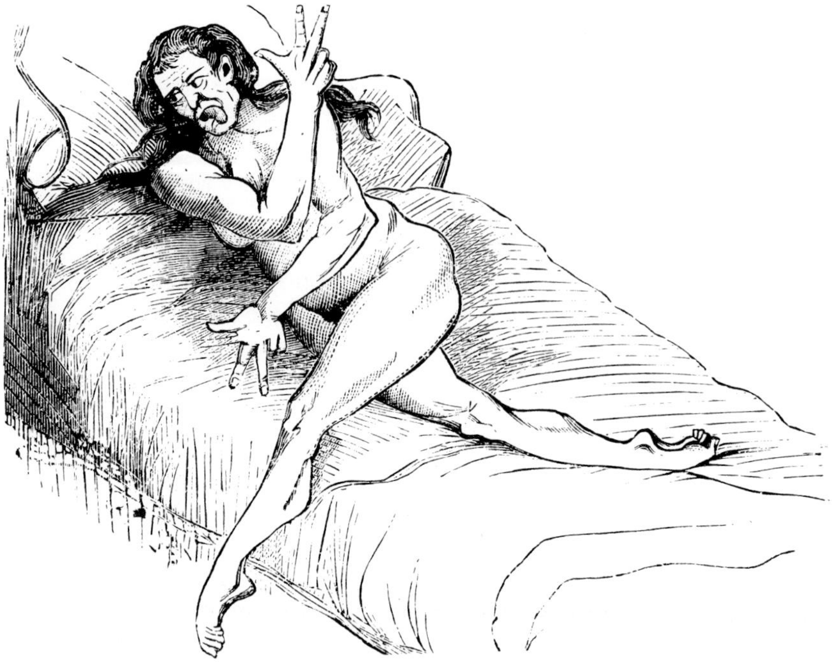

FIG. 153. Hystero-epilepsy; 'from a sketch taken on the spot by Charcot', as one would guess. (After Hammond,[191], Fig. 108, p. 792.)

vascular disorders, meningitis and myelitis, softening, and sclerosis and tumours of the spinal cord.

In Section 3 there are accounts of hydrophobia, epilepsy, catalepsy, ecstasy, chorea, hysteria, multiple cerebrospinal sclerosis, and athetosis. In Section 4 he covers progressive muscular atrophy, glosso-labio-laryngeal paralysis, infantile paralysis, hypertrophy of muscular connective tissue, and functional derangements of motor nerve cells (paralysis agitans, writer's spasm, lead paralysis).

In Section 5, only 28 pages, he deals with facial paralysis, facial spasm and torticollis, cutaneous anaesthesia, and neuralgias (trigeminal, cervical, brachial, intercostal, and sciatic).

There is no account of the anatomy and physiology of the nervous system and his introductory chapter merely lists the instruments he uses – ophthalmoscope, cephalohaemometer, aesthesiometer, thermometer, Becquerel's discs, dynamometer, dynamograph, Duchenne's trocar, and electrical apparatus. Clinical examination is not described and 'reflexes' is not indexed.

In his preface Hammond wrote: 'It rests to a great extent on my own observation and experience, and is therefore no mere compilation. The reader will readily perceive that I have views of my own on every disease considered, and that I have not hesitated to express them.' This forthright approach was taken up by his reviewers. The *Medical Record*[200] said there is 'not a muddy sentence in it. When he is right he is clearly right, when he is wrong he is clearly wrong.' Their reviewer thought the main fault was 'over-positiveness, amounting to recklessness' but that the book was 'an advance on any other single volume'. The *American Journal of Medical Science*[201] gave it a six-page review and thought the book 'the fruit, but not well-ripened fruit, of a large experience ... we do think that a physician with the high scientific attainments and unequalled opportunities of the author owes to the profession a better work than the one under notice'. They also commented on his 'extreme positiveness ... recent theories are stated with the greatest confidence as fixed acquisitions of science'. The reviewer praised his account of aphasia (which *is* good), his advocacy and experience of the ophthalmoscope, and his recognition of athetosis and multiple cerebral sclerosis. But they damned his illustrations:

> The engraver's work is in about the style of a third or fourth class weekly illustrated paper. The lady (p. 364) on whose countenance apprehension and terror are said to be clearly depicted, seems to us to wear an expression of utter vacuity or indifference ... the sketch on p. 704 (of a muscle biopsy in a case of dystrophy) looks like one of Mr Ruskin's pre-Raphaelite drawings.

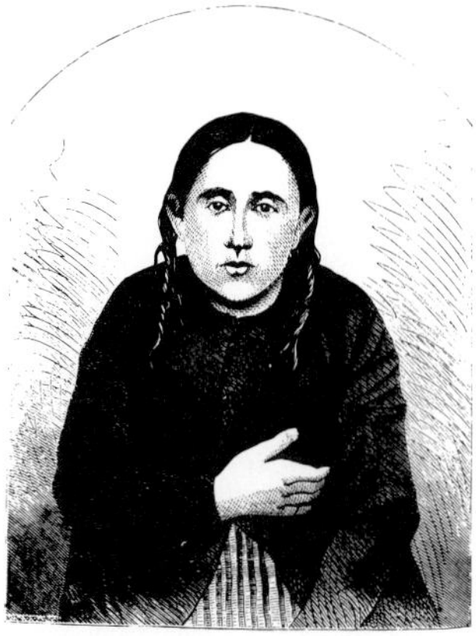

FIG. 154. 'Apprehension and terror', which was scorned by a reviewer. (After Hammond,[191] Fig. 15, p. 364.)

English journals were kinder. The *British Medical Journal*[202] gave it a two-page review and said 'it was a valuable and comprehensive book ... very pleasant reading ... graphic style' and was generally favourable, although on the subject of sclerosis 'it contained a large amount of curious matter'. They did not mention athetosis and questioned 'the specific existence of diffuse and multiple cerebral sclerosis'. Hammond's view that 'very limited paralysis points to cerebral tumour rather than anything else' had not been noted by English writers, 'such as Reynolds and Bastian'.

Hammond's book is often said to have been based largely on the lectures of Charcot. Dana[203] said this in 1928 but he mistakenly gave the year of publication as 1874, not 1871. McHenry[204] says the same. Charcot's famous volumes only began to appear in 1872 although his papers were appearing in French journals from 1858. None of Hammond's reviewers mentioned Charot although the *Medical Record* wrote: 'If the author had taken his inspiration less from the French – of whom Goethe once said "if a thing is not positive, they make it so" – and more from the English, especially from Darwin, he would have done more wisely and made a better and more convincing book.' The *British Medical Journal* reviewer thought that much of the chapters on forms of sclerosis was 'gleaned for the most part from the latest contributions to cerebral pathology by the French and German schools'.

Hammond did not refer to anyone in his preface but in the text he quotes French (Aran, Magendie, Duchenne, Calmeil, Ollivier, Cruveilhier, Landry, Broca, Dax, senior and junior, Trousseau, Bournville, Brown-Séquard, Vulpian, Charcot, and others), German (Rokitansky, Virchow, Romberg, Friedreich, Eulenberg, and others), and British authors (Bell, Marshall Hall, Carswell, Todd, Reynolds, Bennett, Bastian, Lockhart-Clarke, and Hughlings Jackson). He usually gave a reference when he quoted. He referred to Charcot when he discussed cerebral haemorrhage, aphasia, multiple sclerosis, progressive muscular atrophy, bulbar palsy, and neuropathic joints (where he also quoted the observations of Mitchell, father and

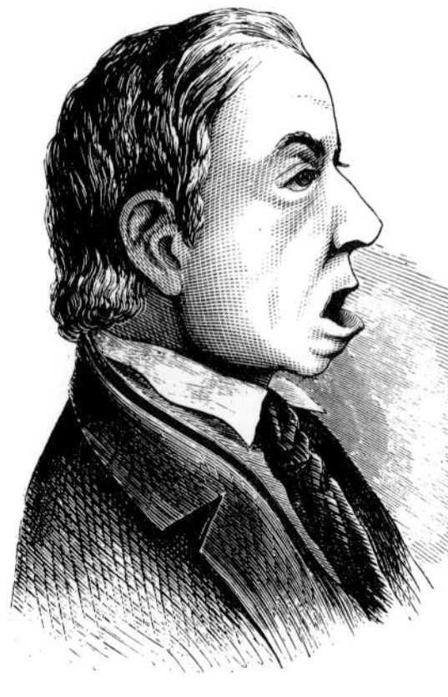

FIG. 155. Bulbar palsy. (After Hammond.[191])

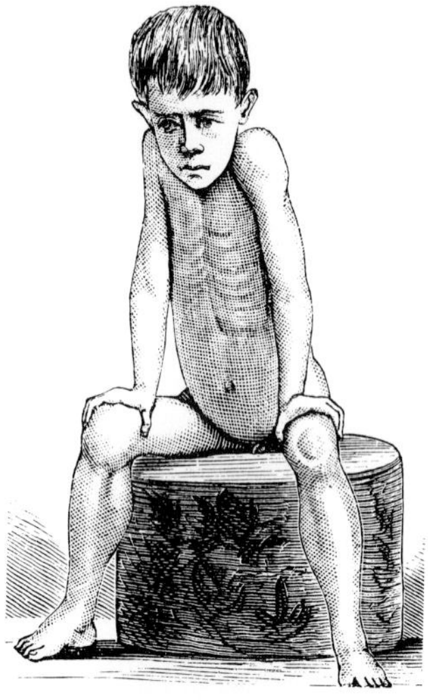

FIG. 156. Muscular dystrophy; 'The remarkable position assumed by the patient as he is about to rise from the sitting position.' (After Hammond,[191] Fig. 54, p. 511.)

son), and to Hughlings Jackson when he was dealing with cerebral haemorrhage and embolism, aphasia, and hemichorea, but not when he considered epilepsy.

The main weakness of Hammond's presentation, which was obviously courageous and well informed, is in the lack of consideration of anatomy and physiology and of methods of clinical examination. Later editions were improved, largely by incorporating text on cerebral localization from a French translation (in 1879) of the book and by including a summary of Nothnagel on topical diagnosis. Hammond saw the difference between static and intention tremor but thought Parkinson had described two different diseases and he is confused about the difference between multiple sclerosis and paralysis agitans. In the latter 'there are no head symptoms, no festination'. He thought that in pseudohypertrophic muscular dystrophy lesions would eventually be shown in the spinal cord, as they had been demonstrated in infantile paralysis, progressive muscular atrophy, and locomotor ataxy. He has an illustration of an affected child, and describes the posture and gait but not the difficulty in rising from a low position. He illustrated this in the seventh edition in 1881 (Gowers described it in 1879).[205] Spinal cord tumour is described as being present in 'hemiparaplegia', after the manner of Brown-Séquard, but the only patient he mentions was one he thought had a gumma compressing the cord. In the seventh edition (in 1881) he asks: 'Who will be the first to attempt the operation?' of 'trephining' for cord tumour. In the brain tumour section he has an illustration of cranial hyperostosis overlying a meningioma.

Although the knowledge of the time could have been better organized and presented the book undoubtedly supplied a need for it went into nine editions and was translated into French, Italian, and Spanish. A study of this historic work reveals how important and dramatic were the developments in the two decades following its publication. With the discoveries of Fritsch and Hitzig, and Ferrier, and the coming of the tendon reflexes, the distinguishing features of paralysis of cerebral and spinal and peripheral origin were gradually recognized.

At the end of the century, Sir William Osler,[206,207] in describing the awakening and progress of medicine in North America, thought he might be accused of being 'visionary' when he said 'At the end of the twentieth century, ardent old-world students may come to this side "as o'er a brook", seeking inspiration from great masters'. Little did he realize how cautious was his prophecy.

A MEMORABLE DECADE 1874–1884

We come to a decade during which the discoveries of three physicians in England were of fundamental importance. These men were David Ferrier, Richard Caton, and J. L. W. Thudichum, pioneers in brain research – in cortical localization, electroencephalography, and brain chemistry, respectively. The fame of the latter two, but not so of Ferrier, was entirely posthumous. When Caton died *The Lancet*[208] mentioned only his educational, civic, religious, classical, and archaeological activities. The *British Medical Journal*[209] ventured only to say that 'he did some original work on localisation of movements in the cerebrum in the seventies'. When Thudichum died the *British Medical Journal*[210] ventured only to say that 'his life-long labours in physiological chemistry do not appear to have borne adequate fruit'. *The Lancet*[211] bequeathed a mere nine lines, saying only that 'he did much work on pathological and physiological chemistry'.

Sir David Ferrier (1843–1928)

'The John Hunter of Neurology',[212] Ferrier had come to London in 1870, after graduating in Edinburgh in 1868, and for three years was a physiologist at King's College Hospital Medical School. He obtained clinical appointments to the Hospital for Epilepsy and Paralysis in Regent's Park in 1872 and to King's College Hospital in 1874. He joined the staff at Queen Square in 1880. His interest in the nervous system had already been demonstrated by his MD thesis on the corpora quadrigemina in various animals, including fishes, a work that was largely carried out in the garden of a country doctor in East Anglia, with whom Ferrier worked for a while in general practice in 1869. For this thesis he was awarded a gold medal.[213–217]

The West Riding lunatic asylum. His first publication was in 1873 in the *West Riding Lunatic Asylum Medical Reports*.[218] He had been invited by his friend, the superintendent Dr (later Sir) James Crichton-Browne, to pursue in his laboratory at Wakefield the work of Fritsch and Hitzig on the effect of galvanism on the brain of the dog.[219] Many eminent men contributed to these now historic reports published annually from 1871 to 1876: they included William Turner, William B. Carpenter, Clifford Albutt, Lauder Brunton, and Hughlings Jackson.

The enlightened superintendent had also inaugurated monthly medical

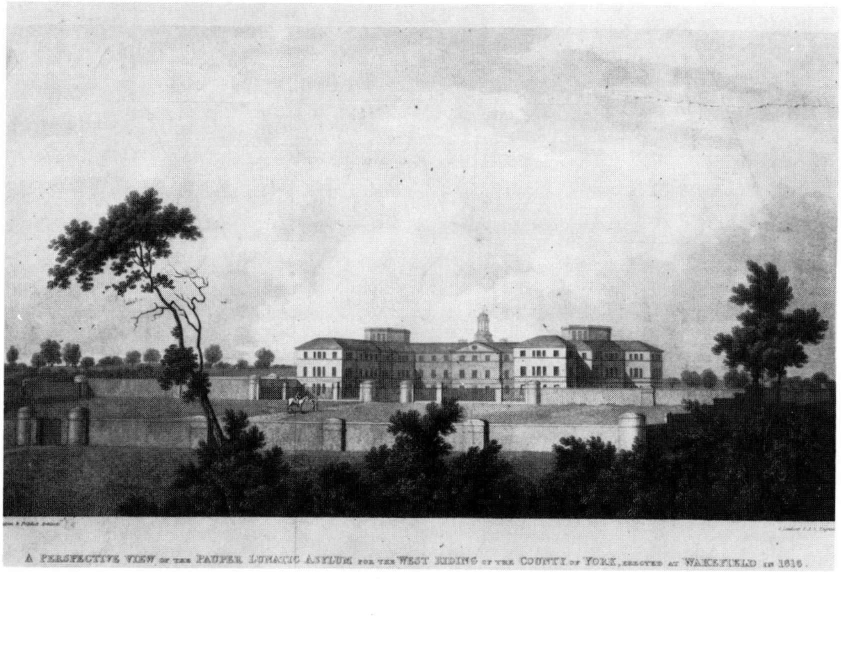
A PERSPECTIVE VIEW of the PAUPER LUNATIC ASYLUM for the WEST RIDING of the COUNTY of YORK, erected at WAKEFIELD in 1816.

FIG. 157. The West Riding Asylum, Wakefield, Yorkshire, where Ferrier began his experimental researches on the brain in 1873.

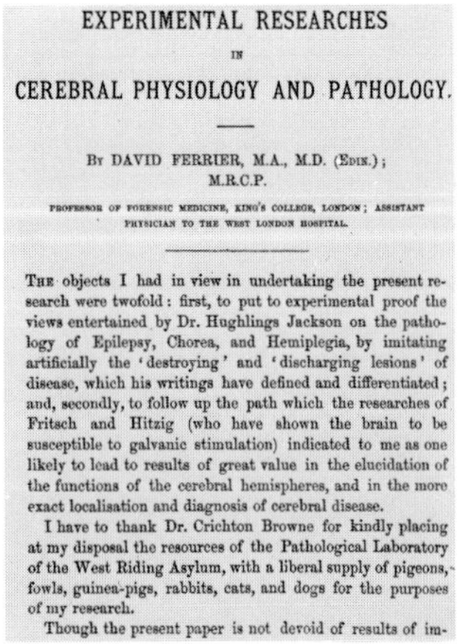

EXPERIMENTAL RESEARCHES

IN

CEREBRAL PHYSIOLOGY AND PATHOLOGY.

By DAVID FERRIER, M.A., M.D. (Edin.); M.R.C.P.

PROFESSOR OF FORENSIC MEDICINE, KING'S COLLEGE, LONDON; ASSISTANT PHYSICIAN TO THE WEST LONDON HOSPITAL.

The objects I had in view in undertaking the present research were twofold: first, to put to experimental proof the views entertained by Dr. Hughlings Jackson on the pathology of Epilepsy, Chorea, and Hemiplegia, by imitating artificially the 'destroying' and 'discharging lesions' of disease, which his writings have defined and differentiated; and, secondly, to follow up the path which the researches of Fritsch and Hitzig (who have shown the brain to be susceptible to galvanic stimulation) indicated to me as one likely to lead to results of great value in the elucidation of the functions of the cerebral hemispheres, and in the more exact localisation and diagnosis of cerebral disease.

I have to thank Dr. Crichton Browne for kindly placing at my disposal the resources of the Pathological Laboratory of the West Riding Asylum, with a liberal supply of pigeons, fowls, guinea-pigs, rabbits, cats, and dogs for the purposes of my research.

Though the present paper is not devoid of results of im-

FIG. 158. Title page of Ferrier's first paper in the *West Riding Lunatic Asylum Medical Reports*.[218]

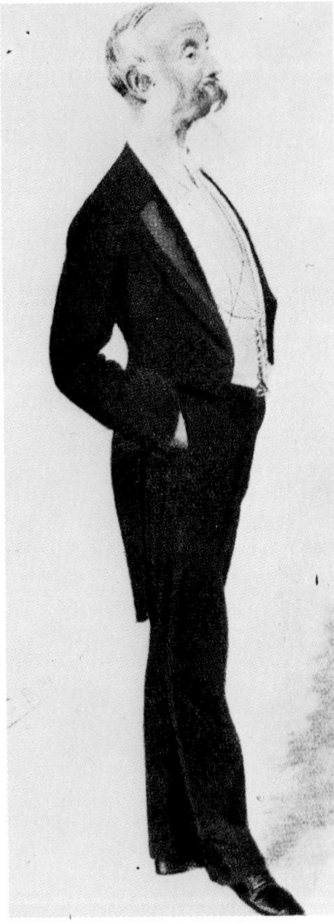

FIG. 159. Sir James Crichton Browne; a cartoon by Spy. He was medical director of the Asylum in 1873 and invited Ferrier to begin his researches there.

conversaziones in the main hall, which was described as 'magnificent and heated by no fewer than six huge open fires'. There were lectures, demonstrations, and opportunities for conversation, then the asylum band provided music (including polkas and gallops) for the occasion and 'suitable refreshments' were served. On 25 November 1873, Ferrier lectured on 'the localization of function in the brain' and Professor Carpenter, of University College, London, on 'the physiological import of Dr Ferrier's experimental investigations into the function of the brain.'[220] For many years Carpenter had taught that consciousness was concerned, not with cortical activity, but with the 'sensory ganglia', notably the optic thalamus, the corpora quadrigemina, and the auditory and gustatory ganglia in the medulla, a view which called forth a scholarly rebuttal in the *Journal of Mental Science* by a chaplain to the Abergavenny Asylum.[221]

Carpenter concluded that Ferrier's results 'entirely harmonise with the view I have long advocated that the cerebrum does *not* act immediately on the motor nerves'. Carpenter was obsessed by the automacity and reflex nature of man's activities and he cited parliamentary reporters who could continue to take down a speech in the House of Commons while they slept for short intervals. John Stuart Mills had also told him that his 'system of logic was in great part mentally constructed during his walks between the India House and his residence at Kensington; and yet he never ran against persons or lampposts'.

After the lectures, visitors to this instructive social event – and they would have included the official Board of Visitors – were able to study such exhibits as 'tumours of the dura mater, atrophy of the left cerebral hemisphere, exostosis of frontal bone, clot in the cerebellum, tumour of the cerebellum, syphilitic disease of the brain, and the brains of monkey, ox, sheep, rabbit, rat, etc.'. There were photographs illustrating 'the physiognomy of different varieties of mental derangements', 'normal and abnormal arrangements of the cerebral convolutions', and there were 'maps showing the geographical distribution of insanity and suicide throughout England and Wales'. They were shown histological preparations of the cerebral convolutions in man and animals and 'injected preparations illustrative of the vascular arrangement in the nervous and other tissues'. One stall exhibited drugs and medicinal preparations and another, scientific and surgical instruments. For the discerning, there were artistic photographs, including some of 'Venice by Moonlight'. The evening, of course, concluded with 'God Save the Queen'.

According to Crichton Browne it was Ferrier who urged that the work which the reports had begun should be continued in some form, after the former's departure for London in 1875. When *Brain* was launched in 1878, the editorial staff consisted of John C. Bucknill, Crichton Browne, Ferrier, and Hughlings Jackson. Ferrier was also a founder member of the Neurological Society in 1886, which took over the management of the journal. Crichton Browne, who held strong views *against* teetotalism, maintaining that no writer had achieved much without alcohol, died in 1938 at the age of 97. He was a fine after-dinner speaker and his Dundreary whiskers were probably the last of an era.

Though Ferrier was never on the staff of the West Riding Lunatic Asylum, Carpenter[220] and J. Shaw Bolton[222] both confirmed that the experiments were performed in that laboratory. Indeed, in his acknowledgements to Crichton Browne, Ferrier[218] mentions 'a liberal supply of pigeons, fowls, guinea pigs, rabbits, cats, and dogs, for the purposes of my research', but he also refers to 'more recent experiments' in which he was helped by Dr Lauder Brunton, the pharmacologist at St. Bartholomew's Hospital in London. He does not make it clear if any of the work was carried out at King's College Hospital Medical School.

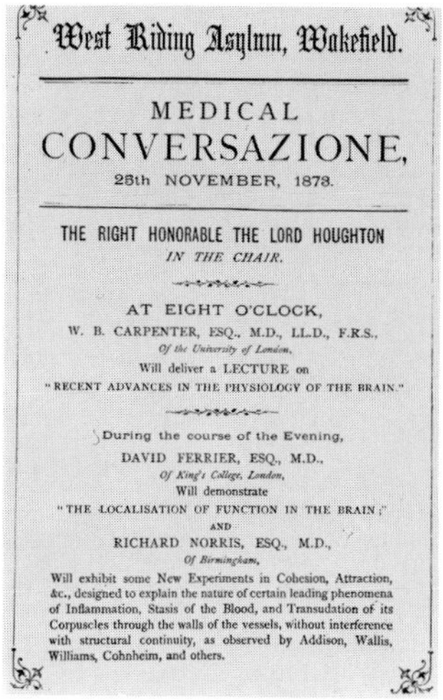
West Riding Asylum, Wakefield.

MEDICAL
CONVERSAZIONE,
28th NOVEMBER, 1878.

THE RIGHT HONORABLE THE LORD HOUGHTON
IN THE CHAIR.

AT EIGHT O'CLOCK,
W. B. CARPENTER, ESQ., M.D., LL.D., F.R.S.,
Of the University of London,
Will deliver a LECTURE on
"RECENT ADVANCES IN THE PHYSIOLOGY OF THE BRAIN."

During the course of the Evening,
DAVID FERRIER, ESQ., M.D.,
Of King's College, London,
Will demonstrate
"THE LOCALISATION OF FUNCTION IN THE BRAIN;"
AND
RICHARD NORRIS, ESQ., M.D.,
Of Birmingham,
Will exhibit some New Experiments in Cohesion, Attraction, &c., designed to explain the nature of certain leading phenomena of Inflammation, Stasis of the Blood, and Transudation of its Corpuscles through the walls of the vessels, without interference with structural continuity, as observed by Addison, Wallis, Williams, Cohnheim, and others.

FIG. 160. Programme of a medical conversazione at the Asylum.

In his 1873 paper, which Ferrier called a 'preliminary statement', his objects were twofold; first, to put to experimental proof the views of Hughlings Jackson on 'destroying' and 'discharging' lesions of the brain, and secondly, to follow up the researches of Fritsch and Hitzig, published in 1870. The latter did not mention the work of Hughlings Jackson. Ferrier was somewhat critical of the researches of the Berlin doctors. Of their attempts at localization of motor function, he wrote, 'their researches in this direction were not carried very far, nor do they, I think, clearly define the nature and signification of the results at which they arrived'. He concluded that convolutional localization was only 'to some extent indicated by the researches of Fritsch and Hitzig' but Carpenter[220] said that Fritsch and Hitzig's experiments 'anticipated those of Ferrier to a greater extent than I was aware of when I delivered my address'.

At first Ferrier used injections of chromic acid into the brain, a technique recommended by Nothnagel, but it was not satisfactory and he proceeded to the use of faradic current and focal ablations. Fritsch and Hitzig began their experiments on unanaesthetized dogs, but Ferrier wrote that 'it may be mentioned here, once and for all, that before and throughout all the following experiments, ether or chloroform was administered'. He was wise to say so in the light of his subsequent abuse by antivivisectionists. In this first paper Ferrier concluded that the anterior portions of the cerebral hemisphere were the chief centres of voluntary motion and the active outward manifestation of intelligence, the individual convolutions were separate and distinct centres, the action of the hemisphere was in general crossed, and that epilepsies were discharging lesions of the different centres in the cerebral hemispheres.

In a paper to the Royal Society in 1874,[223] Ferrier extended his experiments on a variety of animals and concluded that 'the whole brain is regarded as divided into sensory and motor regions ... a scientific phrenology is regarded as possible'. But in this eminent forum there was dissatisfaction that he had not fully acknowledged the work of Fritsch and Hitzig. The referees (Michael Foster and George Rolleston) felt that he had made insufficient reference to their work and T. H. Huxley was called in as a third referee 'for the purpose of ascertaining whether Dr Ferrier has or has not done sufficient justice to the labours of his predecessors in the same field of investigation'.[224] Huxley concluded that he had *not* and Ferrier added a more explicit acknowledgement of their priority in both method and findings. Neither Foster nor Huxley was satisfied, Hitzig complained bitterly, and the referees feared for the reputation of the Royal Society and of English science. Ferrier preferred to omit the experiments on dogs rather than to make the requested changes and consequently only his experiments on monkeys were published. In later years Ferrier was more generous in his acknowledgements to the German workers, writing, in 1883, 'It is not going too far to affirm that [they] inaugurated a new era in cerebral physiology.'[225]

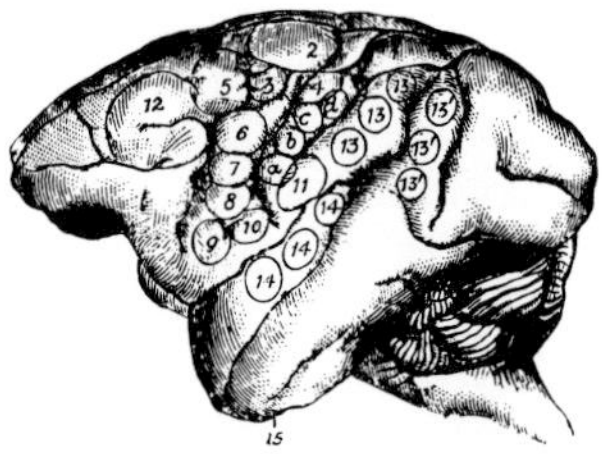

FIG. 161. The left hemisphere of the monkey (after Ferrier,[226] Fig. 29). The numbered and lettered circles indicate sites where electrical stimulation produced contralateral movements. 1 and 2, hind limb; 3, tail; 4, 5, 6, arm; a, b, c, d, hand and fingers; 7–11, face and mouth; 12, 13', 13, eyes and head; 14, ear; 15, lip and nostril of *same* side (inner aspect of temporal lobe).

Two classic monographs: 1876 and 1878. In *The functions of the brain*,[226] his first book, which he dedicated to Hughlings Jackson, Ferrier included two drawings of the cerebral hemispheres of monkey and man in which he had transposed his experimental findings in the monkey on to Ecker's outline of the human brain. An English translation of Ecker's book *On the convolutions of the human brain*, published in 1873, provided a more detailed account than Turner's work of 1866, though the latter had established the fissure of Rolando as the posterior limit of the frontal lobe.

In his introduction Ferrier pointed out the worrying discrepancies that existed concerning brain function as judged by animal experimentation and as a result of observation of disease in man. He thought that the new technique of electrical exploration introduced by Fritsch and Hitzig had given a fresh impetus to the study of brain function and that it was a substantial improvement on the older, ablative methods. He proceeded to review what was known of the functions of the spinal cord, medulla oblongata, mid-brain, and cerebellum and of the different parts of the cerebral hemispheres, including the basal ganglia. He presented a systematic exposition of the bearing of his own experiments on the functions of the brain.

Where Hughlings Jackson utilized the study of focal convulsions and of paralysis resulting from focal lesions, Ferrier employed focal excisions of the cortex and electrical stimulation. His conception with regard to the localization of function in the cortex was that it was primarily 'sensori-motor'. There were areas which responded by way of movements, and outside them, areas which did so by some sensory phenomenon.

It is surprising that Ferrier should have transposed his findings from monkey to man in the light of his statements in this book and in its successor *The localisation of cerebral disease*,[227] which he dedicated to Charcot. Referring to this transposition, he admitted, in the first book, that there existed in different animals great differences in the degree of cerebral organization. There were bound to be marked differences as the result of destruction of cerebral hemispheres. 'An exact correspondence can scarcely be supposed to exist, inasmuch as the movements of the arm and hand are more complex and differentiated than those of the monkey; while, on the other hand, there is nothing in man to correspond with the prehensile movements of the lower limbs and tail in the monkey' (p. 305, Figs. 63 and 64).

He realized the dangers inherent in deductions made from animal experimentation. In his second book he wrote, 'Frog and pigeon physiology has too often been the bane of clinical medicine' (p. 8) ... 'Our electrical stimulation is merely an artificial substitute for that which normally proceeds from the grey matter of the cortex' (p. 18). 'Anatomical homologies must not be pushed too far in support of identity of function' (p. 20). Despite the existence of 'motor' and 'sensory' areas, he emphasized that the functions of the brain were essentially 'sensorimotor'. 'Any system' he wrote, 'which does not take both factors into account must be radically false'. He was not really a party to the exaggerated claims of cerebral localization which came to characterize so much of the literature of brain function in the last quarter of the century. Concerning the organization of cerebral function he wrote, 'Interference at any one point must necessarily tend to general functional disturbance' (p. 2) and again, 'The doctrine of cerebral localization does not assume as Brown-Sèquard would seem to imply, that the symptoms observed in connection with a cerebral lesion are necessarily the result of derangement of function in the part immediately affected. Everyone admits direct and indirect results in cerebral disease' (p. 3).

His general conclusion in 1878 was that 'There are certain regions in the cortex to which definite functions can be assigned; and that the phenomena of cortical lesions will vary according to their seat, and also according to their character – viz. whether "irritative" or "destructive", two classes into which they may all be theoretically reduced' (p. 23). For a decade he increasingly argued that the ultimate object of his studies was the surgical treatment of brain lesions. 'Is there any reason why a surgeon should shrink from opening the cranial cavity, who fearlessly exposes the abdominal viscera?' In 1883[225] he said, 'We are within measurable distance of the successful treatment by surgery of some of the most distressing and otherwise hopeless forms of intracranial disease.' He was encouraged in this outlook by having as a surgical colleague at King's none other than the great Lister.

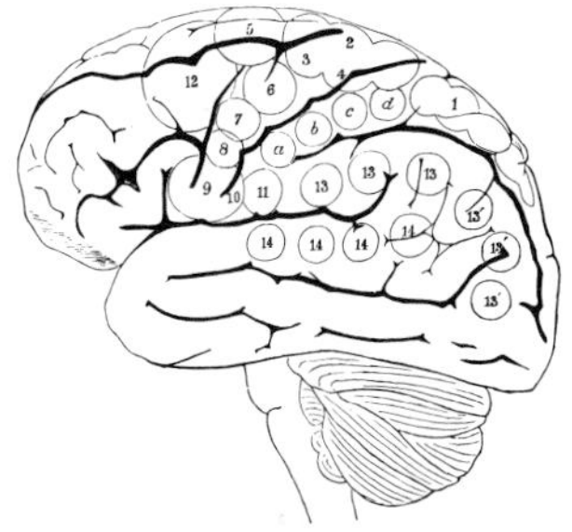

FIG. 162. Human brain (after Ferrier,[226] Fig. 63). His legend stated 'The circles and letters have the same significance as those in the brain of the monkey' depicted in Fig. 161. For Ferrier's comment see p. 390 of the present text.

Ferrier, with brain surgery always in mind, felt obliged to discard many of the older clinico-pathological records of cerebral disease and, with Hughlings Jackson, thought that the study of small localized lesions, especially those that were traumatic, would be more fruitful than that of tumours. One of the first he examined in his book *The localisation of cerebral disease* was the 'American crow bar case ... at one time regarded incredulously as a mere Yankee invention', particulars of which had been given him by Professor Bowditch of Harvard. He reproduced the well-known illustrations of the skull penetrated by the crow bar, still, I believe, preserved in Boston.

Phineas Gage was not the only celebrated American patient quoted by Ferrier in this book. He knew of the case of Mary Rafferty reported in 1874 by Bartholow of Cincinnati.[228] Bartholow quoted the experiments of Fritsch and Hitzig and of Ferrier, and the former's criticism of Ferrier's use of the faradic current, which they maintained stimulated the central ganglia and not the motor cortex. Bartholow was also aware of the criticisms of Dupuy

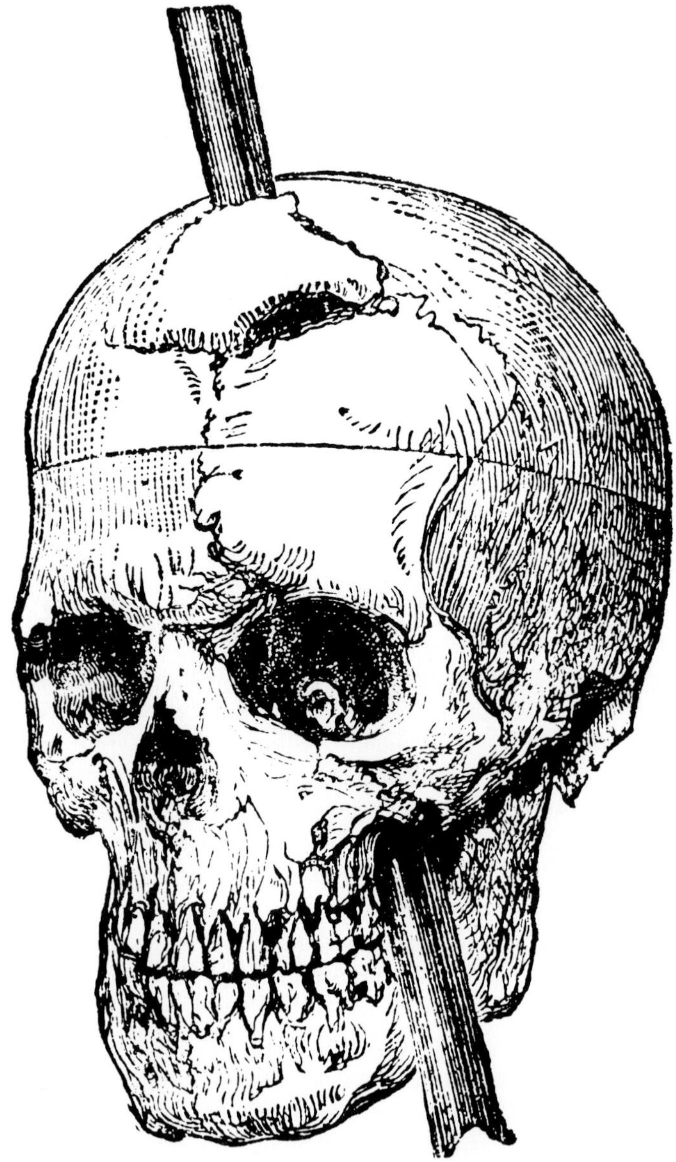

FIG. 163. The American crow bar case of 1848, to which Ferrier referred in both of his classic monographs of 1876 and 1878. Ferrier did not apparently know that the patient, though surviving for 13 years without paresis, did suffer from epilepsy and altered personality. (See Steegman, A. T. in *Surgery* **52**, 952 (1962).)

and his colleagues,[229] whose experiments had been conducted in Vulpian's laboratory. They also thought the faradic current diffused from the cortex through the white matter to the central ganglia, thereby setting up movements. In support of their contention they pointed out that anaesthesia abolished the electrical excitability of the motor cortex but not of the sciatic nerve.

Bartholow's patient suffered from an epithelioma of the scalp which had exposed the posterior parts of each cerebral hemisphere. He found that the dura mater and brain were insensitive to galvanic and faradic currents but managed to produce contralateral sensory and motor responses and, ultimately, convulsions and loss of consciousness. At necropsy the needle tracks were mainly in the parietal lobes and there was suppuration and sinus thrombosis. Bartholow thought 'it most desirable to present the facts as I observed them without comment'. Ferrier thought that his observations were too crude for any topographical deductions but that they confirmed that the human brain reacted similarly to that of the monkey. Kuntz[230] says that 'Bartholow was forced to leave Cincinnati' while Walker[231] said the criticism was levelled at Bartholow for these experiments both in the USA and in Europe. The *British Medical Journal*,[232] in an editorial entitled 'Experiments on the Human Subject', said that Bartholow 'had gone a step beyond Dr Ferrier, and in a direction in which Dr Ferrier is never likely to follow him'. In reply, Bartholow said that 'the patient consented to have the experiments made' (but she was feeble minded), and that the case of Phineas Gage seemed to indicate that puncturing the brain with needles would not be harmful, but he admitted, nevertheless, that his experiments were not really justified.[233]

Ferrier knew of Goltz's views, based on his cerebral experiments on dogs, years before the confrontation in 1881. In *The localisation of cerebral disease* he wrote, 'According to Goltz it is not so much the position as the extent of the injury on which the phenomena of cortical lesions depend. . . . Instead of laying bare a distinct region in the brain, and accurately limiting his destructive lesion he merely trephines in the temporal region and destroys the cerebral substance by squirting it out with a strong stream of water. . . . While Goltz's description of the phenomena themselves resulting from this procedure may be accepted without question, his theory that the effects of cortical lesions depend more on their extent than on their position, must, I think, be unhesitatingly rejected' (p. 121).

The Seventh International Medical Congress: 1881[234–238] The background to the famous and oft-told confrontation between Ferrier and Goltz at the Seventh International Medical Congress in London in 1881 was that of a typical glittering Victorian spectacle. Included among the 120 000 individuals who received invitations were 'all the crowned heads of Europe'. Special steamship passages were arranged and British and French railways offered return tickets from anywhere in France and Italy at the cost of a single fare. A commemorative medal was struck depicting Queen Victoria and Hippocrates.

There were 119 section meetings, 464 written communications, and 360 spoken communications – and some 2400 pages of reports. Sir James Paget presided over the 3000 doctors, who included Pasteur, Lister, Huxley, Virchow, Koch, Wolkmann, Charcot, Jackson, and Gowers. The Prince of Wales read the welcoming address in the presence of his cousin, the Crown Prince of Germany, the Archbishop of York, the Cardinal Archbishop of Westminster, and the Bishop of London. The Congress was 'marked by an unusually abundant series of banquets, receptions and excursions'.

At a conversazione in the Kensington Museum 'lit up by the electric light' there was 'a multitude of languages audible to the visitor which gave a very foreign aspect to the scene'. 'Floral decorations were chaste' at the Guildhall reception, where the 'male and female glee singers delighted the foreigners'. At a dinner for foreign guests at the Star and Garter Hotel in Richmond, Charcot, responding for the guests, poked fun at the hypocrisy of the English in regard to their fox-hunting and vivisection law. There were visits to the famous sewage farm at Croydon, and the Royal Seabathing Infirmary at Margate, Apsley House, and Hampton Court Palace, whence Dr Langdon Down 'conveyed his visitors by river to his residence at Hampton Wick for a garden party'.

Soirées and garden parties. Mr Alfred de Rothschild gave a soirée at his house in Seymour Place; but, alas, there was heavy rain at the garden party given by Baroness Burdett-Coutts in Highgate. There was a visit to John Hunter's house at Earls Court, 'where several human bones recently dug up in the grounds of the great anatomist's former residence, were inspected with great interest by the visitors'. And, to cap it all, 1200 people dined at Crystal Palace and afterwards enjoyed a pyrotechnic display, the original features of which consisted of the 'fire-portraits' of Sir James Paget, Professor Charcot, and Professor Langenbeck (of Berlin). The *British Medical Journal* doubted if the next generation could hope to equal, much less surpass, the advances of the previous 30 or 40 years.[235]

In 1881 Ferrier was 38 and renowned. Goltz, who had been professor of physiology at Strasburg since 1872, was 47.[239] In the chair, for Goltz's paper, was Michael Foster, Sherrington's lecturer at Cambridge.†

Goltz believed that localization of cerebral function could not be studied by electrical stimulation; only by ablation experiments could progress be made.[236]

Fritsch and Hitzig, he explained, 'had already perceived the flaws of the method of stimulus and had attempted a few experiments with extirpation – but only a few experiments'. But Goltz had been 'successful in a large number of experiments ... which would demonstrate the truth of my claims'. Goltz opened a suitcase which lay on the lectern and took from it an obviously damaged skull of a dog with a tiny preserved remnant of brain. This dog, he declared, 'whose skull and brain I have here, survived four major operations and was not killed until a full year had passed after the last operation'. Though 'idiotic' the dog was 'neither deaf nor blind, had lost neither the sense of smell nor of taste, not a muscle of his body was paralysed, not a spot on his hide robbed of sensation ... yet nothing was left in this brain of Ferrier's motor or sensory centres'. He had brought also with him a dog from whose brain he had removed the cortex from both parietal and occipital lobes, in five operations. But it was not paralysed and this would 'prove beyond a shadow of a doubt that Ferrier's theory was ... completely wrong'. Ferrier did not dispute these facts but totally rejected Goltz's conclusions. Ablation experiments on the frog, pigeon, rabbit, or dog could not solve the problem of cerebral localization in man: in such animals the effects of cortical ablation were transient; in monkey and man

† Sherrington, then aged 24, was so impressed by Goltz's decorticated dog, which was on display in Professor Yeo's laboratory at King's College, that he decided to enter the field of neurophysiology and his first paper (with Langley) in 1884 was a study of the medulla and spinal cord of this dog. Sherrington subsequently spent a year in Goltz's laboratory and when he left Strasburg he gave him a gift of three monkeys. Goltz believed this was a hint for him to repeat various experiments on cortical localization, whose implications he still refused to accept.[240]

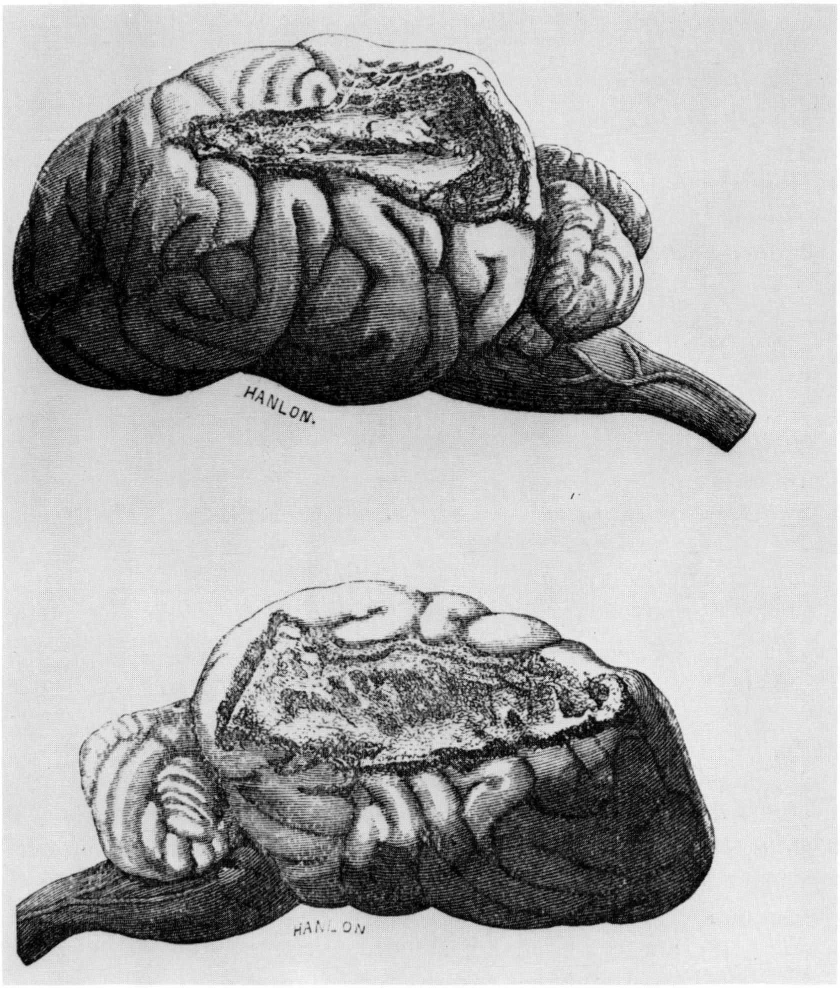

FIG. 164. The brain of the dog which Goltz demonstrated at the Medical Congress of 1881. It was not paralysed although he believed he had extirpated the cortex of both parietal and occipital lobes. Autopsy disproved this (Klein *et al.* *J. Physiol.* 4, 231 (1883) .)

the paralysis was permanent. Goltz's dissections were too crude and Ferrier, with Yeo, had developed more refined techniques.

After the morning's discussions, the decorticated dog was inspected at King's College. It could 'run, jump, see, hear, smell, feel. It does, however, display remarkable deviations from normal in its reactions to sense impressions. Its actions are so aimless and at times so contrary to intelligent behaviour that we must deny it all capacity for reflection and pronounce it a canine imbecile ... providing proof that the theory of localisation was flatly wrong.' An autopsy would show that 'the cerebrum had been almost completely extirpated'.

Ferrier demonstrated two monkeys.† The first was one whose left motor area had been extensively destroyed seven months previously. ('It is a patient!' remarked Charcot when this animal limped into the demonstration room.) The second monkey was one from which, ten weeks previously, the superior temporal convolution had been destroyed in both hemispheres. It was deaf but otherwise normal. Professor Yeo, in summary, at the end of

† In 1883 Ferrier[225] again referred to two monkeys at this demonstration but in his presidential address to the section of neuropathology at the Seventeenth International Congress of Medicine in London, in 1913, he referred to three monkeys. The third monkey had been rendered blind a year previously 'with progressive pallor of the optic discs' but without any other defect, by bilateral 'occipitoangular' ablations. I have not found any contemporary record of this third monkey. Was Ferrier's memory faulty?

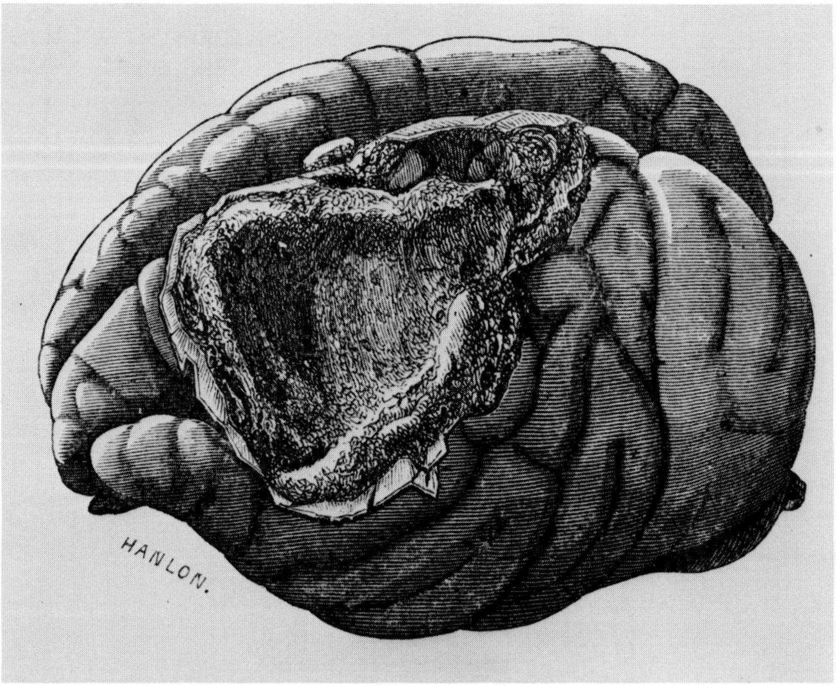

FIG. 165. The brain of the hemiplegic monkey which Ferrier demonstrated at the congress. Confirmation of the ablation of the left motor area. (Klein *et al.* op. cit).

this demonstration, stated, 'having seen these animals I feel sure Professor Goltz would modify his opinion as to the "utter folly" of the view that special parts of the brain are peculiarly associated with certain functional departments'.[241] Subsequently the dog and the hemiplegic monkey were killed and their brains removed.

A committee, which included William Gowers, found that, whereas the lesions in the monkey's brain corresponded exactly to the areas that Ferrier and Yeo had thought they had destroyed, the destruction of the dog's brain was not as extensive as had been thought by Goltz. Clearly the remaining motor and sensory areas, and the lower scale of the differentiation of function in the dog permitted it to retain certain functions. The victory was Ferrier's, but Goltz continued to study the effects of cerebral hemispherectomy in dogs though in 1892 he wrote, 'I am not at all fundamentally opposed to the question of the localisation of cerebral functions.'[242]

Summons at Bow Street. But when the Congress was over Ferrier had to face another contest. He was summoned to appear at Bow Street Police Court under the Cruelty to Animals Act, 1876, for performing 'frightful and shocking experiments' without authority from the Home Secretary. At the outset of the Congress, Virchow had remarked on the then current wave of agitation. 'Persons', he said, 'who unscrupulously exploit the average man's love for animals are at work here in London to convince the populace that the British Vivisection Law of 1876 is inadequate. People who practice methods of hunting which far surpass in cruelty anything that is done in laboratories denounce the Bill which provides that no one in England may experiment on living animals unless he is recognised as a serious scientist and holds a Government licence.'

The prosecution, or persecution as it was called in the medical press, excited world-wide interest. Hughlings Jackson, Lister, Michael Foster, Gerald Yeo, Burdon-Sanderson, Klein, and others attended the hearing. Three defence witnesses were called; Dr MacCormac, Secretary of the physiological section of the Congress, Professor Michael Foster, and the editor of *The Lancet*. It transpired that the account of the demonstration of Goltz's dog and Ferrier's two monkeys in *The Lancet* had been written by Professor Arthur Gamgee of Manchester, but he was not in court.

It was proved that the monkeys had been operated on under general anaesthesia by Professor Yeo, who held a licence under the said Act, and Ferrier was found not guilty 'of an infringement of the Act in having countenanced the subsequent keeping alive of the grieviously injured animals'. It was thought that the Anti-Vivisectionist Society had secured 'a costly but graceless advertisement' and that the whole proceedings were 'a dishonour to the English nation in the eyes of the world'. The *Boston Medical and Surgical Journal*[243] thought that the opening address of counsel was 'the prosiest and poorest twaddle that could have been tolerated in the support of the feeblest case'. The *British Medical Journal*[244] spoke of the growing importance of Ferrier's work and of cases of post-traumatic hemiplegia, post-traumatic focal epilepsy, and cerebral abscess in which patients had been cured by decompressive operations based on Ferrier's researches. The combination of general anaesthesia, Lister's antiseptic surgery, and Ferrier's localization of brain function, heralded a surgery 'of the largest promise'. But curiously no reference at all was made to the possibility of surgical treatment of tumours of the brain. And yet only three years later the first removal of a brain tumour marked the highlight of Ferrier's career.

Brain surgery. Antivivisectionists were as fanatical in their claims as were contemporary phrenologists and in 1884 their activites continued to attract headlines. Bishops, peers, and professors voiced their opinions in language and style which made Victorian public debates so spectacular and acrimonious. On 16 December 1884, readers of *The Times*[246] were informed that a tumour of the brain had been removed for the first time by a London surgeon. This was the heyday of British Imperialism. Readers were also told that the Union Jack had just been raised in Zululand. An expedition to Bechuanaland was being prepared. An Irishman had murdered an English soldier in Ireland.

It was scandalous, said *The Times*, that a British surgeon had to go 'for a few weeks to a foreign country' to conduct some animal experiments, that would clearly benefit his patients, because of the absurd English vivisection law. But the announcement of this surgical event 'absolutely unique in the annals of surgery' took the form of a letter in the correspondence columns. It was entitled 'Brain Surgery' and signed anonymously 'F.R.S.' The author

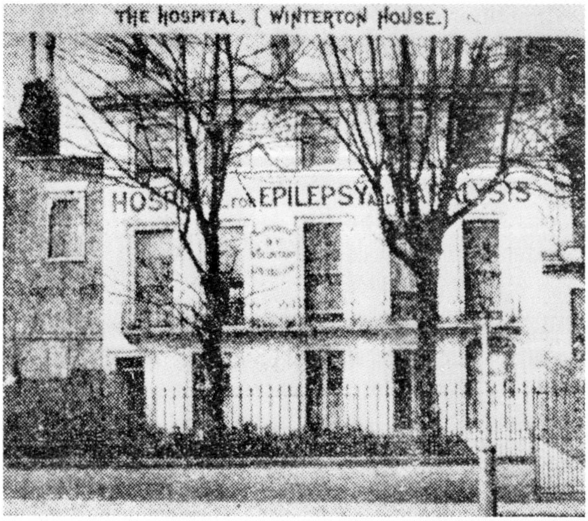

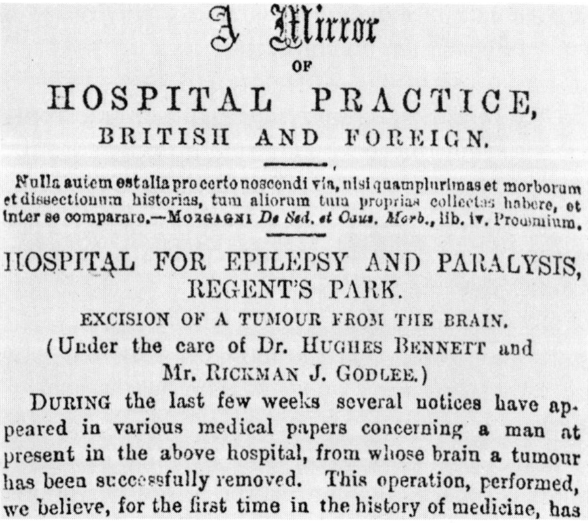

A Mirror
OF
HOSPITAL PRACTICE,
BRITISH AND FOREIGN.

Nulla autem est alia pro certo noscendi via, nisi quamplurimas et morborum et dissectionum historias, tum aliorum tum proprias collectas habere, et inter se comparare.—MORGAGNI *De Sed. et Caus. Morb.*, lib. iv. Proœmium.

HOSPITAL FOR EPILEPSY AND PARALYSIS, REGENT'S PARK.

EXCISION OF A TUMOUR FROM THE BRAIN.

(Under the care of Dr. HUGHES BENNETT and Mr. RICKMAN J. GODLEE.)

DURING the last few weeks several notices have appeared in various medical papers concerning a man at present in the above hospital, from whose brain a tumour has been successfully removed. This operation, performed, we believe, for the first time in the history of medicine, has

FIG. 166 (*left*). The Hospital for Epilepsy and Paralysis, Regent's Park, where a brain tumour was first removed.

FIG. 167 (*right*). *The Lancet* announcement of excision of a tumour of the brain (2, 1090 (1884).) The Latin quotation from Morgagni states that 'There is no short cut to diagnosis; one examines every detail of the anatomy and natural history of the illness. Then one should ascertain the particulars of the disease in question, as well as those of others, and should then compare them with one another.'

was none other than Sir James Crichton Browne. The letter began with these lines:

Sir, – While the Bishop of Oxford and Professor Ruskin were, on somewhat intangible grounds, denouncing vivisection at Oxford last Tuesday afternoon, there sat at one of the windows of the Hospital for Epilepsy and Paralysis, in Regent's Park, in an invalid chair, propped up with pillows, pale and careworn, but with a hopeful smile on his face, a man who could have spoken a really pertinent word upon the subject, and told the right rev. prelate and great art critic that he owed his life, and his wife and children their rescue from bereavement and penury, to some of these experiments on living animals which they so roundly condemned. The case of this man has been watched with intense interest by the medical profession, for it is of a unique description, and inaugurates a new era in cerebral surgery.

His letter which affirmed that this achievement was made possible only as a result of Ferrier's work was followed by a lengthy correspondence, with several fine editorials in *The Times*. At last, it seemed, the criticism was refuted that vivisection had never been of direct benefit to mankind. *The Lancet* article, by Hughes Bennett and Rickman J. Godlee,[247] on this case was published a few days later, on 20 December. For three years, the patient, a Scottish farmer aged 25, named Henderson, had suffered from left-sided focal epilepsy. There was a progressive left hemiparesis and bilateral papilloedema. (No mention was made of the plantar reflex.) The patient died of meningitis 28 days after the operation.

In their short paper they concluded there was a tumour of the brain that involved the cortical substance; it was probably of limited size, and it was situated in the neighbourhood of the upper third of the fissure of Rolando. It proved to be an oligodendroglioma 'about the size of a walnut'. Present at the operation were Hughlings Jackson, Ferrier, Horsley, and, some say, Lister himself. Godlee and Hughes Bennett were both in their mid-thirties at the time; Godlee was a nephew of Lister.[248–250]

Hughes Bennett's father was a well-known professor of medicine at Edinburgh and, when he died after a lithotomy in 1875, a necropsy was performed and a benign parietal brain tumour with overlying hyperostosis was discovered.[251] Edwin Bramwell[252] wrote 'is it not reasonable to suppose that the operability of the tumour in his father's case must have left a vivid impression upon Hughes Bennett's mind, and that in consequence he probably visualized more clearly than most the possibilities of surgery?' Wilfred Trotter and Sir James Crichton Browne agreed with Bramwell that in all probability Bennett, having diagnosed the case and localized the tumour, invited and persuaded Godlee to operate.

Hughes Bennett[253] was on the staff of the Hospital for Epilepsy and Paralysis, Regent's Park, where the operation was performed. He was one of the earliest contributors to *Brain*. He suffered from 'a most painful nervous disorder' which enforced early retirement, and died at the age of fifty-five in 1901. I have failed to discover a photograph of this early neurologist.

Holmes,[254] who knew both Hughlings Jackson and Ferrier, said that when this operation was completed, 'Hughlings Jackson, in his characteristic slow drawl, said to Ferrier, who stood beside him, "awful, awful." "Awful?" said Ferrier, "the operation was performed perfectly." "Yes," replied Jackson, "but he opened a Scotsman's head and failed to put a joke in it."'

It was generally acknowledged in 1884 that the success of this event was largely due to the work of Ferrier. Like many a British neurologist, he lived a long time, dying in 1928 at the age of 86. He had been knighted in 1911. Everyone who knew him commented on his extraordinary energy, amiable manner, and enthusiasm. Kinnier Wilson[255] wrote that 'on the day of Hughlings Jackson's funeral in 1911 I walked away with him from the cemetery and after many minutes of silence, occupied with his own thoughts of his teacher and friend, he suddenly turned and said, "well, when I cease to take an interest in things it will be time for me to go."' Sir Charles Ballance[212] said, 'as Hughlings Jackson is the Socrates of Neurology, so Ferrier may be described as the John Hunter of Neurology'. Sherrington, in 1906, dedicated his classic *The integrative action of the nervous system* to 'David Ferrier, in token of recognition of his many services to the experimental physiology of the central nervous system.'

Richard Caton (1842–1926). The pioneer of electroencephalography[256–259]

Richard Caton had been a medical student with Ferrier at Edinburgh, and they were both founding members of the Physiological Society in 1876. Caton had examined the electrical activity of nerve-muscle preparations and tried to discover whether similar changes in electrical potential occurred in the brain. His experiments were conducted on rabbits and monkeys in Liverpool where he had been appointed lecturer in physiology. He discovered that not only were there changes with sensory stimulation, but that 'feeble currents of varying direction passed through the multiplier when the electrodes are placed on two points of the external surface, or one electrode on the grey matter and one on the surface of the skull. The electric currents of the grey matter appear to have a relation to its function.' In this first publication[260] he noted the electrical changes that occurred when

Ferrier's topographical zones were in action. He sought to demonstrate his results at a meeting of the Royal Society in 1875, but was not successful. It was at that very meeting that Ferrier's own new experiments were demonstrated.

In his second paper in 1877,[261] Caton concluded that 'all the brains examined have shown evidence of the existence of electric currents' and he considered that these currents were related to cerebral activity because they varied with the degree of alertness of the animal, whether it was awake or asleep, and because he noted that the currents were abolished by anaesthesia and ceased at death. Caton was primarily engaged in studying the localization of sensory functions in the brain and he succeeded in noting the effects of visual and probably tactile stimulation, but not with auditory and olfactory stimulation. He observed what is known as intermittent photic stimulation. 'I tried the effect of alternate intervals of light and darkness . . . I found that light caused negative variation almost invariably.' Brazier[259] comments that this was the 'gaslight era' and the mention of flame as a source of light in his experiments exemplifies the skill and degree of success which these Victorian physiologists managed to achieve. Caton thought that 'the study of these currents may prove a means of throwing further light on the function of the hemispheres'. He said, 'I obtained more definite results when experimenting on Ferrier's motor and sensory areas.'

In 1887 Caton attended the Ninth International Medical Congress in Washington, DC, and read a paper on 'Researches on Electrical Phenomena of Cerebral Grey Matter'.[262] He thought 'it was well received but not understood by most of the audience'. Brazier[256] comments that 'this pebble that Caton dropped into the pool in Washington in 1887, was to produce no ripple in this country until 1930, when the first American publication on the electrical activity of the brain appeared'. The Russian journal *Vrach* published an abstract of his paper but, in Brazier's words, 'this abstract was no more successful in catching the eye of Russian and Polish workers than those in the English language were in attracting the attention of Caton's countrymen'.[259]

In 1890, in the pages of the *Centralblatt für Physiologie*, Beck of Cracow and Marxow of Vienna were arguing their case for the priority of the discovery of the electrical activity of the brain. In January 1891 Gotch and Horsley joined in, but all were finally silenced when Caton's letter was published in February, 1891. All were entirely ignorant of Caton's discovery 15 years previously. 'All claimed to have found the potential shift on sensory stimulation but of them only Beck had found the "spontaneous" oscillations of the brain's potentials.'[259] In that same year Caton resigned the Professorship of Physiology in Liverpool, of which he was the first holder, and he was succeeded by Gotch himself. Caton became Lord Mayor of Liverpool in 1907.

When Hans Berger (1873–1941)[263] came to publish his classic paper in 1929 he recalled Caton's work, writing that

> Caton had already (1874) published experiments on the brains of dogs and apes in which bare unipolar electrodes were placed either on the surface of both

hemispheres or one electrode on the cerebral cortex and the other on the surface of the skull. The currents were measured by a sensitive galvanometer. There were found distinct variations in current, which increased during sleep and with the onset of death strengthened, and after death became weaker and then completely disappeared. Caton could show that strong current variations resulted in brain from light shone into the eyes, and he speaks already of the conjecture that under the circumstances these cortical currents could be applied to localisation within the cortex of the brain.

As Lord Cohen[258] remarked, Caton's work might well have remained buried were it not for Hans Berger.

J. L. W. Thundichum (1829–1901). Chemist of the brain[264]

Ludwig Thudichum was a native of Büdingen, who graduated at the nearby University of Giessen in 1851. He was much influenced by the teaching and research of the famous professor of chemistry at that university, von Liebig. Thudichum emigrated to London in 1853 (bringing with him a combustion furnace, a present from von Liebig)[265] and lived there until his death in 1901. He became a naturalized citizen in 1859. He had an original and fertile mind and wrote several books, among which were treatises on the urine, on gallstones, on diseases of the nose (he invented a nasal speculum still sometimes referred to as Thudichum's speculum) – and even published books entitled *The spirit of cookery* (1895) and *A treatise on wines* (1894).

He engaged in clinical practice and from 1865 to 1871 was lecturer on 'pathological and physiological chemistry' in the newly established laboratories of St. Thomas's Hospital Medical School. In 1864 he isolated and identified the normal pigment of the urine, urochrome. In 1869 he wrote a classic paper on 'luteines', pigments originally obtained from the corpora lutea of the ovary and subsequently isolated by him from many animals and plant sources. These substances are now known as carotenoids, precursors of vitamin A.

His studies in various aspects of physiological chemistry attracted the attention of Sir John Simon, then principal medical officer to the Privy Council, who in 1864 engaged him to undertake a series of researches, the results of which were embodied in *Reports on chemical researches to promote and improve identification of disease*.[266] These reports were published as appendices to the reports of the medical officers of the Privy Council and the Local Government Board and appeared at various dates down to 1882. His classic work *The chemical constitution of the brain* was published in 1884.[267]

Thudichum was appointed chemist to the medical department of the Privy Council. It seems that he was originally requested to investigate the effects of typhus on the brain, but his interest was in its chemistry. Leibrich, a German chemist, thought that the brain consisted almost entirely of one single chemical substance containing carbon, hydrogen, nitrogen, and phosphorus, which be named 'protagon.' Thudichum showed that this was actually a mixture of substances: lecithins, cephalins, and myelins. Lecithin and its structure had been discovered in 1867; Thudichum correctly classified the cephalins and myelins as phosphatides.

He identified sphingomyelin, the sulphatides, and cerebrosides in the brain. The classification of these substances was a major achievement and Thudichum bequeathed us several flowery names of Greek derivation for his new brain compounds.[268] He noted the manner in which they were distributed in the grey and white matter but he made no serious attempt to relate his findings to the processes of disease. Nevertheless, he did say, 'I believe that the great diseases of the brain and spine, such as general paralysis, acute and chronic mania, melancholy and others, will be shown to be connected with specific chemical changes in neuroplasm ... in short it is probable that by the aid of chemistry many derangements of the brain and mind, which are at present obscure, will become accurately defineable and amenable to precise treatment, and what is now an object of anxious empiricism, will become one for the proud exercise of exact science.' He thought there should be laboratories of research established in all large hospitals, 'in these the purely chemical diseases, no less than the diseases caused by micro-organisms, should be investigated'.

He was a controversial figure and his researches had little influence in their day and indeed were suspected and criticized.

A notorious review was published by Professor Gamgee in 1877.[269]

Dr Thudichum's paper bristles with new names for old facts, and with the names of numberless new substances which the author discovered at each step of every investigation ... every analysis furnishes the material for a new formula, and every formula the excuse for a new name. No wonder then that in an alphabetical list of chemical educts and products stated to have been found in or produced from the brain of man and animals, there are eighteen marked with an asterisk, indicating that they are 'believed to be now described for the first time as ingredients in gray matter.'

Gamgee continued, 'Dr. Thudichum's researches are always conducted on a large scale' and he went on to say that Thudichum had used over 1000 ox brains in his studies. His discovery of myelin was not accepted – 'it was but impure lecithin'. 'A critical mind fails to make out what cephalin can be, certainly no definite substance. It would be as rational to analyse bread and butter and attribute a formula to it as to do so with cephalin.' Science had gained 'little or nothing' from these researches.

Thudichum himself did not underrate his own achievements and indeed like so many Victorian scientists he spoke proudly of them. 'They are of fundamental importance and all further developments in chemical neurology must start from them as a basis.'

When Thudichum died research of the chemistry of the brain almost came to a halt and his obituary notices reveal that few thought much of his work. Thus, in the *British Medical Journal*,[270] 'It is possible that Thudichum attempted in these researches too much ... the results were not generally considered to correspond adequately to the time and money which they cost ... his views have not been generally accepted by other workers ... and his lifelong labours in physiological chemistry do not appear to have borne adequate fruit.' *Nature*[271] thought that he 'did his best, he was an honest and indefatigable investigator' but that his researches were 'relatively insignificant . . . and gave rise to considerable polemic'. *The Times*[272] thought that 'the knowledge yielded by these researches was hardly commensurate with the time and cost at which it was obtained . . . that his scientific achievements seldom, if ever, realised the expectation which had been formed with regard to them'. But *The Times* also added, 'it is by no means improbable that some of his investigations may yet bear important fruit'.

Certainly Thudichum's fame is entirely posthumous. He was 50 years before his time. Page[273] considers that 'he was the founder of brain chemistry'. Dr Otto Rosenheim,[274] the London biochemist, uncle of the late Lord Rosenheim, thought that 'Thudichum might justly be called the first English biochemist'. In 1930, Dr Rosenheim discovered samples of Thudichum's preparations, many of the highest purity, in the stable of his house. In 1931, largely through Rosenheim's efforts, a Civil List Pension was awarded to each of Thudichum's five daughters who still resided there – at 11 Pembroke Gardens, Kensington.

'THE BIBLE OF NEUROLOGY' OR GOWERS REVISITED

William Richard Gowers (1845–1915), a Londoner by birth and a graduate of University College (where, he said, 'Almost every important step in medical education has first been taken'[275]), was twenty-five years of age when he was appointed to be the first Medical Registrar at the National Hospital, Queen Square.[276, 277] He was forty-three when the second volume of his famous *Manual* was published in 1888. By then he was an experienced writer with over a hundred items in his bibliography including the four books based on his lectures, *Pseudohypertrophic muscular paralysis* (1879), *Diagnosis of diseases of the spinal cord* (1880), *Epilepsy and other chronic*

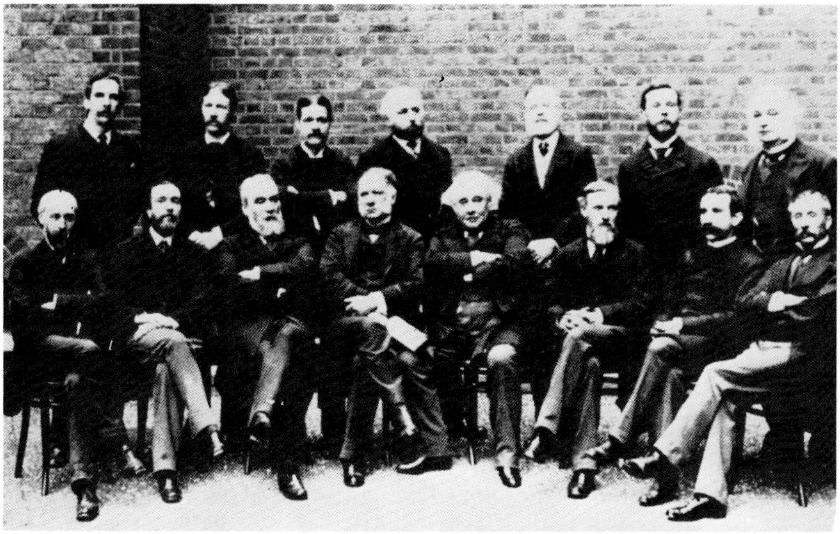

FIG. 168. Medical Staff of the National Hospital, Queen Square, in 1886. Back row, l. to r.; Horsley, Beevor, Cumberbatch, T. Buzzard, B. Carter, Ormerod, Adams. Front row, l. to r.; Marcus Gunn, Bastian, Hughlings Jackson, Ramskill, Radcliffe, Gowers, Semon, Ferrier. (Reproduced by permission of E. Arnold Ltd. from *Queen Square and the National Hospital, 1860–1960* by Sir Ernest Gowers, 1960.)

convulsive diseases (1881), and on *Diagnosis of diseases of the brain* (1887).

Who first dubbed his *Manual*, 'The Bible of Neurology' we do not know. I first heard of it in 1937 from the lips of Foster Kennedy in New York. If I remember rightly he said he had heard it at the National when he was a resident, in 1903. It was still in use there in 1923 when Critchley[278] heard it from F. M. R. Walshe. Just as Charcot at the Salpêtrière used to advise looking up Cruveilhier, at the National, one checked on Gowers. A large work of some 600 000 words, with 341 illustrations, to refer to it as just a 'textbook', seems rather inadequate. Indeed, its reception, the reputation it gained throughout the world, its translation into many languages, and the admiration which it invariably inspires in a neurologist of today when he is fortunate enough to procure a copy – all suggest that we are dealing with an exceptional work of scholarship. As so often happens in such cases, possession would seem to be indicated; occasional, or even periodical, perusal or reference is not enough to bring to light its real worth. It has to be judged in its entirety.

Although comprehensive, it is skilfully organized, never diffuse, remarkably concise and lucid, and with a straightforward, unaffected prose-style, free of those fustian lines and purple patches which characterized so much Victorian writing. It is not without interest that the Treasury, in 1948, should have chosen his son, Sir Ernest, to write *Plain words; a guide to the use of English*.[279]

When dealing with basic topics such as the functional organization of the spinal cord or of the cerebral cortex, Gowers's clarity of thought and powers of exposition are unmistakable. He may not have possessed the winning temperament of an Osler or an Allbutt but as a teacher he must have been commanding. Where Charcot had an audience, Gowers plainly had a class. In an address to medical students at University College in 1884, when emphasizing the distinction between the 'acquisition of facts' and 'the training of the mind' he warned them that 'there is no department of science in which there is so much imperfect observation, hasty generalisation, and fallacious reasoning as there is in medicine'.[275]

Then, there are his own illustrations. 'Charcot-Artiste' is well known but there are few medical texts in which the writer and artist are so well combined as in Gowers's *Manual*. He was an accomplished draughtsman, etcher, and painter. His histological drawings alone display the characteristic thoroughness and attention to detail which is such a feature of his text. At the bedside his enviable ability to make shorthand notes as well as vivid sketches was surely unique.

But there was another factor, besides the talents of the author, that went to making the *Manual* such a landmark in the history of neurology, and that was its timing. In the whole field of neurology the pace of progress had quickened in the sixties and seventies. When Gowers took up his pen there had been, as we have seen, some recent fundamental developments: first, in knowledge of the minute structure of the nervous system; second, in the discoveries concerning the functional organization of the brain and spinal cord; third, in the emergence of the pathological concepts that there were

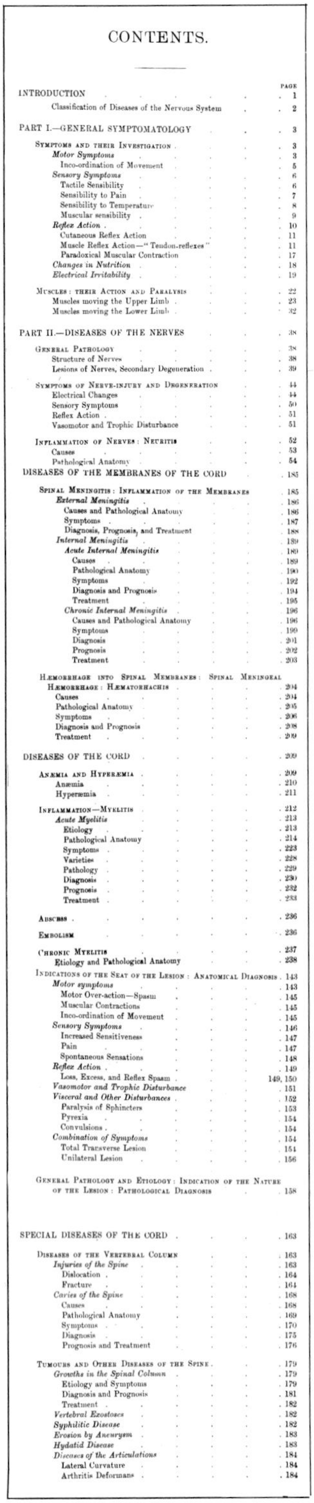

CONTENTS.

'system' diseases within the brain and spinal cord, as well as actual diseases of muscles and nerves; and fourth, the growing realization of the importance of the physical examination of the patient, particularly stimulated by the discovery of the ophthalmoscope and the deep reflexes. When University College Hospital was built – the first especially for teaching purposes – in the eighteen-thirties, physical examination of the patient, if it was similar to that in other London hospitals, was practically non-existent. Newman[280] has recorded that at Guy's the first note on the examination of a patient, under the care of Richard Bright, was not made until 1836.

So, the landscape of neurology was ready, as it were, for survey. And from the belvedere of the National, Gowers peered closely at it in all directions. With accuracy and discernment he set down what it looked like, noting where it was firm and sound, where foundations were likely to remain secure, where it looked fertile and should be cultivated, and where also it appeared sterile and probably unproductive.

Although one anonymous reviewer[281] felt it necessary to point out, in an otherwise laudatory notice, that 'owing to its scope and purpose Dr Gowers' book is more or less of a compilation', the modern reader is left in no doubt that its author had really mastered the contemporary knowledge of the structure and functions of the nervous system and was genuinely experienced in the clinical and pathological manifestations of its diseases. On most pages one senses that he is speaking with that kind of authority which only comes from individual, independent experience and reflection. By modern standards, bibliographical references are few and brief, in footnotes, but, unlike many modern texts, one feels that he is not just quoting, but has carefully sifted the evidence. Mention of other authors is often so passing as to suggest that he expected the reader to realize that he was writing from experience and was familiar with all aspects of the literature. It is a quiet assumption, unproclaimed in preface or text. And it is effective.

The table of contents is comprehensive and informative and is included in these pages (Figs. 169 and 187); it should give the reader who has not seen a copy of the *Manual* a fair idea of its ingredients and arrangement. The index, by modern standards, is not adequate and there is no list of illustrations; each one must be hunted down. As already mentioned, they are, in themselves, worthy of examination and many are here reproduced. The teacher in Gowers may be recognized in a remark he made in the preface to Volume 1. Concerning the illustrations of the topography of the spinal cord he said that the omission of subsidiary letters was intentional, for 'Familiarity with unlettered illustrations facilitates the comprehension of sections of the spinal cord.' In these spinal cord diagrams there is nothing of the 'railway track-and-junction' spectacle which became a feature often in 'technicolour' of many later neurological texts (see C. L. Dana's textbook,[199] 1892, for example).

It is hardly necessary to remind the reader of the meagre nature of the assistance which a clinician of the day, faced with a case of nervous disorder, could expect from the available ancillary diagnostic techniques. There were simple tests for albumen, sugar, and urea in the urine, but very little blood

	PAGE
INFLAMMATION OF NERVES: NEURITIS (*continued*)—	
Symptoms	56
Diagnosis	57
Prognosis and Treatment	58
MORBID GROWTHS IN NERVES: NEUROMA	60
Causes	62
Symptoms	63
Diagnosis, Prognosis, and Treatment	64
DISEASES OF SPECIAL NERVES	65
Phrenic Nerve	65
Nerves of Upper Limb	67
Combined Palsies of the Nerves of the Arm	76
Nerves of the Lower Limb	80
Sciatica	84
Pathological Anatomy and Symptoms	86
Pathology	88
Diagnosis	89
Prognosis and Treatment	90
MULTIPLE NEURITIS	91
Etiology and Pathological Anatomy	92
Symptoms	96
Pathology	99
Diagnosis	100
Treatment	101
Endemic Neuritis	102
Leprous Neuritis	103
PART III.—DISEASES OF THE SPINAL CORD.	
INTRODUCTION—ANATOMY OF THE CORD	105
Structure of the Cord	105
Grey Substance	107
White substance	111
Blood-supply to the Cord	125
FUNCTIONS OF THE SPINAL CORD	126
Motor Conduction	126
Representation of Movements in the Cord	127
Sensory Conduction	130
Reflex Centres	135
Co-ordination of Movement	137
Influence on Nutrition	137
Visceral Control	138
Mutual Relation of Functions	141
Table showing approximate relation to the spinal nerves of the various motor, sensory, and reflex functions of the spinal cord	142
SYMPTOMS OF DISEASE OF THE CORD:	
CHRONIC MYELITIS (*continued*)—	PAGE
Diagnosis	244
Prognosis and Treatment	245
COMPRESSION	246
Causes and Pathological Anatomy	247
Diagnosis	250
Prognosis and Treatment	251
ANTERIOR POLIOMYELITIS: ATROPHIC SPINAL PARALYSIS	251
Acute Atrophic Paralysis (Infantile Palsy)	252
Etiology	253
Symptoms	255
Pathology	263
Diagnosis	266
Prognosis	269
Treatment	270
Subacute and Chronic Atrophic Spinal Paralysis	273
ACUTE ASCENDING PARALYSIS	275
Causes and Symptoms	275
Pathology	277
Diagnosis, Prognosis, and Treatment	279
PARALYSIS FROM INCREASED ATMOSPHERIC PRESSURE—DIVERS' PARALYSIS	280
HÆMORRHAGE INTO SPINAL CORD—HÆMATOMYELIA	281
Etiology and Pathological Anatomy	282
Symptoms	283
Diagnosis	284
Prognosis and Treatment	285
DEGENERATIONS OF CORD	285
LOCOMOTOR ATAXY—TABES DORSALIS	287
History	287
Causes	288
Symptoms	290
Motor	291
Sensory	293
Eye	297
Sphincters	299
Vasomotor and trophic	300
Course and Termination	304
Pathological Anatomy	307
Pathology	314
Diagnosis	319
Prognosis	322
Treatment	323
PRIMARY SPASTIC PARAPLEGIA	327
PRIMARY LATERAL SCLEROSIS:	PAGE
Causes and Symptoms	330
Diagnosis	337
Prognosis and Treatment	339
ATAXIC PARAPLEGIA	341
Causes and Symptoms	341
Pathological Anatomy	343
Pathology	345
Diagnosis	348
Prognosis and Treatment	349
HEREDITARY ATAXY—FRIEDREICH'S DISEASE	349
Symptoms	350
Pathological Anatomy	352
Pathology	354
Diagnosis	355
Prognosis and Treatment	356
CHRONIC SPINAL MUSCULAR ATROPHY:	
PROGRESSIVE MUSCULAR ATROPHY	356
Causes	357
Symptoms	359
Varieties and Complications	366
Course	367
Pathological Anatomy	368
Pathology	375
Diagnosis	378
Prognosis	379
Treatment	380
ARTHRITIC MUSCULAR ATROPHY	381
Pathology	383
Diagnosis	384
Prognosis and Treatment	385
Muscular Atrophy from Over-use	385
IDIOPATHIC MUSCULAR ATROPHY:	

FIG. 169 (pp. 404–6). The contents of Volume 1 of Gowers' *Manual*.

chemistry. The electrical tests developed by Erb were widely used but Duchenne's muscle biopsy procedure had yet to be seriously taken up. For the pathologist, carmine was still the standard stain for nervous tissue in the sixties and seventies. 'Much of the internal anatomy of the brain and spinal cord was worked out by means of it', wrote Rasmussen.[282] The staining techniques of Weigert, Golgi, and Marchi were developed in the eighties, while formaldehyde fixation did not come till the nineties, which also saw the arrival of lumbar puncture and radiology. Gowers's achievement must naturally be judged with such thoughts in mind.

From the table of contents it may be seen that he constructed his book in five parts: I, General Symptomatology; II, Diseases of the Nerves; III, Diseases of the Spinal Cord; IV, Diseases of the Brain; V, General and Functional Diseases. Parts IV and V constitute the second volume. There would be no point in trying to summarize the work, nor even, I think, in trying to write an essay-review. Nor is there much to be gained by drawing attention to such weaknesses as were recognized at the time. One of the most widely praised items was his clinical and pathological account of locomotor ataxy, a disease which has practically disappeared (although one cannot say it will not return). It comprised some forty pages and should be read in its entirety for its historical interest. There is also much in Part V that would interest the reader.

I have had my copy for over thirty years and I shall try and indicate where I have personally found it instructive, where I have come to admire his powers of observation, his reasoning, and, above all, his ability to analyse and explain. A book, even coming from Victorian England, must have had some special stamp and flavour to have won for itself such a lordly sobriquet. What follows is an idiosyncratic view of why this was so.

At the outset there are no windy preliminaries, no advice even about the taking of a clinical history. Presumably he thought the student learned that in hospital. There is no actual section on the 'examination of the patient'. 'Symptoms and their investigation' is the first consideration and that is mainly confined to an account of disorders of movement and sensation, and of reflex action.

He begins by saying that 'The nervous system is almost entirely inaccessible to direct examination; the exceptions to this are trifling'.

Power

The nature of the common defects of motion, sensation, and coordination engage the reader. In thirty-five pages he describes how examination should proceed and what signs should be sought. There is a particularly detailed explanation of the mode of action of the muscles of the limbs and in what manner movements are impaired by individual paralyses. One immediately becomes aware of his patient and punctilious approach. He mentions the difficulties in writing produced by paralysis of the infraspinatus, 'the movement along the lines being by this rotation of the humerus' (p. 26), and by paralysis of the lumbricals and interossei, in which the alternate 'upstroke' and 'downstroke' of the pen is affected. In triceps paralysis a man 'cannot raise his hat in the customary manner' (p. 27). He explains why the toes are 'directed outward' in a gluteal nerve lesion (p. 33) and why walking is possible 'if the leg is not moved forward beyond the vertical position' in a femoral nerve lesion (p. 34). Some two dozen of his fine line drawings illustrate the appearances in the various palsies and are more instructive than some photographs.

In incoordination of movement, when the 'exactly proportioned contraction' of muscles is affected, and there is lack of 'balanced adjustment', 'spontaneous movements' as well as clumsiness occur. 'The irregularity obtains in the fixed as well as in the mobile condition. In the latter it causes ataxy, in the former spontaneous movements' (p. 5).

Sensation

Touch, pain, and temperature must be separately tested, 'since one may be affected and not another' (yet Gowers did not, as we shall see, identify the dissociated sensory loss of syringomyelia). In testing tactile sensation the instrument employed must not give an impression of heat or cold 'lest the patient perceive by the sense of temperature that which he cannot discern by the sense of touch' (p. 6). The patient's ability to 'localise' the touch should be noted. The principal value of the two-point discrimination test was 'for the estimation of changes of sensibility in the same person and the same part than for actual diagnosis' (p. 7). Small weights were useful for examining 'pressure' sensation or one could use 'the instrument contrived for measuring the pressure applied to an artery to ascertain the tension of the pulse'. In testing for pain, too sharp a point 'may here and there be unfelt, although it penetrates the skin', as in the less sensitive parts of the skin the terminal nerve-plexus may be wide. Appreciation of temperature may be perverted, as well as impaired, so that hot feels cold and vice versa. Delay in perception of pain may be accompanied by delay in perception of temperature, but it should be remembered that normally the latter is slower. Hot and cold spoons were useful tools, the use of test-tubes was often only time-consuming.

Ataxia

Gowers commented on the varying ways in which the term 'muscular sense' had been used (pp. 9–10). It will be recalled that Bell referred to movement and posture, weight and resistance, and to pain and fatigue. The nerves 'in the interstitial tissue' of the muscles were thought to explain 'cramp' and the shortening and lengthening of muscle fibres necessary for appreciating weight, posture, and passive movement. Cricket balls with various weights inside were used. Appreciation of weights is not interfered with by simple weakness. On the other hand it was the central innervation, and not the actual muscular contraction, 'that determines the strength of associated movements, and influences the centre concerned in maintaining the equilibrium of the body'. When he discussed the ataxia of tabes dorsalis (pp. 316–18) he concluded that 'we do not at present know to what extent, in any given case, the symptoms are due to the cord disease or to the peripheral nerve lesions'. Either, alone, had been demonstrated to be sufficient.

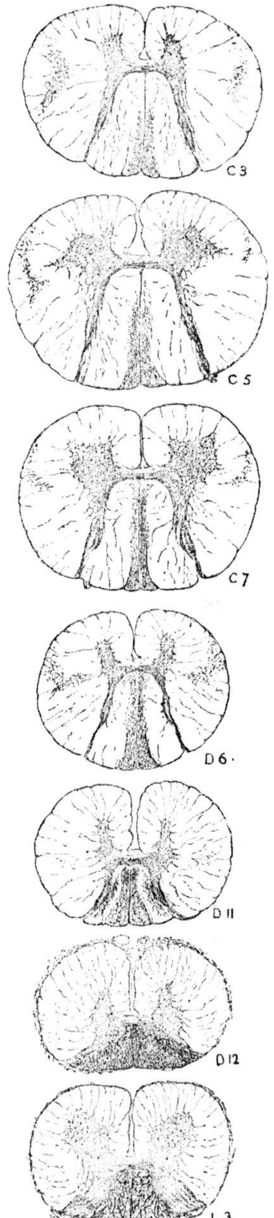

FIG. 170. Locomotor ataxy involving the legs only. The ascending degeneration in the posterior columns becoming limited, in the lower dorsal region, to the root-zone and posterior median columns. The latter only are affected in the upper half of the cord. Ascending degeneration also in the antero-lateral tracts. (After Gowers,[45] Fig. 111.)

... coordination is chiefly an automatic process, depending partly perhaps on muscle-reflex actions, and on the connection of neighbouring sensory structures in the spinal cord, but chiefly on the function of the cerebellum itself, and the connections of the muscles with it, and the interruption of this connection is the chief element in the incoordination of locomotor ataxy (p. 318).

In his book on the spinal cord Gowers had shown that 'the direct cerebellar tract' was afferent, but only degenerated when a lesion of the cord was at, or above, its level of origin at the dorso-lumbar junction. Its function was not known but it not usually degenerate in locomotor ataxia. However, his 'antero-lateral ascending tract', the spinothalamic, which he had also previously described,[283] was sometimes affected in that disease (p. 311). In slight cases he had shown that the degeneration in the posterior columns was often restricted to the 'postero-median' fibres which 'probably constitute the path from these nerves' ('the muscle-nerves' p. 317).

The much-debated 'muscular sense' was discussed by Bastian[284] and others at a meeting of the Neurological Society in 1887. It was generally agreed that it was composed of several different elements but as to what extent 'conscious' and 'unconscious' processes were involved, opinions differed. Gowers did not enjoy meetings and his name is not among those who took part. By the turn of the century 'muscular sense' was giving way to 'position sense' and 'proprioception'. Discrimination of weights was being replaced by tests of the appreciation of passive movements of the digits with the eyes closed, and of placing a finger on a particular part of the body. The tuning fork also came into use.

Reflexes

The reflexes Gowers routinely tested were the cutaneous ones such as the plantar, gluteal, cremasteric, abdominal, and conjunctival, and the knee jerk 'which is probably never absent in health' (p. 319). He now knew that there were nerves in tendons (p. 13) but there is no actual mention of the 'ankle

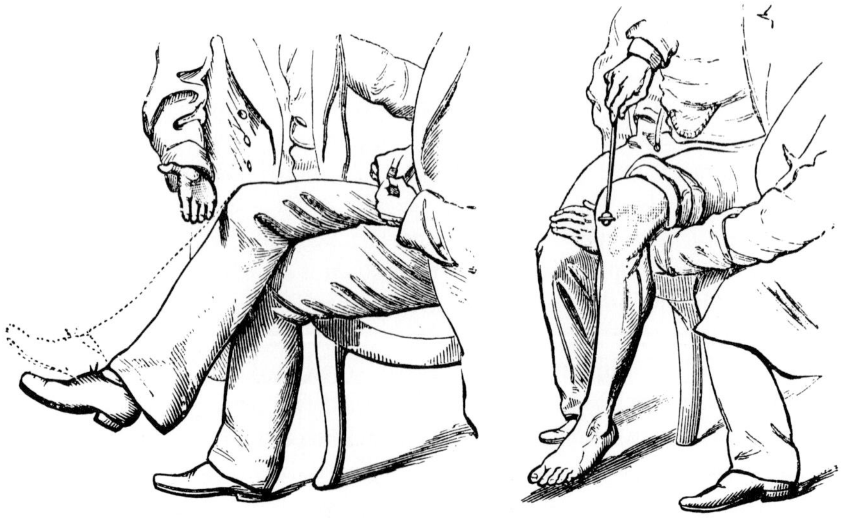

FIG. 171. The knee jerk. 'The blow may be given by the side of the hand, a percussion hammer, or a stethoscope with an india-rubber edge to the ear-piece.' (After Gowers,[45] Figs. 1 and 2.)

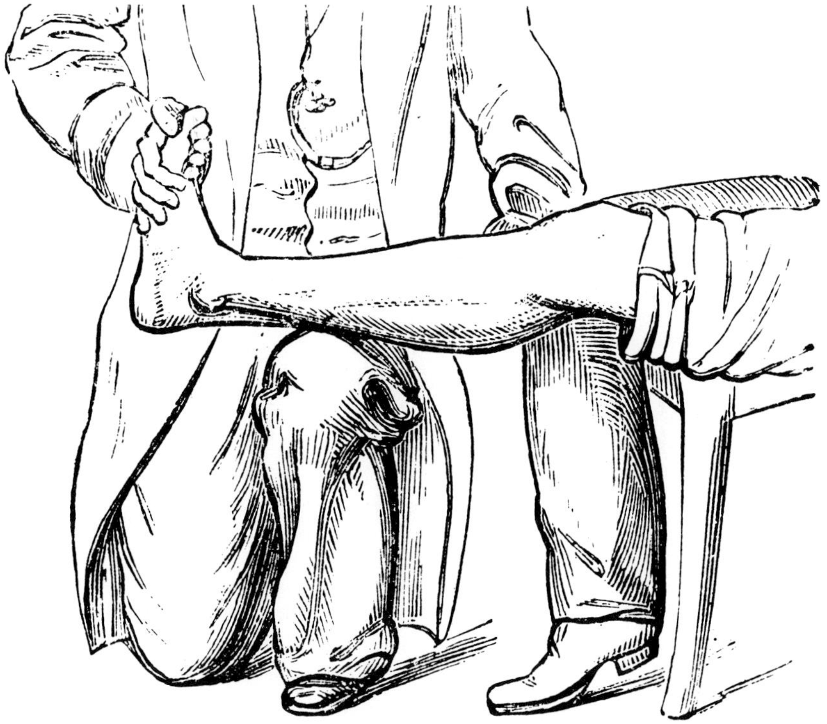

FIG. 172. Method of eliciting the foot-clonus, or 'ankle clonus' or 'foot-phenomenon – Westphal'. (After Gowers,[45] Fig. 3.)

jerk', although he was aware of it, and when he came to write on sciatica (p. 85), made no mention of it although he noted the loss of the knee jerk in femoral nerve lesions. Neither is there any formal mention of what tendon jerks were to be obtained in the upper limbs although, again, there is later mention of the biceps and triceps reflexes being subserved through the sixth and seventh cervical segments (p. 132). In describing nerve lesions the reflexes usually go unmentioned. On page 142 is a table which illustrates the relation between the motor, sensory, and reflex functions and the spinal nerves. In the reflex column the only deep reflex listed is the knee jerk. One's impression is that routinely it was the knee jerk, the plantar reflex, and ankle-clonus on which attention was focused.

As we have seen, Gowers found the term 'tendon jerk' inaccurate. 'The one condition which all have in common is that passive tension is essential for their occurrence, and I have suggested that they be termed *myotatic* contractions ... it is highly probable ... that the condition on which the myotatic irritability depends, is identical with muscular "tone"' (p. 17).

Diseases of nerves

An account of the histological structure of nerve is followed by that of 'secondary degeneration' with appropriate illustrations. He stressed that Ranvier had shown that degeneration 'is not a mere process of death or decay, but an active process, a destruction of the nerve as such by the protoplasm and nuclei of the internodal cells that constitute it' (p. 40). The most common lesion in man was 'neuritis', where the nature of the primary lesion probably influenced the degeneration. The lesion could be acute and focal, or diffuse and chronic.

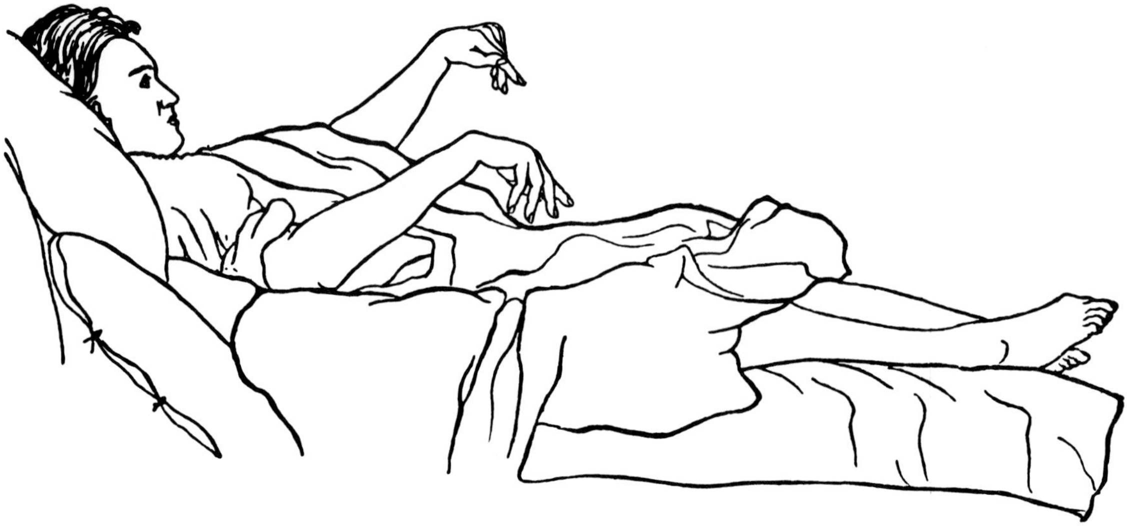

FIG. 173. Multiple alcoholic neuritis. Palsy of extensors of wrist and flexors of ankle. (After Gowers,[45] Fig. 53.)

In lesions of the upper limb he said that 'most movements are related to many spinal roots'. C.4 and 5, the muscles of the shoulder, flexors of the elbow, and supinators; C.6 and 7, the adductors of the arm and extensors of the elbow; C.6–8, pronation; C.5, extension of the wrist; C.8, flexion of wrist, flexion of fingers; C.7 and 8, intrinsic hand muscles; Th.I. (p. 68).

Although he said that 'various morbid processes near the spine and in the neck may cause symptoms in the arms by involving the nerve-roots that enter the plexus' (p. 69), there is no hint of root compression from what we now call cervical sponylosis, nor of the syndrome of costo-clavicular compression. Without radiology these would have been exceedingly difficult to identify. He did however know that paraplegia could result from 'vertebral exostoses' (p. 182).

Individual nerve lesions from injury, compression, and infection were then much commoner in civil life and their features are well described. 'Crutch palsy' most commonly affected the radial nerve, but 'the continental custom of tying together, behind the body, the arms of a prisoner, often causes paralysis of this nerve, sometimes on both sides' (p. 72). In dealing with the median nerve he seems not to have had any suspicions about the carpal tunnel, but in discussing the causes of local atrophy he said that the thenar muscles were sometimes affected. He suspected 'over-use' in one lady from excessive 'illuminating' (p. 385). He warned how a lower cervical lesion may mimic an ulnar one (p. 76). Some of his cases of 'primary neuritis' of the brachial plexus were probably examples of neuralgic amyotrophy, as they were 'rare', 'tedious in their course', 'with pain, acute or burning in character, in the position of the plexus', and followed by 'evidence of organic damage to the nerves that arise from the plexus'.

Cold, wet, draughts, and exposure are not as commonly quoted as in some previous texts but he believed that 'draughty water-closet seats' were to blame for some cases of sciatica (an aetiology also suspected by Charles

Kingsley, writing from his cold Rectory at Eversley). It could also be a consequence of lesions of the spine or cauda equina (p. 89). Alcoholic neuritis was a menace; 'servants are corrupted, and alcohol is often taken in secret, and absolutely denied' (p. 101). In a fourteen-page section on 'multiple neuritis', or 'polyneuritis', he said that the concept 'had profoundly modified many of our conceptions, not only of the processes of disease, but of the range of action of certain morbid influences'. It was 'one of the most important steps in the recent advance of neurology' (p. 91). 'Until recently, indeed, all cases of multiple neuritis were looked upon as spinal' (p. 100). He referred to beriberi and leprosy, as well as alcohol, exposure, septicaemia, 'exhaustion after other maladies', and phthisis, when discussing aetiology. He had never seen alcoholic neuritis in a male, but had notes of eight female cases. 'Alcoholic pseudotabes' or 'alcoholic ataxia', terms suggested by Dreschfeld[285] of Manchester in 1884, could be mistaken for locomotor ataxia.

It will be recalled that Gowers discussed 'acute ascending paralysis' under 'diseases of the spinal cord' but when describing multiple neuritis he said it 'may resemble the most rapid form of multiple neuritis, but, in it, the symptoms ascend the trunk to the arms, and do not begin in the hands and feet at the same time, as does the usual form of multiple neuritis' (p. 100). 'Moreover', he added, 'there is no anaesthesia in the spinal malady'.

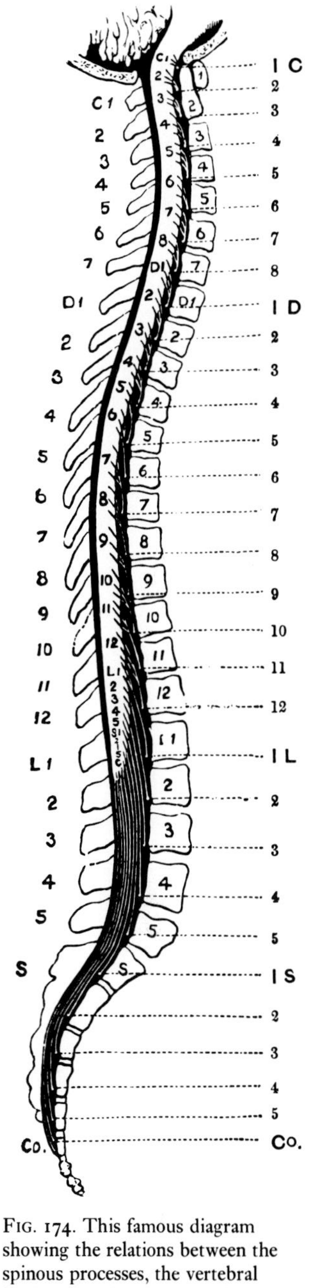

Fig. 174. This famous diagram showing the relations between the spinous processes, the vertebral bodies, and the segments of the spinal cord, first appeared in Gowers' 'Diagnosis of Diseases of the spinal cord' (1880). It was based on dissection made by Victor Horsley. (After Gowers,[45] Fig. 56.)

Diseases of the spinal cord

Characteristically, in Part III, there is a detailed and instructive account of contemporary knowledge of the anatomy and functions of the spinal cord. Among the degenerative disorders listed were 'system-diseases' such as locomotor ataxia, and progressive muscular atrophy; diseases such as chronic myelitis in which the process in the cord was 'random' . . .; and diseases such as 'ataxia paraplegia' and 'hereditary ataxia' in which system involvement was a possibility. Gowers included the myopathies here, not because he did not accept that they were 'primarily muscular', but because 'clinical resemblance may conveniently be allowed to supersede the rules of pathological classification' (p. 386). This must have puzzled some of his readers.

Anatomy and function. Gowers's introductory figures (Figs. 174–176) must have been particularly welcomed by his students. And Fig. 178 depicting 'the element of the motor path' was certainly full of enlightenment. Using terms such as spinal 'segments', 'root-sheaths' and 'root-zone', 'neuroglia', 'ganglion cells', 'glia cells', and 'medullated and non-medullated axis-cylinders' his descriptions carry a modern ring. After describing how the processes of ascending and descending degeneration, and of myelination, had so greatly helped the identification of spinal tracts and the direction of conduction, he added, 'but we cannot affirm that the tracts which do not degenerate through any considerable extent, do not form part of conducting paths' (p. 123). One could be sure only that they did not constitute a *continuous* conducting path, such as the pyramidal.

With regard to the motor tracts he said that 'most movements and muscles are represented in vertical tracts, and the whole anterior grey matter, at any one nerve segment, contains cells that are concerned with different movements. An extensive lesion of small vertical extent may thus weaken many movements, but abolish none' (p. 128). Much more was known of cervical motor representation than of lumbar. Knowledge of the sensory path, Gowers said, was far less definite than that of the motor path – as we have seen. One difficulty in localizing the two sensory paths was 'that the same impression that is felt, may excite a reflex action' (p. 134). For this, afferent root fibres would have to end in the grey matter of the cord. 'Are the two functions subserved by the same or by different fibres?', he asked. There was a similar difficulty in the case of the sensory 'muscle-nerves'. When the cauda equina was diseased there was ascending degeneration of the postero-median column, indicating that those root fibres passed up without interruption. Muscle-reflex action had to be subserved by other fibres.

Clinical features. 'The symptoms of diseases of the spinal cord consist in derangement of its functions; the loss of some, the exaltation and perversion of others' (p. 143). The combination of symptoms indicated the seat of the lesion; its *nature* was inferred from its mode of development and other considerations. The commonly bilateral character of the clinical features depended on two causes; the close proximity of the structures in the two halves of the cord in the case of focal lesions, and the fact that degenerative system lesions were usually bilateral.

As far as loss of power was concerned, the effect was the same whether the lesion was in the upper or lower segment of the motor path, 'but the other symptoms that accompany the loss of power differ very much according as the interruption is in the upper or lower segment' (p. 144). The latter formed part of the reflex arc and influenced muscle nutrition, so that when diseased there was loss of reflexes and wasting of muscles. In a lesion of the

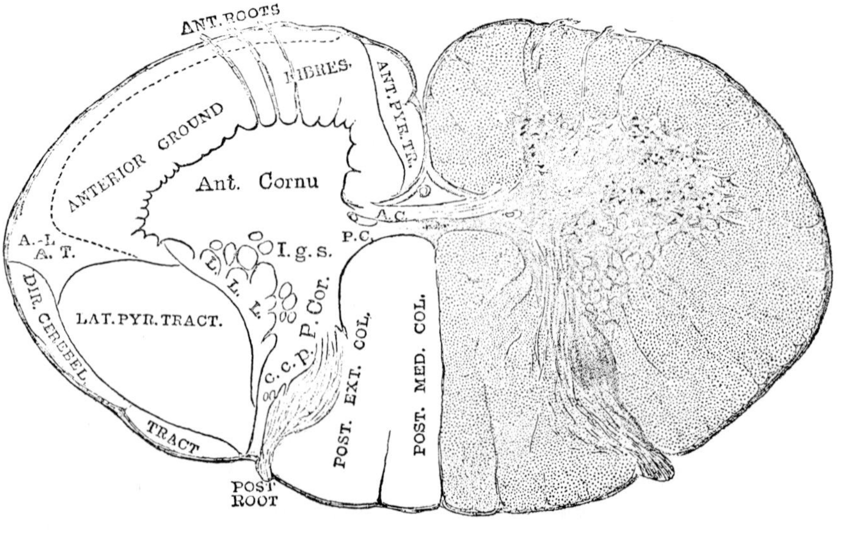

FIG. 175. Diagram of a transverse section of the spinal cord in the cervical region (After Gowers,[45] Fig. 57.)

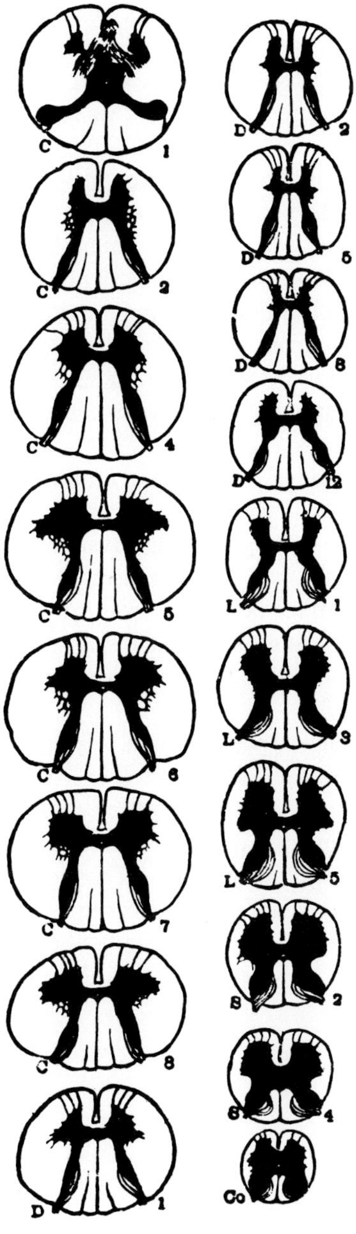

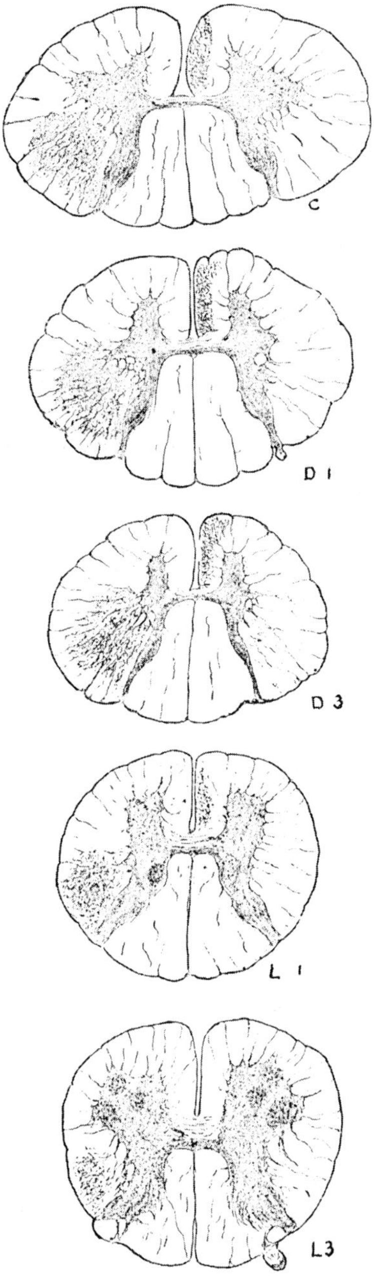

FIG. 176 (*left*). Diagram showing the relative size and shape of the cord and its grey matter at different levels. (After Gowers,[45] Fig. 58.)

FIG. 177 (*right*). Descending degeneration of the pyramidal tracts in a case of hemiplegia from disease of the right cerebral hemisphere. Anterior tract on the same side; lateral tract on the opposite side. (After Gowers,[45] Fig. 65.)

FIG. 178 (*below*). Diagram of an element of the motor path. C, C, cortical cell; S. C. spinal cell; A, C. anterior cornua; S, path from sensory roots. Dotted line indicates junction between upper and lower segments. Gowers said 'This conception of the motor path conduces to clearer ideas of many phenomena of disease . . .' (p. 116), a statement which generations of teachers and students have verified. (After Gowers,[45] Fig. 66.)

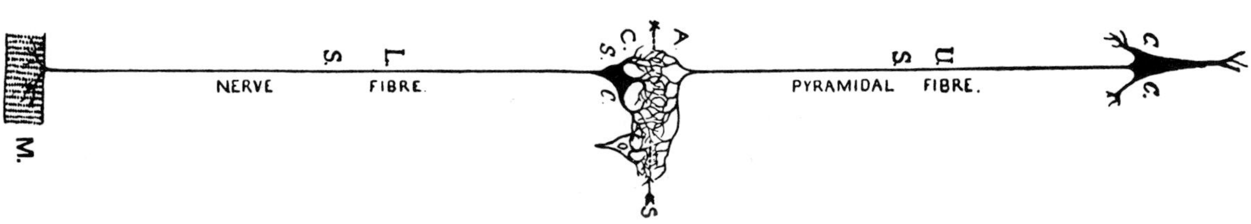

upper segment there was no wasting, and reflex action was commonly increased. In a cervical lesion both segments may be involved so that the signs in the upper limbs may be very different from those in the lower limbs. How familiar these lines must sound to the modern reader recalling his initial introduction to the subject.

Spasm, in acute lesions, might be due to 'direct irritation of motor centres', but in chronic lesions the mechanism was different and probably dependent on 'over-action of the reflex centres, due, not to irritation, but to deficient control' (p. 145). Muscular contractions, or shortening of muscles, occurred in three different ways: (1) as a result of long-continued irritation of motor fibres, chiefly of the nerve roots; (2) from long continued spasm, common in the flexors of the hip and knee; and (3) whenever one group of muscles is much more paralysed than its opponents, the latter becoming contracted, although spasm is absent.

Loss of sensation was common but occurred less readily than motor loss. There was no clear evidence that there was a division of the sensory path into upper and lower segments but it was certainly conceivable. Interruption of the posterior sensory roots, but not of the sensory tracts, caused loss of reflexes. A focal lesion may damage both, as in compression. In sensory testing, therefore, it was important to examine the trunk as well as the limbs below; loss in the former might be present when there was none in the legs.

In *spastic paraplegia* there was 'tonic extensor spasm' which was said to have a 'clasp-knife' character because 'when near full extension the spasm suddenly comes on and completed the movement, as the blade of a pocket knife moves under the influence of the spring' (p. 150). Clonic spasm superficially resembled Brown-Séquard's 'spinal epilepsy'. The central mechanisms operating in spasm were probably also 'those concerned in the reflex act of standing. The spasm often enables a patient to stand, when his voluntary power is quite insufficient for the act' (p. 151). All very Sherringtonian.

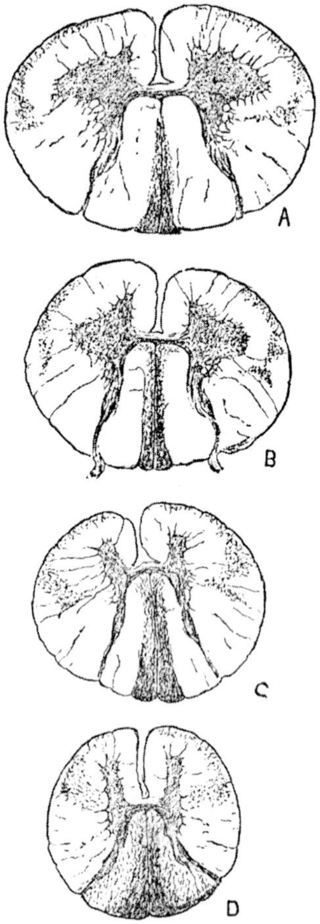

FIG. 179. Ascending degeneration in the postero-median columns and the antero-lateral ascending tract. The cord was crushed at L.1. (After Gowers,[45] Fig. 67.)

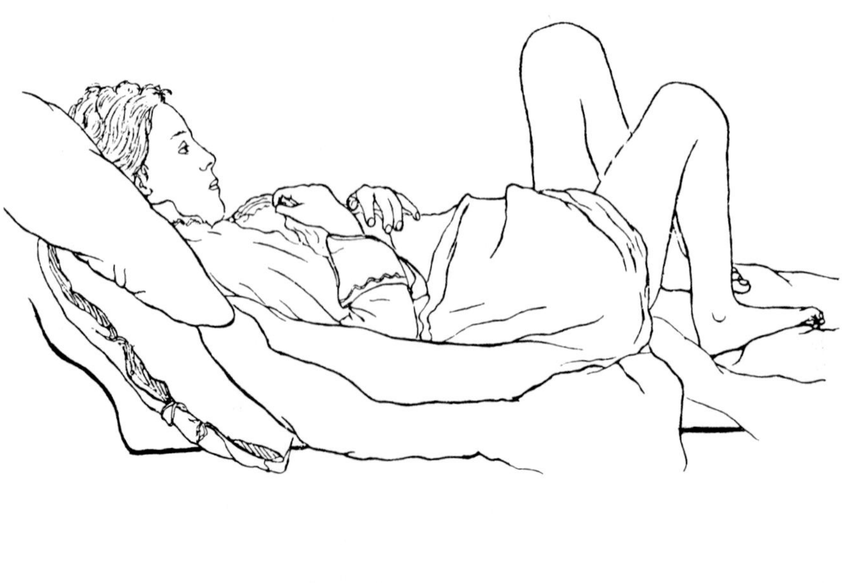

FIG. 180. Flexion contraction of legs in myelitis of dorsal region. (After Gowers,[45] Fig. 93.)

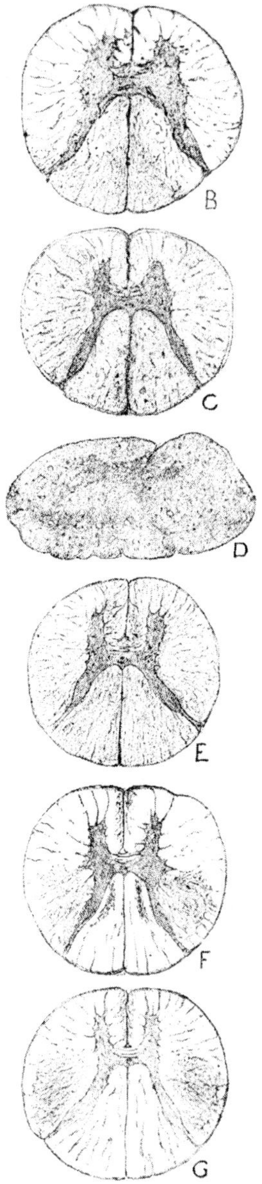

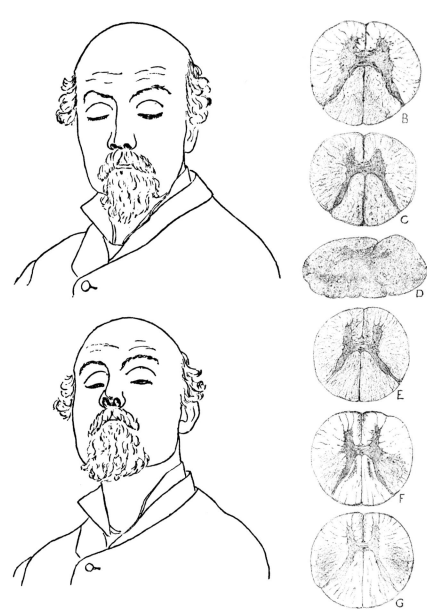

FIG. 181 (*left*). Double tabetic ptosis. The patient was not a Shakespearian-looking Englishman, but one of Charcot's patients. (After Gowers,[45] Fig. 106.)

FIG. 182 (*right*). Compression of the spinal cord and 'pressure-myelitis' in a case of caries of the spine. D, compression in mid-dorsal region; C and E, myelitis. B, ascending degeneration in posterior columns; F and G, descending degeneration in anterior and lateral pyramidal tracts. F, 'comma-shaped descending degeneration in the anterior part of the post-external column'. (After Gowers,[45] Fig. 98.)

Convulsions, Gowers thought, *had* been known to occur in lesions of the cervical cord, recalling Brown-Séquard's epileptic guinea pigs.

The speed of onset was an important factor in diagnosis. Vascular lesions were sudden or acute, inflammation could be acute, subacute, or subchronic; degeneration was subchronic (six weeks to six months) or chronic (more than six months).

In *ataxic paraplegia* (p. 341) the sclerosis in the posterior columns differed from that in locomotor ataxy in two respects. It did not primarily affect the lumbar region nor the posterior root-zones. He did not know of any case in which the peripheral nerves had been examined and there is no mention of

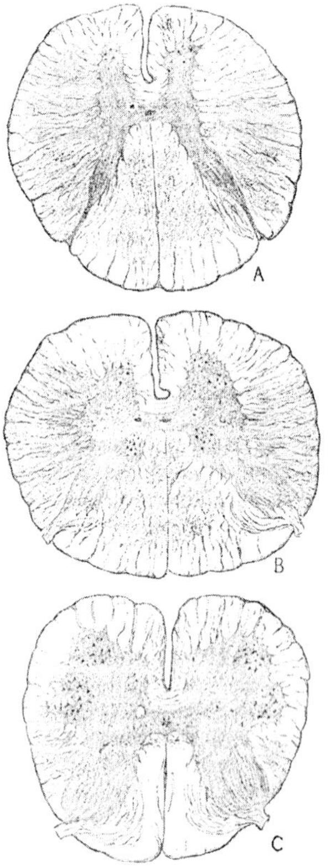

FIG. 183. Ataxic paraplegia; combined lateral and posterior sclerosis. A, upper dorsal; B, twelfth dorsal; C, mid-lumbar; The posterior column degeneration is practically confined to B and A. Pyramidal degeneration is greater in A and B. (After Gowers,[45] Fig. 121.)

paraesthesiae. He thought the mechanism of the ataxia lay, not in the involvement of the sensory 'muscle-nerves', but of the posterior columns or, possibly, of the direct cerebellar tracts. However, there was sometimes loss of sensation in the legs and absent knee jerks. 'If the knee jerk is lost as in tabes, it is not restored by degeneration of the pyramidal tracts' (p. 347). The disorder seemed to be 'allied to system-diseases'. Duration or pallor are not mentioned. Did his haemoglobinometer hold the key? Probably only superficial sensation was tested. Passive movements of the toes and the arrival of the tuning fork later assisted the identification of subacute combined sclerosis, but it is difficult to believe that all Gowers's cases were of that nature.

In *hereditary ataxy*, Gowers did mention that 'the sense of posture', as well as that of touch, pain, and temperature, were normal. Since Friedreich's publication of 1863, Gowers said that there had been about sixty-five cases recorded. He had found an affected family in 1880 (Charcot in 1884). He referred to it as an 'hereditary ataxic paraplegia' and, clinically and pathologically, it occupied a position between 'ataxic paraplegia' and 'simple tabes'. The early age of onset, the scoliosis and talipes, the nystagmus, the defective articulation, and the jerky tremors of the head and arms served to distinguish it clinically, but the cerebellar origin of the latter features were yet to be traced. The sclerosis of the posterior columns was intense and the 'cervical root-zones never escape'. The degeneration of the lateral columns was not limited to the pyramidal paths; it also involved the direct cerebellar tracts. The pons and medulla were sometimes shrunken and degeneration had been noted in the restiform bodies. But actual cerebellar changes are not mentioned.

In *progressive muscular atrophy*, he wondered whether injury or over-use of a limb played any aetiological role. He suspected the former might do so, as in paralysis agitans, but the disease affected all classes of society so that manual labour was not a likely factor. Gowers did not often state the average duration of a degenerative disease but he mentions a case where the course neared its end in nine months and another in which it remained confined to one arm for seven years. He also thought he had seen its progress arrested. Sensations and aching pains were felt but he did not mention cramps. The face, except for the lips, was not affected and there was a curious tendency for the uppermost part of the trapezius, and the levator anguli scapulae to escape. Lordosis in the erect posture disappears when the patient sits down, something which he had checked with a plumb-line, but without mentioning Duchenne's account and diagram. He observed that 'fibrillation' often preceded wasting and that the latter involved the subcutaneous tissues as well as the muscles. In one case, which he previously reported in *Brain*, he described the 'doll's eye' phenomenon.

> I have once met with a remarkable reflex fixation of the eyeballs in a case of advanced progressive muscular atrophy. If the patient, looking to one side, was suddenly told to look at an object on the other side, his head was instantly turned towards the second object, while the eyes remained fixed on the first, by a movement

corresponding to that of the head, but in the opposite direction, and then, after a few seconds, they were slowly moved towards the second object. The phenomenon continued to the end of the patient's life (pp. 365–6).

This, he said, was evidence of a normal reflex mechanism in the fixation of the eyes that was, as it were, 'isolated by disease, which lessened voluntary control over it'.

In his detailed examination of the pathological evidence in progressive atrophy, Gowers concluded that 'the only adequate explanation of the facts is that the degeneration of the upper and lower segments is simultaneous, or if not simultaneous, at least so far independent that neither is the cause or consequence of the other'. There was a decay of the whole motor path from the cortex of the brain to the muscles. 'I have not met with a single case of progressive muscular atrophy in which the pyramidal tracts were unaffected' (p. 373). He did not think Charcot's introduction of the term 'amyotrophic lateral sclerosis' very helpful, with its implication that the primary lesion was the degeneration of the pyramidal tracts, and that the atrophy of the anterior horn cells was secondary or 'deuteropathic'. 'Charcot's distinction is in effect giving a new name to an old disease' (p. 378). The clinical manifestations were determined by the timing, extent, and severity of the degeneration in the upper and lower segments of the motor path.

In the ten pages devoted to *syringomyelia*, nine are taken up in describing the various cavities seen in the spinal cord, mainly in children (hydromyelia), and usually symptomless. He thought that those in adults were not fundamentally different. Both were developmental in origin. There was probably defective closure of the central canal and alterations taking place in any persistent embryonal tissue. Gliomatosis was a feature and tumours were common. But simple closure of part of a central canal did not cause distension of the part above. It was often difficult to be certain whether a central cavity was really the central canal; an epithelial lining was no criterion. In some cases there was internal hydrocephalus and an absent cerebellum (p. 436).

The clinical syndrome in the adult was 'seldom suspected during life' because it resembled other more common maladies. There was muscular atrophy, loss of sensibility, and trophic changes in the upper limbs, often accompanied by weakness and spasticity in the lower limbs. The disease might terminate in two or three years. 'The cutaneous anaesthesia usually involves the same region as the muscular wasting, but extends beyond the limits of the latter.' Gowers did not mention any particular modality of sensation, nor burn scars; possibly too much of the altered appearance in the hands was attributed to trophic lesions. A few years later he did appreciate that the sensory loss was in fact dissociated.[286]

Gowers recognized two types of *muscular dystrophy*, the pseudo-hypertrophic and the atrophic, although there were 'intermediate' cases. He had seen forty-three cases of the former and considered the latter to be rare. The hereditary factors were obvious in both. In the pseudo-hypertrophic form 'the disease is transmitted by mothers who are not themselves its

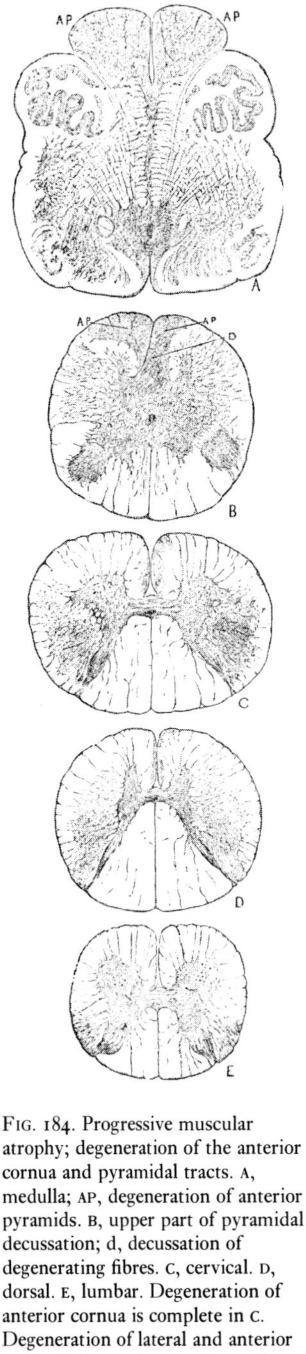

FIG. 184. Progressive muscular atrophy; degeneration of the anterior cornua and pyramidal tracts. A, medulla; AP, degeneration of anterior pyramids. B, upper part of pyramidal decussation; d, decussation of degenerating fibres. C, cervical. D, dorsal. E, lumbar. Degeneration of anterior cornua is complete in C. Degeneration of lateral and anterior pyramidal tracts is conspicuous in C and D. In E the anterior pyramidal tract has ceased. (After Gowers,[45] Fig. 135.)

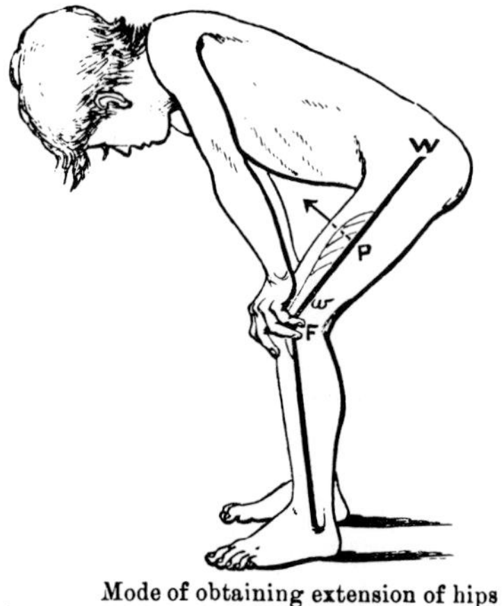

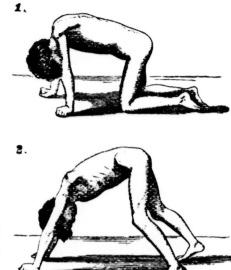

Mode of obtaining extension of hips in pseudo-hypertrophic paralysis. F, fulcrum of the lever formed by the femur. P, mean position at which the power is applied by contraction of the quadriceps femoris. W, position of weight in the ordinary mode of rising. w, the place to which part is transferred by putting hands on knees.

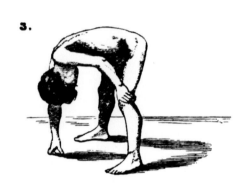

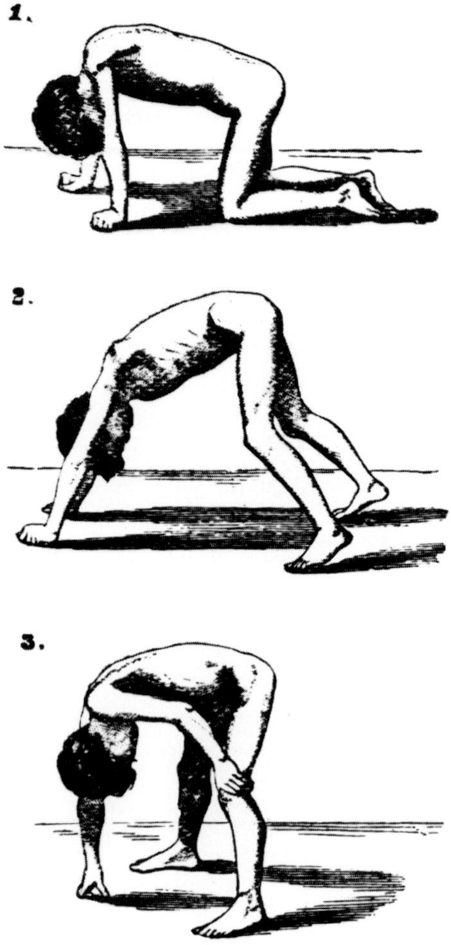

FIG. 185 (*left*). Pseudohypertrophic paralysis; mode of obtaining extension of hips. (After Gowers,[45] Fig. 142.)

FIG. 186 (*right*). Pseudo-hypertrophic paralysis; mode of rising from the ground. Later to be known as Gowers's sign. (After Gowers,[45] Fig. 143.)

subjects' and it was four times commoner in the male. It began in childhood and although it varied in its course and in the amount and distribution of the hypertrophy, its cardinal features were fairly uniform. The atrophic type affected both sexes equally, it was rarely confined to one generation, as sometimes occurred in the first type, and it was more variable, and started later in life. In both, the lower half of the pectoralis major and the latissimus dorsi were very susceptible to atrophy, whereas the face was not affected in the pseudo-hypertrophic type but often involved in the atrophic type. In smiling, elevation of the lips, without the angles of the mouth, gave rise to that appearance he was later to describe in myasthenia, a malady not described in his *Manual*.

In the pseudo-hypertrophic form he commented on the not infrequent wasting of only the clavicular part of the sterno-mastoid muscle, and how hypertrophy most commonly affected the calf muscles and the spinati. The latter, in the atrophic type, rarely wasted. Mental deficiency sometimes complicated the pseudo-hypertrophic type.

Although the appearance of the 'myopathic face', with its dull expression and pouting lips, was often quite striking, the contour of the face was little affected, and actual wasting might not be apparent. The tongue muscles were not affected and the ocular extremely rarely. He had seen one case in which there was slowly progressive bilateral ptosis with ophthalmoplegia, followed by facial weakness (p. 406). He wondered whether it was myopathic or neuropathic. His 'distal' type of myopathy, which I have never seen, was described later, in 1902.[287]

Diseases of the brain

The first three hundred pages of the second volume deal with the structure and function of the brain, the symptoms of brain disease, the cranial nerves, and a summary of the localization of cerebral disease. It is a *tour de force* which, published today in paperback, would still provide a sound and readable introduction for students. Like the remainder of the text, there are no frills, it is dense with information, facts and theories are clearly distinguished, and Gowers pays great attention to terminology. Indeed, concerning the latter, his footnotes reveal, occasionally in an amusing fashion, his striving for accuracy. Terms such as 'supra-marginal', 'monoplegia', 'hemianopia', 'illusions' called for comments. Even the use of 'anterior' and 'posterior' in relation to the pons and crura is questioned as their direction 'is nearer the horizontal than the vertical'. When he came to 'aphasia' he said that it owed its currency to Trousseau 'who summoned it from a slumber of two thousand years' seemingly unaware of its antiquity, and believing that it was 'invented' for him in 1861, by a M. Chrysaphis. But it was an improvement on 'aphemia' which meant not 'speechlessness' but 'infamy'. Gowers did not welcome the word 'dysphasia', nor did he think it would come into use. It did not have the merit of 'unimpeachable exactness', and in any case it sounded too much like 'dysphagia'.

The cortex. Concerning his sketch of the layers of the cortex (Fig. 188) he said that it seemed that the three superficial layers, and the deepest layer, were fairly uniform over the greater part of the cortex; it was the intervening elements which showed the greatest variation. When Bevan Lewis [288, 289] identified the Betz cells in Meynert's fourth layer he had suggested a division of the cortex into six layers, as shown in Gowers's right column in his sketch.

'The evidence we possess', he said, 'regarding the cortical centres in the human brain is derived solely from the comparison of the effects of disease, observed during life, with its position ascertained after death' (p. 13). But he thought there was 'a general correspondence' between man and monkey. As with the spinal cord more was known of the localization of motor than of sensory functions. His diagrams (Figs. 189 and 190) were intended to be guides; 'we need not therefore conceive that these parts subserve no other function'. There were reasons for believing that there were sensory functions in motor areas. There was the sensory aura of the epileptic motor spasm, and the slight blunting of sensibility in the extremity of a hemiplegic limb, to explain.

The exact position of the visual centres in the occipital lobes was not

CONTENTS.

FIG. 187. Contents of Volume 2 of Gowers' *Manual*.[195] Diseases of the Brain and Cranial Nerves; General and Functional Diseases of the Nervous System.

known, but complete hemianopia was most frequently produced by a lesion of the apex of the lobe and especially of the cuneus. There was some suggestion that the upper quadrant of a half-field was represented anteriorly, and the lower quadrant posteriorly. In so-called 'crossed-amblyopia' there was a dimness of sight in the opposite eye with field constriction. This possibly arose from lesions involving 'a higher visual centre', near where Ferrier had visualized it in the angular gyrus. Loss of recognition of words and objects may occur from such lesions, without loss of sight.

Deafness from a lesion of the first temporal convolution was usually temporary; each auditory nerve must be connected with both hemispheres.

In dealing with speech (pp. 101–16) Gowers joined the band of Head's 'Diagram Makers', headed by his colleague at University College, Bastian (1837–1915), famous for the diagram which showed how different word centres were interconnected by subcortical paths. What Head[290] later described as 'Chaos', in a chapter heading of his book on *Aphasia*, was almost certainly not what one of Gowers's students would have felt. Looking back, it may have been too simplified, but it must have been a godsend. Not that Gowers did not appreciate the difficulties of understanding what was involved in the cortical representation of speech. 'The subject abounded in difficulty', he said; there was 'an abundance of theory ... and precise knowledge was scanty'. He also commented on 'how much deficiency of fact a clear diagram may hide'.

Gowers adopted the terms proposed by Wernicke in 1881 – motor aphasia, sensory aphasia, conduction aphasia, and total aphasia. The terms 'agraphia', 'alexia', 'word-deafness', and 'word-blindness' were used and explained. Gowers said that he had only once seen a patient rendered 'absolutely wordless' by a stroke. 'Amnesic aphasia' was not a satisfactory term, as 'there is more than one memory for words'. At the end of his sixteen-page section on aphasia, he added what must be one of the most concise summaries on the history of this subject.

The faculty of language was first attributed to the frontal lobes by Bouillaud, in 1825, and to the left hemisphere, near the island of Reil, by Dax, in 1836. The title of Dax's paper is worth preserving. It was 'Lesions of the Left Half of the Brain coinciding with Loss of Memory of the Signs of Thought'. The function was further limited to the third frontal by Broca in 1861. The localisation of the auditory centre in the first temporal is due to Meynert and Wernicke, and to the latter belongs also the credit of the localisation of word-deafness to this region of the left hemisphere (p. 116). (*Pace* to Gall; 'phrenology' is not indexed.)

The central ganglia. There were considerable differences in the connections of the thalamus and the corpus striatum with the rest of the brain, so their functions were probably fundamentally different. But 'we are still almost entirely in the dark as to the nature of their function' (p. 36). The most important thalamic connections were with the cortex, the optic tracts, and the tegmentum of the crus. There was still much difference of opinion about the extent of its connection with the fillet. 'It was doubtful whether the corpus striatum has any connection with the cortex and the old hypothesis

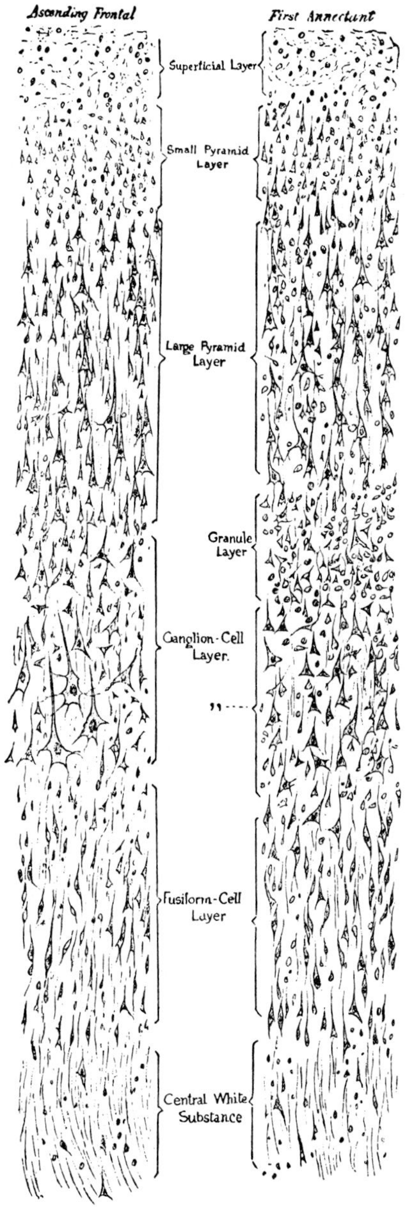

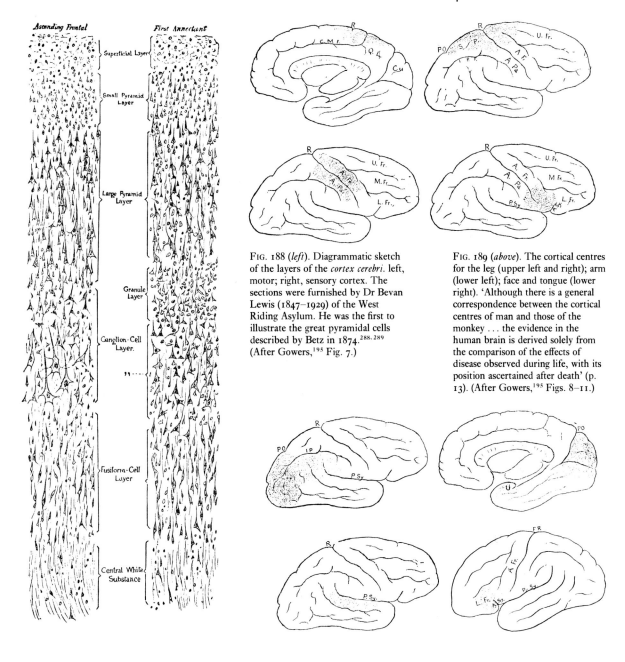

FIG. 188 (*left*). Diagrammatic sketch of the layers of the *cortex cerebri.* left, motor; right, sensory cortex. The sections were furnished by Dr Bevan Lewis (1847–1929) of the West Riding Asylum. He was the first to illustrate the great pyramidal cells described by Betz in 1874.[288, 289] (After Gowers,[195] Fig. 7.)

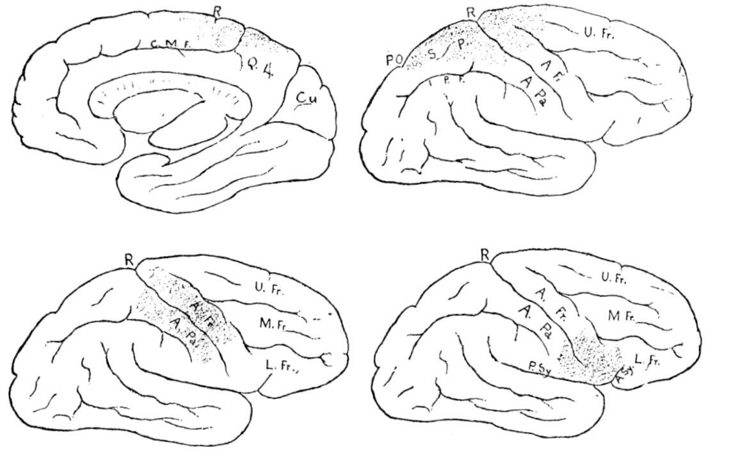

FIG. 189 (*above*). The cortical centres for the leg (upper left and right); arm (lower left); face and tongue (lower right). 'Although there is a general correspondence between the cortical centres of man and those of the monkey . . . the evidence in the human brain is derived solely from the comparison of the effects of disease observed during life, with its position ascertained after death' (p. 13). (After Gowers,[195] Figs. 8–11.)

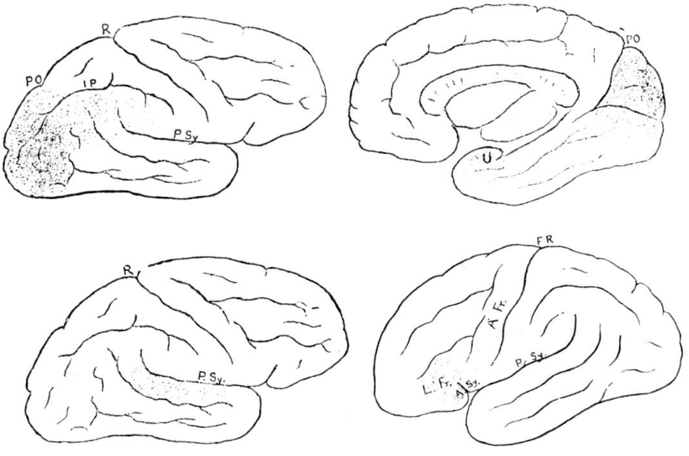

FIG. 190. The cortical centres for vision (upper left and right); hearing (lower left); motor speech (lower right). (After Gowers,[195] Figs. 12, 13, 17, 18.)

that its cells interrupt the fibres which conduct motor impulses seems to be altogether wrong' (p. 37). When the cerebellum was absent the corpus striatum was reduced to a third of its normal size.

As to the corpora quadrigemina, 'we have no direct evidence of the function of these ganglia', but their relations with the optic nerves and oculo-motor muscles, and some experimental data, suggested that they were concerned with the adjustment of ocular movements to visual impressions (p. 38).

The cerebellum. There was a three-layered, uniform cortex with central grey masses but the connections of the fibres in the white matter had been difficult to trace, unaided as they were by secondary degenerations. Some of the fibres of the inferior peduncle coursed to the dentate nucleus and possibly connected it with the olivary body. Others went to the middle lobe, including fibres from the direct cerebellar tract. The fibres of the middle peduncle connected the grey matter of the pons with the cortex of the cerebellar hemisphere. Most of those from the superior peduncle radiated widely, some crossing the mid-line. Cerebellar function had long been a source of mystery, but now

> There is, however, abundant evidence, experimental and pathological, to show that this part of the brain is in some way connected with the co-ordination of movement, and especially with those muscular actions which maintain the equilibrium of the body. It appears, however, that this function is confined to the middle lobe. (p. 52)

Disease of the hemispheres did not affect this function unless there was compression of the middle lobe. The function of the latter must include a mechanism which 'combined and harmonised' centripetal impulses from the limbs, trunk, eyes, and ears. But the function of the hemisphere was still 'mysterious'. They lessened in size as you descended the scale of animals, until they disappeared in birds, where there was only the middle lobe. Connections were with those parts of the cortex 'which subserved psychical processes'. There were no recognizable features associated with loss of the cerebellar hemispheres. It was thus possible that 'the old theory' which related them to 'psychical processes' might be correct (p. 53).

The symptoms of brain disease. It was not so much the pathological character of the lesion, but its seat, and the effect on the neural elements, which determined the symptoms. Function was disturbed, subjectively or objectively; it was 'impaired' or 'increased', sometimes both. Increased action was sometimes the effect of 'irritation', at other times, of 'inhibition'. Destruction, compression, inflammation, arrest of blood supply, or 'wasting of nerve elements' were the five most important forms of structural damage. The effects could be focal or diffuse, or both.

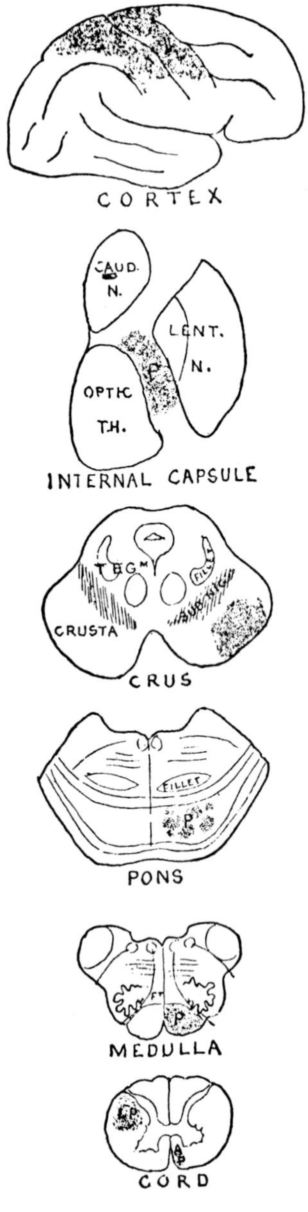

Fig. 191. Diagram of the course of the pyramidal tract of the right hemisphere. 'Our knowledge of the course of the motor path is more complete than any other set of fibres' (p. 25). (After Gowers,[195] Fig. 21.)

The commonest motor symptoms were *hemiplegia* and *convulsions.* Cortical lesions could cause more discrete paralysis than elsewhere in the brain. 'Movements are represented exclusively in the opposite hemisphere in proportion as they are unilateral, in both hemispheres in proportion as they are bilateral' (p. 69). The connection between the hemisphere and the muscles of the same side was not yet known. Bilateral degeneration in the lateral columns can occur with a unilateral cerebral lesion. Certain movements toward one side may be produced by the action of muscles situated on both sides – as in turning of the head or eyes. As 'conjugate deviation of the eyes' was usually transient in hemiplegia, two facts could be deduced. First, that 'movements, rather than muscles, are represented in the cerebral hemispheres and are lost in disease'. Second, that lateral movements by muscles of both sides are represented in both hemispheres, but that in a normal state they are chiefly effected by the opposite

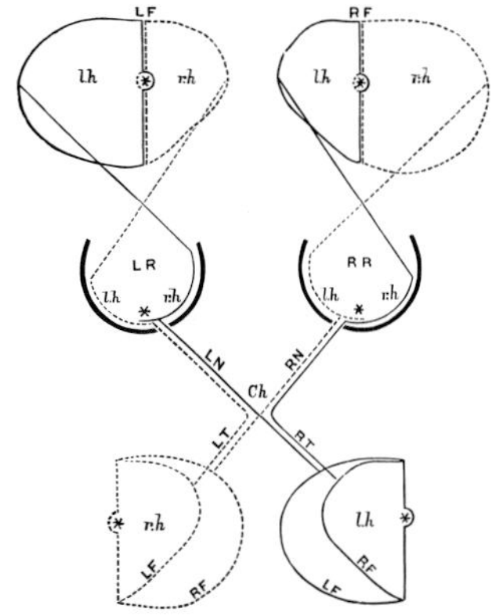

FIG. 192. Diagram of the relation of the fields of vision, retina, and optic tracts. The asterisk is at the macula lutea. Below the optic tracts are the superimposed halves of the fields from which impression pass by each optic tract. (After Gowers,[195] Fig. 41.)

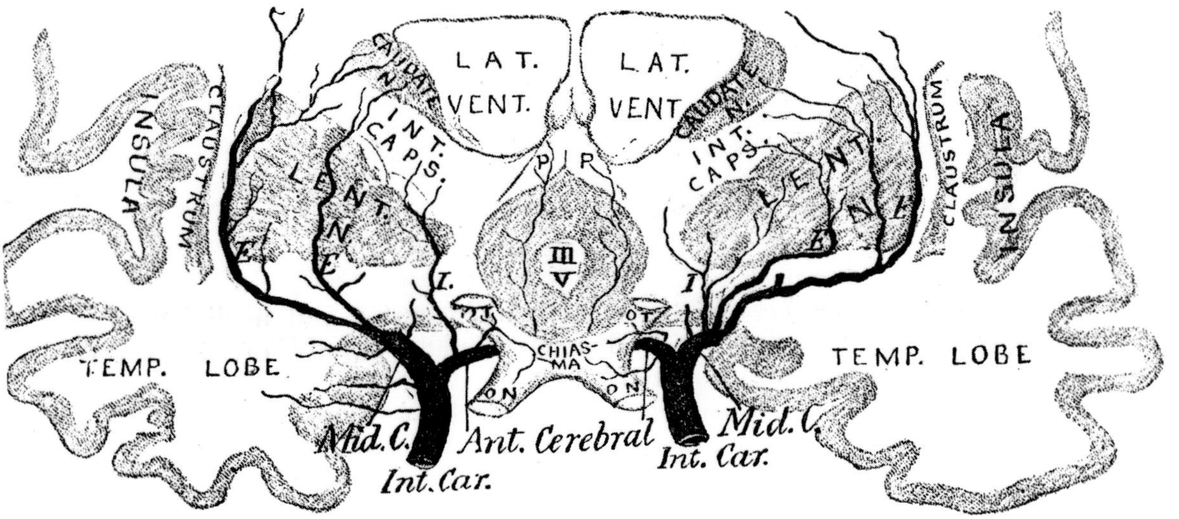

FIG. 193. Diagram of the blood supply to the central ganglia by the lenticulo-striate arteries.

hemisphere. Previously existing, but unused, mechanisms come into action in unilateral disease, so that an effect may be temporary.

Gowers showed with photographs the difference between the voluntary and emotional movements of the face after hemiplegia, and although the upper half of the face was usually little affected, sometimes, for a time, the eye on the palsied side cannot be closed. The varieties of hemiplegia depended on the differences in the seat of the lesion. In addition to complete hemiplegia the common partial varieties were brachial, crural, and brachio-facial monoplegias. Another variety was determined by the level of the lesion in the motor pathway. The face escapes in a medullary lesion; with a lesion in the lower pons the face is affected, on the side of the lesion, while one in the upper pons affects the other side. In the crus, there may be a unilateral third nerve palsy.

Post-hemiplegic rigidity, of the early and late varieties, first described by Todd, evidently depended 'on the over-action of the spinal centres' that were normally concerned with 'tone'. A knee jerk may be lost for a few days after a stroke.

Gowers classified post-hemiplegic disorders of movement according to whether they were fine or coarse, quick or slow, rhythmic or jerky, and continuous or irregular. Little was known of their pathological basis but he observed two points. First, they were far more frequent after cerebral softening from vascular occlusion than after haemorrhage. Second, they were much more common after hemiplegia in infancy or childhood than when it occurred in adult life. In the latter the lesion was usually in or near the thalamus or in the posterior part of the internal capsule. But a lesion limited to the cortex could also give rise to these movements.

'The great characteristic of the *convulsions* of organic brain disease is their local commencement' (p. 86). Not that it did not occur in idiopathic epilepsy, but on the whole, a visceral aura *suggested* idiopathic, and local

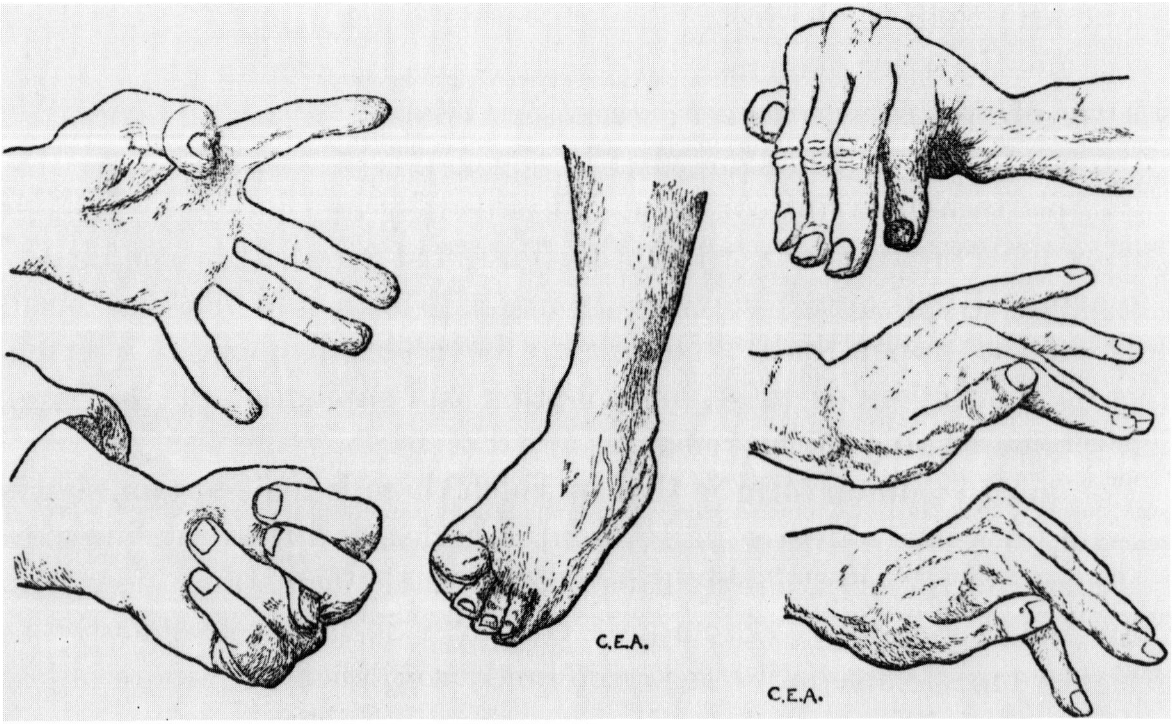

FIG. 194. Post-hemiplegic mobile spasm (athetosis). Left: four months after hemiplegia; right; six years. Centre: same case as on left; 'the foot was habitually inverted, and the great toe often over-extended'.

commencement *suggested* epilepsy from an organic lesion. As in hemiplegia, the bilateral representation of certain muscles had clinical effects, permitting their escape in one case and ensuring their involvement in the other. The spread of a local fit may be to bilaterally innervated muscles, such as the thoracic, before it involved those of an opposite limb. And, as also in hemiplegia, there were muscles on the two sides that could be involved in a convulsion, which, together, normally had a unilateral action. The muscles of the head and eyes, in a unilateral convulsion, usually turned them to the side of the convulsion. When the convulsion spreads to the opposite side, and is subsiding on the first side, the head and eyes may then turn to the second side.

In idiopathic epilepsy special sense aurae were commoner than in symptomatic epilepsy, but in the latter they were then of localizing significance.

Sensory loss and *sensory irritation* of unilateral distribution were less common than motor symptoms. Sensory loss from a cortical lesion was rarely extensive, but from a capsular lesion it could be quite marked. Although sensory fibres probably went to the thalamus, and possibly also to the lenticular nucleus, it was unlikely that their activity influenced consciousness, or that their disease caused any loss of sensation.

Appreciation of posture and the ability to recognize the nature of objects when the eyes were closed may be impaired, despite normal tactile sense. Gowers had encountered this both in cortical and deep lesions of the hemisphere. Typically, sensory loss mainly affected only the extremities of limbs, and were often associated with tingling and formication. Pain in hemiplegic limbs also occurred and in one case of hemiparesis it was severe, persisting for years, and associated with hemianopia; there was 'little loss of cutaneous sensibility'. Gowers envisaged the lesion to be in the posterior extremity of the internal capsule. When Dejerine (1849–1917) and Roussy (1874–1948)[300] came to identify the thalamic syndrome in 1906, one of their three patients had a hemianopia, and the posterior portion of the internal capsule was involved in all three. The thalamic portion of the syndrome in Gowers's patient was not suspected (p. 88).

In analysing the source of the *headache* of intracranial disease, and the role of the meninges and brain substance, he said 'It should be remembered that the normal sensibility of the peritoneum would not prepare us for the intense pain of peritonitis' (p. 90). As for the *mental symptoms*, he said, 'With the much disputed question of the relation of mind to brain the physician has nothing to do' (p. 91). Psychology had already given him terms that were unsatisfactory. The physician knew that it was 'cerebral processes' and not 'mental processes' which mattered. 'Consciousness' and its loss, 'memory' and its loss were terms he also discussed. Like Jackson, he did not think there was any 'special faculty of memory'. The retrograde amnesia of concussion had not been studied but he mentioned a published case in which there was a progressive and complete shrinking of a three-day retrograde amnesia (p. 100).

In *apoplexy* (p. 92), loss of consciousness could not be due to pressure, because it could follow laceration, or embolism. It was a consequence of the 'suddenness of the lesion'.

The cranial nerves. The 150 pages devoted to disorders of the cranial nerves was probably the best of its day. (In my copy there still remains a sheet of notepaper, dated 'November 22, 1893, Moorfields', on which, in elegant, small script, someone described the symptoms, signs, and analysis, with a diagram showing the disposition of the images, red and white, of a candle, in a case of left external rectus palsy.) I have little doubt that even a 'one-off' such exercise today would be more valuable to a student than many textual descriptions.

The optic nerve. In addition to ophthalmoscopy, and tests for acuity and colour vision, Gowers used the perimeter and published many examples of typical field defects. The Bjerrum type of screen came later. He asked why do more fibres cross to the opposite optic tract than pass to the tract of the same side? He explained that the prominence of the nose reduced the *functional* size of the temporal half of the retina, so that fewer fibres would emerge from it – and they did not cross. He used the method now termed 'confrontation' but did not employ the many-sized and coloured hat-pins at his disposal, now cherished by many, but white and coloured paper squares, of side one-third of an inch, on pen-holders. Reflex closure or non-closure of the eyes on lateral threat was used.

He knew that in hemianopia the patient might be unaware of his visual

FIG. 195. Paralysis of left external rectus. Coloured glass over the right eye. Primary deviation on looking toward an object (O) on the left. Position of double images. Secondary deviation of the right eye when the screen (S), obstructing the fixation of * by this eye, compels fixation by the weak muscle. When the screen is removed, the right eye, in fixing, moves back to the position of the dotted outline of the cornea. (After Gowers,[195] Fig. 86.)

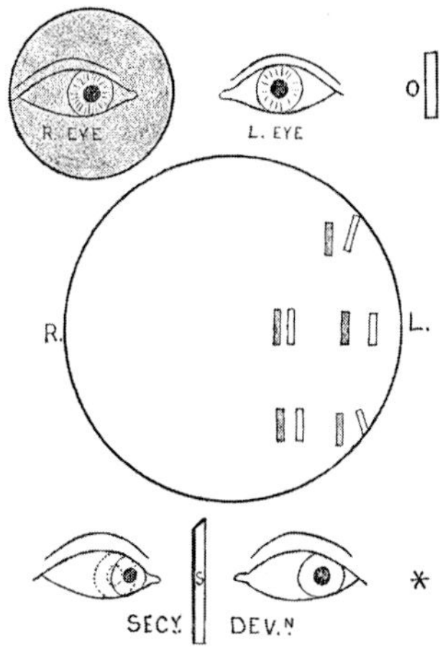

defect and mentioned one patient in whom the loss was only discovered by the nurse who noticed that he never ate his potatoes, which were always placed on one side of the plate. At that time it was not known that all the optic tract fibres concerned in vision terminated in the lateral geniculate bodies. Gowers regarded the pulvinar of the thalamus as the 'intermediate visual centre' (p. 50). Unawareness of hemianopia could not therefore imply its suprageniculate nature.

Whether or not there was sparing or inclusion of the fixation point did not depend on the position of the lesion; it could occur in those of the tract, thalamus, or hemisphere and in homonymous and bitemporal hemianopia. He thought it depended on individual variations in the decussation of the nerves. The 'vertical' meridian was not always vertical and the line was not always sharp. In partial hemianopia, lower quadrants seemed to be lost more frequently than the upper. Quadrantic defects were rare in tract lesions. The significance of what we call 'congruous' and 'incongruous' effects was not established. Altitudinal hemianopia, but not so-named, was 'very rare'. Gowers mentioned a case report, but its anatomical basis had yet to be explained.

Varieties of visual disorientation were beginning to be described, and Gowers referred to Munk's term of 'mind-blindness', in which visual memory appeared to be lost, especially for faces and places. Inattention hemianopia and defective localization in a half-field were not mentioned by Gowers. The parieto-occipital regions were coming under suspicion – an area, Gowers noted, which 'exceeds in size the whole brain of the monkey'.

FIG. 196. Partial paralysis of left third nerve. Defective movement upward from weakness of the superior rectus, and downward from weakness of the inferior rectus (After Gowers,[195] Fig. 91)

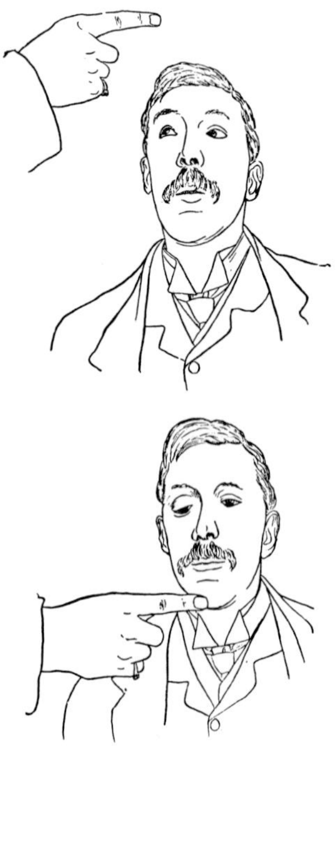

Ocular palsies. There were five signs here (p. 159): limitation of movement, squint, secondary deviation of the normal eye, erroneous projection, and diplopia – an outline still standard. There were accompanying sketches and diagrams (see Figs. 195 and 196). He commented on the difficulty of detecting a fourth nerve palsy. Paralyses of conjugate deviation, upward, downward, and laterally, were described. Upward gaze in one of his published cases was subsequently found to be due to a small mid-line quadrigeminal tumour. In paralysis of lateral conjugate deviation, the internal rectus may still contract during convergence. Two good diagrams (Figs. 94 and 95 in his text) accompany his explanations.

Nuclear ophthalmoplegias were acute or chronic. Hutchinson (1828–1913) had introduced the terms 'external' and 'internal'. Gowers thought Wernicke's term of 'acute polio-encephalitis superior' to denote his cases, in contradistinction to a similar affection of the bulbar nuclei which had been termed 'polio-encephalitis inferior', quite inaccurate. He had no comment to make on the possible aetiology of Wernicke's three cases. He wondered whether acute multiple neuritis ever involved the ocular nerves in other cases. Syphilis was the main suspicion in most cases but in the chronic variety there were patients who went for many years without developing further lesions. He did not query the possibility of ocular myopathy.

There were cases in which 'the weakness may be less in the morning than in the evening' (p. 184) and in many chronic cases the diplopia subsided.

When the internal ocular muscles remained unaffected, the nerve trunks could not be the seat in bilateral cases. Although he had previously mentioned 'reflex ocular fixation' he did not consider the possibility of 'pseudo-ophthalmoplegia' or supra-nuclear palsy. The one case he described of ophthalmoplegia, in which there was ocular nuclear degeneration resembling that seen in progressive muscular atrophy, was a syphilitic one, who also had optic atrophy, mental change and limb weakness. The passing of neurosyphilis, the recognition of myasthenia, and the advent of ocular myopathy are developments which have made a diagnosis of primary nuclear ophthalmoplegia nowadays highly suspect and rare.

Nystagmus. There were four varieties (p. 193): eye disease from early life; in albinism; in miners; and in diseases of the nervous system 'of the most varied seat and character'. It was seen in disseminated sclerosis, cerebellar tumour, and 'in many diseases of the brain, diffuse and focal', and also in diffuse degeneration of the cord. It was usually horizontal, rotatory, or vertical – and bilateral, also usually rhythmical and regular, but alternate movements could be quick and slow. No visual disturbance resulted when it dated from infancy, and usually in adults it was not accompanied by any sensation of the movement of objects.

It was difficult to explain. Its bilateral symmetry suggested a central origin. It could be induced by rotation of the body. He did not mention its occurrence in railway passengers. But pressure on the ear in otitis had caused it: therapeutic irrigation of the ears is not mentioned; investigative irrigation of labyrinthine function came later, with Barany (1876–1936). But it was associated with vertigo so that the semicircular canals were involved in the mechanisms. 'The wide variation in the position of organic disease that may cause nystagmus is scarcely surprising when we consider how wide and various must be the total connections of the functions of vision, of movement of the eyes, and of the maintenance of equilibrium; and that we can trace a connection between nystagmus and these' (p. 196). In a footnote on page 195 he mentions a cerebellar case with ocular and pharyngo-laryngeal nystagmus. 'The rate of movement was the same as in the ocular muscles, 180 per minute'.

The practical value of nystagmus, Gowers concluded, was not that it possessed localizing value, but that it so often appeared quite early in degenerative diseases of the nervous system.

Gowers expertly forged ahead with the remaining cranial nerves, describing in detail and explaining with clarity the various symptoms and signs which followed their involvement in disease. One can only choose a few samples to illustrate his approach.

The trigeminal. In four pages on taste he analysed the evidence concerning its pathway and concluded that 'the fibres that reach the facial by the chorda tympani must leave the nerve again, and the opinion is probably correct which assumes that they pass from the geniculate ganglion of the facial, by the Vidian nerve, to the sphenopalatine ganglion. Thus again reaching the fifth nerve, they seem to ascend in the second division to its root and the brain' (p. 210). He used electrical stimulation of the tongue in testing taste.

Serial clonic spasms of the jaw may be an isolated disability, chronic and often nocturnal. I have seen this as the sole manifestation for up to twenty years in adults who finally had a generalized convulsion.

The facial. Here he takes up twenty-five pages, half of which are used in a model account of facial palsy, based on his own notes of 100 cases. 'The two sides of the face present a strange incongruity, and the smile or frown, deprived of half its range, loses more than half its character, so that it is difficult to recognise the expressional difference of the distorting contractions of cheek and brow which occur on the unaffected side' (p. 217). In the young, the altered appearance may be slight, 'but it is otherwise when time has scored the face with furrows'. The sense of smell may appear to be impaired on the affected side when the nostril fails to expand, and actually narrows, on sniffing. Some return of power to orbicularis oris may merely be due to its being a circular muscle with innervation which could cross the mid-line.

The auditory. 'Exact aural diagnosis stops at the middle ear, and its present state resembles that of the diagnosis of affections of the eye before the invention of the ophthalmoscope' (p. 238). He complained that the term 'nervous deafness' was no better than 'amaurosis'. As yet the distinction between deafness from lesions of nerve and labyrinthine could not be made. The meatus should be inspected; an ophthalmoscope, with a three-inch lens and speculum, enabled one to see the ear drum. He used the tuning fork and assumed that the vibrations passed directly from bone to labyrinth. If it could not be heard longer through the air than through the bone there was impaired conduction through the meatus or middle ear. (Humour rarely peeps through but he allowed himself to comment that if a stethoscope is applied to one meatus, sounds entering the other ear can be distinctly heard; giving truth to the old adage 'in one ear and out the other'). 'If a watch is heard through bone, it is not likely that the tuning fork will reveal impairment'. Tinnitus should not be confused with the murmur from an intracranial aneurysm; the latter could also be heard through a stethoscope. He found nothing wrong with a lady who for twenty years had heard 'the sound of music'. Clonic spasms of palate, face, or near the Eustachian tube may produce audible clicking sounds.

The vagus. 'In excision of an enlarged thyroid, both recurrent laryngeals have been repeatedly divided, from the time of Galen down to the present' (p. 253).

The laryngeal muscles must act in very complex combinations, for 'The different fibres of each muscle have not all the same direction and cannot have the same action' (p. 258). The actions may be simple in opening and closing the glottis but not in producing 'the infinite variety of vocal sounds'. 'Spastic dysphonia', spasm excited by attempts to speak, a recently introduced German term, had been allied to 'writer's cramp'. A patient who had suffered from the latter developed laryngeal spasms on learning to play the flute at the age of fifty. Gowers was usually pretty critical of many modes of therapy but he had found that laryngeal spasms could often be relieved by a 'necklet of ice'; the ice was enclosed in 'tube of gutta-percha tissue, the edges being stuck together by means of chloroform' (p. 272).

The hypoglossal. 'In paralysis of one hypoglossal nerve the tongue at rest is in its normal position in the mouth, but its root is higher on the paralysed side than on the unparalysed side, in consequence of the loss of the tonic contraction of the posterior fibres of the hyoglossus' (p. 275). Isolated protrusor spasms of the tongue affected some individuals (non-iatrogenic!). Customarily averse to many newly-minted, pseudo-classical terms, he allowed entry of the word 'aphthongia' (p. 277) which had been coined in connection with spasm of the tongue and muscles attached to the hyoid bone, on attempts at speaking. Strange that he should discourage 'dysphasia' and not forcibly reject this unlovely neologism. The author of *Plain words* would not have liked it.

The localization of cerebral disease

In a dozen pages, before beginning a description of actual diseases of the nervous system, Gowers summarized the main features by which localization of lesions of the brain might be identified. He referred again to the necessary precautions which the physician must keep in mind. An acute lesion often had diffuse effects; so had the effects of pressure, disturbed circulation, irritation, and inhibition.

Cortical lesions. In the *central* region motor and sensory 'spasms' and paresis were the cardinal symptoms 'with local commencement' their chief characteristic. Local paralysis was of more importance than local convulsion, because in the former the centre concerned must be involved, while in the latter the centre may be adjacent. Sensory loss, mainly in the extremities, was usually slight, tactile sensibility being more affected than that of pain. Hemianaesthesia did not occur, but postural loss did, although it was of little localizing value for it occurred in capsular lesions.

Prefrontal. Aphasia, adversive attacks, and foot involvement in upper lesions, occurred, but on the whole the absence of motor and sensory paralysis was the main feature. In some cases, especially in bilateral lesions, there might be 'considerable mental change', 'various in character, but sufficiently frequent to be of some significance'.

Parietal. In the parieto-occipital area there may be no motor or sensory signs. Extensive parietal disease did cause sensory loss but no mention was made of its nature.

Occipital. Hemianopia.

Temporal. Transient deafness, auditory or olfactory aurae.

Subcortical lesions. Convulsions were less common but many lesions involved grey and white matter so that convulsions with symptoms resulting from involvement of communicating and ascending and descending fibre tracts were likely to occur.

Centrum ovale. The symptoms and signs largely depended on how much the lesion approached the cortex and the internal capsule.

Corpus callosum. 'We do not yet know of any symptoms that are the result of the damage to the callosal fibres' (p. 285).

Internal capsule. At the anterior end no definite symptoms were known. At the angle, the motor path for the face and tongue passed; that for the arm in the anterior, and that for the leg in the middle third of the posterior limb of the capsule. Sensory fibres passed in the posterior third of the posterior limb and behind them the optic fibres. But the actual limitations of the palsy in even small lesions was slight.

Corpus striatum. Acute lesions of the caudate of lenticular nuclei were usually accompanied by hemiplegia because of the involvement of the internal capsule. Lesions confined to these nuclei caused no persistent motor or sensory symptoms, but in a few cases of chronic lesions mobile spasm and chorea had been described.

Thalamus. Paresis, mobile spasm, incoordination of the opposite hand might occur but sensation is not impaired. Hemianopia may be found in lesions of the pulvinar.

Corpora quadrigemina. Impairment of vision and loss of pupillary reflex activity; paresis of upward gaze.

Crus cerebri. Hemiplegia involving the lower part of the face, with a third nerve palsy on the side of the lesion.

Pons. Alternate hemiplegia with involvement of the fifth, sixth, and seventh nerves according to its site and extent. Loss of conjugate movement to the side of the lesion. Small pupils in acute lesions.

Medulla. Acute and chronic forms of bulbar palsy.

Cerebellum. Lesions of the middle lobe – a reeling gait, ataxia of the legs (but rarely of the arms). The unsteadiness is not necessarily related to vertigo. A hemisphere lesion *per se* could not be recognized. The knee jerk was sometimes lost or variable, and difficult to obtain. Convulsions were rare. In lesions of the middle cerebellar peduncle, vertigo and forced movements of head or trunk when the patient is lying or standing may be observed. The eyes may not be on the same horizontal plane.

It was with such facts, meagre yet basic, and not dependent on any actual theory, that the scene was set for the dramatic entry of brain surgery. There were still large gaps in this field of cerebral localization and it is not without interest that some of them – the effects of cerebellar lesions, the nature of cortical sensory loss, and the cortical representation of vision – were the subjects of notable contributions by a physician whom Gowers brusquely dismissed when he came looking for a post at the National[301a]. Holmes (1876–1965) actually resembled Gowers in his method of approach and thoroughness, in his talents as a clinician and teacher, and in his literary style. He, too, could be brusque. His rejection of my first submission to *Brain*, of which he was then editor, certainly singed my thalamus.

Intracranial tumours

When he came to deal with these Gowers confessed that with regard to localization, only 'the general region in which the growth is placed may be determined in the majority of instances'. He devoted forty pages to this topic and found that a classification based on the structures in which they originated was of little practical value. He grouped them according to their frequency. Tuberculomata and gummata headed the list; gliomata and carcinoma came next; and parasitic cysts was his last category. There were neuromata, psammomata, cholesteatomata, etc. It must have been a satisfying experience to witness the disappearance of headache, vomiting, optic neuritis, and recent paralytic symptoms after a course of potassium iodide and mercury (p. 490). He did not discuss meningiomas as such, nor the differential diagnosis between infiltration and compression, but he described the involvement of the cranial nerves in basal tumours, illustrated the displacement of the falx, explained the likelihood of internal hydrocephalus when the aqueduct was compressed. Symptoms were therefore general and local.

Mental failure and 'emotional mobility' might nevertheless be the sole signs of a tumour 'in any situation'. Pronounced mental changes were most often seen in tumours of the anterior portion of the frontal lobe. But he warned that errors arise in such forms of presentation. Tumour 'like every other form of brain disease may evoke in predisposed persons the manifestations of hysteria' (p. 472). After reading of how so much was made of hysteria in the female throughout the years, it is good to hear Gowers say of it, in relation to tumour diagnosis, that it was often diagnosed 'without a shadow of excuse, merely because the patient is of the female sex' (p. 486). In a young woman convulsion or paralysis from tumour might excite quite understandable nervous symptoms. Who has not had to be reminded of that at some time or other in his career?

The convulsive attacks of tumour were of four chief forms. Generalized; brief episodes like *petit mal*; focal; and tetanic, as in some cerebellar cases. Focal fits could be very frequent and continue for long periods of time. He had one patient with focal fits beginning in face, arm, or foot on the same side, which occurred at a frequency of 100 to 150 each day for eleven months; '17,000 fits (carefully recorded)' (p. 476).

He was cautious about the prospects for brain surgery. Probably only 'a small proportion' would be suitable; those near the surface, or in an occipital or temporal lobe perhaps. If a tumour in a cerebellar hemisphere could be identified, that, too, might be removed. Whenever there was the remotest suspicion of syphilis, the appropriate treatment should first be tried.

Aneurysms. Gowers distinguished between the miliary aneurysms of Charcot, so important in the aetiology of cerebral haemorrhage, and found on small intracerebral arteries, and the larger ones on the carotid, basilar, and vertebral vessels and their main branches. The second type presented as tumours, but rarely caused convulsion. Before rupture they may or may not have exerted local effects by compression. They were common at all ages.

Paroxysmal headache was one symptom. A murmur was rarely heard. An aneurysm of the internal carotid, within the cavernous sinus, compressed the optic nerve and the nerves in the wall of the sinus. The third nerve suffered earliest, and corneal sensation was impaired. When the aneurysm was on the anterior cerebral artery, the ocular nerves escaped compression, but loss of sight and smell might occur on that side. No identifiable symptoms could be associated with the anterior communicating artery. A third nerve palsy was the characteristic feature of an aneurysm on the posterior communicating artery.

He referred to a published case, with illustration, of a vertebral artery aneurysm which compressed the facial nerve and presented with facial spasm (p. 230). The basilar artery was a common site for aneurysms, and symptoms, if they occurred, were sometimes bilateral, with pressure on the pons, and perhaps the development of hydrocephalus. Occipital headache and giddiness were often prominent.

The difficulties of diagnosis of aneurysm did not cease with life; the haemorrhage which followed rupture often destroyed the evidence of its origin. Spontaneous cures, from clotting, undoubtedly did occur, as signified by the sudden subsidence of headache and skull murmur, with the slow healing of ocular palsy. But the prognosis was grave. Ligation of the common carotid had been successful in some cases, but for basilar aneurysm, the vertebral artery would have to be ligated. And Dr Alexander's ligation of this artery for the treatment of epilepsy was in itself a risky procedure.

In this account of intracranial aneurysms one feels uncertain to what extent it was based on personal experience. At times it appears that he might be analysing the manifestations of the unruptured sac on the basis of its anatomical relations with adjacent nerve structures at the base of the brain. He included a good illustration (p. 499, Fig. 140) of a dissection to show the relation of vessels and nerves. He also analysed the distribution of 154 published cases of aneurysms. Generally speaking, he suspected an aneurysm when there was evidence of 'tumour' located 'in the position of a vessel'. He does not actually cite specific cases of his own, and Symonds[301b] and other earlier writers on the subject of the unruptured aneurysm do not usually mention Gowers. Cushing[301b] said the diagnosis was seldom made before 1923.

Cerebrovascular disorders

'Of all regions of cerebral pathology, that of congestion of the brain is perhaps the most obscure' (p. 341). An extensive symptomatology had been elaborated around the notion of 'congestion', with little foundation. There was 'scarcely any pathological anatomy of congestion of the brain' (p. 344). Perhaps transient symptoms such as 'confusion', 'vague giddiness', 'tingling in the extremities' might be considered as symptoms of congestion. Paroxysms of coughing could induce sudden, brief loss of consciousness, with or without clonic spasms (cough syncope), and throbbing vessels were sometimes seen and felt. But to what degree such symptoms could be attributed to congestion was not precisely known.

Better understood now, Gowers thought, was the sequence of events which lead up to cerebral haemorrhage, and softening from thrombosis and haemorrhage.

There was nothing in the old story of an 'apoplectic build', but age and heredity were obvious factors. The miliary aneurysms on small vessels which Charcot had discovered were due to degeneration of the muscular coat of the vessel. It was not an 'arteritis', although it had been so called by some. Larger vessels were affected by 'atheroma' and had only an indirect connection with haemorrhage. These changes in the small and large vessels might co-exist, but each could be found without the other. Disease of the kidney had been found in about one-third of all cases of cerebral haemorrhage, and whatever the nature of Bright's disease, degeneration of small arteries was a feature and hypertrophy of the heart a common finding.

It was doubtful whether symptoms such as transient vertigo, weakness or tingling in the limbs, mental confusion, or slight affection of speech should be called 'prodromata of haemorrhage'. They could just as well result from atheroma causing 'interference with the blood supply to certain parts of the brain'. Such symptoms were 'indicators, not of the cause of the cerebral haemorrhage, but of an associated condition' (p. 364).

Acute softening of the brain resulted from arterial occlusion by thrombosis or embolism. The source of an embolus 'must be somewhere between the lungs and the brain – in the pulmonary veins, the left side of the heart, the commencement of the aorta, or the large arteries of the neck' (p. 388). He cited the well-known sources in valvular disease, but he did not actually say whether he had ever seen occlusive disease in the carotid or vertebral arteries in the neck. The characteristic distribution of atheromatous plaques in the intracranial carotid and vertebro-basilar systems was well recognized. Syphilitic arteritis was common.

As in the case of cerebral haemorrhage, premonitory symptoms in embolism were 'not true prodromata', but consist of slighter attacks of the same character, due to the obstruction of small vessels by small emboli' (p. 398). Such symptoms were more common in cerebral thrombosis.

The role of raised blood pressure was not yet established, though it was suspected. The instrument for measuring it did not exist, but disease of the great arteries of the neck could have been disclosed by dissection.

Disseminated or insular sclerosis

Charcot had described 'Sclerose en Plaques Disseminées' over twenty years before; in Germany it was called 'Multiple Sclerosis'. The term 'Insular' had been proposed, said Gowers, by Dr Moxon, 'who first described the disease in this country'. Gowers said that 'little can be added to the description given by Charcot'. What was so striking about the clinical features was the frequency of nystagmus, the peculiar 'scanning' speech, the 'jerky incoordination' of the arms in a patient, who, although gravely disabled, often remained 'happy and cheerful'. Then, there was the varying course, sometimes progressive and fatal within a year or so, and at other times chronic or remitting. Lastly, the lesions themselves were quite distinctive – 'islets of sclerosis', mainly in the white matter of the brain and spinal cord. As Charcot had shown, despite the disintegration of the myelin sheaths, the axis cylinders often persisted for some time. Secondary degeneration did not develop if they were preserved.

The peculiar 'jerky irregularity' of voluntary movements had suggested to Charcot that it might be due to 'irregular resistance to conduction in the nerve-fibres at sclerosed spots', but Erb and others believed it must be due to the particular location of certain islets, which interfered with coordinating mechanisms.

In Gowers's experience the duration varied between two and fifteen years. In some cases of optic atrophy there was no clinical or ophthalmoscopic evidence of a prior neuritis. It appeared to be a primary atrophy, like that in tabes. In other cases the posterior columns appeared to suffer exclusively. And was the disease related in any way to those forms of 'subacute myelitis' in which the brain was not affected, and which did not recur? Such observations led him to suggest that the disease 'seems to occupy an intermediate position between the subacute and syphilitic inflammations, on the one hand, and the system-scleroses on the other'.

Diffuse sclerosis. Under this title (p. 519) Gowers said there were patients, usually children, with 'simple mental defect', in whom at autopsy there was a 'primary' sclerosis of certain regions of the brain. Sometimes it affected a whole hemisphere. It might be limited to the cortex and subjacent white matter or involve only a part of the white substance. He had seen one adult case. He doubted whether it could be recognized during life but it sounds as if it could be grouped with that type of demyelinating disorder Schilder (1886–1940) described in 1912.

Miliary sclerosis. Gowers used this term, which he acknowledged was not accurate, to report a case of a man of fifty who died after an illness of ten weeks in which there was progressive paralysis and rigidity, a few convulsions, unintelligible speech, and coma. Throughout both hemispheres and mainly at the junction of the cortical grey and white matter, but also in the central grey matter, there were 'minute reddish-grey spots'. There were none in the white matter. He drew them (p. 521, Fig. 142) and said he had not heard of any similar case. It may have been an example of subacute spongioform encephalopathy.

General and functional diseases (Part V)

Tetanoid chorea. If the two preceding disorders are questionably recognizable, it is certainly not so with what he called 'tetanoid chorea'. Kinnier Wilson[302] wrote of hepato-lenticular degeneration, which he described in 1912, that in his textbook Gowers reported 'the cases of a brother and sister under the title "Tetanoid Chorea, Associated with Cirrhosis of the Liver"'. Gowers's clinical description of the one case he saw was certainly characteristic of Wilson's disease. But he did not see the second case, a brother not a sister, and at autopsy made no mention of the liver, or any other organ for that matter, either in his title or text in his book. He said he had not been able to find any record of a similar case and described it as follows.

The patient was a boy aged ten. A brother was said to have died from some affection similar to that from which this child was suffering. There was a history of three other relations having suffered from maladies resembling chorea. In the patient the symptoms commenced gradually, seven months before death. They consisted of tonic spasm, which was continuous, and varied by paroxysmal attacks of similar, but more intense spasm. The face was involved on both sides, so as to cause a constant peculiar smile. The tongue was pressed back against the palate in such a manner as to impede swallowing and prevent speech. The arms were extended, pronated, and rotated inwards, so as to bring the back of the forearm outwards, while the fingers were generally slightly flexed at all joints, but at times were extended, and slowly moved in the irregular way characteristic of athetosis. The legs were extended at all the joints, the feet being over-extended in talipes equino-varus, and the toes were flexed. At times the spasm at the hip became flexor, so that the extended legs were raised off the bed. The muscles of the trunk were also involved in the spasm. At first, the left side was the more severely affected, but afterwards the spasm became equal on the two sides. The electric irritability of the muscles was normal, and there was no mechanical excitability of the nerves. There

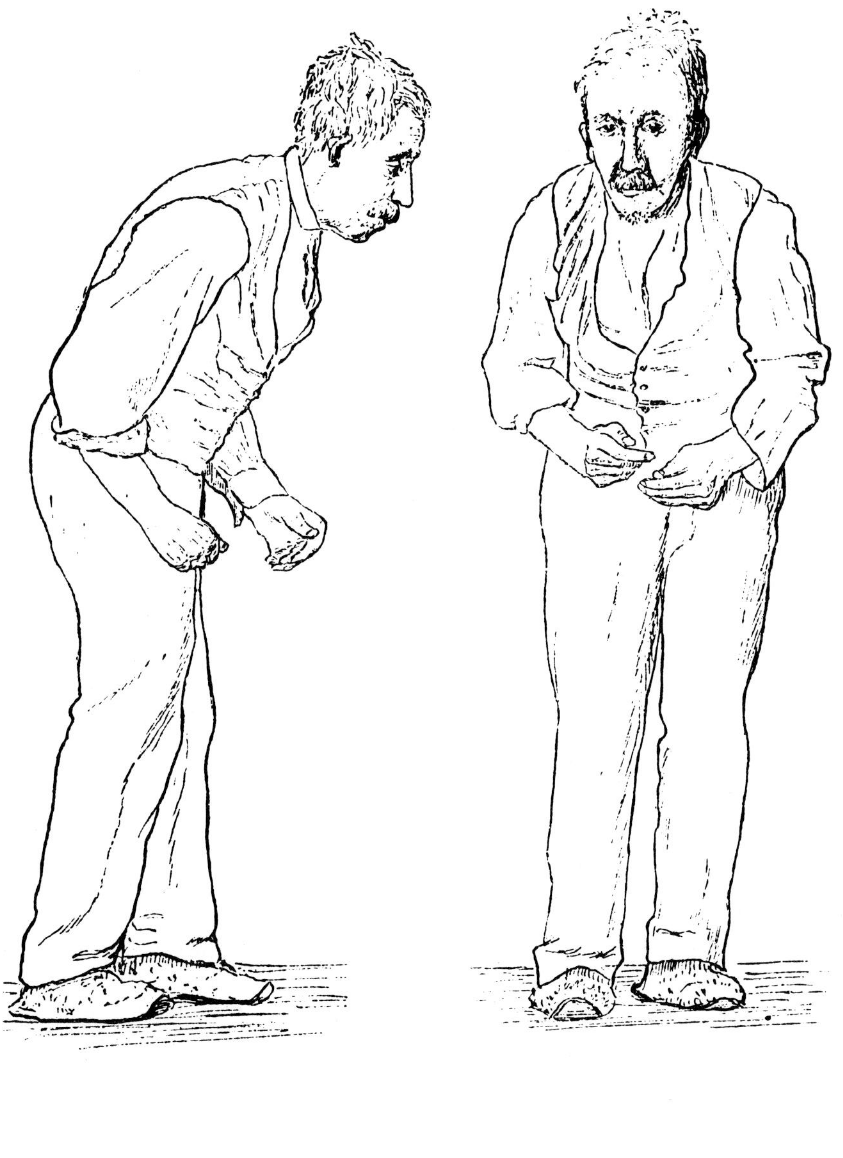

FIG. 197. Paralysis agitans. The 'movement of the fingers at the metacarpo-phalangeal joints is similar to that by which Orientals beat their small drums' (p. 593). (After Gowers,[195] Fig. 145.)

was considerable pyrexia during the more severe stage of the disease. The boy steadily emaciated, and died from exhaustion. The whole central nervous system appeared normal to the naked eye, and no distinct morbid appearances could be discovered on microscopical examination (Vol. 2, p. 656).

Experience in later years led Gowers to associate tetanoid chorea with cirrhosis of the liver.[303] The boy's liver had actually been 'hard, lobular, light in colour' but its cirrhotic nature had not been recognized. A sister also developed the disease and proved to have cirrhosis but there was no microscopical examination.

The original account of tetanoid chorea occupied less than a page in that section of the book, of some one hundred pages, in which he dealt with diseases in which there were involuntary movements of one kind or another. Familiar ones, such as *chorea*, *paralysis agitans*, and *spasmodic*, *torticollis*, and rare ones such as *Dubini's electric chorea*, *myocionus multiplex*, and *saltatoric spasm*. The description of *paralysis agitans*, as expected, is excellent and his sketch of a patient (Fig. 197) is, in my opinion, superior to that of Richer's in Charcot's *Iconographie*. He used myograph tracings to study tremors of various kinds. He mentioned the recently (1872) recorded cases of *hereditary chorea* described by Huntington, in Long Island, noting that there was an account of an affected family in England in 1887. He did not say whether he had actually seen the disorder.

Myoclonus of various types were described, with their typical 'shock-like muscular contractions' – epidemic in Lombardy, sporadic in England. Some, no doubt, a manifestation of subacute encephalitis or encephalopathy. In some of his cases of *spasmodic torticollis* the disorder spread to the trunk and limbs as in the disorder which later came to be called *dystonia musculorum deformans* by Oppenheim (1858–1919).

The humble clerk is a familiar figure in the literature of that time, working long hours over his ledgers, in ill-lit draughty offices, and with his mittened hands holding the new steel pen. He must have experienced many complaints, but none was more tormenting than 'writer's cramp' to which Gowers devoted some twenty pages. The coming of the typewriter, the features of the different varieties of which he discussed, has more or less banished the disorder, but I have included a couple of pages in facsimile of his account, because of its interest. Described by one reviewer of his *Manual* as 'unsatisfactory' and by a modern authority as 'a masterpiece'[304] it still makes enjoyable reading. Like many of his other clinical descriptions it was based on a close analysis of a stated number of cases, his own and those of others. Thus, in writer's cramp, 135 cases; in epilepsy, 1450 cases; in Menière's disease, 106 cases.

In the chapter on epilepsy he summarized his book of 1881, concluding that it was unquestionably a disease of the grey matter of the brain, especially of the cortex. Of the '*nature* of the change in the grey matter' it was necessary to remember that we had direct evidence only of the *liberation* of energy. Within nerve cells there must be a capacity for restraint as well as for action, and in epilepsy we were probably seeing the consequences of 'instability' between these functions. 'The view that it is the resistance

SYMPTOMS. 663

the two last fingers of the right. For a time these devices give a little help, but the spasm gradually increases in degree, and overcomes the fixing help, or it spreads to the muscles of the upper arm.

Although the onset is gradual in almost all cases, in very rare instances the affection comes on in an acute manner. In the cases of this character, pain has generally been a permanent symptom, and some slight symptoms have usually preceded the acute onset. One patient, who had noticed a slight " crampy " feeling in his fingers after writing for a long time, one day wrote rapidly for several hours and then the hand suddenly became so stiff that he could scarcely move it. He gave up, but next day was no better, and when I saw him, ten days later, he could only write two words, and that with extreme slowness and effort, and the attempt caused much pain. Another patient, who had been conscious for some time of a little more fatigue in writing than was usual, sat down one day to write a number of letters on a subject that vexed her much. After writing for about two hours, she felt a sudden pain around the wrist, passing down to the knuckles, and up the forearm to the elbow. The hand then slowly closed in spasm. She forced the fingers back and went on writing for a short time with much pain and difficulty. Subsequently, for some years, as soon as she attempted to write, the same pain came on, followed by spasm. Other acts, after a time, also excited the pain, although much less readily than writing.

The spasm is almost always tonic in character; and, although it may now and then be varied by a slight start or jerk, there is very seldom actual clonic spasm. I have only seen one case with such clonic spasm; in this, as soon as the patient attempted to write, the first finger and thumb became flexed at all joints by clonic spasm, and slipped off the pen. The affection had existed for five years, and was at first limited to writing; afterwards any action in which the fingers were flexed would bring on the spasm. But tonic spasm is often accompanied by some tremor, and occasionally the tremor is the most conspicuous symptom. The letters are "shaky" and the lines are varied here and there by angular zigzags. As soon as the attempt to write is relinquished, the tremor usually ceases. It is rare to meet with tremor only; in most cases spasm is associated with it; there may be at first simple spasm and afterwards some tremor in addition, or tremor may at first occur alone and afterwards tonic spasm as well as tremor. Occasionally, in old standing cases, there is slight tremor in the hand when the patient is not writing, and when this is the case there is often some tremor in the left hand as well as in the right.

The spasm may be limited to the act of writing, and other actions, even such as involve delicate muscular co-ordination, may be performed without the slightest difficulty. It is not uncommon, for instance, for the patient to be able to shave himself or to play the piano with perfect facility. In slight cases the spasm may be limited even to the act of

664 WRITERS' CRAMP.

difficulty.* I have known a patient to be able to paint without difficulty, although he could scarcely write. A still more curious limitation has been observed; printing characters could be traced with a pen, although an attempt to write in the ordinary manner at once brought on spasm.

But absolute limitation to the act of writing is seldom met with, except in cases of very slight degree. In most severe cases the patient experiences some difficulty in actions requiring delicate co-ordination of the same muscles. One patient, for instance, had no difficulty in any other action except in shaving himself. Another, at the end of twelve years, could do everything except draw and scratch out with a penknife. The extent to which the spasm spreads to other actions thus varies much in different cases. It is greatest in cases in which flexor spasm predominates. Occasionally, in such cases, the spasm comes on when any action is attempted, and I have known one case in which spasm, at first confined to the act of writing, ultimately not only extended to all other actions but became spontaneous, so that when the hand was at rest the fingers and wrist gradually became flexed.

Power in the hand may be quite unimpaired. Sometimes the grasp is a little weaker than it should be, and it is not uncommon, as Poore has pointed out, to find definite slight weakness of certain muscles of the hand. Occasionally there is considerable loss of power and inability to sustain effort. There may in rare cases be slight wasting of certain muscles, but this is altogether exceptional in cases of true writers' cramp.

The electric irritability of the nerves and muscles may be perfectly normal, or may present, a slight change, increase or diminution, chiefly in cases that have lasted for some time. The change is usually the same to faradaism and voltaism, and the degree of irritability is similar in both muscles and nerves. It is often found in all the nerves which are accessible to examination. It is thus to be regarded as a primary change in nerve irritability, not of muscle irritability; the change in the irritability of the muscles depends on the motor nerve-endings they contain.† It may be remembered that all three nerves of the arm, radial (musculo-spiral), ulnar, and median, supply muscles employed in writing. Several cases I have seen show that increased irritability is the earlier change of the two and that the diminution of irritability succeeds it.

Sensory symptoms are seldom entirely absent, and are often very prominent. The tonic spasm is accompanied by a painful sense of fatigue in the muscles, and by definite, dull pain, often referred to the

* Partly because he can press more firmly on the pencil, and thus steady the hand (see Poore, 'Med.-Chir. Trans.,' vol. lxi, p. 127).

† At the same time it would be wrong to lay much weight on this consideration, because it is possible that an abnormal irritability of the muscular fibres may cause them to respond more readily to a given stimulation of the nerve-fibres. We can only judge of the stimulation of the motor nerves by the effect on the muscular fibres. It is, however, customary to regard a change in muscular effect of stimulation of the nerves as evidence of a change in the nerve-fibres themselves.

FIG. 198. Writer's cramp; text of pages 663–4. (After Gowers.[195])

which is unstable, enables us to understand the phenomena of inhibition which sometimes occur as part of the attack' (p. 700). He enlarged his description of the many minor forms of epilepsy, and the ways in which a convulsion may be evoked (e.g. musicogenic) in the second edition of his book on epilepsy, in 1901. And in *The border-land of epilepsy* in 1907 he described the experiences of patients with other episodic disorders such as syncope, migraine, and those which disturbed sleep (including 'sleep paralysis'). In his account of *narcolepsy* in the *Manual*, he mentioned vivid dreams, but not sleep paralysis or cataplexy.

Bromides, introduced in the 1860s, Gowers thought must exert their therapeutic effect in epilepsy, by direct action on nerve cells. It is curious that, like lumbar puncture, and 'local medication of the cord', bromides were first used to reduce sexual desire and the habit of masturbation. The

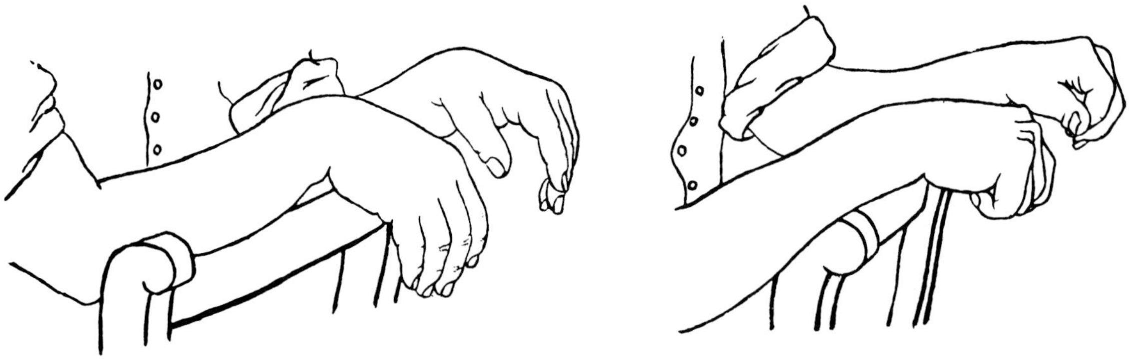

FIG. 199. Wrist-drop from lead poisoning. Left: maximum extension of wrists and fingers. Right: extension by the proper extensors of the wrist when the fingers are flexed. (After Gowers,[195] Figs. 169, 170.)

suggestion came from Sir Charles Locock (1799–1875), physician-accoucher to Queen Victoria.[305] Such factors operating in young women at the time of the menses might excite convulsion.

In the concluding sections of the *Manual* there are accounts of *neuralgia* and *headache* which, although admirable, might be more interesting to the modern reader if, in them, he had unearthed a reference to syndromes which have emerged in recent years. But there is nothing to suggest such afflictions as cluster headache, cranial arteritis, polymyalgia, or polymyositis. 'Neuralgia', of necessity, before radiology, often included various joint lesions and entrapment syndromes, not to mention the effects of metastases in malignant disease. Gowers's account of trigeminal neuralgia is not particularly good; it is more an analysis of the distribution of pain in the three divisions than a picture of such a unique neuralgia.

A modern neurologist might be surprised to find a full account of *exophthalmic goitre* in a textbook of neurology. But that was not uncommon in those days, when the function of the thyroid was not known, and when toxic goitre caused such 'nervous' symptoms as protruding eyes, rapid pulse, tremors, agitation, and sometimes, actual mania. It was often fatal but no lesion in the nervous system could be found (p. 816). Yet 'The paralysis of the ocular muscles sometimes goes on to complete ophthalmoplegia, and is then more than a functional affection; it seems to be due to degeneration of the muscular fibres' (p. 814). As for the thyroid gland itself, extirpation sometimes caused 'mental weakness' so that 'the organ has a mysterious influence on the nervous system, and an opposite influence is at least conceivable, if equally mysterious' (p. 818).

Lastly, there was that old world malady, *hysteria*, of ancient vintage, and a fresh one from the new world, *neurasthenia*. Gowers said that he based his account of hysteria 'chiefly on its manifestations in the English race' (p. 903). In France it 'reaches a higher degree'; 'It is said that French hysterics bite their tongues during attacks' (p. 702). Such variations, he said, were probably determined by differences in nervous constitution that are recognized in the expression 'national temperament'.

As for neurasthenia, which he left to the very last page, and the cursory treatment of which so annoyed the American reviewer of the *Manual*, it was spoken of 'as a definite disease . . . books have even been written about it, and it has been divided into various classes according to the character of the symptoms that are present'. You might just as well try to classify 'debility'. The closing sentence in his book was the following.

It is often better not to gratify the craving for nomenclature that is manifested by many patients, but rather to explain to them that to give their ailments a definite name would involve more error than truth.

The *Manual* may not have amounted to a Bible but it was certainly a New Testament. We can be sure that good Thomas Willis would have counted it 'An Exact Neurology or Doctrine of the Nerves'.

REFERENCES

INTRODUCTION

[1] Walsh, J. Galen's writings and influences inspiring them. *Ann. Med. Hist.* **6**, 1 (1934).

[2] Singer, C. Galen as a modern. *Proc. R. Soc. Med.* **42**, 563 (1949).

CHAPTER 1

[1] Edelstein, L. The development of Greek anatomy. *Bull. Inst. Hist. Med.* **3**, 235 (1935).

[2] Clarke, E. Aristotelian concepts of the form and function of the brain. *Bull. Hist. Med.* **37**, 1 (1963).

[3] Keynes, Sir Geoffrey. *The life of William Harvey*. Clarendon Press, Oxford (1966). p. 101.

[4] Hippocrates. On the *sacred disease. Med. Class.* **3**, 366 (1938–9). Hippocrates. *Works*. With English translation. Ed. W. H. S. Jones and E. T. Withington. 4 vols. Heinemann (1923–31); Loeb Classical Library. Vol. 2, p. 139. See also *Med. Class.* **3**, 366 (1938–9); and Clarke, E. and O'Malley, C. D. in *The human brain and spinal cord*. University of California Press (1968). p. 4.

[5] Dobson, J. F. Herophilus of Alexandria. *Proc. R. Soc. Med.* **18**, 19 (1925).

[6] Dobson J. F. Erasistratus. *Proc. R. Soc. Med.* **20**, 21 (1927).

[7] Clendening, Logan. *Source book of medical history*. Dover Medical Publications, New York (1960). p. 50.

[8] Clarke, E. and O'Malley, C. D. *The human brain and spinal cord*. University of California Press (1968). p. 462.

[9] Prendergast, J. S. The background of Galen's life and activities, and its influence on his achievements. *Proc. R. Soc. Med.* **23**, 1131 (1930).

[10] Finlayson, J. Bibliographic demonstrations of classical medical writers; Galen. *Br. Med. J.* **i**, 573, 730 (1892).

[11] Neuburger, M. *History of medicine*, (Translated by E. Playfair.) Oxford University Press, London (1910). Vol. 1. p. 246.

[12] Siegel, R. E. *Galen on psychology, psychopathology, and function and diseases of the nervous system*. Karger, Basle (1973). p. 261.

[13] Parkinson, J. An essay on the shaking palsy. Sherwood, Neely and Jones, London. (1817). p. 23.

[14] Temkin, O. *The falling sickness; a history of epilepsy from the Greeks to the beginnings of modern neurology* (2nd edn.). Johns Hopkins University Press (1971). p. 60.

[15] Siegel, R. E. *Galen's system of physiology and medicine; An analysis of his doctrines and observations on blood flow, respiration, humours and internal diseases*. Karger, Basle (1968). p. 308.

[16] Anonymous. Discovery of the nine missing books of Galen's principal anatomical work. *Lond. Med. Gaz.* **35**, 329 (1844).

[17] Coxe, J. R. *The writings of Hippocrates and Galen epitomized from the original Latin translations*. Lindsay and Blackiston, Philadelphia (1846).

[18] Singer, C. *Ann. Med. Hist.* **1**, 433 (1917).

[19] Brock, A. J. *Galen on the natural faculties*. (With an English translation.) Heinemann, London (1916). p. 321.

[20] Walzer, R. *Galen on medical experience*. Oxford University Press (1944).

[21] Singer, C. *Galen on anatomical procedures*. Oxford University Press (1956).

[22] Duckworth, W. L. H. *Galen on anatomical procedures* (the later books). (Eds. M. C. Lyons and B. Towers.) Cambridge University Press (1962).

[23] May, Margaret Talmadge. *Galen on the usefulness of the parts of the body*, 2 vols. Cornell University Press, Ithaca, New York (1968).

[24] Wilder, W. H. De locis affectis. In *Selected readings in pathology*. (Ed. E. R. Long.) Bailliere Tindall and Cox (1929). p. 18.

[25] Fulton, J. F. On the motion of muscles (De motu musculorum). In *Selected readings in the history of physiology* (2nd edn.). Thomas, Springfield, Illinois (1966).

[26] Goss, C. M. On the anatomy of muscles for beginners, by Galen of Pergamon. *Anat. Rec.* **145**, 477 (1963).

[27] Goss, C. M. On the anatomy of nerves by Galen of Pergamon. *Am. J. Anat.* **118**, 327 (1966).

[28] Smith, Emilie Savage. Galen's account of the cranial nerves and the autonomic nervous system. *Clio Medico* **6**, 77, 173 (1971).

[29] Walsh, J. Galen's writings and the influences inspiring them. *Ann. Med. Hist.* **8**, 176 (1926); *ibid.* N.S. **6**, 1, 143 (1934); *ibid.* N.S. **7**, 428, 570 (1935); *ibid.* N.S. **8**, 65 (1936); *ibid.* N.S. **9**, 34 (1937); *ibid.* N.S. **11**, 525 (1939).

[30] Sarton, G. *Galen of Pergamon*. University of Kansas Press (1954). p. 52.

[31] Siegel, R. E. *Galen on sense perception; his doctrines, observations, and experiments on vision, hearing, smell, taste, touch and pain, and their historical background*. Karger, Basle (1970). p. 60.

[32] Temkin, O. *Galenism; rise and decline of a medical philosophy*. Cornell University, Press (1973).

[33] Singer, C. op. cit. 21, p. xxii.

[34] May, M. T. op. cit. 23, Vol. 2, p. 505.

[35] Clendening, L. op. cit. 7, p. 49.

[36] Singer, C. op. cit. 21, p. 226.

[37] May, M. T. op. cit. 23, Vol. 2, p. 620.

[38] Brock, A. J. op. cit. 19, p. 321.

[39] Siegel, R. E. op. cit. 15, p. 86.

[40] May, M. T. op. cit. 23, Vol. 2, p. 573.

[41] May, M. T. op. cit. 23, Vol. 2, p. 684.

[42] May, M. T. op. cit. 23, Vol. 2, p. 703 and 709.

[43] May, M. T. op. cit. 23, Vol. 2, p. 532.

[44] May, M. T. op. cit. 23, Vol. 1, p. 72.

[45] May, M. T. op. cit. 23, Vol. 2, p. 524.

[46] May, M. T. op. cit. 23, Vol. 1, p. 101.

[47] May, M. T. op. cit. 23, Vol. 1, p. 103.

[48] May, M. T. op. cit. 23, Vol. 1, p. 106.

[49] May, M. T. op. cit. 23, Vol. 1, p. 107

[50] May, M. T. op. cit. 23, Vol. 1, p. 109.

[51] May, M. T. op. cit. 23, Vol. 1, p. 148.

[52] May, M. T. op. cit. 23, Vol. 1, p. 151.

[53] May, M. T. op. cit. 23, Vol. 1, p. 154.

[54] May, M. T. op. cit. 23, Vol. 1, p. 162.

[55] May, M. T. op. cit. 23, Vol. 1, p. 164.

[56] Singer, C. op. cit. 21, p. 32.

[57] Choulant, L. *History and bibliography of anatomic illustration in its relation to anatomic science and the graphic arts*. (Trans. and ed. M. Frank.) University of Chicago Press. (1920) p.88.

[58] Fulton, J. F. A note on Francesco Gennari and the early history of cytoarchictectural studies of the cerebral cortex. *Bull. Hist. Med.* **5**, 895 (1937).

[59] May, M. T. op. cit. 23, Vol. 1, p. 427.

[60] May, M. T. op. cit. 23, Vol. 1, p. 415.

[61] Woollam, D. H. M. The historical significance of the cerebrospinal fluid. *Med. Hist.* **1**, 91 (1957).

[62] Woollam, D. H. M. Concepts of the brain and its function in classical antiquity. In *The history and knowledge of the brain and its functions*. (Ed. F. N. L. Poynter.) Blackwell Scientific, Oxford (1958). p. 5.

[63] May, M. T. op. cit. 23, Vol. 1, p. 421.

[64] May, M. T. op. cit. 23, Vol. 1, p. 410.

[65] Siegel, R. E. op. cit. 15, p. 118.

[66] May, M. T. op. cit. 23, Vol. 1, p. 387.

[67] Woollam, D. H. M. op. cit. 62, p. 14.

[68] Duckworth, W. L. H. op. cit. 22, p. 10.

[69] O'Malley, C. D. *Andreas Vesalius of Brussels 1514–1564*. University of California Press (1964). p. 320.

[70] Duckworth, W. L. H. op. cit. 22, p. 181.
[71] Duckworth, W. L. H. op. cit. 22, p. 186.
[72] Duckworth, W. L. H. op. cit. 22, p. 187.
[73] Goss, C. M. op. cit. 27, p. 328.
[74] Siegel, R. E. op. cit. 12, p. 89.
[75] Duckworth, W. L. H. op. cit. 22, 89.
[76] Duckworth, W. L. H. op. cit. 22, p. 102.
[77] Duckworth, W. L. H. op. cit. 22, p. 163.
[78] French, R., The origins of the sympathetic nervous system from Vesalius to Riolan. *Med. Hist.* **15**, 45 (1971).
[79] Duckworth, W. L. H. op. cit. 22, p. 81.
[80] Clarke, E. and O'Malley, C. D. op. cit. 8, p. 151.
[81] Walsh, J., op. cit. 29 (1926).
[82] Singer, C. *A short history of anatomy and physiology from the Greeks to Harvey*. Dover Publications, New York (1957). p. 59.
[83] Duckworth, W. L. H. op. cit. 22, p. 85.
[84] Walsh, J., op. cit. 29 (1937).
[85] May, M. T. op. cit. 23, Vol. 1, p. 391.
[86] May, M. T. op. cit. 23, Vol. 1, p. 397.
[87] May, M. T., op. cit. 23, Vol. 1, p. 403.
[88] May, M. T. op. cit. 23, Vol. 2, p. 463.
[89] May, M. T. op. cit. 23, Vol. 2, p. 483.
[90] May, M. T. op. cit. 23, Vol. 2, p. 484.
[91] May, M. T. op. cit. 23, Vol. 2, p. 477.
[92] May, M. T. op. cit. 23, Vol. 2, p. 491.
[93] May, M. T. op. cit. 23, Vol. 2, p. 494.
[94] May, M. T. op. cit. 23, Vol. 2, p. 493.
[95] May, M. T. op. cit. 23, Vol. 2, p. 495.
[96] May, M. T. op. cit. 23, Vol. 2, p. 501.
[97] Foster, Sir Michael. *Lectures on the history of physiology during the 16th, 17th and 18th centuries*. Dover, New York (1970). p. 273.
[98] Gutierrez-Mahoney, C. G. de and Schecher, M. M. The myth of the *rete mirabile* in man. *Neuroradiology* **4**, 141 (1972).
[99] May, M. T. op. cit. 23, Vol. 1, p. 430.
[100] Siegel, R. E. op. cit. 15, p. 110.
[101] May, M. T. op. cit. 23, Vol. 1, p. 425.
[102] Duckworth, W. L. H. op. cit. 22, p. 4.
[103] Woollam, D. H. M. op. cit. 62, p. 15.
[104] May, M. T. op. cit. 23, Vol. 2, p. 570.
[105] May, M. T. op. cit. 23, Vol. 2, p. 573.
[106] May, M. T. op. cit. 23, Vol. 2, p. 572.
[107] May, M. T. op. cit. 23, Vol. 2, p. 603.
[108] Duckworth, W. L. H. op. cit. 22, p. 223.
[109] Siegel, R. E. op. cit. 12, p. 578.
[110] Duckworth, W. L. H. op. cit. 22, p. 253.
[111] Duckworth, W. L. H. op. cit. 22, p. 185.
[112] May, M. T. op. cit. 23, Vol. 2, p. 704.
[113] Fulton, J. F., *Selected readings in the history of physiology* (1st edn.). Thomas, Springfield, Illinois (1930). p. 184.
[114] Sherrington, Sir Charles S. Notes on the history of the word tonus as a physiological term. In *Contributions to medical and biological research dedicated to Sir William Osler*. Hoeber, New York (1919). Vol. 1, p. 261.
[115] Clarke, Edwin. The doctrine of the hollow nerve in the 17th and 18th centuries. In *Modern science and culture, historical essays in honour of Owsei Temkin*. (Eds. Lloyd G. Stevenson and R. P. Multhauf.) Johns Hopkins University Press (1968). p. 123.
[116] Temkin, O. and Temkin, C. L. Some extracts from Galen's 'Anatomical Procedures'. *Bull. Hist. Med.* **4**, 466 (1936).
[117] Duckworth, W. L. H. op. cit. 22, p. 15.
[118] Duckworth, W. L. H. op. cit. 22, p. 12.
[119] Singer, C. op. cit. 21, p. 230.
Duckworth, W. L. H. op. cit. 22, p. 19.
[121] Clarke, E. and O'Malley, C. D. op. cit. 8, p. 16.
[122] May, M. T. op. cit. 23, Vol. 1, p. 418.
[123] Hippocrates 'On the articulations'. *Med. Class.* **3**, 247 (1938–39).
[124] Duckworth, W. L. H. op. cit. 22, p. 21.
[125] Duckworth, W. L. H. op. cit. 22, p. 23.
[126] Duckworth, W. L. H. op. cit. 22, p. 25.
[127] Clarke, E. and O'Malley, C. D. op. cit. 8, p. 294.
[128] Siegel, R. E. op. cit: 12, p. 61.
[129] Singer, C. op. cit. 82, p. 61, Fig. 30.
[130] Sherrington, Sir Charles S. *Man on his Nature*. Cambridge University Press (1941). p. 243.
[131] Singer, C. op. cit. 21, p. 183.
[132] Cooke, J. *A treatise on nervous diseases*. Wells and Lilly; Carey and Lea, Philadelphia (1824). p. 6.
[133] Siegel, R. E. op. cit. 12, p. 87.
[134] Sarton, G. op. cit. 30, p. 91.
[135] Garrison, F. H. *An introduction to the history of medicine* (2nd edn.). Saunders, Philadelphia (1917). p. 98.
[136] Allbutt, Sir Clifford T. *Greek medicine in Rome*. Macmillan, London (1921). p. 289.
[137] Brazier, Mary A. B. The evolution of concepts relating to the electrical activity of the nervous system; 1600 to 1800. In *The brain and its functions*. (Ed. F. N. L. Poynter.) Blackwell, Oxford (1958). p. 198.
[138] Soury, J. *Le systeme nerveux central, structure et fonctions; histoire critique des théories et doctrines*. Carre et Naud, Paris (1899). p. 305.
[139] Souques, A. Les connaissances neurologiques de Galien. (Apercu critique.) *Rev. Neurol.* **1**, 296 (1933).
[140] Singer, C. Galen as a modern. *Proc. R. Soc. Med.* **42**, 563 (1949).
[141] Cole, F. J. *A history of comparative anatomy from Aristotle to the 18th century*. Macmillan, London (1949). p. 42.
[142] King, Lester S. *The growth of medical thought*. University of Chicago Press (1963). p. 46.
[143] Clarke, E. and O'Malley, C. D. op. cit. 8, p. 15.
[144] Langley, J. N. Sketch of the progress in the 18th century as regards the autonomic nervous system. *J. Physiol.* **50**, 225 (1915–16).
[145] Sherrington, Sir Charles S. op. cit. 130, pp. 40, 111.
[146] Temkin, O. op. cit. 32, p. 191.
[147] Farrington B. *Greek science; its meaning for us*. Penguin, Harmondsworth (1969). p. 294.

CHAPTER 2

[1] Singer, C. *A short history of science to the 19th century*. Clarendon Press, Oxford (1941). p. 154.
[2] Lind, L. R. *Studies in pre-Vesalian anatomy; biography, translations, documents*. The American Philosophical Society, Philadelphia (1975). p. 159.
[3] O'Malley, C. D. *Andreas Vesalius of Brussels, 1514–1564* University of California Press (1964). p. 319.
[4] Keynes, Sir Geoffrey. *The life of William Harvey*. Clarendon Press, Oxford (1966). p. 179.
[5] Castiglione, A. The Medical School at Padua and the Renaissance of Medicine. *Ann. Med. Hist.* **7**, 214 (1935); Andreas Vesalius; Professor at the Medical School of Padua. *Bull. N.Y. Acad. Med.* **19**, 766 (1943). Andreas Vesalius and the 'Fabrica'; 1543–1943. *J. Am. Med. Ass.* **121**, 582 (1943).
[6] Lind, L. R. op. cit. 2, p. 17.
[7] Singer, C. How medicine became anatomical. *Br. Med. J.* ii, 1499 (1954).
[8] Anonymous. The Luther of anatomy. *Br. Med. J.* **ii**, 383 (1911).

[9] Eriksson, Ruben, *Andreas Vesalius's first public anatomy at Bologna, 1540. An eyewitness report by Baldasar Heseler.* Almquist and Wilksells, Uppsala (1959).
[10] Wiegand, W. Marginal notes by the printer of the Icones. In *three Vesalian essays to accompany* The Icones Anatomicae *of 1934*. Macmillan, New York (1952).
[11] Singer, C. Some Vesalian problems. *Bull. Hist. Med.* **17**, 425 (1945).
[12] Singer, C. and Rabin, C. *A prelude to modern science, being a discussion of the history, sources and circumstances of the 'Tabulae Anatomicae Sex' of Vesalius.* Cambridge University Press (1946).
[13] Anonymous. Two forerunners; our debt to Copernicus and Vesalius; the passing of medieval science. *Times Literary Supplement* 29 May, 1943. p. 258.
[14] O'Malley, C. D. op. cit. 3, p. 160.
[15] O'Malley, C. D. op. cit. 3, p. 162.
[16] O' Malley, C. D. op. cit. 3, p. 253.
[17] O'Malley, C. D. op. cit. 3, p. 156.
[18] O'Malley, C. D. op. cit. 3, p. 170.
[19] Straus, W. L. and Temkin, O. Vesalius and the problem of variability. *Bull. Hist. Med.* **14**, 609 (1943).
[20] O'Malley, op. cit. 3, p. 170.
[21] French, R. The origins of the sympathetic nervous system from Vesalius to Riolan. *Med. Hist.* **15**, 45 (1971).
[22] Singer, C. Some Galenic and animal sources of Vesalius. *J. Hist. Med.* **1**, 6 (1946).
[23] Spencer, W. G. Vesalius; his delineation of the framework of the human body in the *Fabrica* and *Epitome. Brit. J. Surg.* **10**, 382 (1923).
[24] Meyer, Alfred, *Historical aspects of cerebral anatomy.* Oxford University Press (1971). p. 10.
[25] Ivins, W. M. What about the *Fabrica* of Vesalius? In *Three Vesalian essays to accompany* The Icones Anatomicae *of 1934*. Macmillan, New York (1952).
[26] Herrlinger, Robert, *History of medical illustration from antiquity to AD 1600.* Pitman Medical Publications, London (1970). p. 42.
[27] Choulant, Ludwig. *History and bibliography of anatomic illustration in its relation to anatomical science and the graphic arts* (1852, Leipzig). (Translated and edited by M. Frank.) University of Chicago Press (1920). p. 172.
[28] Sigerist, H. E. Albanus Torinus and the German edition of the *Epitome* of Vesalius. *Bull. Hist. Med.* **14**, 653 (1943).
[29] Wiegand, W. op. cit. 10.
[30] Lambert, Samuel W. The fabric of the human body by Andreas Vesalius. In *Source book of medical history* by Logan Clendening. Dover, New York (1960). p. 143.
[31] Lambert, Samuel W. op. cit. 30, p. 144.
[32] Garrison, Fielding H. Selections from Vesalius, showing the improvements introduced into the second edition of the *Fabrica* (1555). *Ann. Med. Hist.* **4**, 100 (1922).
[33] Wightman, W. P. D. Wars of ideas in neurological science – from Willis to Bichat and from Locke to Condillac. In *The history and philosophy of knowledge of the brain and its functions,* (Ed. F. L. N. Poynter) Blackwell Scientific, Oxford (1958). p. 144.
[34] Singer, C. *Vesalius on the human brain.* Oxford University Press (1952). p. 13.
[35] Singer, C. op. cit. 34, p. 5.
[36] Singer, C. op. cit. 34, p. 6.
[37] Pagel, Walter. Medieval and Renaissance contributions to knowledge of the brain and its functions. In *The brain and its functions.* (Ed. F. L. N. Poynter.) Blackwell Scientific, Oxford (1958). p. 114.
[38] Singer, C. op. cit. 34, p. 39.
[39] Foster, Sir Michael, *Lectures on the history of physiology during the 16th, 17th and 18th centuries.* Dover, New York (1970). p. 259.
[40] Foster, Sir Michael op. cit. 39, p. 255.
[41] Sherrington, Sir Charles S. *Man on his nature.* Cambridge University Press (1941). p. 40.
[42] Foster, Sir Michael op. cit. 39, p. 257.
[43] Clarke, Edwin and O'Malley, C. D. *The human brain and spinal cord; a historical study illustrated by writings from antiquity to the twentieth century.* University of California Press (1968). p. 155.
[44] O'Malley, C. D. op. cit. 3, p. 378.
[45] O'Malley, C. D. and Saunders, J. B. de C. M. Vesalius as a clinician. *Bull. Hist. Med.* **14**, 594 (1943).
[46] O'Malley, C. D. op. cit. 3, p. 378.
[47] O'Malley, C. D. op. cit. 3, p. 383.
[48] O'Malley, C. D. op. cit. 3, p. 390.
[49] O'Malley, C. D. op. cit. 3, p. 393.
[50] O'Malley, C. D. op. cit. 3, p. 396.
[51] Fisch, Max H. Vesalius in the English State Papers. *Bull. Med. Libr. Ass.* **33**, 231 (1945).
[52] O'Malley, C. D. op. cit. 3, p. 297.
[53] O'Malley, C. D. The Vesalian influence in England. *Acta Med. Hist. Patav.* **10**, 11 (1964).
[54] Crummer, LeRoy, The copper plates in Raynalde and Geminus. *Proc. R. Soc. Med.* **20**, 53 (1926).
[55] Singer, C. op. cit. 34, p. xii.
[56] Edelstein, Ludwig. Andreas Vesalius the humanist. *Bull. Hist. Med.* **14**, 547 (1943).
[57] Cullen, G. M. The passing of Vesalius. *Edin. Med. J.* **13**, 324, 388 (1918).
[58] Farrington, B. The preface of Andreas Vesalius to *De fabrica corporis humani 1543. Proc. R. Soc. Med.* **25**, 1361 (1932).
[59] Hotchkiss, W. P. Preface of The fabric of the human body. In *Source book of medical history* by Logan Clendening. Dover, New York (1960). p. 128.
[60] Cushing, Harvey. *A bio-bibliography of Andreas Vesalius.* Schuman, New York (1943).
[61] Singer, C. and Rabin, C. op. cit. 12.
[62] Lind, L. R. *The* Epitome *of Andreas Vesalius.* (Translated from the Latin with preface and introduction. Anatomical notes by C. A. Asling.) Macmillan, New York (1949).
[63] Saunders, J. B. de C. M. and O'Malley, C. D. *Illustrations from the works of Andreas Vesalius.* World Publishing, Cleveland (1950).
[64] Singer, C. op. cit. 34.
[65] Eriksson, R. op. cit. 9.
[66] Singer, C. Eighteen years of Vesalian studies. *Med. Hist.* **5**, 210 (1961).
[67] O'Malley, op. cit. 3.
[68] Castiglione, A. Andreas Vesalius and the *Fabrica. J. Am. Med. Ass.* **121**, 582 (1943).
[69] Foster, Sir Michael. op. cit. 39, p. 20.
[70] O'Malley, op. cit. 3, p. 139.
[71] Singer, C. op. cit. 34, p. xii.
[72] Sherrington, C. S. *Goethe on nature and science* (2nd edn.). Cambridge University Press (1949). p. 19.
[73] O'Malley, C. D. Studies of the brain during the Italian Renaissance. In *Essays on the history of Italian neurology; Proceedings of the International Symposium on the History of Neurology, Varenna, August 30th–September 1, 1961.* (Ed. L. Belloni.) Instituto di Storia della Medicina, Università degli Studi, Milano. Elli and Pagani, Milan (1963). p. 31.

CHAPTER 3

[1] Singer, C. *A short history of science to the nineteenth century.* Clarendon Press, Oxford (1941). p. 185.
[2] Gilbert, William. *De magnete* etc. (Translation by the Gilbert Club.) Chiswick Press, London (1900). p. 35.
[3] Bacon, Sir Francis. The advancement of learning, 1605. In *The works of Francis Bacon.* (Eds. J. Spedding, R. L. Ellis, and D. E. Heath). Longmans, London (1857). Vol. 3,

p. 253.
[4] Bacon, Sir Francis, op. cit. 3, p. 283.
[5] Bacon, Sir Francis, op. cit. 3, p. 358.
[6] Bacon, Sir Francis. op. cit. 3, p. 370.
[7] Bacon, Sir Francis. op. cit. 3, p. 371.
[8] Bacon, Sir Francis. op. cit. 3, p. 374.
[9] Bacon, Sir Francis. op. cit. 3, p. 375.
[10] Bacon, Sir Francis. op. cit. 3, p. 332.
[11] Bacon, Sir Francis. op. cit. 3, p. 292.
[12] Singer, C. *A short history of anatomy and physiology from the Greeks to Harvey*. Dover, New York (1957). p. 171.
[13] Medawar, Sir Peter, *The art of the soluble; creativity and originality in science*. Penguin, Harmondsworth (1969). p. 21.
[14] Dewhurst, K. An Oxford medical quartet; Sydenham, Willis, Locke and Lower. *Br. Med. J.* **ii**, 857 (1963).
[15] Dewhurst, K. *John Locke (1632–1704). Physician and philosopher. A medical biography*. The Wellcome Historical Medical Library, London (1963).
[16] Viets, H. R. A. A patronal festival for Thomas Willis with remarks by Sir William Osler, Bart., FRS. *Ann. Med. Hist.* **1**, 118 (1917).
[17] Keevil, J. J. The 17th century English medical background. *Bull. Hist. Med.* **31**, 523 (1957).
[18] Debus, Allen G. (Ed.) *Medicine in 17th century England*. University of California Press (1974).
[19] Hoff, E. C. and Hoff, P. M. The life and times of Richard Lower. *Bull. Hist. Med.* **4**, 517 (1936).
[20] Keynes, Sir Geoffrey. *The life of William Harvey*. Clarendon Press, Oxford (1966).
[21] Gunther, R. T. *Early medical and biological science*. Oxford University Press (1926). p. 21.
[22] Gibson, W. C. *The medical interests of Christopher Wren*. W. Andrews Clark Memorial Library, Los Angeles (1969); *The biomedical pursuits of Christopher Wren. Med. Hist.* **14**, 331 (1970).
[23] Dewhurst, K. Willis in Oxford; some new mss. *Proc. R. Soc. Med.* **57**, 682 (1964).
[24] Dewhurst, K. Some letters of Dr. Thomas Willis. *Med. Hist.* **16**, 63 (1972).
[25] Dewhurst, K. *Thomas Willis as a physician*. W. Andrews Clark Memorial Library, Los Angeles (1964).
[26] Miller, W. S. Thomas Willis (1621–1675). *Bull. Hist. Med.* **3**, 215 (1923).
[27] Dow, R. S. Thomas Willis as a comparative neurologist. *Ann. Med. Hist.* **2**, 181 (1940).
[28] Symonds, Sir Charles. The circle of Willis. *Br. Med. J.* **i**, 119 (1955).
[29] Symonds, Sir Charles, Thomas Willis F.R.S (1621–1675). In *The Royal Society, its origins and founders*. (Ed. H. Hartley.) The Royal Society, London (1960). p. 91.
[30] *The Royal Society; a brief guide to its activities*. The Royal Society, London (1978). p. 3.
[31] Stensen, Niels, Discours sur l'anatomie du cerveau, 1665. In *Steno and brain research in the 17th century*. (Ed. G. G. Scherz.) Pergamon Press, Oxford (1968).
[32] O'Malley, C. D. *Andreas Vesalius of Brussels, 1514–1564*. University of California Press (1964). p. 239.
[33] King, Lester, S. The transformation of Galenism. In *Medicine in 17th century England*. (Ed. Allen G. Debus.) University of California Press (1974). p. 7.
[34] King, Lester, S. *The road to medical enlightenment 1650–1695*, MacDonald, London (1970).
[35] Russell, Bertrand. *History of western philosophy*. George Allen and Unwin, London (1957). p. 558.
[36] Isler, Hansruedi, *Thomas Willis 1621–1675; doctor and scientist*. Hafner, New York (1968). p. 48.
[37] *Thomas Willis, The anatomy of the brain and nerves* (tercentenary edn.) (Ed. William Feindel.) McGill University Press (1965). 2 vols.
[38] Keele, K. D. Thomas Willis on the brain; an essay review. *Med. Hist.* **6**, 194 (1965).
[39] Morton, L. T. *A medical biography (Garrison and Morton)*. (3rd edn.). Andre Deutsch, New York (1970). p. 577, No. 5020.
[40] Morton, op. cit. 39, p. 539, No. 4673.
[41] Hierons, R. Willis's contributions to clinical medicine and neurology. *J. Neurol. Sci.* **4**, 1 (1967).
[42] Creighton, C. *A history of epidemics in Britain*. Frank Cass, London (1965). Vol. 1, p. 568.
[43] Crookshank, F. G. *Influenza; essays by several authors*. W. Heinemann, London (1922). p. 88.
[44] Creighton, op. cit. 42, Vol. 1, p. 568.
[45] Garrison, Fielding H. *An introduction to the history of medicine*. W. B. Saunders & Co., Philadelphia and London (1917). (2nd edn.) p. 254.
[46] Rolleston, Sir Humphry. Thomas Willis. *Med. Life* **41**, 177 (1934).
[47] Hippocrates. Of the Epidemics. *Med. Class.* **3**, 116 (1938–39).
[48] Morton, L. T. op. cit. 39, p. 374, No. 3166.
[49] Hierons, R. op. cit. 41.
[50] Miller, W. S. Thomas Willis and his *De phthisi pulmonari. Am. Rev. Tuberc.* **5**, 934 (1922).
[51] Miller, W. S. op. cit. 26.
[52] Hierons, R. op. cit. 41.
[53] Major, Ralph H. *Classic descriptions of disease* (3rd edn.). Blackwell Scientific, Oxford (1948).
[54] Hierons, R. op. cit. 41.
[55] Liveing, E. *On megrim, sick-headache and some allied disorders*. J. and A. Churchill, London (1873). pp. 336, 363.
[56] Willis, T. *Practice of physick. Being the whole works of that renowned and famous physician*. (English Translation by S. Pordage.) London (1684). S. B. Of the headache, p. 110.
[57] Critchley, M. *The malady of Anne, Countess of Conway; a case for commentary. King's Coll. Hosp. Gaz* **16**, 44 (1937).
[58] Critchley, M. idem. *Trans. Med. Soc. Lond.* **67**, 92 (1952).
[59] Symonds, Sir Charles. op. cit. 28.
[60] Willis, T. op. cit. 56, S.B. Of the headache, p. 119.
[61] Willis, T. op. cit. 56, S.B. Of the vertigo, p. 145.
[62] Willis, T. op. cit. 56, S.B. Of the sight, p. 81.
[63] Willis, T. op. cit. 56, S.B. Of the sense of smelling, p. 89.
[64] Willis, T. op. cit. 56, S.B. Of hearing, p. 73.
[65] Willis, T. op. cit. 56, S.B. Of hearing, p. 73.
[66] Willis, T. op. cit. 56, S.B. Of Coma etc p. 139.
[67] Critchley, M. The pre-dormitum. *Rev. Neurol.* **93**, 101 (1955).
[68] Willis, T. op. cit. 56, S.B. Of coma etc., p. 139.
[69] Willis, T. op. cit. 56, S.B. Of sleeping and waking, p. 88.
[70] Willis, T. op. cit. 56, S.B. Of the lethargy, p. 135.
[71] Lennox, W. G. Willis on narcolepsy. *Arch. Neur. Psych.* **41**, 348 (1939).
[72] Willis, T. op. cit. 56, S.B. Other sleepy distempers, p. 134.
[73] Willis, T. op. cit. 56, S.B. Other sleepy distempers, p. 134.
[74] Willis, T. op. cit. 56, S.B. Other sleepy distempers, p. 134.
[75] Lennox, W. G. op. cit. 71.
[76] Willis, T. op. cit. 56, S.B. Other sleepy distempers, p. 135.
[77] Adams, E. W. Thomas Willis M.A., M.D. (1621–1675). *Quart. Med. J. (Sheffield)* **11**, 136 (1902).
[78] Willis, T. op. cit. 37, A.B. p. 100.
[79] Willis, T. op. cit. 56, C.D. p. 3.
[80] Willis, T. op. cit. 56, C.D. p. 5.
[81] Willis, T. op. cit. 56, C.D. Of the epilepsie, p. 11.
[82] Willis, T. op. cit. 56, C.D. p. 7.

[83] Willis, T. op. cit. 56, C.D. Chapter III, p. 14.
[84] Willis, T. op. cit. 56, C.D. Of the epilepsie, p. 11.
[85] Willis, T. op. cit. 56, C.D. p. 2.
[86] Willis, T. op. cit. 56, C.D. Of the epilepsie, p. 13.
[87] Willis, T. op. cit. 56, C.D. p. 7.
[88] Hierons, R. op. cit. 41.
[89] Willis, T. op. cit. 56, C.D. p. 7.
[90] Willis, T. op. cit. 56, C.D. p. 10.
[91] Willis, T. op. cit. 56, S.B. Part 2, Chapter 9, p. 161.
[92] Willis, T. op. cit. 56, S.B. Part 2, Chapter 9, p. 162.
[93] Willis, T. op. cit. 56, S.B. Part 2, Chapter 9, p. 163.
[94] Willis, T. op. cit. 56, S.B. Part 2, Chapter 9, p. 163.
[95] Guthrie, L. G. Myasthenia gravis in the 17th century. Lancet **i**, 330 (1903).
[96] Willis, T. op. cit. 56. S.B. Part 2, Chapter 9, p. 167.
[97] Willis, T. op. cit. 56, S.B. Part 2, Chapter 9, p. 167.
[98] Keynes, Sir Geoffrey. The history of myasthenia gravis. *Med. Hist.* **5**, 313 (1961).
[99] Wilks, Sir Samuel. On cerebritis, hysteria and bulbar paralysis. *Guy's Hosp. Rep.* **22**, 7 (1877).
[100] Willis, T. op. cit. 56, S.B. Part 2, Chapter 8, p. 153.
[101] Willis, T. op. cit. 56, S.B. Part 2, Chapter 8, p. 154.
[102] Willis, T. op. cit. 56, S.B. Part 2, Chapter 8, p. 155.
[103] Dewhurst, K. op. cit. 14.
[104] Dewhurst, K. op. cit. 25, p. 16.
[105] Payne, J. F. *Thomas Sydenham.* J. Fisher Unwin, London (1900). p. 151
[106] Dewhurst, K. *Dr. Thomas Sydenham (1621–1675); his life and original writings.* University of California Press (1966).
[107] Rather, L. J. Pathology at mid-century; a reassessment of Thomas Willis and Thomas Sydenham. In *Medicine in 17th century England.* (Ed. Allen G. Debus.) University of California Press (1974). p. 111.
[108] Zilboorg, G. and Henry, G. *A history of medical psychology.* Norton, New York (1941). p. 178.
[109] Cranefield, P. F. A 17th century view of mental deficiency and schizophrenia; Thomas Willis on stupidity or foolishness. *Bull. Hist. Med.* **35**, 291 (1961).
[110] Vinchon, J. and Vie, J. Un Maitre de la neuropsychiatrie XVII siècle; Thomas Willis. *Anns. méd.-psychol.* **12**, 109 (1928).
[111] Zilboorg, G. and Henry, G. op. cit. 108, p. 527.
[112] Morton, L. T. op. cit. 39, p. 551, No. 4793.
[113] Hare, E. H. The origin and spread of dementia paralytica. *J. Ment. Sci.* **105**, 594 (1959).
[114] Willis, T. op. cit. 56, S.B. Part 2, Chapter 9. p. 163.
[115] Willis, T. op. cit. 56, S.B. Part 2, Chapter 9. p. 164.
[116] Willis, T. op. cit. 56, S.B. Part 2, Chapter 13, p. 212.
[117] Zilboorg, G. and Henry, G. op. cit. 108, p. 550.
[118] Lord Brain, The concept of hysteria in the 17th century. In *Doctors past and present.* Pitman, London (1964). p. 46.
[119] Willis, T. op. cit. 56, C.D. p. 69.
[120] Willis, T. op. cit. 56, C.D. p. 72.
[121] Willis, T. op. cit. 56, C.D. p. 69.
[122] Willis, T. op. cit. 56, S.B. Part 2, Chapters 11 and 12; Of melancholy and madness, p. 188.
[123] Willis, T. op. cit. 56. S.B. Part 2, Chapter 13; Of stupidity or foolishness, p. 209.
[124] Cranefield, P. F. op. cit. 109.
[125] Meyer, A. Emergent patterns of the pathology of mental disease. *J. Ment. Sci.* **106**, 785 (1960).
[126] Singer, C. op. cit. 12, p. 171.
[127] O'Malley, C. D. The Vesalian influence in England. *Acta Med. Hist. Patav.* **10**, 11 (1964).
[128] O'Malley, C. D., Poynter, F. N. L. and Russell, K. F., *Lectures on the whole of anatomy; William Harvey.* University of California Press (1961).
[129] Whitteridge, Gweneth. *The anatomical lectures of William Harvey.* E. and S. Livingstone, Edinburgh (1964).
[130] Keynes, Sir Geoffrey. op. cit. 20, p. 108.
[131] Hunter, R. A. and Macalpine, I. William Harvey; his neurological and psychiatric observations *J. Hist. Med.* **12**, 126 (1957).
[132] Keynes, Sir Geoffrey. op. cit. 20, p. 296.
[133] Lord Brain, op. cit. 118, p. 44.
[134] Willis, T. op. cit. 56. Preface to *Of fevers.* p. 45.
[135] Meyer, A. and Hierons, R. Observations on the history of the circle of Willis. *Med. Hist.* **6**, 119 (1962).
[136] Meyer, A. and Hierons, R. A note on Thomas Willis's views on the corpus striatum and internal capsule. *J. Neurol. Sci.* **1**, 547 (1964).
[137] Meyer, A. and Hierons, R. On Thomas Willis's concepts of neurophysiology. *Med. Hist.* **9**, 1, 142 (1965).
[138] Hierons, R. and Meyer, A. *Some priority questions arising from Thomas Willis's work on the brain. Proc. R. Soc. Med.* **55**, 287 (1962).
[139] Hierons, R. and Meyer, A. Willis's place in the history of muscle physiology. *Proc. R. Soc. Med.* **57**, 687 (1964).
[140] Clarke, Edwin and O'Malley, C. D. The human brain and spinal cord; a historical study illustrated by writings from antiquity to the twentieth century. University of California Press (1968).
[141] Isler, Hansruedi. op. cit. 36.
[142] Willis, T. op. cit. 37, A.B. p. 96.
[143] Clarke, Edwin and O'Malley, C.D. op. cit. 140, p. 724.
[144] Willis, T. op. cit. 37, A.B. p. 99.
[145] Willis, T. op. cit. 37, A.B. p. 107.
[146] Willis, T. op. cit. 37, A.B. p. 91.
[147] Willis, T. op. cit. 37, A.B. p. 61.
[148] Willis, T. op. cit. 37, A.B. p. 110.
[149] Willis, T. op. cit. 37, A.B. p. 121.
[150] Willis, T. op. cit. 37, A.B. p. 108.
[151] Willis, T. op. cit. 37, A.B. p. 87.
[152] Willis, T. op. cit. 37, A.B. p. 74.
[153] Willis, T. op. cit. 37, A.B. p. 88.
[154] Willis, T. op. cit. 56, S.B. Part 1, Chapter 11, Of the senses, p. 61.
[155] Willis, T. op. cit. 37, A.B. p. 102.
[156] Willis, T. op. cit. 37, A.B. p. 96.
[157] Willis, T. op. cit. 56, S.B. Part 1, Chapter 11, Of the senses, p. 60.
[158] Willis, T. op. cit. 37, A.B. p. 102.
[159] Willis, T. op. cit. 37, A.B. p. 111.
[160] Sherrington, Sir Charles S. *The integrative action of the nervous system.* Cambridge University Press (1947). p. 346.
[161] Dewhurst, K., op. cit. 106, p. 65.
[162] Willis, T. op. cit. 37, A.B. p. 129.
[163] Willis, T. op. cit. 37, A.B. p. 132.
[164] Willis, T. op. cit. 56, M.M. p. 48.
[165] Willis, T. op. cit. 56, p. 37.
[166] Willis, T. op. cit. 56, S.B. Part 1, Chapter 11, p. 61.
[167] Willis, T. op. cit. 37, A.B. p. 96.
[168] Brazier, Mary A.B. The historical development of neuro-physiology. In *Handbook of physiology, Vol. 1, Neurophysiology.* (Eds. J. Field, H. W. Magoun, and V. E. Hall.) American Physiological Society, Washington, D.C. (1959). p. 31.
[169] Foster, Sir Michael. *Lectures on the history of physiology during the 16th, 17th and 18th centuries.* Dover, New York (1970). p. 268.
[170] Foster, Sir Michael. op. cit. 169, p. 278.
[171] Sherrington, Sir Charles S. *Man on his nature.* Cambridge University Press (1941). p. 159.
[172] Sherrington, Sir Charles S. *The endeavour of Jean Fernel.* Cambridge University Press (1946). p. 83.
[173] Liddell, E. G. T. *The discovery of*

reflexes. Clarendon Press, Oxford. (1960). p. 98.
[174] Meyer, A. and Hierons, R. op. cit. 137, p. 142.
[175] Fearing, F. Reflex action. (Reprint.) (1964). Hafner, New York (1964). p. 58.
[176] Fulton, J. F. *Muscular contraction and the reflex control of movement*. Williams and Wilkins, Baltimore (1926). p. 17.
[177] Fulton, J. F. *Selected readings in the history of physiology*. (1st edn.). Thomas, Springfield, Illinois (1930). p. 257.
[178] Fulton, J. F. *Physiology of the nervous system*. Oxford University Press (1938). p. 54.
[179] Fulton, J. F. The historical contribution of physiology to neurology. In *Science, medicine and history; essays on the evolution of scientific thought and medical practice*. (Ed. E. A. Underwood.) Oxford University Press (1953). Vol. 2, p. 539.
[180] Hoff, H. E. and Kellaway, P. The early history of the reflex. *J. Hist. Med.* 7, 211 (1952).
[181] Liddell, E. G. T. op. cit. 173.
[182] Canghuilhem, G. *La formation du concept de réflexe aux XVIIe et XVIIIe siècles*. Presse Université de France, Paris (1955).
[183] Sheehan, D. Discovery of the autonomic nervous system. *Arch. Neurol. Psych.* **35**, 1081 (1936).
[184] Meyer, A, and Hierons, R. op. cit. 137.
[185] Willis, T. op. cit. 37, A.B. p. 146.
[186] Willis, T. op. cit. 37, A.B. p. 151.
[187] Willis, T. op. cit. 37, A.B. p. 152.
[188] Willis, T. op. cit. 37, A.B. p. 155.
[189] Willis, T. op. cit. 37, A.B. p. 157.
[190] Willis, T. op. cit. 37, A.B. p. 161.
[191] Willis, T. op. cit. 37, A.B. p. 169.
[192] Willis, T. op. cit. 56, Ph. Rat. p. 116.
[193] Meyer, A, and Hierons, R. op. cit. 135.
[194] Simmer, Hans H. The beginnings of endocrinology. In *Medicine in 17th century England*. (Ed. Allen G. Debus.) University of California Press (1974). p. 215.
[195] Adams, E. W. op. cit. 77.
[196] Rolleston, Sir Humphry D. *The endocrine organs in health and disease with an historical review*. Oxford University Press (1936). p. 12.
[197] Willis, T. op. cit. 56, C.D. p. 16.
[198] Miller, W. S. op. cit. 26.
[199] Rolleston, Sir Humphry D. op. cit. 46.
[200] Rolleston, Sir Humphry D. op. cit. 196.
[201] Symonds, Sir Charles. op. cit. 28.
[202] Symonds, Sir Charles. op. cit. 29.
[203] Feindel, W. Thomas Willis; the founder of neurology. *Canad. Med. Ass. J.* **87**, 289 (1962).
[204] Feindel, W. op. cit. 37, Vol. 1, p. 13.
[205] Isler, Hansruedi. op. cit. 36, p. 68.
[206] Hierons, R. op. cit. 41.
[207] Willis, T. op. cit. 56, S.B. Part 1, p. 30.
[208] Isler, Hansruedi. op. cit. 36, p. 103.
[209] Simmer, Hans H. op. cit. 194, p. 235.
[210] Willis, T. op. cit. 37, A.B. p. 70.
[211] Willis, T. op. cit. 37, A.B. p. 71.
[212] Willis, T. op. cit. 37, A.B. p. 85.
[213] Willis, T. op. cit. 37, A.B. p. 104.
[214] Willis, T. op. cit. 37, A.B. p. 105.
[215] Cushing, Harvey. Neurophysiological mechanisms from a clinical standpoint. *Lancet*, **ii**, 119, 175 (1930).
[216] Willis, T. op. cit. 37, A.B. p. 86.
[217] Simmer, Hans H. op. cit. 194, p. 235.
[218] Tjomsland, A. Niels Stensen; his tercentenary. *Ann. Med. Hist* **10**, 491 (1938).
[219] Scherz, G. G. *Steno and brain research in the 17th century*. Pergamon Press, Oxford (1968).
[220] Foster, Sir Michael. op. cit. 169, p. 280.
[221] Fulton, J. F. op. cit. 176, p. 19.
[222] Hierons, R. and Meyer, A. op. cit. 139.
[223] Foster, Sir Michael. op. cit. 169, p. 279.
[224] Ridley, H. *Anatomy of the brain*. S. Smith and B. Walford (1695).
[225] Rasmussen, A. T. *Some trends in neuroanatomy*. Brown, Dubuque (1947). p. 12.
[226] Meyer, A. *Historical aspects of cerebral anatomy*. Oxford University Press (1971). p. 12.
[227] Ridley, H. op. cit. 224, p. 21.
[228] Ridley, H. op. cit. 224, p. 29.
[229] Ridley, H. op. cit. 224, p. 64.
[230] Ridley, H. op. cit. 224, p. 160.
[231] Freind, J., *History of physick; from the time of Galen to the beginning of the sixteenth century*. J. Uralther, London (1725–26). 2 vols.
[232] Morton, L. T. op. cit. 39, p. 736, No. 6378.
[233] Greenwood, M. On John Freind. *Janus*, **37**, 193 (1933).
[234] Hutchinson, B. *Biographica medica*. J. Johnson, London (1799). Vol. 2, p. 481.
[235] McHenry, Lawrence C. *Garrison's history of neurology*. Thomas, Springfield, Illinois (1969). p. 271.
[236] Pettigrew, T. J. *Biographical memoirs of the most celebrated physicians and surgeons*. Fisher, Son & Co., Whittaker & Co. (1838–40). 4 vols.
[237] Choulant, Ludwig, *History and bibliography of anatomic illustration in its relation to anatomical science and the graphic arts (1852)*. (Translated and edited by M. Frank.) University of Chicago Press (1920).
[238] Morton, L. T. op. cit. 39, p. 737, No. 6395.
[239] Withington, E. T. *Medical history from the earliest times*. Scientific Press, London (1894). (Reprinted 1964).
[240] Neuburger, Max. *Die historische Entwicklung der experimentellen Gehirn- und Ruckenmarksphysiologie vor Flourens*. Verlag von F. Enke, (Stuttgart) (1897).
[241] Neuburger, Max. op. cit. 240, p. 33.
[242] Soury, J. *Le système nerveux central; structure et et fonctions; histoire critique des théories et des doctrines*. Carré et Naud, Paris (1899).
[243] Soury, J. op. cit. 242, p. 434.
[244] Soury, J. op. cit. 242, p. 428.
[245] Liddell, op. cit. 173, p. 98.
[246] O'Malley, C. D. in Preface to Foster, op. cit. 169.
[247] Foster, Sir Michael (1836–1907). Obituary notice in *Proc. R. Soc.* **B. LXXX**, lxxii (1908).
[248] Symonds, Sir Charles. op. cit. 28.
[249] Foster, Sir Michael. op. cit. 169, p. 270.
[250] Foster, Sir Michael. op. cit. 169, p. 277.
[251] Foster, Sir Michael. op. cit. 169, p. 271.
[252] Foster, Sir Michael. op. cit. 169, 247.
[253] MacNalty, Sir A. S. *A biography of Sir Benjamin Ward Richardson; 1828–1896*. Harvey and Blythe, London (1950).
[254] Richardson, Sir B. W. *Disciples of Aesculapius*. Hutchinson, London (1900). Vol. 2, pp. 592–602.
[255] Ackerknecht, E. H. In Isler, Hansruedi. op. cit. 36.
[256] Meyer, A. Karl Friedrich Burdach and his place in the history of neuroanatomy. *J. Neurol. Neurosurg. and Psychiat* **33**, 553 (1970).
[257] Meyer, A. Karl Friedrich Burdach on Thomas Willis. *J. Neurol. Sci.* **3**, 109 (1966).
[258] Sherrington, Sir Charles S. op. cit. 171, p. 245.
[259] Sigerist, H. E. *The great doctors; a biographical history of medicine*. Dover, New York (1971).
[260] Power, Sir D'Arcy. *British masters of medicine*. Medical Press and Circular, London (1936).
[261] Poynter, F. N. L. (Ed.) *The history and philosophy of knowledge of the brain and its functions*. An Anglo-American Symposium, London, 1957. Blackwell Scientific, Oxford (1958).
[262] Medawar, Sir Peter B. Two conceptions of science. In *The art of*

the soluble. Penguin, Harmondsworth (1967). p. 134.
[263] Medawar, Sir Peter B. op. cit. 262, p. 132.
[264] Trevelyan, G. M. Bias in history. In *An autobiography and other essays*. Longmans, Green, London (1949). p. 81.

CHAPTER 4

[1a] Sullivan, J. W. N. *Isaac Newton*. Macmillan, London (1938). p. 33.
[1b] King, Lester S. *The medical world of the eighteenth century*. University of Chicago Press (1958).
[2] Frost, Robert. *The poetry of Robert Frost*. (Ed. Edward Connery Lathem.) Holt, Rinehart and Winston, New York (1969). p. 362.
[3] Le Fanu, W. R. The lost half-century in English medicine; 1700–1752. *Bull. Hist. Med.* **46**, 319 (1972).
[4] Lindeboom, G. A. *Herman Boerhaave, the man and his work*. Methuen, London (1968). p. 286.
[5] King, Lester S. *The growth of medical thought* (1963). University of Chicago Press, Midway reprint (1973).
[6] Jackson, Stanley W. Force and kindred notions in eighteenth century neurophysiology and medical psychology. *Bull. Hist. Med.* **44**, 397 (1970).
[7] Prochaska, G. A dissertation on the functions of the nervous system. In *Unzer and Prochaska on the nervous system*. (Translated by T. Laycock.) The Sydenham Society, London (1851). p. 430.
[8] Meyer, Alfred. *Historical aspects of cerebral anatomy*. Oxford University Press (1971). p. 128.
[9] Clarke, Edwin. The doctrine of the hollow nerve in the 17th and 18th centuries. In *Medicine, science and culture*. (Eds. Lloyd G. Stevenson and Robert P. Multhauf.) Johns Hopkins University Press (1968). p. 123.
[10] Rather, L. J. Some relationships between eighteenth century fibre theory and nineteenth century cell theory. *Clio Medica* **4**, 191 (1969).
[11] Jarcho, Saul. Giovanni Battista Morgagni; his interests, ideas and achievements. *Bull. Hist. Med.* **22**, 503 (1948).
[12] Stensen, Niels. Discours sur l'Anatomie du cerveau, 1665. In *Steno and brain research in the seventeenth century*. (Ed. G. G. Scherz. Pergamon Press, Oxford (1968).
[13] Clarke, E. and Bearn, J. G. The brain 'glands' of Malpighi elucidated by practical history. *J. Hist. Med.* **23**, 309 (1968).
[14] Hazen, A. T. Johnson's life of Frederic Ruysch. *Bull. Hist. Med.* **7**, 324 (1939).
[15] McHenry, Lawrence C. Dr. Samuel Johnson's medical biographies. *J. Hist. Med.* **14**, 298 (1959).
[16] Clarke, E. and Bearn, J. G. op. cit. 13.
[17] Meyer, Alfred. op. cit. 8, p. 122.
[18] Clarke, Edwin and O'Malley, C. D. *The human brain and spinal cord*. University of California Press (1968). p. 32.
[19] Monro. I. Alexander. *The works of Alexander Monro M.D.* (collected by his son). Elliot, Edinburgh (1781). p. 319.
[20] Clarke, E. and O'Malley, C. D. op. cit. 18, p. 36.
[21] Meyer, Alfred. op. cit. 8, p. 162.
[22] Lesky, Erna. *The Vienna Medical School of the nineteenth century*. Johns Hopkins University Press, Baltimore (1976). p. 7.
[23] Fulton, J. F. A note on Francesco Gennari and the early history of the cytoarchitechtural studies of the cerebral cortex. *Bull. Hist. Med.* **5**, 895 (1937).
[24] Schiller, Francis. The rise of the 'Enteroid Processes' in the 19th century. *Bull. Hist. Med.* **39**, 326 (1965).
[25] Clarke, E. and O'Malley, C. D. op. cit. 18, p. 390.
[26] Meyer, Alfred. op. cit. 8, p. 19.
[27] Clarke, E. and O'Malley, C. D. op. cit. 18, p. 643.
[28] Coiter, V. Externarum et internarum principalium humani corporis partium tabulae etc. (1572). Reprinted in *Opusc. selecta Neerl. Arte med.* **18**, (1955). (Eds. B. W. Th. Nuyens and A. Schierbeek.) With introduction, biography, bibliography, and English translation.
[29] Blasius, G. Anatome medullae spinalis, et nervorum inde provenientium. Amstelodami, C. Crommelinus (1666). Quoted by Schulte, B. P. M. and Endtz, L. J. in *A short history of neurology in the Netherlands*. Amsterdam (1977). Published on the occasion of the Eleventh International Congress of Neurology, September, 1977. p. 12.
[30] Thomas, H. M. Decussation of the pyramids – an historical inquiry. *Johns Hopkins Hosp. Bull.* **21**, 304 (1910).
[31] Haller, A. *First lines of physiology*. With a new introduction by Lester S. King. Johnson Reprint, New York (1966). Vol. 1, p. 225.
[32] Monro, II, Alexander. *Observations on the structure and function of the nervous system*. Creech and Johnson, Edinburgh (1783).
[33] Haller, A. op. cit. 31, Vol. 1, 197.
[34] Haller, A. op. cit. 31, Vol. 1, 219.
[35] Haller, A. op. cit. 31, Vol. 1, 221.
[36] Woollam, David H. M. The historical significance of the cerebrospinal fluid. *Med. Hist.* **1**, 91 (1957).
[37] Squires, Alden W. Emanuel Swedenborg and the cerebrospinal fluid. *Ann. Med. Hist.* **2**, 52 (1940).
[38] Woollam, D. H. M. op. cit. 36.
[39] Maudsley, H. Emanuel Swedenborg. *J. Ment. Science* **15**, 169, 417 (1869–70).
[40] Swedenborg, E. *Brain considered anatomically, physiologically and philosophically*. 2 vols. (Translated by R. L. Tafel.) J. Speirs, London (1882–1887). Reprinted by the Swedenborg Society, 1935.
[41] Swedenborg, E. *Three transactions on the cerebrum; a posthumous work of Emanuel Swedenborg*. (Edited and translated by A. Acton.) The Swedenborg Scientific Association, Philadelphia, Vol. 1 (1938); Vol. 2 (1940).
[42] Swedenborg, E. op. cit. 40, Vol. 2, p. 713.
[43] Swedenborg, E. op. cit. 40, Vol. 2, p. 380.
[44] Swedenborg, E. op. cit. 40, Vol. 2, p. 291.
[45] Swedenborg, E. op. cit. 40, Vol. 2, p. 399.
[46] Swedenborg, E. op. cit. 40, Vol. 1, xxii.
[47] Cotugno, D. F. A. *A treatise on the nervous sciatica, or nervous hip gout*. (Translated by H. Crantz.) J. Wilkie, London (1775). p. 8.
[48] Cotugno, D. F. A. op. cit. 47, p. 26.
[49] Baas, J. H. *Outlines of the history of medicine and the medical profession*. (English translation by H. E. Handerson.) Vail, New York (1889). p. 692.
[50] Henry, Thomas. *Memoirs of Albert de Haller, M.D.* J. Johnson, London (1783).
[51] Coxe, W. Biographical and literary anecdotes of Haller. In *Travels in Switzerland*. T. Cadell, London (1789). Vol. 2.
[52] Foster, Sir M. *Lectures on the history of physiology during the 16th, 17th and 19th centuries*. Dover, New York (1970). p. 205.
[53] Hemmeter, J. C. Albrecht von Haller; scientific, literary and poetical activity. *Bull. Johns Hopkins Hosp.* **19**, 65 (1908).
[54] Sigerist, Henry E. Albrecht von Haller. In *Great doctors, a bibliographical history of medicine*. (Translated by E. and C. Paul.) George Allen and Unwin, London

(1933). p. 191.
55 Klotz, Oskar. Albrecht von Haller (1708–77). *Ann. Med. Hist.* **8**, 10 (1936).
56 King, Lester S. Some aspects of Haller's life. In *First lines of physiology* by Albrecht von Haller (1786). Johnson Reprint, New York (1966).
57 Haller, A. op. cit. 56.
58 Seller, W. Memoir of the life and writings of Robert Whytt. *Trans R. Soc. Edin.* **23**, 99 (1864).
59 Haller, A. A dissertation on the sensible and irritable parts of animals. (1753). (English translation 1755.) *Bull. Hist. Med.* **4**, 651 (1936). With an introduction by Oswei Temkin.)
60 Temkin, O. The classical roots of Glissons's doctrine of irritation. *Bull. Hist. Med.* **38**, 297 (1964).
61 Haller, A. op. cit. 59, p. 658.
62 Haller, A. op. cit. 59, p. 659.
63 Haller, A. op. cit. 59, p. 677.
64 Haller, A. op. cit. 59, p. 690.
65 Haen, Anton De. *Difficulties in the modern system of physic with respect to the sensibility and irritability of the parts of the human body, proposed to the medical world* (1761). English translation in *The Medical Museum* **1**, 156, 185, 341 (1763).
66 Haller, A. op. cit. 59, p. 692.
67 Haller, A. op. cit. 31, Vol. 1, p. 223.
68 Haller, A. op. cit. 59, p. 671.
69 Foster, Sir Michael op. cit. 52, p. 294.
70 Foster, Sir Michael op. cit. 52, p. 298.
71 Haller, A. op. cit. 31, Vol. 1, 217.
72 Haller, A. op. cit. 31, Vol. 1, 216.
73 Haller, A. op. cit. 31, Vol. 1, 218.
74 Haller, A. op. cit. 31, Vol. 1, 221.
75 Sigerist, A. op. cit. 54.
76 Coxe, W. op. cit. 51.
77 Haller, A. op. cit. 59, p. 695.
78 Baas, J. H. op. cit. 49.
79 Seller, W. op. cit. 58.
80 Comrie J. D. An eighteenth century neurologist. *Edin. Med. J.* **32**, 755 (1925).
81 Carmichael, L. Robert Whytt; a contribution to the history of physiological psychology. *Psychol. Rev.* **34**, 287 (1927).
82 French, R. K. *Robert Whytt, the soul and medicine.* Wellcome Institute of the History of Medicine (1969).
83 Whytt, R. *The works of Robert Whytt, M.D.* (published by his son) (3rd edn.) Balfour, Auld and Smellie, Edinburgh. (1768)
84 Whytt, R. An essay on the vital and other involuntary motions of animals. (1751). op. cit. 83, pp. 1–208.
85 Whytt, R. Observations on the sensibility and irritability of the parts of men and other animals (1755). op. cit. 83, pp. 255–306.
86 Whytt, Robert. Observations on the nature, causes and cure of those disorders which have been commonly called nervous, hypochondriac or hysteric; to which are prefixed some remarks on the sympathy of nerves (1764). op. cit. 83, pp. 487–714.
87 Whytt, Robert. Observations on the most frequent species of the hydrocephalous internus, viz. the dropsy of the ventricles of the brain. (published for the first time in the *Works*). op. cit. 83, pp. 725–45.
88 Whytt, R. op. cit. 83, p. 9.
89 Whytt, R. op. cit. 83, p. 11.
90 Whytt, R. op. cit. 83, p. 11.
91 Whytt, R. op. cit. 83, p. 12.
92 Whytt, R. op. cit. 83, p. 12.
93 Whytt, R. op. cit. 83, p. 133.
94 Whytt, R. op. cit. 83, p. 134.
95 Whytt, R. op. cit. 83, p. 65.
96 Whytt, R. op. cit. 83, p. 70.
97 Whytt, R. op. cit. 83, p. 63.
98 Whytt, R. op. cit. 83, p. 75.
99 Whytt, R. op. cit. 83, p. 64.
100 Whytt, R. op. cit. 83, p. 102.
101 Whytt, R. op. cit. 83, p. 122.
102 Whytt, R. op. cit. 83, p. 126.
103 Whytt, R. op. cit. 83, p. 132.
104 Whytt, R. op. cit. 83, p. 153.
105 Whytt, R. op. cit. 83, p. 205.
106 Whytt, R. op. cit. 83, p. 290.
107 O'Malley, C. D. and Saunders, J. B. de C. M. *Leonardo da Vinci and the human body.* Schuman, New York (1952). p. 352.
108 Stuart, Alexander. *Dissertatio de structura et motu musculari.* S. Richardson, London (1738). (English translation in *Three lectures on muscular motion.* Woodward, London (1739).
109 Liddell, E. G. T. *The discovery of reflexes.* Clarendon Press, Oxford (1960). p. 61.
110 Whytt, R. op. cit. 83, p. 284.
111 Whytt, R. op. cit. 83, p. 285.
112 Whytt, R. op. cit. 83, p. 203.
113 French, R. K. op. cit. 82, p. 113.
114 Sherrington, C. S. In *Textbook of physiology.* (Ed. E. A. Schafer.) 2 vols. Young and Pentland (1900). Vol. 2, p. 811.
115 Whytt, R. op. cit. 83, p. 303.
116 Whytt, R. op. cit. 83, p. 489.
117 Whytt, R. op. cit. 83, p. 505.
118 Whytt, R. op. cit. 83, p. 505.
119 Hoff, H. E. and Kellaway, P. The early history of the reflex. *J. Hist. Med.* **7**, 211 (1952).
120 Whytt, R. op. cit. 83, p. 521.
121 Whytt, R. op. cit. 83, p. 287.
122 Whytt, R. op. cit. 83, p. 288.
123 Whytt, R. op. cit. 83, p. 512.
124 Unzer, J. A. The principles of physiology. In *Unzer and Prochaska on the nervous system.* (Translated and edited by Thomas Laycock.) The Sydenham Society, London (1851). p. 69.
125 Prochaska, G. op. cit. 124, p. 430.
126 French, R. K. op. cit. 82, p. 63.
127 Comrie, J. D. op. cit. 80.
128 Hippocrates. Aphorisms. *Med. Class.* **3**, 305 (1938–39).
129 Canghuilem, G. *La formation du concept de réflexe aux XVIIe et XVIIIe siècles.* Presse Université de France, Paris (1955). p. 93.
130 Foster, Sir Michael op. cit. 52, p. 281.
131 Fontana, F. The laws of irritability. A literal translation of the memoir 'De Irritabilitis Legibus' (1767) by J. F. Marchand and Herbel Edward Hoff *J. Hist. Med.* **10**, 197, 302, 399 (1955).
132 Whytt, R. op. cit. 83, p. 539.
133 Whytt, R. op. cit. 83, p. 532.
134 Whytt, R. op. cit. 83, p. 630.
135 Whytt, R. op. cit. 83, p. 508.
136 Whytt, R. op. cit. 83, p. 523.
137 Whytt, R. op. cit. 83, p. 598.
138 Whytt, R. op. cit. 83, p. 526.
139 Withering, W. An account of the foxglove (1785). *Med. Class.* **2**, 295 (1937–38).
140 Swedenborg, E. op. cit. 40, Vol. 1, p. xii.
141 McHenry, L. C. *Garrison's history of neurology.* Thomas, Springfield, Illinois (1969). p. 107.
142 Rasmussen, A. T. *Some trends in neuroanatomy.* Brown, Dubuque, Iowa (1947). p. 10.
143 Neuburger, M. Swedenborg on the spinal cord. Transactions International Swedenborg Congress, London, July 4–8. Swedenborg Society, London (1910). p. 50.
144 Ramstrom, M. Emanuel Swedenborg as an anatomist. *Br. Med. J.* **ii**, 1153 (1910).
145 Schwedenberg, T. H. The Swedenborg manuscripts. *Arch. Neurol.* **2**, 407 (1960).
146 Akert, K. and Hammond, M. P. Emanuel Swedenborg and his contributions to neurology. *Med. Hist.* **4**, 255 (1962).
147 Swedenborg, E. op. cit. 40, Vol. 1, p. xx.
148 Swedenborg, E. op. cit. 40, Vol. 1, p. 85.
149 Swedenborg, E. op. cit. 41, Vol. 1, p. 40.
150 Swedenborg, E. op. cit. 40, Vol. 1, p. 73.
151 Swedenborg, E. op. cit. 40, Vol. 1, p. 57.
152 Swedenborg, E. op. cit. 40, Vol. 1, p. 58.
153 Retzius, G. The principles of the

minute structure of the nervous system as revealed by recent investigations. *Proc. Soc. Lond. Ser. B* **80**, 414 (1908).
[154] Swedenborg, E. op. cit. 40, Vol. 1, p. 770.
[155] Swedenborg, E. op. cit. 40, Vol. 2, p. 323.
[156] Swedenborg, E. op. cit. 40, Vol. 2, p. 324.
[157] Swedenborg, E. op. cit. 40, Vol. 2, p. 324.
[158] Swedenborg, E. op. cit. 40, Vol. 2, p. 325.
[159] Swedenborg, E. op. cit. 41, Vol. 1, p. 1024.
[160] Neuburger, M. op. cit. 143.
[161] Swedenborg, E. op. cit. 40, Vol. 1, p. 642.
[162] Swedenborg, E. op. cit. 40, Vol. 2, p. 132.
[163] Swedenborg, E. op. cit. 40, Vol. 2, p. 105.
[164] Swedenborg, E. op. cit. 41, Vol. 1, p. 1074.
[165] Swedenborg, E. op. cit. 40, Vol. 1, p. 86.
[166] Rabagliati, A. *Brain* **6**, 404 (1883–84).
[167] Unzer, J. A. op. cit. 124.
[168] Prochaska, G. op. cit. 124.
[169] Unzer, J. A. op. cit. 124, p. 24 and 359.
[170] Prochaska, G. op. cit. 124, p. 446.
[171] Hoff, Herbel E. Galvani and the pre-Galvanian electro-physiologists. *Ann. Sci.* **1**, 157 (1936).
[172] Walker, W. C. Animal electricity before Galvani. *Ann. Sci.* **2**, 84 (1937).
[173] Brazier, Mary A. B. The evolution of concepts relating to the electrical activity of the nervous system. In *The brain and its functions.* (Ed. F. N. L. Poynter.) Blackwell Scientific, Oxford (1958). p. 191.
[174] Brazier, Mary A. B. The historical development of neurophysiology. In *Handbook of physiology, Vol. 1, Neurophysiology.* (Eds. J. Field, H. W. Magoun, and V. E. Hall.) American Physiological Society Washington, D.C. (1959). p. 1.
[175] Galvani, Luigi. *De Viribus electricitatis in motu musculari commentarius.* Licht, Cambridge, Massachusetts (1953). (Translation by R. M. Green.)
[176] Galvani, Luigi. *Commentary on the effects of electricity on muscular motion.* A translation by Margaret G. Foley, with notes and critical introduction by I. Bernard Cohen. Together with a facsimile of Galvani's *De viribus electricitatis in motu musculari commentarius* (1791) and a bibliography of the editions and translations of Galvani's book prepared by J. F. Fulton and M. D. Stanton. Burndy Library Publ. No. 10, Norwalk, Connecticut (1953).
[177] Galvani, L. op. cit. 175, p. 24.
[178] Brazier, Mary A. B. The electrophysiology of muscle and nerve in man from the pre-galvanic era to about 1930. In *Neuromuscular diseases, Handbook of electroencephalography and clinical neurophysiology.* (Ed. J. A. Simpson.) Elsevier, Amsterdam (1973). Vol. 16, p. 16B–5.
[179] Priestley, J. *The history and present state of electricity with original experiments.* J. Dodsley, J. Johnson, and J. Payne, and T. Cadell. (3rd edn.) 2 vols. (1775).
[180] Priestley, J. *A familiar introduction to the study of electricity.* (1st edn.) J. Dodsley, J. Johnson, and J. Payne, and T. Cadell (1768).
[181] Gray, Stephen. Experiments concerning electricity. *Phil. Trans.* **37**, 18 (1731).
[182] Licht, S. The history of electrodiagnosis. *Bull. Hist. Med.* **16**, 450 (1944).
[183] Whytt, R. op. cit. 83, p. 14.
[184] Kellaway, P. The part played by electric fish in the early history of bio-electricity and electrotherapy. *Bull. Hist. Med.* **20**, 112 (1946).
[185] Walsh, J. On the electrical property of the torpedo. *Phil. Trans.* **63**, 461 (1773).
[186] Walsh, J. Of torpedos found on the coast of England. *Phil. Trans.* **64**, 464 (1774).
[187] Hunter, J. Anatomical observations on the torpedo. *Phil. Trans.* **63**, 481 (1773).
[188] Cavendish, H. An account of some attempts to imitate the effects of the torpedo by electricity. *Phil. Trans.* **66**, 196 (1776).
[189] Boerhaave, H. *Academical lectures on the theory of physic.* 6 vols. W. Innys, London (1743–1757). Vol. 3, p. 290.
[190] Haller, A. op. cit. 31, Vol. 1, p. 222.
[191] Monro I, Alexander. op. cit. 19.
[192] Monro I, Alexander. op. cit. 19, p. 317.
[193] Monro I, Alexander. op. cit. 19, p. 333.
[194] Clarke, Edwin and O'Malley, C. D. op. cit. 18, p. 175.
[195] Wright, R. E. St. Clair. *Doctors Monro; a medical saga.* The Wellcome Historical Library, London (1964). p. 42.
[196] Clark-Kennedy, E. A. *Stephen Hales D.D., F.R.S. An eighteenth century biography.* Cambridge University Press (1929).
[197] Hales, Stephen. *Statical essays containing haemostaticks.* (3rd edn.). 2 vols. W. Innys and R. Manby (1769). Vol. 2, p. 57.
[198] Whytt, R. op. cit. 83, p. 125.
[199] Whytt, R. op. cit. 83, p. 305.
[200] Fontana, F. *Traité sur le venin de la Vipère sur les poisons Americains ...* etc. 2 vols. Florence (1781). Vol. 2, p. 207.
[201] Fontana, F. op. cit. 200, Vol. 2, p. 244.
[202] Monro II, A. op. cit. 32.
[203] Monro II, A. *Experiments on the nervous system ... with a view to determining the nature and effects of animal electricity.* W. Creech, Edinburgh (1793).
[204] Monro II, A. *Three treatises; on the brain, the eye, and the ear.* (1797).
[205] Prochaska, G. op. cit. 124, p. 390.
[206] Swammerdam, J. Experiments on the specific movements of the muscles in the frog. 1738. Reprinted in *Opusc. selecta Neerl. Arte med.* **1**, (1907).
[207] Liddell, E. G. T. op. cit. 109, p. 32.
[208] Schulte, B. P. M. and Endtz, L. J. *A short history of neurology in the Netherlands.* Published by Abbédon/Klop Ltd, Katwijk on the occasion of the Eleventh International Congress of Neurology, September, 1977, Amsterdam (1977). p. 16.
[209] Licht, S. op. cit. 182.
[210] Brazier, Mary A. B. op. cit. 174, p. 13.
[211] Brazier, Mary A. B. op. cit. 174, p. 17.
[212] Martyn, J. and Chambers, E. *History and memoirs of the Royal Academy of Science, Paris.* (Translated and abridged.) Knapton, London (1742). p. 187.
[213] Priestley, J. op. cit. 179, Vol. 2, p. 179.
[214] French, R. K. op. cit. 82, p. 74.
[215] O'Malley, C. D. In review of translation of Galvani's *Commentary* by Margaret G. Foley (op. cit. 176). *J. Hist. Med.* **9**, 475 (1954).
[216] Pupilli, G. C. In introduction to R. M. Green's translation of Galvani's *Commentary* (op. cit. 175).
[217] Volta, A. An account of some discoveries made by Mr. Galvani of Bologna with experiments and observations on them. *Phil. Trans.* **83**, 10 (1793).
[218] Volta, A. On the electricity excited by the mere contact of conducting substances of different kinds. *Phil. Trans.* **90**, 403 (1800).
[219] Monro II, A. op. cit. 203.
[220] Aldini, J. *An account of the Galvanic experiments performed on the body of a malefactor executed at Newgate, January 17th 1803.* Cuthell and

Martin, Holborn (1803).
[221] Morgagni, G. B. *The seats and causes of diseases investigated by anatomy*. 3 vols. (Translated by B. Alexander.) A. Millar and T. Cadell, London (1769).
[222] Morgagni, G. B. Selections from *De sedibus Med. Class.* **4**, 628 (1940).
[223] Morgagni, G. B. *The seats and causes of diseases investigated by anatomy*. 3 vols. Hafner, New York (1960).
[224] Virchow, R. Morgagni and the anatomical concept (1894). (Translated from the original German by R. E. Schlueter and J. Auer.) *Bull. Hist. Med.* **7**, 975 (1939).
[225] Long, E. R. *A history of pathology*. Baillière, Tindall and Cox, London (1928). p. 113.
[226] Jarcho, S. Giovanni Battista Morgagni; his interests, ideas and achievements *Bull. Hist. Med.* **22**, 503 (1948).
[227] Benassi, E. quoted by Jarch, S op. cit. 226.
[228] Morgagni, G. B. op. cit. 222, p. 673.
[229] Allbutt, Sir Clifford. *Greek medicine in Rome* Macmillan, London (1921). p. 533.
[230] Baillie, Matthew. *The morbid anatomy of some of the most important parts of the human body*. J. Johnson and G. Nicol, London (1794).
[231] Wardrop, J. *The works of Matthew Baillie* 2 vols. Longman, Hurst, London (1825). Vol. 1, p. 1.
[232] Wardrop, J. op. cit. 231, Vol. 1, p. 9.
[233] Wardrop, J. op. cit. 231, Vol. 1, p. 232.
[234] Wardrop, J. op. cit. 231, Vol. 2, p. 453.
[235] Comrie, J. D. An eighteenth century consultant. *Edin. Med. J.* **32**, 17 (1925).
[236] Cullen, William. *Nosology or a systematic arrangement of diseases*. (Translated from the Latin by C.S.) Bell and Bradfute, Edinburgh (1810).
[237] Allbutt, Sir Clifford T. *Medicine in 1800. Br. Med. J.* **ii**, 1848 (1900).
[238] Cullen, William. op. cit. 236, p. 97.
[239] Cooke, J. *A treatise on nervous diseases*. Longman, London (1820–23).
[240] Riese, W. History and principles of classification of nervous diseases. *Bull. Hist. Med.* **18**, 465 (1945).

CHAPTER 5

[1] Cooke, J. *A treatise on nervous diseases*. Wells and Lilly, Boston, Mass. (1824).
[2] Munk, W. *The roll of the Royal College of Physicians of London* (2nd edn.). Royal College of Physicians, London (1878). p. 53.
[3] McHenry, L. C. *Garrison's history of neurology*. Thomas, Springfield, Illinois (1969). p. 271.
[4] Cooke, J. op. cit. 1, p. 72.
[5] Romano, J. and Merritt, H. H. The singular affection of Gaspard Vieusseux; an early description of the lateral medullary syndrome. *Bull. Hist. Med.* **9**, 72 (1941).
[6] Pott, P. *Further remarks on the useless state of the lower limbs in consequence of a curvature of the spine; being a supplement to a former treatise on that subject*. Johnson, London (1782). Reprinted in *Med. Class.* **1**, 271 (1936).
[7] Rath, G. Neural pathology. A pathogenetic concept of the 18th and 19th centuries. *Bull. Hist. Med.* **33**, 526 (1959).
[8] Cheyne, J. *An essay on hydrocephalus acutus or dropsy in the brain*. Mundell, Doig and Stevenson, Edinburgh (1808). p. 23.
[9] Quin, C. W. *Dropsy of the brain*. J. Murray, Dublin (1790).
[10] Cheyne, J. *Cases of apoplexy and lethargy with observations upon the comatose diseases*. T. Underwood, London (1812).
[11] Long, Esmond R. *A history of pathology*. Baillière Tindall and Cox, London (1929).
[12] Schiller, F. Strokes before and after Virchow. *Med. Hist.* **14**, 115 (1970).
[13] McHenry, L. C. op. cit. 3, p. 249.
[14] Cheyne, J. A case of apoplexy, in which the fleshy part of the heart was converted into fat. *Dublin Hosp. Rep.* **2**, 216 (1818).
[15] Stokes, W. *Diseases of the heart and the aorta*. Hodges and Smith, Dublin (1854). p. 324.
[16] Marshal, A. *The morbid anatomy of the brain in mania and hydrophobia*. S. Sawrey, London (1815).
[17] Hooper, R. *The morbid anatomy of the human brain*. Longman, London (1826).
[18] Courville, C. B. The ancestry of neuropathology; Robert Hooper's morbid anatomy of the human brain. *Bull. Los Angeles Neur. Soc.* **10**, 155 (1945).
[19] Abercrombie, J. *Pathological and practical researches on diseases of the brain and spinal cord*. Waugh and Innes, Edinburgh (1828).
[20] Bright, R. *Reports of medical cases. Vol. 2 Diseases of the brain and nervous system*. Longman, London (1831).
[21] Bright, R. Cases illustrative of the effects produced when the arteries and brain are diseased. *Guy's Hosp. Rep.* **1**, 9 (1836).
[22] Swan, J. *A treatise on diseases and injuries of the nerves*. Longman, London (1834).
[23] Denmark, A. An example of symptoms resembling Tic Doulereux produced by a wound in the radial nerve. *Med. Chir. Trans.* **4**, 48 (1813).
[24] Swan, J. *A demonstration of the nerves of the human body*. Longman, London (1830).
[25] Swan, J. in *The concise dictionary of national biography*. Oxford University Press (1930). p. 1267.
[26] Carswell, R. *Illustrations of the elementary forms of disease*. Longman, London (1838).
[27] Carswell, Sir Robert. In *The dictionary of national biography*. Macmillan, London (1887). Vol. 9, p. 191.
[28] Courville, C. B. The ancestry of neuropathology; Sir Robert Carswell, Dean of the English atlas-makers. *Bull. Los Angeles Neur. Soc.* **13**, 143 (1948).
[29] Ackerknecht, E. H. *Medicine at the Paris Hospital 1794–1848*. Johns Hopkins University Press (1967).
[30] Guillain, G. *J-M. Charcot 1825–1893. His life – his work*. (Edited and translated by Pearce Bailey.) Paul B. Hoeber, New York (1959). p. 35.
[31] Cruveilhier, J. *L'Anatomie pathologique du corps humain; descriptions avec figures lithographiées et coloriées; diverses alterations morbides dont le corps humain est susceptible*, 2 vols. Baillière, Paris (1829–42).
[32] Rosen, G. Hospitals, medical care and social policy in the French Revolution. *Bull. Hist. Med.* **30**, 124 (1956).
[33] Corvisart, J-N. *Essai sur les maladies et les lésions organiques du coeur et des gros vaisseaux* (2nd edn.) Vol. 1, p. xv. Mequignon-Marvis, Paris (1811).
[34] Ollivier d'Angers, C. P. *De la moelle epinière et de ses maladies*. Crevot, Paris (1824). p. viii.
[35] Holmes, O. W. *Medical essays 1842–1882*. Houghton, Mifflin, Boston, Massachusetts (1883). p. 420.
[36] Osler, W. *An Alabama student and other biographical essays*. Clarendon Press, Oxford (1908). p. 8.
[37] Ackerknecht, E. H. op. cit. 29, p. 9.
[38] Ackerknecht, E. H. op. cit. 29, p. 141.
[39] Rostan, Leon. *Recherches sur le ramollisement du cerveau. Ouvrage dans lequel on s'efforce de distinguer les diverses affections de ce viscère par des signes caractéristique*. (2nd edn.). Béchet, Paris (1823).
[40] Lallemand, Francois. *Recherches anatomico-pathologiques sur l'encéphale et des dépendances*. Baudouin Frères, Paris (1820–24).
[41] Bouillaud, J-B. *Traité clinique et*

physiologique de l'encéphalite ou inflammation du cerveau et de ses suites. Baillière, Paris (1825).
[42] Bouillaud, J-B. *Recherches cliniques propres à démontrer que la perte de la parole correspond à la lésion des lobules antérieurs du cerveau, et à confirmer l'opinion de M. Gall, sur le siège de l'organe du langage articulé. Arch. Gén. Méd.* **8**, 25 (1825).
[43] Ackerknecht, E. H. op. cit. 29, p. 105.
[44] Andral, Gabriel. *Clinique médicale ou choix observations recueillies à l'hôpital de la charité (clinique de M. Lerminier)*, 4 vols. Librairie de Deville Cavellin, Paris (1823–27).
[45] Andral, Gabriel. *The clinique medicale; or reports of medical cases.* (Condensed and translated by Daniel Spillan, M.D.) Renshaw, London (1836).
[46] Andral, Gabriel. *Cours de pathologie interne.* Librairie des sciences médicales. De Just Rouvier et E. Lebouvier, Paris (1836).
[47] Andral, Gabriel. op. cit. 46, Vol. 1, p. xiv.
[48] Andral, Gabriel. op. cit. 46, Vol. 1, p. xix.
[49] Andral, Gabriel. op. cit. 44, tome V, *Maladies de l'encéphale* (2nd edn.). (1833). p. 734.
[50] Andral, Gabriel. op. cit. 49, p. 355.
[51] Andral, Gabriel. op. cit. 45, p. 109.
[52] Rosen, G. An American doctor in Paris in 1828. Selections from the diary of Peter Solomon Townsend. *J. Hist. Med.* **6**, 64 (1951).
[53] Andral, Gabriel. op. cit. 45, p. 250.
[54] Andral, Gabriel. op. cit. 45, p. 82.
[55] Rullier, M. Destruction d'une grande partie de la moelle épinière avec contracture des bras, et mobilité parfaite des membres inférieurs. *J. Physiol. Exp. Path.* **3**, 173 (1823).
[56] Delhoume, L. *L'Ecole de Dupuytren; Jean Cruveilhier.* 1937. Baillière, Paris, p. 171.
[57] Charcot, J.-M. *Lectures on diseases of the nervous system.* (Translated by G. Sigerson.) The New Sydenham Society, London (1877). Vol. 1, p. 158.
[58] Lasègue, C. Cruveilhier; sa vie scientifique et ses oeuvres. *Arch. Gén. Méd.* **23**, 594 (1874).
[59] Flamm, Eugene S. The neurology of Jean Cruveilhier. *Med. Hist.* **17**, 343 (1973).
[60] McMenemey, W. H. Neurological investigation in Britain from 1800 to the founding of the National Hospital. *Proc. R. Soc. Med.* **53**, 605 (1960).
[61] Waring, J. I. William Middleton Michel in Paris 1842–1846; A vignette of Cruveilhier. *J. Hist. Med.* **23**, 349 (1968).
[62] Soury, J. *Le système nerveux central, structure et fonctions; histoire critique des théories et des doctrines.* Carré et Naud, Paris (1899). p. 528.
[63] Cushing, H. *Tumours of the nervus acusticus and the syndrome of the cerebellopontile angle.* Saunders, Philadelphia (1917). p. 4.
[64] Cushing, H. and Eisenhardt, L. *Meningiomas; their classification, regional behaviour, life history and surgical end results.* Thomas, Springfield, Illinois (1938). p.5.
[65] Cruveilhier, J. Sur la paralysie musculaire, progressive, atrophique. *Bull. Acad. Méd. (Paris)* **18**, 490, 536 (1852–53).
[66] Luys, J. B. Atrophie musculaire progressive.; lésions histologiques de la substance grise de la moelle épinière. *Gaz. Méd. (Paris)* **15**, 505 (1860).
[67] Bell, C. *Letters of Sir Charles Bell. Selected from his correspondence with his brother, George Joseph Bell.* Murray, London (1870). p. 117.
[68] Bell, Whitfield J. *The Colonial physician and other essays.* Scientific Historical Publications, New York (1975). p. 228.
[69] Bell, C. op. cit. 67, p. 128.
[70] Bell, C. op. cit. 67, p. 170.
[71] Bell, C. *Idea of a new anatomy of the brain submitted for the observations of his friends.* Strahan and Preston, London (1811). Reprinted in (a) Fulton, J. F. *Selected readings in the history of physiology.* C. C. Thomas, Springfield, Illinois (1930) and (1966). (b) *Med. Class.* **1**, 105 (1936). (c) Walker, A. *Documents and dates of modern discoveries in the nervous system.* (1839). Facsimile reprint, with introduction by Paul F. Cranefield. Scarecrow Reprint, Metuchen, New Jersey (1973). p. 37. (d) Cranefield, P. F. *The way in and the way out; Francois Magendie, Charles Bell, and the roots of the spinal nerves.* Futura, Mt Kisco, New York (1974). (e) Gordon-Taylor, G. and Walls, E. W. *Sir Charles Bell. His life and times.* Livingstone, London (1958). (f) Facsimile reprint by Dawsons of Pall Mall, London (1966).
[72] Gordon-Taylor, Sir G. and Walls, E. W. *Sir Charles Bell. His life and times.* Livingstone, London (1958). p. 108.
[73] Walker, A. op. cit. 71c, p. 30.
[74] Sherrington, C. S. In *Textbook of physiology* (Ed. E. A. Schäfer), Y. J. Pentland, Edinburgh (1900). Vol. 2, pp. 787, 793.
[75] Cranefield, P. F. op. cit. 71d.
[76] Gordon-Taylor, Sir G. and Walls, E. W. op. cit. 72, p. 109.
[77] Cranefield, P. F. op. cit. 71d, p. 45.
[78] Magendie, F. Expériences sur les fonctions des racines des nerfs rachidiens. *J. Physiol. exp. path.* **2**, 276 (1822).
[79] Walker, A. op. cit. 71c, p. 87.
[80] Magendie, F. Expériences sur les fonctions des racines des nerfs qui naissent de la moelle épinière. *J. Physiol. Exp. Path.* **2**, 366 (1822).
[81] Olmsted, J. M. D. *Francois Magendie; pioneer in experimental physiology and scientific medicine in XIX century France.* Schuman, New York (1944). p. 36.
[82] Walker, A. op. cit. 71c, p. 92.
[83] Müller, J. *Elements of physiology.* 2 vols. (Translated by W. Baly.) Taylor and Walton, London (1838–42). Vol. 1, p. 643.
[84] Bell, C. On the nerves; giving an account of some experiments on their structure and functions, which lead to a new arrangement of the system. *Phil. Trans.* **111**, 398 (1821). Reprinted in *Med. Class.* op. cit. 71b, p. 123.
[85] Bell, C. On the nerves which associate the muscles of the chest, in the actions of breathing, speaking and expression. Being a continuation of the paper on the structure and function of the nerves. *Phil. Trans.* **112**, 284 (1822).
[86] Bell, C. On the nerves of the face, being a second paper on the subject. *Phil. Trans.* **119**, 317 (1829). Reprinted in *Med. Class.* op. cit. 71b, p. 155.
[87] Mayo, H. *Anatomical and physiological commentaries.* Underwood, London (1822–23).
[88] Gordon-Taylor, Sir G. and Walls, E. W. op. cit. 72, p. 131.
[89] Bell, C. On the motions of the eye, in illustration of the uses of the muscles and nerves of the orbit. *Phil. Trans.* **113**, 166 (1823). Reprinted in *Med. Class.* op. cit. 71b, p. 173.
[90] Bell, C. *The nervous system of the human body.* Longmans, London (1830).
[91] Bell, C. *The nervous system of the human body.* Duff Green, Washington, D.C. (1833).
[92] Bell, C. *Physiologische and pathologische untersuchungen des Nervensystems.* (Translated by M. H. Romberg.) Stuhr, Berlin (1836).
[93] Pichot, A. *Sir Charles Bell; histoire de sa vie et de ses travaux.* M. Lévy Frères, Paris (1859).
[94] Darwin, C. *The expression of the emotions in man and animals.* Murray, London (1872). p. 2.
[95] Bell, C. On the nervous circle which

connects the voluntary muscles with the brain. *Phil. Trans.* **116**, 163 (1826).
[96] Bell, C. *The hand, its mechanisms and vital endowments, as evincing design.* Pickering, London (1833). p. 197.
[97] Bell, C. Of the eyelids; as indicating different affections of the nerves. *Lond. Med. Gaz.* **1**, 110 (1827).
[98] Bell, C. Clinical lecture on partial paralysis of the face. *Lond. Med. Gaz.* **1**, 747 (1827). Affections of portio dura. *Lond. Med. Gaz.* **13**, 921 (1834).
[99] Bell, C. Tic douloureux. *Lond. Med. Gaz.* **17**, 874 (1835).
[100] Bell, C. *The nervous system of the human body* (3rd edn.). Longmans, London (1836).
[101] Gall, F. J. and Spurzheim, J. C. *Recherches sur le système nerveux en général, et sur celui du cerveau en particulier.* Schoell and Nicholle, Paris (1809).
[102] Anon. Report on a memoir of Drs. Gall and Spurzheim relative to the anatomy of the brain. *Edin. Med. Surg. J.* **5**, 36 (1809).
[103] Spurzheim, J. G. *The anatomy of the brain with a general view of the nervous system.* (Translated by R. Willis.) Highley, London (1826). pp. ix–x.
[104] Gall, F. J. and Spurzheim, J. C. *Anatomie et Physiologie du système nerveux en général, et du cerveau en particulier, avec des observations sur la possibilité de reconnaître plusieurs dispositions intellectuelles et morales de l'homme et des animaux, par la configuration de leurs têtes.* 4 vols. with Atlas of 100 plates. Schoell, Paris (1810–19).
[105] Gall, F. J. and Spurzheim, J. C. op. cit. 104, Vol. 4, p. 68.
[106] Young, Robert M. *Mind, brain and adaptation in the nineteenth century.* Clarendon Press, Oxford (1970). p. 44.
[107] Gall, F. J. and Spurzheim, J. C. op. cit. 104, Vol. 2, p. 263.
[108] Gall, F. J. and Spurzheim, J. C. op. cit 104, Vol. 4, p. 76.
[109] Rolleston, J. D. Jean-Baptiste Bouillaud (1796–1881). A pioneer in cardiology and neurology. *Proc. R. Soc. Med.* **24**, 1253 (1930–31).
[110] Flourens, P. Détermination des propriétés du système nerveux, ou recherches physiques sur l'irritabilité et la sensibilité. *J. Physiol, Exp. Path.* **2**, 372 (1822).
[111] Flourens, P. Recherches physiques sur les propriétés et les fonctions du système nerveux dans les animaux vertébrés. *Arch. Gén. Méd.* **2**, 321 (1823).
[112] Flourens, P. *Recherches experimentales sur les propriétés et les fonctions du système nerveux dans les animaux vertebres* (2nd edn.). Crevot, Paris (1842).
[113] Benton, A. L. and Joynt, R. J. Early descriptions of aphasia. *Arch. Neurol.* **3**, 205 (1960).
[114] Andral, G. op. cit. 45, p. 119.
[115] Dax, Marc. Lésions de la moitié gauche de l'encéphale coincidant avec l'oubli des signes de la pensée. (Lu a Montpellier en 1836).) *Gaz. Hebdom.* **2**, 259 (1865).
[116] Dax, G. Sur le même sujet. *Gaz. Hebdom.* **2**, 260 (1865).
[117] Broca, P. Perte de la parole. Ramollisement chronique et destruction partielle du lobe antérieur gauche du cerveau. *Bull. Soc. Anthrop.* **2**, 235, 301 (1861).
[118] Broca, P. Remarques sur le siège de la faculté du langage articulé; suivies d'une observation d'aphemie. *Bull. Soc. Anatom.* **6**, 330 (1861).
[119] Swedenborg, E. *The brain considered anatomically, physiologically, and philosophically.* 2 vols. (Edited and translated by R. L. Tafel.) Speits, London (1882 and 1887). Vol. 1, p. 94.
[120] Combe, G. *Essays on phrenology.* Bell and Bradfute, Edinburgh (1819). p. 142.
[121] Hammond, W. A. The physiology and pathology of the cerebellum. *Quart. J. Psych. Med. Med. Jurisprudence* **3**, 14 (1869).
[122] Ferrier, D. *The functions of the brain.* Smith, Elder, London (1876). Reprinted by Dawsons, London (1966). p. 121.
[123] Holmes, G. A form of familial degeneration of the cerebellum. *Brain* **30**, 466 (1907).
[124] Anon. *Recent discoveries in the physiology of the nervous system. Edin. Med. Surg. J.* **21**, 142 (1824).
[125] Anon. *Postscript to the Historical Sketch. Lond. Med. Phys. J.* **50**, 66 (1823).
[126] Fadiga, E. The first Italian contributions to the study of cerebellar functions and the work of Luigi Luciani. In *Essays on the history of Italian neurology.* (Ed. L Belloni.) Elli and Pagani, Milano (1963).
[127] Rolando, L. *Saggio sopra la verra struttura del cervelo dell'uomo e degl'animali, e sorpa le funzioni del sistema nervosa.* Sassari (1809). English translation of extracts from the French translation by Flourens, in *J. Physiol. Exp. Path.* **3**, 95 (1823). *Lond. Med. Phys. J.* **50**, 66 (1823).
[128] Rolando, L. op. cit. 127. *Lond. Med. Phys. J.* **50**, 72 (1823).
[129] Soury, J. op. cit. 62. p. 529.
[130] Dow, R. S. and Moruzzi, G. *The physiology and pathology of the cerebellum.* University of Minnesota Press (1958). p. 5.
[131] Anon. op. cit. 125, p. 76.
[132] Olmsted, J. M. D. Pierre Flourens. In *Science, medicine and history.* (Ed. E. A. Underwood.) Oxford University Press (1953). Vol. 2, p. 290.
[133] Fritsch, G. and Hitzig, E. The electrical excitability of the cerebrum. (Translated by Gerhardt von Bonin.) In *Some papers on the cerebral cortex.* Thomas, Springfield, Illinois (1960). p. 73.
[134] Magendie, F. op. cit. 125, p. 77.
[135] Magendie, F. Memoire sur les fonctions de quelque parties du système nerveux. *J. Physiol. Exp. Path.* **4**, 399 (1824).
[136] Bouillaud, J-B. Recherches clinique tendant a réfuter l'opinion de M. Gall sur le fonction du cervelet etc. *Arch. Gén. Méd.* **15**, 225 (1827).
[137] Riese, W. and Hoff, E. C. A history of the doctrine of cerebral Localisation. *J. Hist. Med.* **5**, 50 (1950); *ibid.* **6**, 439 (1951).
[138] Hall, Charlotte. *Memoirs of Marshall Hall, by his widow. A biographical memoir of Dr. Marshall Hall.* Bentley, London (1861). p. 88.
[139] Hall, M. On the reflex functions of the medulla oblongata and medulla spinalis. *Phil. Trans.* **123**, 635 (1833).
[140] Bettany, G. T. *Eminent doctors, their life and their work.* 2 vols. Glogg, London (1885). Vol. 1, p. 264.
[141] Hale-White, Sir William. *Great doctors of the 19th century.* Arnold, London (1935). p. 85.
[142] Green, J. H. S. Marshall Hall (1790–1857); a biographical study. *Med. Hist.* **2**, 120 (1958).
[143] Jefferson, Sir Geoffrey. Marshall Hall, the grasp reflex and the diastaltic spinal cord. In *Science, medicine and history.* 2 vols. (Ed. E. A. Underwood.) Oxford University Press (1953). Vol. 2, p. 303.
[144] Hall, M. *On the diseases and derangements of the nervous system.* Baillière, London (1841). p. vii.
[145] Hall, M. *Synopsis of the diastaltic nervous system.* J. Mallet, London (1850). pp. 1 and 10.
[146] Hall, M. *Memoirs on the nervous system.* Sherwood, Gilbert and Piper, London (1837).
[147] Hall, M. *New memoir on the nervous system.* Baillière, London (1843).
[148] Hall, M. op. cit. 144, pp. 226, 232.
[149] Hall, M. *Synopsis of cerebral and spinal seizures*, etc. J. Mallet, London

(1851).
[150] Hall, M. *Synopsis of apoplexy and epilepsy....* J. Mallett, London (1852).
[151] Hall, M. op. cit. 149, p. 12.
[152] Fulton, J. F. *Selected readings in the history of physiology.* (2nd edn.). Thomas, Springfield, Illinois (1966). p. 291.
[153] Fearing, F. *Reflex action. A study in the history of physiological psychology.* Williams and Wilkins, Baltimore (1930). p. 140.
[154] Riese, W. History and principles of classification of nervous diseases. *Bull. Hist. Med.* **18**, 465 (1945).
[155] Hoff, H. E. and Kellaway, P. The early history of the reflex. *J. Hist. Med.* **7**, 211 (1952).
[156] Jefferson, Sir Geoffrey. op. cit. 143, p. 308.
[157] Canguilhem, G. *La formation du concept de réflexe aux XVIIe et XVIIIe siècles.* Presse Université de Paris (1955). p. 169.
[158] Liddell, E. G. T. *The discovery of reflexes.* Clarendon Press, Oxford (1960). pp. 63–73.
[159] Clarke, Edwin and O'Malley, C. D. *The human brain and spinal cord; a historical study illustrated by writings from antiquity to the twentieth century.* University of California Press, Los Angeles (1968). p. 347.
[160] Sherrington, Sir Charles. *The integrative action of the nervous system.* Cambridge University Press (1947). p. 319.
[161] Hall, M. *An essay on the symptoms and histories of diseases considered chiefly in their relation to diagnosis.* Longman, London (1822).
[162] Jefferson, Sir Geoffrey. op. cit. 143, p. 320.
[163] Bernard, C. *An introduction to the study of experimental medicine.* (1865). (Translated into English by L. J. Henderson in 1926.) Dover, New York (1957). p. 200.
[164] Bernard, C. op. cit. 163, p. 146.
[165] Bernard, C. op. cit. 163, p. 100.
[166] Grande, F. and Visscher, M. B. *Claude Bernard and experimental medicine.* Schenkman, Cambridge, Massachusetts (1967). (Includes first English translation of Bernard's *Cahier rouge* by H. H. Hoff, L. Guillemin and R. Guillemin). p. 101 of *Cahier rouge.*
[167] Bernard, C. op. cit. 163, p. 19.
[168] Bernard, C. op. cit. 163, p. 193.
[169] Bernard, C. op. cit. 163, p. 105.
[170] Bernard, C. op. cit. 163, p. 111.
[171] Bernard, C. op. cit. 163, p. 114.
[172] Bernard, C. op. cit. 163, p. 115.
[173] Bernard, C. *La science expérimentale* (2nd edn.). Baillière, Paris (1878).
[174] Bernard, C. op. cit. 163, p. 92.
[175] Bernard, C. *Leçons de physiologie expérimentale appliqué a la médicine.* Baillière, Paris (1855–56). Vol. 2.
[176] Cranefield, P. F. op. cit. 71d, p. 52.
[177] Bernard, C. op. cit. 166, *Cahier rouge,* p. 44.
[178] Bernard, C. op. cit. 166, *Cahier rouge,* p. 114.
[179] Bernard, C. Recherches anatomique et physiologique sur la corde du tympan, pour servir à l'histoire de l'hémiplégie faciale. *Ann. Méd. Psych.* **1**, 408 (1843).
[180] Bernard, C. Recherches expérimentales sur les fonctions du nerf spinal, ou accessoire de Willis; etudié spécialement dans ses rapports avec le pneumo-gastrique. *Arch. Gén. Méd.* **4**, 397 (1844); *ibid.* **5**, 51 (1844).
[181] Bernard, C. Bibliography of writings. In *Medical classics.* Williams and Wilkins, Baltimore (1938–39). Vol. 3, p. 518.
[182] Bernard, C. Influence de la section des nerfs pneumogastriques sur les contractions du coeur. *C.R. Soc. Biol.* **1**, 13 (1849).
[183] Bernard, C. Paralysie de l'oesophage par la section des deux nerfs pneumogastriques. op. cit. 182, p. 14.
[184] Bernard, C. Expériences sur le tournoiement. op. cit. 182, p. 13.
[185] Bernard, C. Influence de la section des pedoncules cerebelleux moyens sur la composition de l'urine. op. cit. 182, p. 14.
[186] Bernard, C. Sur l'indépendance de l'élément moteur et de l'élément sensitif dans les phénomènes du système nerveux. op. cit. 182, p. 15.
[187] Brown-Séquard, C. E. Des rapports qui existent entre la lésion des racines motrices et des racines sensitives. op. cit. 182, p. 15.
[188] Bernard, C. Action physiologique des venins (Curare). *C.R. Soc. Biol.* **1**, 90 (1849).
[189] Bernard, C. Action du curare et de la strychnine sur les grenouilles. *C.R. Soc. Biol.* **2**, 68, 85 (1875).
[190] Bernard, C. Analyse physiologiques des propriétés des systèmes musculaires et nerveux au moyen du curare. *C.R. Acad. Sci.* **43**, 825 (1856).
[191] Bernard, C. *Sur l'emploi du curare dans le traitement du tetanos. C.R. Acad. Sci.* **49**, 333, 823 (1859).
[192] Griffith, H. R. and Johnson, G. E. The use of curare in general anaesthesia. *Anesthesiology* **3**, 418 (1942).
[193] Fessard, A. *Claude Bernard and the physiology of junctional transmission.* op. cit. 166, p. 105.
[194] Foster, M. *Claude Bernard.* Fisher Unwin, London (1899). p. 100.
[195] Olmsted, J. M. D. and Olmsted, E. H. *Claude Bernard and the experimental method in medicine.* Abelàrd-Schuman, New York (1952). p. 81.
[196] Foster, M. op. cit. 194, p. 104.
[197] Schiller, F. Benedict Stilling (1810–1879) In *The founders of neurology* (2nd edn.). (Eds. W. Haymaker and F. Schiller.) Thomas, Springfield, Illinois (1970). p. 81.
[198] Bernard, C. Influence du grand sympathique sur la sensibilité et sur la calorification. *C.R. Soc. Biol.* **3**, 163 (1851).
[199] Bernard, C. De l'influence du système nerveux grand sympathique sur la chaleur animale. *C.R. Acad. Sci.* **34**, 472 (1852).
[200] Bernard, C. Expérience sur les fonctions de la portion céphalique du grand sympathique. *C.R. Soc. Biol.* **4**, 155 (1853).
[201] Budge, J. L. and Waller, A. Recherches sur le système nerveux. I. Action de la partie cervicale du nerf grand sympathique et d'une portion de la moelle epinière sur la dilatation de la pupille. *C.R. Acad. Sci.* **30**, 379 (1851).
[202] Bernard, C. Sur les effets de la section de la portion céphalique du grand sympathique. *C.R. Soc. Biol.* **4**, 168 (1853).
[203] Bernard, C. De l'influence de deux ordres de nerfs qui determinent les variations de couleurs du sang veineux des organes glandulaires à l'état de fonction et à l'état de repos. *C.R. Acad. Sci.* **47**, 393 (1858).
[204] Brown-Séquard, E. Experimental researches applied to physiology and pathology. *Med. Exam. (Phila.)* **8**, 481 (1852).
[205] Budge, J. L., De l'influence de la moelle epinière sur la chaleur de la tête. *C.R. Soc. Biol.* **36**, 377 (1853).
[206] Waller, A. V. Neuvieme mémoire sur le système nerveux. *C.R. Acad. Sci.* **36**, 378 (1853).
[207] Bernard, C. *Leçons sur la physiologie et la pathologie du système nerveux,* 2 vols. Baillière, Paris (1858).
[208] Bernard, C. op. cit. 163, p. 217.
[209] Bernard, C. op. cit. 166, p. 93 of *Cahier rouge.*
[210] Jackson, J. H. *Selected writings.* (Ed. J. Taylor.) Hodder and Stoughton, London (1931). Vol. 1, p. 184.
[211] Olmsted, J. M. D. *Charles Edouard Brown-Séquard.* Johns Hopkins University Press (1946).
[212] Schiller, J. Claude Bernard and Brown-Séquard; The chair of general

physiology and the experimental method. *J. Hist. Med.* **21**, 260 (1966).
[213] Brown-Séquard, C. E. Recherches expérimentales sur la physiologie et la pathologie des capsules surrénales. *C. R. Acad. Sci.* **43**, 422 (1856).
[214] Brown-Séquard, C.E. *Course of lectures on the physiology and pathology of the central nervous system.* Collins, Philadelphia (1860). p. 2.
[215] Brown-Séquard, C. E. op. cit. 214, p. 54.
[216] Brown-Séquard, C. E. De la transmission des impressions sensitives par la moelle épinière. *C.R. Soc. Biol.* **1**, 192 (1849).
[217] Bell, C. *Anatomy and physiology of the human body* (6th edn.). (1826). p. 29; quoted by J. M. D. Olmsted, in The aftermath of Charles Bell's famous 'Idea'. *Bull. Hist. Med.* **13**, 341 (1943).
[218] Bell, C. *On the decussation of the posterior columns of the Crus Cerebri.* 1834–35, Lond. Med. Gaz., 15, 626.
[219] Brown-Séquard, C.E. Mémoire sur la transmission des impressions sensitives dans la moelle épinière. *C.R. Acad. Sci.* **31**, 700 (1850).
[220] Brown-Séquard, C.E. op. cit. 214, p. 29.
[221] Brown-Séquard, C.E. op. cit. 214, Preface.
[222] Schiller, F. and Haymaker, W. *The founders of neurology* (2nd edn.). Thomas, Springfield, Illinois (1970). p. 258.
[223] Schiff, M. *Lehrbuch der physiòlogie des Menschen.* Lahr *Verlag* Von M. Schauenburg (1858–59). Vol. 1, p. 235.
[224] Keele, K. D. *The anatomies of pain.* Blackwell, Oxford (1957). p. 102.
[225] Brown-Séquard, C. E. Experimental researches applied to physiology and pathology. *Med. Exam. (Phila.)* **8**, 481 (1852).

CHAPTER 6

[1] Bell, C. *The nervous system of the human body* (2nd edn.). Longman Rees, London (1830). p. iii.
[2] Schwann, T. *Microscopical researches into the accordance in the structure and growth of animals and plants* (1839). (Translated by Henry Smith.) New Sydenham Society, London (1847). p. 142.
[3] Kölliker, A. *Manual of human histology.* 2 vols. (Translated by G. Busk and T. Huxley.) New Sydenham Society, London (1853). Vol. 1, p. 494.
[4] Sydenham, T. Of acute diseases in general. *Med. Class.* **4**, 313 (1939–40).
[5] Riese, W. History and principles of classification of nervous diseases. *Bull. Hist. Med.* **18**, 465 (1945).
[6] Romberg, Moritz Heinrich, *A manual of the nervous diseases of man*, 2 vols. (Translated and edited by E. H. Sieveking.) (The New Sydenham Society, London (1853).
[7] Romberg, Moritz Heinrich, *Lehrbuch der nervenkrankheiten des menschen.* Duncker, Berlin (1840–46).
[8] Viets, Henry R. The history of neurology in the last hundred years. *Bull. N. Y. Acad. Med.* **24**, 772 (1948).
[9] Viets, Henry R. Moritz Heinrich Romberg (1795–1873). In *The founders of neurology* (2nd edn.). (Compiled and edited by Webb Haymaker and Francis Schiller.) Thomas, Springfield, Illinois (1970). p. 506.
[10] Rомber, Moritz Heinrich, *De rachidite congenita.* Berolini (1817). *typ. C.A. Plateni.* English translation, The New Sydenham Society, London (1853).
[11] Soemmerring, S. T. Abbildungen und Beschreibungen einiger Misgeburten die sich ehemals auf dem anatomischen Theater zu Cassel befanden (Mayence, Universitatsbuchhandlung, 1791). In *Classic description of disease* (3rd edn.) by Ralph H. Major. Blackwell, Oxford (1945). p. 297.
[12] Romberg, Moritz Heinrich, op. cit. 6, Vol. 1, p. viii.
[13] Obituaries in *Br. Med. J.* **i**, 111 (1860); *Lancet* **i**, 151 (1860); *Med. Times & Gaz.* (1860), **1**, 147; *Proc. R. Soc.* **11**, xxxii (1862); *The Times*, 6 February 1860; *Illustr. London News* **36**, 156 (1860).
[14] Cartwright, F. F. Robert Bentley Todd's contributions to medicine. *Proc. R. Soc. Med.* **67**, 893 (1974).
[15] McIntyre, Neil. Robert Bentley Todd; 1809–1860. *King's Coll. Hosp. Gaz.* **35**, 79, 184 (1956).
[16] Todd, R. B. Physiology of nervous system. In *The cyclopaedia of anatomy and physiology*, 4 vols. (1835–59). Vol. 3 Longman, Brown, Green, Longmans & Roberts, London (1847), pp. 585–723.
[17] Todd, R. B. *The descriptive and physiological anatomy of the brain, spinal cord and ganglions and of their coverings, adapted for the use of students.* Sherwood, Gilbert and Piper, London (1845).
[18] Todd, R. B. *Clinical lectures on paralysis, certain diseases of the brain, and other affections of the nervous system* (2nd edn.). Churchill, London (1856).
[19] McIntyre, Neil. op. cit. 15, p. 90.
[20] Kirkes, W. S. On some of the principal effects resulting from the detachment of fibrinous deposits from the interior of the heart, and their mixture with the circulating blood. *Med. Chir. Trans.* **35**, 281 (1852).
[21] Jackson, J. H. *Selected writings*, 2 vols. (Ed. J. Taylor.) Hodder and Stoughton, London (1931). Vol. 2, p. 8.
[22] Jackson, J. H. op. cit. 21, Vol. 2, p. 56.
[23] Todd, R. B. On the pathology and treatment of convulsive diseases. *Lond. Med. Gaz.* **8**, 661, 724, 815 (1849).
[24] Burton, H. On a remarkable effect upon the human gums produced by the absorption of lead. *Med. Chir. Trans* **23**, 63 (1840).
[25] Jefferson, Sir Geoffrey. The prodromes to cortical localisation. *J. Neurol. Neurosurg. Psychiat.* **16**, 59 (1953).
[26] Collier, J. *Inventions and the outlook in neurology, being the Harveian Oration at the Royal College of Physicians, London, October 1934.* Clarendon Press, Oxford (1934). (In *Lancet* **ii**, 855. (1935).)
[27] Obituary, Sir John Russell Reynolds, Bart. *Lancet* **ii**, 1582 (1896).
[28] Lord Brain, FRS. The neurological tradition of the London Hospital. In *Doctors past and present.* Pitman, London (1964). p. 108.
[29] Lasègue, C. Duchenne (De Boulogne); sa vie scientifique et ses oeuvres. *Arch. Gén. Méd.* **26**, 687 (1875).
[30] Lhermitte, Jean. Duchenne de Boulogne et son temps. *Bull. Acad. Med. Paris.* **130**, 745 (1946).
[31] Guilly, P. *Duchenne (de Boulogne).* Baillière, Paris (1936).
[32] Duchenne de Boulogne, G. B. A. *De l'électricisation localisée, et son application à la pathologie et à la therapeutique.* Baillière, Paris (1855).
[33] Duchenne de Boulogne, G.B.A. *Selections from the clinical works of Duchenne (De Boulogne).* (Translated and edited by G. V. Poore.) The New Sydenham Society, London (1883).
[34] Gull, William. Cases of paraplegia *Guy's Hosp. Rep.* **2**, 143 (1856).
[35] Gull, William, Cases of paraplegia. *Guy's Hosp. Rep.* **4**, 169 (1858).
[36] Gull, Sir William Withey. Anorexia nervosa (apepsia hysterica, anorexia hysterica). *Trans. Clin. Soc. Lond.* **7**, 22 (1874).
[37] Gull, Sir William Withey. On a cretinoid state supervening in adult life in women. *Trans. Clin. Soc. Lond.*

7, 180 (1874).
[38] Gull, William. Cases of aneurysms of the cerebral vessels. *Guy's Hosp. Rep.* **5**, 281 (1859).
[39] Gull, Sir William Withey. *A collection of the published writings of W. W. Gull MD, FRS.* (Edited and arranged by T. D. Acland.) The New Sydenham Society, London Vol. 1, 1894; Vol. 2, 1896).
[40] Gull, W. W. op. cit. 39, Vol. 1, 109.
[41] Gull, Sir W. W. Case of progressive atrophy of the muscles of the hands; enlargement of the ventricle of the cord in the cervical region, with atrophy of the gray matter (*Hydromyelus*). *Guy's Hosp. Rep.* **8**, 244 (1862).
[42] Brown-Séquard, C. E. *Course of lectures on the physiology and pathology of the central nervous system.* Collins, Philadelphia (1860).
[43] Brown-Séquard, C. E. Lectures on the physiology and pathology of the nervous system. *Lancet*, **ii**, 593, 659, 755, 821 (1868).
[44] Keele, K. D. *Anatomies of pain.* Blackwell, Oxford (1957).
[45] Gowers, W. R. *A manual of diseases of the nervous system.* 2 vols. Churchill, London (1886–88). Vol. 1, p. 131.
[46] Gowers, W. R. op. cit. 45, Vol. 1, p. 134.
[47] Zotterman, Yngve. Thermal sensations. In *Handbook of physiology, Vol. 1, Neurophysiology.* American Physiological Society, Washington, D.C. (1959). Chapter 18, p. 435.
[48] Ferrier, D. *The functions of the brain.* Smith, Elder, London (1876). Reprinted for Dawsons of Pall Mall, London (1966). p. 17.
[49] Westphal, C.F.O. Uber einige durch mechanische Ein-wirkung auf Sehnen und Muskeln hervorgebrachte Bewegungs-Erscheinungen. *Arch. Psychiat. Nervenkr.* **5**, 803 (1875).
[50] Erb, W. H. Ueber Sehnenreflexe bei Gesunden und Ruckens-kranken. *Arch. Psychiat. Nervenkr.* **5**, 792 (1875).
[51] Schiller, F. The reflex hammer; in memoriam Robert Wartenberg (1887–1956). *Med. Hist.* **11**, 75 (1967).
[52] Gowers, W. R. A study of the so-called tendon-reflex phenomena. *Lancet* **i**, 156 (1879).
[53] Waller, A. On the physiological mechanisms of the phenomenon termed tendon reflex. *J. Physiol.* **11**, 387 (1890).
[54] Foster, M. *A textbook of physiology* (7th edn.). Part III. The central nervous system. Macmillan, London (1897). p. 999.
[55] Wartenberg, R. Studies in reflexes. History, physiology synthesis and nomenclature. *Arch. Neur. Psych.* **51**, 113, (1944); *ibid.* **52**, 341, 359 (1944).
[56] Wilks, Sir S. *Lectures on diseases of the nervous system delivered at Guy's Hospital.* Churchill, London (1878).
[57] Wilks, Sir S. Observations on the pathology of some of the diseases of the nervous system. *Guy's Hosp. Rep.* **12**, 152 (1866).
[58] Wilks, Sir S. Drunkard's or alcoholic paraplegia. *Med. Times Gaz.* **2**, 470 (1868).
[59] Wilks, Sir S. On cerebritis, hysteria and bulbar paralysis, as illustrative of arrest of function of the cerebrospinal centres. *Guy's Hosp. Rep.* **22**, 7 (1877).
[60] McHenry, Lawrence C. *Garrison's history of neurology.* C. C. Thomas, Springfield, Illinois (1969). p. 443.
[61] Critchley, Macdonald, *Sir William Gowers, 1845–1915*; A *biographical appreciation.* Heinemann, London (1949). p. 48.
[62] Charcot, J. M. *Lectures on the diseases of the nervous system* (2nd series. (Translated and edited by G. Sigerson.) New Sydenham Society, London (1881). A facsimile edition by Hafner, New York (1962). pp. 192, 341.
[63] Charcot, J. M. *Lectures on the localisation of cerebral and spinal diseases.* (Translated by W. B. Hadden.) The New Sydenham Society, London (1883). p. 317.
[64] Erb, W. On a characteristic site of injury in the brachial plexus. In *Neurological classics* by R. H. Wilkins and I. A. Brody. Johnson Reprint, New York (1973). p. 114.
[65] Hammond, W. A. *A treatise on diseases of the nervous system* (7th edn.). Appleton, New York (1893). p. 373.
[66] Beevor, C. E. A case of amyotrophic lateral sclerosis with clonus of the lower jaw. *Brain* **8**, 516 (1885–6).
[67] Jackson, J. H. op. cit. 21, Vol. 2, p. 56.
[68] Gowers, W. R. op. cit. 45, Vol. 2, p. 688.
[69] Heine, J. von. Beobachtungen über Lähmungszustände der untern Extremitäten und deren Behandlung. Köhler, Stuttgart (1840).
[70] Little, W. J. Course of lectures on the deformities of the human frame. Lecture IX. *Lancet* **i**, 350 (1843–44).
[71] Little, W. J. On the influence of abnormal parturition difficult labour, premature birth, and asphyxia neonatorum, on the mental and physical condition of the child, especially in relation to deformities. *Trans. Obstetric. Soc. Lond.* **3**, 293 (1861).
[72] Marie, Pierre. *Lectures on diseases of the spinal cord.* (Translated by M. Lubbock.) The New Sydenham Society, London (1895). p. 85.
[73] Erb, W. On spastic spinal paralysis. (Translated by R. Saundby.) *Lond. Med. Rec.* **5**, 435, 477 (1877).
[74] Gowers, W. R. op. cit. 45, Vol. 1, p. 341.
[75] Marie, Pierre. op. cit. 72, p. 410.
[76] Russell, J. S. R., Batten F. E. and Collier, J. S. Subacute combined degeneration of the spinal cord. *Brain* **23**, 39 (1900).
[77] Gowers, W. R. and Horsley, Victor. A case of tumour of the spinal cord. Removal; recovery. *Med. Chir. Trans* **71**, 377 (1888).
[78] Smith, Logan Pearsall. *Unforgotten years.* Constable, London (1938). p. 168.
[79] Leyden, Ernst von. Ueber poliomyelitis and neuritis. *Z. klin. Med.* **1**, 387 (1879–80).
[80] Bontius, J. *De medicina indorum* (1642). (English translation 1769.) Chapter 1, Book IV, Concerning a certain type of paralysis which the natives call beriberi. Reprinted in *Classic descriptions of disease* (3rd edn.) by Ralph H. Major. Blackwell, Oxford (1945). p. 605.
[81] Lettsom, J. C. Some remarks on the effects of lignum quassiae amarae. *Mem. Med. Soc. Lond.* **1**, 128 (1787).
[82] Jackson, J. On a peculiar disease resulting from the use of ardent spirits. *New Eng. J. Med. & Surg.* **11**, 351 (1822).
[83] Anon. *J. Nerv. Ment. Dis.* **5**, 571 (1878).
[84] Graves, R. J. *Clinical lectures on the practice of medicine* (2nd edn.). Reprinted by New Sydenham Society, London (1884). p. 574.
[85] Chomel, A.-F. De l'épidémie actuellement régnante à Paris. *J. Hebd. de Méd.* **1**, 333 (1828).
[86] Graves, R. J. op. cit. 84, p. 579.
[87] Gowers, W. R. op. cit. 45, vol. 1, p. 91.
[88] Viets, Henry R. History of peripheral neuritis as a clinical entity. *Arch. Neur. Psychiat.* **32**, 377 (1934).
[89] Trousseau, A. op. cit. 84, p. ix.
[90] Landry, O. Note sur la paralysie ascendante aigue. *Gaz. Hebd. de Méd.* **6**, 472, 486 (1859).
[91] Haymaker, W. In *The founders of neurology* (2nd edn.). (Eds. W. Haymaker and F. Schiller.) C. C. Thomas, Springfield, Illinois (1970). p. 468.
[92] Duménil, L. Paralysie périphérique du mouvement et du sentiment

portant sur les quatre membres. Atrophie des rameaux nerveux des parties paralysées. *Gaz. Hebd. de Méd.* 1, 203 (1864).

[93] Duménil, L. Contributions pour servir a l'histoire des paralysies périphériques, et specialement de la névrite. *Gaz. Hebd. de Méd.* 3, 51, 67, 84 (1866).

[94] Buzzard, T. On some forms of paralysis dependent upon peripheral neuritis. *Lancet* ii, 983 (1885).

[95] Gowers, W. R. op. cit. 45, Vol. 1, p. 275.

[96] Ross, J. and Bury, J. S. *On peripheral neuritis; a treatise.* Griffin, London (1893).

[97] Wilson, S. A. Kinnier. *Neurology*, 2 vols., Arnold, London (1940). Vol. 1, p. 209.

[98] Remlinger, P. J. B. Octave Landry (1826–1865). *Presse Méd.* **41**, 227 (1933).

[99] Stewart, T. G. On paralysis of hands and feet from disease of nerves. *Edin. Med. J.* **26**, 865 (1881).

[100] Joffroy, A. De la névrite parenchymateuse spontanée généralisée ou partielle. *Arch. de Physiol.* **6**, 172 (1878).

[101] Victor, M. and Yakovlev, P.I. S.S. Korsakoff's Psychic Disorder in conjunction with peripheral neuritis. *Neurology* **5**, 394 (1955).

[102] Jackson, J. H. Ophthalmology in its relation to general medicine. *Br. Med. J.* **i**, 575, 605, 672, 703, 804 (1877). Reprinted in *Selected writings of Hughlings Jackson.* (Ed. J. Taylor.) Hodder and Stoughton, London (1932). Vol. 2, p. 300.

[103] Sorsby, A. *A short history of ophthalmology.* Bale Sons & Danielsson, London (1933).

[104] Heberden, Sir William. Of the night-blindness or nyct-alopia. *Med. Trans. Coll. Phys., Lond.* **1**, 60 (1768).

[105] Huddart, J. An account of persons who could not distinguish colours. *Phil. Trans. R. Soc.* **67**, 260 (1777).

[106] Dalton, J. Extraordinary facts relating to the vision of colours. *Mem. Lit. Phil. Soc. Manchester* **5**, Pt. 1, 28 (1798).

[107] Brisseau, M. *Traité de la cataracte et du glaucoma.* L. d'Houry, Paris (1709).

[108] Helmholtz, H. *Description of an ophthalmoscope for the investigation of the retina in the living eye.* English translation of Helmholtz's *Beschreibung eines Augenspiels* (1851, Berlin) by T. H. Shastid, Cleveland Press, Chicago (1916).

[109] Pagenstetcher, E. H. and Genth, C. P. *Atlas der pathologischen Anatomie des Augapfels.* Kriedel, Wiesbaden (1873–75).

[110] Allbutt, T. C. *On the use of the ophthalmoscope in diseases of the nervous system and of the kidneys; also in certain other general disorders.* Macmillan, London (1871).

[111] Gowers, W. R. *A manual and atlas of medical ophthalmoscopy* (2nd edn.). Churchill, London (1882).

[112] Chance, B. Short studies on the history of ophthalmology. *Arch. Ophth.* **1**, 13, 348 (1935); **11**, 14, 203 (1935); **111**, 17, 241 (1937); Hughlings Jackson, the neurological ophthalmologist, with a summary of his works.

[113] Jackson, J. H. On the use of the ophthalmoscope in affections of the nervous system. *Med. Times Gaz.* **2**, 359 (1863).

[114] Williamson-Noble, F. A. Hughlings Jackson and the Ophthalmoscope. *Post. Grad. Med. J.* **11**, 163 (1935).

[115] Jackson, J. H. Observations of defects of sight in brain disease. *R. Lond. Ophth. Hosp. Rep.* **4**, 10, 389 (1863); *ibid.* **5**, 51, 251 (1866).

[116] Jackson, J. H. Lecture on optic neuritis from intracranial disease. *Med. Times Gaz.* **1**, 241, 341, 581 (1871). Reprinted in *Selected writings of Hughlings Jackson.* Vol. 2, p. 251.

[117] Jackson, J. H. Observations on defects of sight in diseases of the nervous system. *R. Lond. Ophth. Hosp. Rep.* **5**, 51 (1866).

[118] Graefe, A. von. About the complication of inflammation of the optic nerve with diseases of the brain (1860). English translation of von Graefe's paper in *Neurosurgical classics*, compiled by R. H. Wilkins. Johnson Reprint, New York (1965). p. 293.

[119] Jackson, J. H. Ophthalmology and diseases of the nervous system (Bowman Lecture). *Br. Med. J.* **ii**, 945 (1885), *Lancet* **ii**, 935 (1885). Reprinted in *Selected writings of Hughlings Jackson.* Vol. 2, p. 346.

[120] Paton, W. L. and Holmes, G. The pathology of papilloedema. *Brain* **33**, 389 (1911).

[121] Garrison, Fielding H. *An introduction to the history of medicine.* (2nd edn.). Saunders, Philadelphia (1929). p. 379.

[122] Bailey, Pearce. The past, present and future of neurology in the United States (1950). *Neurology* I, I.

[123] Burr, A. R. B. *Weir Mitchell, his life and letters.* Duffield, New York (1929).

[124] Earnest, E. *Silas Weir Mitchell, novelist and physician.* University of Pennsylvania Press, Philadelphia (1950).

[125] Brecht, V. B. In Introduction to *Hugh Wynne, free Quaker, sometime Brevet Lieutenant-Colonel on the staff of his Excellency General Washington* (school edn.). By S. Weir Mitchell. Century, New York (1922). p. ix.

[126] Shryock, R. H. *Medicine in America; historical essays.* Johns Hopkins University Press, Baltimore (1966). p. 90.

[127] Mitchell, S. W., Morehouse, G. R., and Keen, W. W. *Gunshot wounds and other injuries of nerves.* Lippincott, Philadelphia (1864) p. 40.

[128] Mitchell, S. W. *Injuries of nerves and their consequences.* Lippincott, Philadelphia (1872). Republished with introduction by Lawrence C. McHenry, Jr. American Academy of Neurology Reprint Series. Dover, New York (1965).

[129] Mitchell, S. W. The medical department in the Civil War. *J.A.M.A.* **62**, 1444 (1914).

[130] Middleton, W. S. Turner's Lane Hospital. *Bull. Hist. Med.* **40**, 14 (1966).

[131] Keen, W. W. Surgical reminiscences of the Civil War. In *Addresses and other papers.* Saunders, Philadelphia (1905). p. 437.

[132] Keen, W. W. *The treatment of war wounds.* Saunders, Philadelphia (1918).

[133] Adams, G. W. *Doctors in blue; The medical history of the Union Army in the Civil War.* Abelard Schuman, New York (1952).

[134] Griffiths, D. L. Medicine and surgery in the American Civil War. *Proc. R. Soc. Med.* **59**, 204 (1965).

[135] Beard, G. M. Neurasthenia or nervous exhaustion. *Boston Med. & Surg. J.* **3**, 217 (1869).

[136] Freeman, D. S. *South to posterity; an introduction to the writing of Confederate history.* Scribner's, New York (1939). p. 4.

[137] Rosen G. Nostalgia; a 'forgotten' psychological disorder. *Psychol. Med.* **5**, 340 (1975).

[138] Sachs, B. Review of W. R. Gowers' *A manual of diseases of the nervous system. J. Nerv. Ment. Dis.* **14**, 123 (1887).

[139] Richards, R. L. Causalgia; a centennial review. *Arch. Neurol.* **16**, 339 (1967).

[140] Mitchell, S. W. The relations of pain to weather, being a study of the natural history of a case of traumatic neuralgia. *J. Nerv. Ment. Dis.* **73**, 305 (1877).

[141] Richards, R. L. The term 'Causalgia'. *Med. Hist.* **11**, 97 (1967).

[142] Bean, W. B. Robley Dunglison, M.D. *Arch. Int. Med.* **115**, 375 (1965).
[143] Tinel, J. *Les blessures des nerfs.* Masson, Paris (1916).
[144] Meredith, Roy. *Mr. Lincoln's camera man; Mathew Brady.* Scribner's, New York (1946).
[145] Seddon, Sir H. *Surgical disorders of peripheral nerves.* Churchill-Livingstone, London (1972). p. 33.
[146] Paget, J. Clinical lecture on some cases of local paralysis. *Med. Times Gaz.* **1**, 331. (1864).
[147] Vulpian, E. F. A. In preface to *Des lésions des nerfs et leurs consequences,* par le Docteur S. Weir Mitchell. (Traduit et annoté par M. Dastre.) Masson, Paris (1874).
[148] Brieger, Gert. H. American surgery and the germ theory of disease. *Bull. Hist. Med.* **40**, 135 (1966).
[149] Mitchell, John K. *Remote consequences of injuries of nerves and their treatment.* Lea, Philadelphia (1895).
[150] Mitchell, John K. *On a new practice in acute and chronic rheumatism. Am. J. Med. Sci.* **8**, 55 (1831).
[151] Mitchell, John K. Further cases and observations relative to rheumatism. *Am. J. Med. Sci.* **12**, 360 (1833).
[152] Mitchell, S. W. Spinal arthropathies. *Am. J. Med. Sci.* **69**, 339 (1875).
[153] Kelly, M. John Kearsley Mitchell (1793–1858) and the neurogenic theory of arthritis; a reappraisal. *J. Hist. Med.* **20**, 151 (1965).
[154] Jackson, J. H. *Selected writings.* (Ed. J. Taylor.) Hodder and Stoughton, London (1932). Vol. 1, p. 55.
[155] Jackson, J. H. op. cit. 154, Vol. 2, pp. 397, 440.
[156] Fulton, J. F. Neurology and War. *Trans. & Stud. Coll. Phys. Phila.* **8**, 157 (1940).
[157] Mitchell, S. W., Morehouse, G. R., and Keen, W. W. *Reflex paralysis.* Circular No. 6. Surgeon General's Office (1864). Reprinted with an introductory note by John F. Fulton Historical Library, Yale University School of Medicine (1941).
[158] Haymaker, W. In *The founders of neurology.* (Eds. W. Haymaker and F. Schiller. C. C. Thomas, Springfield, Illinois (1970). p. 482.
[159] Sunderland, S. *Nerves and nerve injuries.* Williams and Wilkins, Baltimore (1968).
[160] Walter, R. D. *S. Weir Mitchell, M.D. – neurologist. A medical biography.* C. C. Thomas, Springfield, Illinois (1971).
[161] Mitchell, S. W. Researches on the physiology of the cerebellum. *J. Nerv. Ment. Dis.* **57**, 320 (1869).
[162] Hammond, W. A. The physiology and pathology of the cerebellum. *Quart. J. Psych. Med. & Med. Jur.* **3**, 14 (1869).
[163] Mitchell, S. W. Post-paralytic chorea. *Am. J. Med. Sci.* **68**, 342.
[164] Osler, W. *The cerebral palsies of children; a clinical study from the Infirmary for Nervous Diseases.* Blakiston, Philadelphia (1889).
[165] Osler, W. *On chorea and choreiform affections.* Blakiston, Philadelphia (1894).
[166] Bannister, H. M. Diagnostic significance of the tendon reflex. *J. Nerv. Ment. Dis.* **5**, 656 (1878).
[167] Mitchell, S. W. and Lewis, M. J. Physiological studies of the knee jerk. *Med. News* **48**, 169, 198 (1886).
[168] McHenry, L. C. *Garrison's history of neurology.* C. C. Thomas, Springfield, Illinois (1969). p. 348.
[169] Mitchell, S. W. Ailurophobia and the power to be conscious of the cat as near, when unseen and unheard. *Am. Med.* **9**, 851 (1905); *Trans. Assoc. Am. Phys.* **20**, 4 (1905).
[170] Mitchell, S. W. On a rare vasomotor neurosis of the extremities and on the maladies with which it may be confounded. *Am. J. Med. Sci.* **76**, 17 (1878).
[171] Mitchell, S. W. Clinical lecture on certain painful affections of the feet. *Phila. Med. Times* **3**, 81, 113 (1872).
[172] Mitchell, S. W. *Clinical lessons on nervous diseases.* Lea, Philadelphia (1897).
[173] Lewis, T. Clinical observations and experiments relating to burning pain in the extremities, and to so-called 'Erythromelalgia' in particular. *Clin. Sci.* **1**, 175 (1933).
[174] Smith, L. A. and Allen, E. V. Erythermalgia (Erythromelalgia) of the extremities; a syndrome characterised by redness, heat and pain. *Am. Heart J.* **16**, 175 (1938).
[175] Catchpole, B. N. Erythromelalgia. *Lancet* **i**, 909 (1964).
[176] Babb, R. B., Alarcon-Segovia, D., and Fairbairn, J. F. Erythermalgia; review of 51 cases. *Circulation* **29**, 136 (1964).
[177] Abramson, D. I. *Vascular disorders of the extremities.* (2nd edn.). Harper and Row, Baltimore (1974). p. 248.
[178] McHenry, L. C. op. cit. 128, p. xi.
[179] Mitchell, S. W. Remarks on the effects of Anhelonium Lewinii (the mescal button). *Br. Med. J.* **ii**, 1625 (1896).
[180] McHenry, L. C. op. cit. 128, p. xx.
[181] Mills, C. K. Silas Weir Mitchell; his place in neurology. *J. Nerv. Ment. Dis.* **41**, 65 (1914).
[182] Mitchell, S. W. Address at the semi-centennial meeting of the American Medico-psychological Association. *J. Nerv. Ment. Dis.* **21**, 413 (1894).
[183] Osler, Sir William. Obituary notice to S. W. Mitchell. *Br. Med. J.* **i**, 120 (1914).
[184] Cushing, Harvey. In *Neurological biographies and addresses.* Foundation volume to commemorate opening of the Neurological Institute of McGill University. Oxford University Press (1936). p. 27.
[185] Tilney, F. and Jelliffe, S. E. *Semi-centennial anniversary volume of the American Neurological Association, 1875–1924.* Boyd, Albany (1924).
[186] Duncan, L. C. The days gone by; the strange case of Surgeon-General Hammond. *Military Surgeon* **64**, 98, 252 (1929).
[187] McHenry, L. C. Surgeon-General William Alexander Hammond. *Military Medicine* **128**, 1199 (1963).
[188] Haymaker, W. and Schiller, F. *The founders of neurology* (2nd edn.). C. C. Thomas, Springfield, Illinois (1970). p. 445. (p. 295 in 1953 edn.).
[189] Hammond, W. A. and Mitchell, S. W. Experimental researches relative to Corroval and Vao; two new varieties of Woorar,pa, the South American arrow poison. *Am. J. Med. Sci.* **38**, 2 (1859).
[190] Tilney, F. and Jelliffe, S. E. op. cit. 185, p. 437.
[191] Hammond, W. A. *A treatise on diseases of the nervous system.* Appleton, New York and Lewis, London (1871).
[192] Denny-Brown, D. *Diseases of the basal ganglia and subthalamic nuclei.* Oxford University Press (1946). p. 272.
[193] Gowers, W. R. On athetosis and post-hemiplegic disorders of movement. *Med. Chir. Trans.* **59**, 271 (1876).
[194] Gowers, W. R. On some symptoms of organic brain disease. *Brain* **1**, 48 (1878).
[195] Gowers, W. R. *A manual of diseases of the nervous system.* Churchill, London (1886). Vol. 2, p. 82.
[196] Hammond, G. M. Athetosis; its treatment and pathology. *J. Nerv. Ment. Dis.* **13**, 731 (1886).
[197] Hammond, G. M. Pathology of the original case of athetosis. *J. Nerv. Ment. Dis.* **15**, 555 (1890).
[198] Charcot, J. M. *Lectures on diseases of the nervous system* (2nd ser.). (Translated by G. Sigerson.) The New Sydenham Society, London (1881). Hafner, New York (1962). p. 390.

[199] Dana, C. L. *A textbook of nervous diseases.* Wood, New York (1892). p. 19.

[200] *Med. Record* **6**, 353 (1871).

[201] *Am. J. Med. Sci.* **63**, 123 (1872).

[202] *Br. Med. J.* **i**, 172 (1873).

[203] Dana, C. L. Early neurology in the United States. *J. Am. Med. Ass.* **90**, 1421 (1928).

[204] McHenry, L. C. *Garrison's history of neurology.* C. C. Thomas, Springfield, Illinois (1969). p. 327.

[205] Gowers, W. R. Pseudo-hypertrophic muscular paralysis. *Lancet* **ii**, 1, 37, 73, 113 (1879).

[206] Osler, Sir William. British Medicine in Greater Britain. Address at British Medical Association Meeting in Montreal *Br. Med. J.* **2**, 576 (1897).

[207] Osler, Sir William. British Medicine in Greater Britain. British Medical Association (1897). Reprinted in *Aequanimatas and other addresses* by H. K. Lewis, London (1948). p. 163.

[208] *Lancet* **i**, 102 (1926).

[209] *Br. Med. J.* **i**, 71 (1926).

[210] *Br. Med. J.* **ii**, 726 (1901).

[211] *Lancet* **ii**, 746 (1901).

[212] Ballance, Sir Charles. The late Sir David Ferrier. *Br. Med. J.* **i**, 574 (1928).

[213] *The Provincial Medical Journal* **4**, 321 (1885).

[214] Stewart, T. G. *J. Ment. Sci.* **74**, 375 (1928).

[215] Viets, H. R. West Riding; 1871–1876. *Bull. Hist. Inst. Med.* **6**, 477 (1935).

[216] Critchley, E. Sir David Ferrier; 1843–1928. *King's Coll. Hosp. Gaz.* **36**, 243 (1957).

[217] Clarke, E. David Ferrier. *Dictionary of Scientific Biography* **4**, 593 (1971).

[218] Ferrier, D. Experimental researches in cerebral physiology and pathology. *West Riding Lunatic Asylum Med. Rep.* **3**, 30 (1873).

[219] Sherrington, Sir Charles. Sir David Ferrier. *Proc. R. Soc Lond. Ser B,* **103** VIII (1928).

[220] Carpenter, W. B. On the physiological import of Dr. Ferrier's experimental investigations into the functions of the brain. *West Riding Lunatic Asylum Med. Rep.* **4**, 1 (1874).

[221] Davies, The Rev. W. G. Consciousness and 'unconscious cerebration'. *J. Ment. Sci.* **19**, 202 (1873).

[222] Bolton, J. Shaw, *Lancet* **i**, 786 (1928).

[223] Ferrier, D. The localisation of function in the Brain. *Proc. R. Soc Lond.* **22**, 229 (1874).

[224] Young, R. M. *Mind, brain and adaptation in the nineteenth century.* Clarendon Press, Oxford (1970). p. 237.

[225] Ferrier, D. The progress of knowledge in the physiology and pathology of the nervous system. *Br. Med. J.* **ii**, 805 (1883).

[226] Ferrier, D. *The functions of the brain.* Smith, Elder, London (1876). Reprinted for Dawsons of Pall Mall, London (1966).

[227] Ferrier, D. *The localisation of cerebral disease.* Smith, Elder, London (1878).

[228] Bartholow, R. Experimental investigations into the functions of the human brain. *Am. J. Med. Sci.* **67**, 305 (1874).

[229] Dupuy, C. Examen de quelques points de la physiologie du cerveau (1873). Quoted by W. J. Dodds in On the localisation of the functions of the brain; being an historical and critical analysis of the question. *J. Anat. Physiol.* **12**, 340, 454, 636 (1878).

[230] Kuntz, A. In *The founders of neurology* (2nd edn.). (Eds. W. Haymaker and F. Schiller.) C. C. Thomas, Springfield, Illinois (1970). p. 231.

[231] Walker, A. Earl. The development of the concept of cerebral localisation in the 19th century. *Bull. Hist. Med.* **31**, 99 (1957).

[232] *British Medical Journal.* Editorial. Experiments on the human subject. *Br. Med. J.* **i**, 687 (1874).

[233] Bartholow, R. Experiments on the functions of the human brain. *Br. Med. J.* **i**, 727 (1874).

[234] *British Medical Journal.* The festivities of the Congress. *Br. Med. J.* **ii**, 303 (1881).

[235] *British Medical Journal.* Medicine at the Congress. *Br. Med. J.* **ii**, 784 (1881).

[236] Thorwald, J. *The triumph of surgery.* (Translated from the German by R. and C. Winston.) Thames and Hudson, London (1960). pp. 3–40.

[237] Liddell, E. G. T. *The discovery of reflexes.* Clarendon Press, Oxford (1960). p. 105.

[238] Wilkins, R. *Neurosurgical classics.* Johnson Reprint, New York and London (1965). p. 119.

[239] Haymaker, W. In *the founders of neurology* (2nd edn.). (Eds. W. Haymaker and F. Schiller.) C. C. Thomas, Springfield, Illinois (1970). p. 217.

[240] Cohen of Birkenhead, Lord. *Sherrington; Physiologist, philosopher and poet.* Liverpool University Press (1958). p. 37.

[241] Transactions of the International Medical Congress, 1881, 4 vols. (Ed. Sir W. W. MacCormac.) Kolckmann, London (1881). See vol. 1, pp. 228 et seq.

[242] Clarke, E. and O'Malley, C. D. *The human brain and spinal cord.* University of California Press (1968). p. 564.

[243] *The Boston Medical and Surgical Journal* **2**, 552 (1881).

[244] *The British Medical Journal* **ii**, 822 (1881).

[245] *The Times*, 21 December 1884.

[246] *The Times*, 16 December 1884.

[247] Bennett, A. H. and Godlee, R. J. Excision of a tumour from the Brain. *Lancet* **ii**, 1090 (1884).

[248] Bennett, A. H. and Godlee, R. J. *Sequel to the case of excision of a tumour from the brain. Lancet* **i**, 13 (1885).

[249] Bennett, A. H. and Godlee, R. J. Case of cerebral tumour (abstract) with discussion by Jackson, Ferrier, Macewen, and Horsley. *Br. Med. J.* **i**, 988 (1885).

[250] Trotter, W. A landmark in modern neurology. *Lancet* **ii**, 1207 (1934).

[251] Cadge, W. The case of the late Professor Hughes Bennett. *Br. Med. J.* **ii**, 453 (1875).

[252] Bramwell, E. Alexander Hughes Bennett and the first recorded case in which an intracranial tumour was removed by operation. *Edin. Med. J.* **42**, 312 (1935).

[253] *British Medical Journal* **ii**, 1444 (1901).

[254] Holmes, Sir Gordon. *The National Hospital, Queen Square; 1860–1948.* Livingstone, Edinburgh (1954). p. 72.

[255] Wilson, S. A. Kinnier. *Br. Med. J.* **i**, 526 (1928).

[256] Brazier, Mary A. B. The rise of neurophysiology in the nineteenth century. *J. Neurophysiol.* **20**, 212 (1957).

[257] Brazier, Mary A. B. The historical development of neurophysiology. In *Handbook of physiology.* American Physiological Society, Washington, D.C. (1959). Vol. 1, p. 49.

[258] Cohen of Birkenhead, Lord. Richard Caton (1842–1926); Pioneer electrophysiologist. *Proc. R. Soc. Med.* **52**, 645 (1959).

[259] Brazier, Mary A. B. History of the electrical activity of the brain. Pitman, London (1961). Chapter 2, pp. 4–25.

[260] Caton R. The electric currents of the brain. *Br. Med. J.* **ii**, 278 (1875).

[261] Caton, R. Interim report on investigation of the electrical currents of the brain. *Br. Med. J. Suppl.* **i**, 62 (1877).

[262] Caton, R. Researches on electrical phenomena of cerebral grey matter. *Trans. Ninth Intern. Med. Congr.* **3**, 246 (1887).

[263] Berger, J. Über das Elektrenkephalogramm des Menschen (1929). Quoted by Cohen, op. cit. 258.

[264] Drabkin, David L. Thudichum, chemist of the brain. University of Pennsylvania Press, Philadelphia (1958).

[265] Castiglione, A. *A history of medicine*. (Translated from the Italian and edited by E. B. Krumbhaar.) (2nd edn.) Knopf, New York (1947). p. 793.

[266] Thudichum, J. L. W. On researches intended to promote an improved chemical identification of diseases. *10th Rep. Med. Offr Privy Council* (1867).

[267] Thudichum, J. L. W. *A treatise on the chemical constitution of the brain.* Baillière, Tindall and Cox, London (1884).

[268] Tower, Donald B. Origins and development of neurochemistry. *Neurology* **8**, *Suppl. 1*, 3 (1958).

[269] Gamgee, S. Thudichum on the chemistry of the brain. *Brit. & Foreign Med-Chir. Rev.* **60**, 1 (1877).

[270] *British Medical Journal* **ii**, 726 (1901).

[271] *Nature* **64**, 527 (1901).

[272] *The Times*, 10 September 1901.

[273] Page, Irvine H. *Chemistry of the brain.* Baillière, Tindall and Cox, London (1937). p. 3.

[274] Rosenheim, O. Quoted by Drabkin, D. L. op. cit. 264.

[275] Gowers, W. R. Introductory lecture delivered at University College, London. *Lancet* **ii**, 582 (1884).

[276] Critchley, Macdonald. *Sir William Gowers. 1845–1915; A biographical appreciation.* Heinemann, London (1949).

[277] Gowers, Sir Ernest. *Queen Square and the National Hospital 1860–1960.* Arnold, London (1960).

[278] Critchley, Macdonald. Personal communication.

[279] Gowers, Sir Ernest. *Plain words; a guide to the use of English.* H.M.S.O., London (1948).

[280] Newman, C. *The evolution of medical education in the 19th century.* Oxford University Press (1957). p. 91

[281] Anonymous. *Br. Med. J.* **ii**, 824 (1886).

[282] Rasmussen, A. T. *Some trends in neuroanatomy.* Brown, Dubuque, Iowa (1947). p. 36.

[283] Gowers, W. R. Diagnosis of diseases of the spinal cord. *Med. Times Gaz.* **2**, 524, 575, 657, 683 (1879).

[284] Bastian, H. C. The 'muscular sense'; its nature and cortical localisation. *Brain* **10**, 1 (1887).

[285] Dreschfeld, J. On alcoholic paralysis. *Brain* **7**, 200 (1884); *ibid.* **8**, 433 (1885).

[286] Gowers, W. R. A clinical lecture on a case of syringomyelia. *Clin. J.* **2**, 65 (1893). See also *Clinical lectures on diseases of the nervous system.* Churchill, London (1895). p. 175; *Manual* (2nd edn). Vol. 1, p. 574.

[287] Gowers, W. R. On myopathy and a distal form. *Br. Med. J.* **ii**, 89 (1902).

[288] Lewis, W. Bevan. On the comparative structure of the cortex cerebri. *Brain* **1**, 79, (1878).

[289] Lewis, W. B. and Clarke, H. The cortical lamination of the motor area of the brain. *Proc. R. Soc.* **27**, 38 (1878).

[290] Head, H. Aphasia and kindred disorders of speech, 2 vols. Cambridge University Press (1926). Vol. 1, p. 77.

[300] Dejerine, J. and Roussy, G. Le syndrome thalamique. *Rev. Neurol.* **14**, 521 (1906).

[301] Symonds, Sir Charles. *Studies in neurology.* Oxford University Press (1970). a, p. 3; b, p. 28.

[302] Wilson, S. A. Kinnier. *Neurology*, 2 vols. Arnold, London (1940). Vol. 2, p. 806.

[303] Gowers, W. R. On tetanoid chorea and its association with cirrhosis of the liver. *Rev. Neur. Psych.* **4**, 249 (1906).

[304] Critchley, M. op. cit. 276, p. 49.

[305] Locock, Sir Charles. In discussion on a paper by E. H. Sieveking, entitled 'Analysis of 52 cases of epilepsy observed by the author'. *Lancet* **i**, 528 (1857).

NAME INDEX

SUBJECT INDEX